Preventive Therapy in Complimentary Medicine

Preventive Therapy in Complimentary Medicine

Volume I

To liberate Humankind from the
pain and furffering of synthetic and
chemicalized medications

Dr. Lumumba Umunna Ubani

Library of Congress Control Number: 2011907351
ISBN: Hardcover   978-1-4628-7686-0
                   Softcover   978-1-4628-7685-3
                   Ebook   978-1-4628-7687-7

This book was printed in the United States of America.

To order additional copies of this book, contact:
Xlibris Corporation
0-800-644-6988
www.XlibrisPublishing.co.uk
Orders@XlibrisPublishing.co.uk
301803

Contents

Dedication

I dedicate this book to my two sons, younger son Ugochukwu Ubani and elder son Ezewuiro Ubani. I also dedicate this book to two of my lady confidantes: Ngozi Lorreta Amaefule and Ngozi Victoria Ashwood, both of London. I also dedicate this book to my late mother, Madam Eunice Igbemma Ubani, for her devotion and never-ending love for all her ten children. May her soul rest in perfect peace! Last and not the least, this book stands for the complete devotion to all the women of African origin who gave their love, their sweat, and their life so that we may survive and continue from where they stopped.

I have in mind, in particular, the following African women, who are alive: Dr Joy Degruy, who is a nationally and internationally renowned educator, author, TV presenter, and ambassador for social justice. She is an associate professor at Portland State University in the United States of America. Another person in my mind is our African queen Madam Oprah Winfrey, an African-American television host, an actress, a TV producer, and a philanthropist. She is a multi-award winner talk show presenter. The most impressive part of her life is her humble family background to her present noble position. May the good Lord continue to guide her humble life.

FOREWORD

Who is this Nigerian crying in the wilderness? No! Dr Ubani is a world traveler, now living in the heart of busy London.

He knows both sides of our modern society the under nourished and the over fed. And the folly of both these cultures. Both cultures say "That's how life is. They have both so much to learn that KNOWLEDGE IS LIFE. Proper knowledge gives the good life and length of days. Where do we start? At birth NO! Much—much earlier than that. Both parents must be in prime condition. Today's parents are not in prime condition. Dr. Ubani has noticed all these in his travels to many countries and noticed their various ways of life. Some have good points that we should copy, others have cultures that we must avoid.

Dr. Ubani 's findings should be an eye opening to many of us. Our requirements are Good food—but where can we get it.? Pure air-but where can we get it?

Pure water But where can we get it?. Peace of mind—But where can we get it? In Dr. Ubani's training with the AA.I. of D. therapy He has taken on the motto:

KEEP HELPING THE SICK OF THIS WORLD! You will notice this theme in all chapters of his book and in his own life style. Cultures have changed. Laws have changed and People have changed. At one time we were all convinced that the world was FLAT. WE must change as knowledge comes to the fore. More so as we learn more, about the human body and our involvement with the season. If this is a new field for you, progress slowly. Don't jump words because you think you know what they mean. Lots of new words come with any new science. Words mean different things to different people with different background. Most medical words come from very old cultures and have been semi-adopted and the meanings have changed. An example is Homoeopathy, who would have thought that less means more. I had to get my wife to read it to me several times before I started to understand and believe.

Always test and prove to yourself that a thing is true. Some things I don't know. How does a brown cow just by eating green-grass manage to produce white milk, which can be made into yellow butter. And if left long enough will turn green with mould. Nature understands that is why we must work with Mother Nature. She is the boss not us fickle humans, Who think we know every thing.A wise man said "We have much to learn". May this book expand your mind and your list of happy healthy friends

I salute you, Dr. J. Carson-Dunlop
Dean, Anglo-American Institute of Drugless
Therapy Scotland, United Kingdom.

ACKNOWLEDGEMENT

T his book is the product of many hard days and nights of efforts and the fruit of group-supporting endeavour. As Martin Miles puts it in his book titled *Homoeopathy & Human Evolution*, without the roots of a plant, working below the dark soil of the earth, we would not have the flower. Indeed, without the honest cooperation of my professional colleagues, the completion of this book would not have been possible.

I would like to extend my gratitude to the following people: First, Dr Victor Nkom, a medical specialist in London for his continuous support and moral courage; and second, Dr John Carson-Dunlop, the president of British Guild of Drugless Medicine and the principal of Anglo-American Institute in Scotland for his endless support and affection throughout my postgraduate study there. My thanks also go to the staff of London College of Holistic Medicine for their continued cooperation and support; to Dr Lily of Oru Medical Centre and Maternity; and finally, to my professional elder homeopath Dr Gibson Anukuru of Healthier Green in South East London, who had devoted much of his time and energy in supporting and exposing me to homoeopathy and various learning resources during the period of my initial training in complementary medicine. I would also like to extend my gratitude to the following people whose articles I have used to enrich my body of knowledge in this book: Madam Dounne Alexander, MBE FRSA, a writer and the director of her own business called GRAMMA's; Dr Subhuti Dharamanand an international consultant at the Portland Institute of Traditional Medicine, Oregon, USA; and the late Prof. Charles Ssali, the director of Mariandina Nutritional Health Products—I remain grateful for all his suggestions and ideas he gave me during one of his health seminars held in London a few months before his death; and Dr Llaila O. Afrika, a historian, an author, and an international consultant on addictionology and naturopathic medicine. He read the entire manuscript of this book during the launching of his book *The Nutricide* in London and said that it was far-reaching. Finally,

I thank Dr Jalath Anyanwu, a homeopathic practitioner in Port Harcourt, River State of Nigeria, who was the first person to encourage me to set up St. Luke's Natural Medical Health Centre in Umuaghara Ogbe, Imo State of Nigeria.

PREFACE

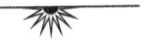

I n the former European colonies, wonderful and enviable legacies of the cleanest standards were established. Both in civil and educational institutions, they left good examples of the cleanest people in the world. What we saw as the Europeans' high standard of hygiene and personal health care has dropped and is nowhere to be found today in both Britain and Africa. One wonders why and what has gone wrong? In countries like Switzerland, Germany, and France, we are told that a high standard of hygiene still prevails. We often hear the slogan that we are going back to the basics. It was thought that going back to basics would include revamping the individual and collective dirty habits one finds in Britain. It is surely not true that taking bath often will kill the many bacteria protecting the skin. If the average person had an idea of the nature and the quantity of the bacteria that colonises the unlearnt areas of our bodies, such as unclean anuses, armpits, ears, noses, and many other parts of our bodies, he or she will do everything to wash and keep such areas of the body in constant cleanliness. The term 'hygiene' is becoming old-fashioned these days. But in the process of preventive health therapy, we are called upon to devote both time and attention to the matter of personal, food, clothes, and environmental hygiene.

Dirty habits are one of the major sources of contamination and unhealthy lifestyle. Preventive health care measure must pay attention to the above factors. Most people indulge in much use of deodorants, perfumes, and breath sweeteners just to camouflage and hide the unpleasant dirty smell and odour to the detriment of their own health. Thank goodness for the banning of smoking in many public places in Britain! Indeed, this is one of the far-reaching legislations ever passed to protect the public. As a major part of campaign for preventive therapy in the practice of complementary medicine, practitioners must, as a matter of urgency, begin to practise extensive personal hygiene, personal environmental health care habits, nutrition, and dietary personal health care, and personal health care lifestyle and behaviour. These habits will generate a new physical outlook and will certainly support and motivate our patients to look, listen, and follow our new direction towards preventive therapy. General information on casual internal bodily cleanliness is not sufficient. For example, a newborn baby hardly exhibits such an obnoxious odour nor does he or she have the need for breath sweeteners, perfumes, or extensive deodorants. As we grow in age, our adult life habits, thoughts, learned behaviour towards our feeding habits and style, our internal and physical hygiene, all these account for the type of body, clothes, and smell which we mute out. But constant cleanliness will go a long way towards minimising the dangers to health resulting from lapses in these areas.

The British Holistic Medical Association defined holistic medicine as a whole person's approach to health care. Holistic practitioners aim at treating their patient or client as a whole person with psychological, spiritual, emotional, social, and physical needs. Practitioners believe that by recognising health and illness at these levels, they can give better health care and can help people use their own capacity for self-healing. Thus, natural health practitioners must intervene at the most appropriate level or levels in each individual case. Preventive medicine in the orthodox medical profession is very extensive. This book concentrates on preventive therapy in complementary medicine. The points raised in the chapters of this book are only but a scratch in an otherwise extensive area. But the information outlined here will help complementary practitioners to pay added attention to every stage in their practice.

There are many other aspects of health care therapies essential for the prevention of unhealthy lifestyles included in this book, such practices as the effects of thought (state of mind) on health and the body. In this book, practitioners are strongly advised to recognise that no matter the attention to every other aspect of the health care treatment, without adequate attention to the state of human mind as the 'propeller' (mind and boy mind), balanced health may not be achieved. The next important aspect is the practice of taking in deep breaths from time to time. Sexual life is also therapeutic in the practice of preventive therapy. Many very relevant areas are covered under this topic. The importance of nutrition functions, mineral substances, and the vital functions of water in the body are very much stressed. The attention of complementary health care practitioners is being drawn to the vital matter of nourishing the human soul (spiritual food); this is as important as the applied physical food, nutrition-mineral and vitamin intake to the body for preventive therapy.

In this book, I have included important issues such as malaria fever and its associated illnesses. To understand the sources of this kind of illness, it is essential to give a brief explanation of how mosquitoes breed and behave. Once that is understood, we can then do our possible best to control and, if possible, prevent the spread of such diseases. Another important matter is the problem of sexual dysfunctionalities. These can refer to abnormality in sexual relationships or the inability of sexual response. Most of the cases are male biased. In this book, herbal-dietary supplementation sources of remedies are presented for the purpose of prevention. Probably most sexual dysfunctionalities have their origins in the brain, so finding out how attractions and arousal work has the potential of providing medical answers finally someday.

The primary purpose of covering extensive areas of complementary medicine is to explore various aspects and to show the nature of the practices that are in existence almost throughout the world. In doing so we are able to ascertain the different approaches of preventive therapy that may be suitable for our own application. The book also delves into some non-medical aspects of life, such as soul nourishment (spiritual) and sexual joy as the satisfaction of the inner spiritual essence in the humans. It is presented here that lack of inner satisfaction of these may lead to physical depression and restlessness resulting in psychosomatic disorders. The book stresses strongly on applied hygiene, human nutrition, and applied food supplementation therapy.

Dr Lumumba U. Ubani

INTRODUCTION

Reflecting on natural health and beauty, we realise that in the early part of the twentieth century, a fascination with science and technology and the discoveries of various miracle drugs created supreme confidence in medical science. We became detached from the principles of natural health previously enshrined in cultures all over the world.

When you consider the vast chemical cocktail we are all now exposed to, it is no great surprise that autoimmune and other degenerative diseases are spiralling out of control; even at the turn of the twentieth century, heart diseases and cancer were extremely rare. We can still find tribes of extremely long-living peoples who live a healthy life and enjoy excellent nutrition as Mother Nature intended. These include the Vilcabamba tribe of Ecuador who have an average cholesterol count of eighty points lower than the U.S. average; heart disease, cancer, and diabetes are virtually unknown. The Hunza in Pakistan also live virtually disease-free and are often seen working hard in the fields at the age of 120! The more and more we understand the importance of treating the whole person, the more we know that our bodies have an innate ability to heal themselves when treated in a holistic way. The mainstream medical profession tends to treat symptoms in isolation, usually with synthetic, toxic substances that cause considerable damage to the immune system.

This book is written for you men and women from all walks of life now engaged in one aspect or the other of complementary medicine. For you who are so engaged in this most wonderful profession and involved in the perpetual efforts of trying to set mankind free from the suffering of ill health, I say to you (*GIDE nkeji*), 'Hold on to your own.' In writing a book of this nature, the knowledge of natural medicine—homeopathy, African phytomedicine, nutrition and dietary therapy—has compounded to enable me explain the need and importance of the focus on preventive therapy. With due respect to the noble profession of orthodox medicine, only a few general practitioners possess the knowledge of nutrition and dietary requirement in health care. Even the pharmacists' training programme hardly deals with nutrition and dietary subjects at all. The only reference the training programmes make to human nutrition is in relation to deficiency diseases. For the practitioners in complementary health care, the knowledge and application of nutrition and dietary therapy must form the cardinal prerequisite of an efficient and effective practice.

Most books on complementary medicine concentrate mainly on the practice of dos and don'ts of the old school. The primary purpose of this book is to expose both the students of complementary medicine and the practitioners to the validity and importance of preventive therapy. The saying is that 'prevention is always better than cure'. This book is not just another text on the principle of complementary medicine nor is it an instruction manual. It is rather a reference book essential for the efficient practice of preventive therapy in complementary medicine. It must form an important book of reference for both students and practitioners of natural medicine no matter the aspect involved.

The period of the past 200 years was full of struggle by many masters in the field of complementary medicine, such as Dr Hahnemann, Dr Kent, and Dr Herring. Most of the practitioners in the field had concentrated principally on remedies whose major actions were based on stimulating the human immune system to deal with diseases more effectively. An ever-changing world presents to us ever-changing health care problems and demands. A successful approach to the challenges of ill health in our patients in modern time must strengthen our knowledge and equip us for the future. Artistic application of holistic and individualistic principles on complementary medicine demands continuous research, education, learning, and experience.

We must continue to increase our professional knowledge and skills, to increase our awareness of the ever-changing world, and to update ourselves about the demands and the needs of our patients. To say that we are going to continue doing something in a certain way because that is the way it has always been done is not sufficient reason to continue that way. In her book *What is the Alternative*, Hazel Courtney expressed her thanks to all for 'the swinging winds of change' that are beginning to blow towards the alternative direction. The struggle of many years of efforts for the snail-speed recognition and acceptance of the complementary health care has only begun to be given attention here in the Western societies. We should not raise ourselves up and congratulate ourselves. This commencing of our recognition must never be seen as the end of the battle but as the beginning of the end itself. It is one thing to win a battle but another thing to keep and maintain the territories won.

The term 'alternative medicine' is rather too strong a term to describe the complementary nature of the new age therapy. The suggestion that we are in competition with the conventional medical practice is a misleading one. Complementary medicine is in no way aiming at the replacement of the conventional medical practice nor can it ever. The term *complementary* is more harmonious and forward-looking. The British Institute of Complementary Medicine has defined the word 'complementary medicine' as meaning to complement the needs of the patient at the level of mind, body, and spirit. The institute has outlined its mission as a focal point of learning and helping for those concerned with the future of humanity and the future of health care and the way people are educated and trained in their profession and personal development. It is also the meeting point to share in the deeper understanding of the philosophies of life and living. They maintain that complementary medicine is holistic in practice. This means the caring of the whole person and not just a part.

Classification of Complementary Medicine

From the list of practices of medicines given by the British Institute of Complementary Medicine, some of them are as follows:

- Homeopathy
- Herbalism
- Naturopathy
- Chromotherapy
- Aromatherapy
- Osteopathy
- Hypnotherapy
- Reflexology
- Remedial massage
- Indian medicine—Ayurveda
- African traditional medicine
- Electrotherapy

- Fitness and bio-alignment therapy
- Nutrition and dietary therapy
- Chinese traditional medicine
- Hydrotherapy

An attempt will be made to describe the nature of each of the above practices. In whichever complementary medicine we are involved, the concept of holistic approach to natural medicine is a cardinal prerequisite for an effective and efficient practice. The understanding and full appreciation of the biochemistry of the organisms we are called upon to help is a major factor in our professional natural health care. The principal aim of this book is to draw the attention of all the practitioners in every division of complementary medicine to begin to re-evaluate their individual professional stand on the issue of preventive therapy as a major part of the remedial treatments which pervade their current practice.

The major aim of this book is to draw the attention of the complementary health care practitioners towards the urgent need for us to begin to re-evaluate in greater detail our health care remedial treatment. Our approach must now focus principally on functional complementary medicine based on the philosophy of 'holism' with preventive therapy as a cardinal point of attention. For some of the complementary practices, the pattern has been 'orthodox' in approach, for example, setting up a clinic or health centre with the expectation of sick people trooping in and out for treatment. This 'never-ending' expectation of people with illness, in fact, negates the concept of holistic medicine. In our quest for complementary preventive therapy, we must aim at 'Nature's Materia Medica' consisting of the following conditions of life:

- Sunshine
- Fresh air and pure clean water
- Nutritionally balanced food
- Adequate temperature
- Sufficient light
- Exercise
- Sufficient rest
- Sufficient sleep
- Occasional fasting
- Cleanliness of both internal and external parts of the body

- Positive orderly state of mind
- Clean and peaceful environment

Disease is usually caused by violation of the law and the conditions of life. In our efforts towards preventive therapy, we must consider some vital factors of health. For example, you have a beautiful plant in a box placed on your window pavement. It is healthy and of a rich green colour. Its flowers are of delicate tints. You have seen to it that the soil in the box meets all of its needs, that it receives an adequate supply of water at proper intervals including adequate ventilation and is not destroyed by cold, and that it receives adequate supply of sunshine. Were you to neglect to supply its water needs for two weeks, it would wither and die; were you to deprive it of sunshine, it would wither and lose its green colouring and ultimately die; were the soil be deficient in any of its needs, it would fail and die. Its need for air is equally as urgent as yours. These are the natural needs of human beings, and lack of their completeness of the public whom we are called upon to care for holistically is the reason for my criticism of most of the complementary health care practitioners who go by the name of 'holistic medicine practitioners'. It is also the reason for my writing this book. Views of this nature I am sure are not new. But their emphasis is almost dying away slowly. Practitioners tend to behave in ways that seem to suggest that once people hear such terms as 'holistic health care', they will be rest assured that all have been taken care of in their lives. But do you know something? No functional terms are of any use at all, unless they are describing an operational functionality that goes to remedy the imbalance in the people's health condition. If you like to use the highest phrase to describe your practice, if the health imbalance in your patients is not remedied, you have failed as a practitioner! It will also be regarded as a count against your profession.

The fundamental basis of preventive therapy must be nutrition and dietary measure, which aims at the application of wholeness. If we look around us, it is already evident that the orthodox approach to nutrition is based primarily on quantitative factors, in terms of daily requirements of calories, minerals, carbohydrates, fats, and protein differentiation. Complementary preventive therapy must, in addition to taking into account these, be concerned with the genesis that food be eaten near to its natural state as possible, given the correct quantity and the correct quality in the correct mix to arrive at the balanced meal for each person.

Our understanding is that the refinement and processing of foods will always result in the loss of their essential vitamins, minerals, and trace elements; hence, the balance and interaction cannot be satisfactorily replaced by any synthetic substitute.

Although an individual has the greatest personal control over his or her daily food intake, as a matter of fact, the dietary habits, lifestyle, eating behaviour of people, and their social attitudes tend to place a barrier in the way towards a healthy label for their well-being. Preventive complementary therapy is for the practitioners to become skilful in the requirements of healthy dieting for maintaining the bio-active body function and optimum resistance to diseases. In our search for preventive therapy, dietetic control and knowledge of applied nutrition must be used to stimulate and potentiate the body's recuperative energies in states of acute or chronic illness. In the logic for basing complementary health care preventive therapy on nutrition and dietary supplementation, we must, as a matter of great concern, maintain our stand on healthy processes of food production. These include non-chemical additives and non-preservative toxins which render foods dangerous and poisonous. The principle of wholeness is also critical to the programme of preventive therapy at every level/stage of food chain: starting from the planting, growing, harvesting, processing, packaging, transporting, storage, delivery, preparations, washing, cooking, warming, freezing, serving to the consumption plate. The major objective must be to ensure that food fulfils its optimal bio-availability to the body. These requirements call for a continuous counselling and guiding of the patients by the practitioners. As complementary medicine practitioners, we must be able to

- read the research findings relating to herbs and other forms of therapeutic nature,
- extract such information and interpret the relevant report,
- use the relevant matters that relates to a given health problems(s),
- understand their uses for the prevention purposes and/or for treatment.

Some of the times those involved in complementary therapy demonstrate signs of apathy against research reports about health and herbal usage. But we do not have a choice in the matter; if we cannot support the use of the materials we are using with an authentic research evidence, our practices will be open to doubt.

Complementary Medicine in Different Countries of the World

While writing this book within the limit of the information available, I have researched into the existence, the nature, the type, and the scope of complementary medicines that operate within the following regions:

- Europe
- African Continent
- Asia
- America
- The Arab world
- Chinese region
- The Caribbean region
- Canada

The aim of this survey is to know about the availability and the nature of the preventive practice that may or may not exist in each of these places.

CHAPTER 1

In this chapter, an attempt is made to preset a brief definition of traditional medicine and harmonise this with the term 'herbal medicine' and many other practices that go by or with the name. Thereafter, there is an elucidation of the health care crisis in America and in Great Britain; it draws from the statistics of various diseases and the factors that degrade and debilitate human health in the societies of both countries. This chapter raises the important question as to why so many people–civilised people–would knowingly indulge in such a habit which they know too well to degrade the qualities of their lives. This chapter concludes by pointing out how even the medical practitioners themselves also indulge in such unhealthy habits. A more broader definition of traditional medicine by the World Health Organisation is also given here.

1.1 Traditional Medicine

The brief definition of traditional medicine finds expression in the following order:

> Traditional medicine (also known as indigenous or folk medicine) comprises medical knowledge systems that were developed over generations within various societies before the era of modern medicine. Traditional medicine is an ancient medical practice that existed in human societies before the application of modern science to health. It has evolved to reflect different methods and approaches. Traditional Chinese medicine system is at least twenty-three centuries old. It aims to prevent or heal disease by maintaining or restoring yin-yang. The system includes a range of traditional medicine practices originating in China. Although well accepted in the

mainstream of medical practice, traditional medicine (TM) refers to the knowledge, skills, and practices based on the theories, beliefs, and experiences indigenous to different cultures, used in the maintenance of good health care. Herbal medicine is a plant or a part of a plant used for its scent, flavour, or therapeutic properties. Herbal medicine products are dietary supplements that people take to improve their health. Ordinarily, when we say herbal medicine, it also refers to botanical medicine or phytomedicine, and it refers to using a plant's seeds, berries, roots, leaves, bark, or their flowers to produce therapeutic prevention or treatment. Traditional medicine is a practice of protecting and restoring health that existed before the relatively recent arrival of modern medicine. It often serves as one component of a comprehensive system of medicine that may involve the use of plant-, animal-, and mineral-based medicines; spiritual therapies; regulation of diet and exercise; and manual techniques (like acupuncture or massage) not only to maintain health but also to prevent and treat illnesses.

1.2 The World Health Organisation's Definition of Traditional Medicine

Traditional medicine is the sum total of knowledge, skills, and practices based on the theories, beliefs, and experiences indigenous to different cultures that are used to maintain health as well as to prevent, diagnose, improve, or treat physical and mental illnesses. Traditional medicine that has been adopted by other populations (outside its indigenous culture) is often termed alternative or complementary medicine. Herbal medicines include herbs, herbal materials, herbal preparations, and finished herbal products that contain parts of plants or other plant materials as active ingredients.

Who Uses Traditional Medicine?

In some Asian and African countries, 80 per cent of the population depends on traditional medicine for primary health care. In many developed countries, 70-80 per cent of the population has used some form of alternative or complementary medicine (e.g. acupuncture). Herbal treatments are the most popular form of traditional medicine and are highly lucrative in the international marketplace. Annual revenues in Western Europe reached $5 billion in 2003-4. In China, sales of products totaled $14 billion in 2005. Herbal medicine revenue in Brazil was $160 million in 2007. So you see this is not a profession that can be brushed aside for any reason. However, it is hoped that each society within the developing nations should refine and organise its own traditional medical practice to the extent of at least that of the Chinese system.

Challenges and International Diversity

Traditional medicine has been used in some communities for thousands of years. As traditional medicine practices are adopted by new populations there are challenges. Traditional medicine practices have been adopted in different cultures and regions without the parallel advance of international standards and methods for evaluation. These are the very current challenges being faced by this aspect of health care system.

National Policy and Regulation

Not many countries have national policies for traditional medicine. Regulating traditional medicine products, practices, and practitioners is difficult due to variations in definitions and categorisations of traditional medicine therapies. A single herbal product could be defined as a food, a dietary supplement, or a herbal medicine, depending on the country. This disparity in regulations at the national level has implications for international access and distribution of the products.

Safety, Effectiveness, and Quality

Scientific evidence from tests done to evaluate the safety and effectiveness of traditional medicine products and practices is limited. While evidence shows that acupuncture, some herbal medicines, and some manual therapies (e.g. massage) are effective for specific conditions, a further study of products and practices is needed. Requirements and methods for research and evaluation are complex. For example, it can be difficult to assess the quality of finished herbal products. The safety, effectiveness, and quality of finished herbal medicine products depend on the quality of their source materials (which can include hundreds of natural constituents) and how the elements are handled from the hastering, the procurement through to the production processes, the preservation to their administration for human application/consumption.

Knowledge and Sustainability: Patient Safety and Use

Herbal materials for products are collected from wild plant populations and cultivated medicinal plants. The expanding herbal product market could drive overharvesting of plants and threaten biodiversity. Poorly managed collection and cultivation practices could lead to the extinction of endangered plant species and the destruction of natural resources. Efforts to preserve both plant populations and knowledge on how to use them for medicinal purposes is needed to sustain traditional medicine. Many people believe that because medicines are herbal (natural) or traditional they are safe (or carry no risk for harm). However, traditional medicines and practices can cause harmful, adverse reactions if the product or therapy is of poor quality or it is taken inappropriately or in conjunction with other medicines. Increased patient awareness about safe usage is important, as well as more training, collaboration, and communication among providers of traditional and other medicines.

WHO Response

WHO and its member states cooperate to promote the use of traditional medicine for health care. The collaboration aims to support and integrate traditional medicine into national health systems in combination with national policy and regulation for products, practices, and providers to ensure safety and quality; ensure the use of safe, effective, and quality products and practices, based on available evidence; acknowledge traditional medicine as part of primary health care; to increase access to care and preserve knowledge and resources; and ensure patient safety by upgrading the skills and knowledge of traditional medicine providers.

Key Facts

a) In some Asian and African countries, as stated before, 80 per cent of the population depend on traditional medicine for primary health care. Herbal medicines are the most lucrative form of traditional medicine, generating billions of dollars in revenue. Traditional medicine can treat various infectious and chronic conditions: New anti-malarial drugs were developed from the discovery and isolation of artemisinin from Artemisia annua L., a plant used in China for almost 2000 years. Counterfeit, poor quality, or adulterated herbal products in international markets are serious patient-safety threats. More than 100 countries have regulations for herbal medicines.

b) According to the World Health Organisation (WHO), up to 80 per cent of people living in developing countries still rely primarily on traditional medicine for their health care. The use of them in industrialised countries is also spreading rapidly, where they are often referred to as alternative medicines or complementary medicines or even as herbal dietary supplements or natural health products. Systems of traditional medicine that are widely used in national health care systems around the world include traditional African medicine, Ayurvedic medicine, traditional Chinese medicine, traditional Unani medicine, and traditional Western herbal medicine. Others include traditional Japanese Kampo medicine and traditional Tibetan Buddhist medicine.

c) While many of these systems of medicine are taught in medical schools with a well-defined written herbal materia medica and formulary, there are also non-written systems of traditional medicine that are passed on through the oral tradition, such as the traditional Native American medicine of various tribes throughout North and South America and other Shamanic healing systems that involve the use of medicinal plants.

In this book, I will delve into various traditional medicine herbal practices that exist in many countries and see how we can use some of their methods for preventive therapy.

1.3 Health Crisis in UK and USA

According to Dr Roger Newman Turner, the healing power of most of the therapeutic techniques in complementary medicine such as acupuncture, homoeopathy, naturopathy, and Ayurveda, all focus attention on the body's ability to heal itself. Following these natural therapies, some other practices talk of their enabling the human body in its natural efforts towards self-regulation and healing. They all state an involvement in the holistic approach to health care. The earlier physician's observation of human body in disease and health saw that it was an integral part of nature and universe, which depended on harmonious symbiosis. These were found to present the basis of established essentials of life, such as air, *light*, food, movement, and rest. But in pursuing the fine analysis, we have tended to lose sight of the most cardinal factors in maintaining a harmonious body, mind, and spirit. Be it in the conventional orthodox medical practice or in the practice of complementary therapies, most of our attention and focus is on 'medicine, medicine, and medicine'. This myopic approach to human health care came to a head with the emergence of industrial revolution, the discovery, and the application of technology in the pharmaceutical industry. This is even made worse by the commercialisation of health care services hence our concentration and focus on 'treatment, treatment, and nothing but treatment'.

Reading through the numerous textbooks and professional magazines including the health care national statistics, the grim picture painted of the medical profession's failure to preserve lives is disconcerting. But the practitioners still go about their daily business with all impunity. One thing is certain, and that is, it was the 'consumers' (the clients)' choice that elevated the orthodox medical practitioners to the supreme career which they had enjoyed for a very long period of time. It is the same consumers who have now started to divert their attention to complementary medicine. If we take them for granted, it will be them who will drag us down in no time. This fact needs to be drummed constantly into the complementary medicine professionals' ears from time to time. Let us now look at some of the sad information about the health crisis in both the United States of America and the United Kingdom. The entire medical profession including the complementary medicine therapies do have a case to answer about the health care and life-saving profession in which they have found themselves. We have both moral and ethical obligation for the health care and the preservation of people's life. The recent shift of emphasis, which believes that the individual members of the society have responsibility to take care of their own lives, is a half-truth. As health care practitioners, we owe it to our clients to not only examine and diagnose to determine the actual mood of treatment or therapy but also guide, counsel, and educate them about their health and how to go about caring for it.

According to the official publication of the American Public Health Service, nearly 99 per cent of the American population suffers from health problem of one kind or the other. Yet the U.S. medical profession including the complementary practitioners, in that country, has the heart to boast that America is the best-fed and among the healthiest nations in the world and that her health care is unexcelled anywhere in the world. In the UK, both the media and National Health Service are publicising the individual's responsibility for his or her own health with such speed and impunity, and it is beginning to sound like an abdication of responsibility. While it is obvious that the citizenry should be responsible for their own health care and well-being, we owe it as a duty to provide comprehensive health care education and information at all levels of the society. The UK Office of National Statistics Report has shown that circulatory diseases now account for 45 per cent of all deaths in Britain and that 57 per cent of all circulatory diseases are due to ischemic heart diseases. In the USA, the Public Health Service recognises just only 3,600,000 of over 240,000,000 people being healthy. This is only 1.85 per cent of the population of the nation. Nearly 50 per cent of Americans suffer from diseases, and over 50,000,000 suffer from severe heart diseases. Recent estimates suggest that 2 per cent of the population in the UK has some persistent neurological disability, approximately 1,100,000 people. The autopsies of the most fit young men who died in the Korean war showed that 77 per cent of them died of heart diseases. About 1,250,000,000 visits are made to the family doctors annually in America. Another 250,000,000 visits are made to the emergency departments of the hospitals and clinics. In Britain, almost 500,000 people consult their GPs each year with complaints of indigestion, and over 25 per cent of them are considered to be very serious. Cancer is one of the main causes of death each year and over 140,000 people die, that is, one in four of all deaths throughout the nation.

In America, cancer is the number one cause of death among the children. In many countries of the world, almost no cancer exists. Arthritis and rheumatic complaints affect 30,000,000. Over 60 per cent of the American population suffers from defective vision. Eyeglasses are the usual remedy, which infect and worsen the problem. In Britain, the number of people with osteoarthritis and rheumatoid arthritis is continuing to rise. Arthritis and Rheumatism Council and Epidemiology Research Unit have estimated that lifetime prevention of soft tissue rheumatism is close to 50 per cent of the middle and older age groups.

Over 50,000,000 Americans will spend some time in the hospital each year. About 50 per cent of American population suffer from chronic digestion disorder due to wrong diet and dietary practices. About $2 billion are spent annually in America on deodorants and a lot more on perfumes, colognes, breath sweeteners, etc. Body odours and foul smells are evidence of foul body conditions. These habitual maladies have gradually found their way into Britain. In the 1960s, Britain was the cleanest nation in the world apart from Switzerland. But today, with the emergence of hippies, scruffiness and dirty living have become the order of the day. Some $600 billion will be spent in 1999 in America on health care (on diseases). This means that an average American has an annual disease bill of over $2,500. The fact is that people spend less on their health and more on diseases. The same condition would apply to Britain if and when the NHS is abolished. There are almost about 12,000,000 asthmatic sufferers in America and a relatively large percentage in Britain. Although complementary medicine therapies like homeopathy, Hebraism, and naturopathy can and do help most sufferers to recover completely, a higher per cent preventative therapy should and must be found on a much more permanent basis. There are over 15,000,000 diabetics or near diabetics in America and a similar relatively large number in Britain. Except where there is severe atrophy in the UK, homeopathy will always restore normal health without the use of insulin or chemical drugs. But we are now challenged to come up with a more preventive measure.

There are almost 50,000,000 people suffering from insomnia in America and a substantial per cent of this in the UK as well. Most of the sleeplessness is caused by a myriad of drugs, foods, drinking, thoughts, and habits which can and should be prevented. Over 100,000,000 Americans drink alcohol and consume narcotic drugs, and over 15,000,000 people are chronic alcoholics. Approximately 60, 000,000 Americans are narcotised from digestive leucotomies and irregular heartbeat; whether it is in the United States or in the United Kingdom, these conditions are largely the result of a pathogenic diet or cooked foods; drug habits; and processed, prepared, and improper food habits including many abnormal health hazard practices. Complementary health care therapy must, as of necessity, indulge in finding more reliable preventative measure. Over 200,000,000 Americans and a relatively astonishing number of people in the UK are hooked in one or more drug habits. The most frequently used drugs are caffeine (present in coffee and soft drinks), salt in tinned foods, nicotine, alcohol, aspirin, Teenier (in tea), the brain (in cocoa), chocolate, and vinegar.

Apart from the shattering effects of the powerful inducement of advertisements, which plays on the psychology of the public, homeopathy, Hebraism, and naturopathy can succeed in reducing significantly most of the above health hazard habits. However, we must continue our efforts towards the reduction and eventual elimination of the craving for coffee, salt, alcohol and soft drinks, painkillers, cocoa, chocolate, and all other health hazard/damaging condiments. This calls for increased public health care education and awareness through continuous seminars, workshops, simulations, conventions, and information communication in schools, public libraries, and post offices and through radio and TV programmes. We must increase our knowledge of nutrition and dietary therapy. We must also begin to study the components and production factors of the dietary supplements and holistically concern ourselves with the dietary habits and intakes of our clients. Preventative therapy must aim at the whole person approach or nothing. About 90,000,000 aspirins are taken daily in America. Relatively similar quantities are also consumed in Britain. In USA, this amounts to about 36,000 tons of aspirins yearly. Over 5 billion sleeping pills are consumed annually in America. An estimated 13 billion of habituates and amphetamine pills are taken annually. Tranquillisers are a way of life for 15,000,000 Americans. Nearly 25,000,000 of Americans go through the surgical operation each year. While the surgical operation may remove the flesh impression of a disease's effects, the underlying causes remain. For us in complementary medicine, prevention will always be better than the cure.

Almost every baby born in America has been drugged long before birth, either by the physician or by drugs in the mother's bloodstream when she is drugged herself. But at birth, drugging children is a routine. Most of the American population, about 98 per cent of them, have had false teeth. About 31,000,000 people have no teeth of their own. Fillings, dental cavities, decays, and deformed teeth are so prevalent that they are considered normal. The *Washington Post* has stated that despite thousands of tons of cartons of toothpaste, mouthwashes, fluoridated water, etc., an average American child still has six cavities filled before reaching the school age. Bad teeth are symptomatic of bad health whether this is in America or in Britain. These statistics are really very frightening. If such a number of men, women, and children, young and old, are in such an agonising suffering state of ill health through causes attributable to individual behaviour, lifestyle, habit, and ignorance of medical profession, both orthodox and complementary practitioners must be ashamed of themselves. The point I am making can be summarised in the following paragraph:

Prosperity may shower its brightest gifts on men and women; wealth and art may combine to beautify and embellish his or her home; Science and good literature may elevate his or her understanding and refine his or her tastes; the good and the wise may count his or her society, he or she may be exalted to the highest position to which his or her country may elevate his or her but to what avail are all these if his or her body is weakly and wracked with pain, and his/her home a scene of corroding anxiety and humiliating mortification caused by feeble, sickly or defective children? Health next to life, is man's most precious possession and without it, his life is not likely to amount to much (Dr Herbert M. Sheldon, *New York Herald of Health*, October 1862.)

The above quotation remains as lively and truthfully today as it was during the days of its writing in the previous century. In the present-day health care system, the wind of change is blowing everywhere. It is blowing harder on conventional medical practices, but it certainly will not leave the complementary therapies untouched if we are already not being touched by this wind of change; we must begin to revamp our 'modus operandi, our techniques, our skills, and our approach to holistic health care. The wind of change, which is blowing, can be so profuse towards any direction. It is far-reaching than most people would care to imagine. The fact is that some of the orthodox medical practitioners are already joining. If we cannot improve on the preventative therapy to save our patients from this age-old malady of tooth decay, the difference between the conventional medical practice and us is not clear at all. Over 8,000,000 children are mentally retarded, disturbed, defective, or otherwise seriously handicapped because of brain problems in America. Most of the deficiencies result from the child being drugged via the mother during pregnancy. We thank God that complementary medicine, such as homeopathy, Hebraism, naturopathy, Chinese traditional medicine, and others, has no hand in this wholesale practice of mass destruction in the use of chemical 'zed' drug. But we have both the moral and legal duties to ensure that the clients who come our way are inculcated with the principle of complementary health care preventive therapy.

Americans consume up to 250 billion cups of coffee a year, and in the United Kingdom, a similar large number is being consumed too

Caffeine is known to be one of the deadly drugs to which most people are addicted. A survey and health evaluation programme has revealed that in America physicians were sicker and more diseased than the average American. It is an eye-opener to know that health specialists suffer more heart attacks in their relative youth—in their forties and fifties. I regret that I have no relevant statistics to make a comparison between US and the UK in this respect. In complementary health care, we must take note of this situation. The worst drug offenders in America are the physicians; the number of physicians on so-called hard drugs (heroin, opium, cocaine, etc.) is about nineteen times greater than among the general public addicted to the same drugs. This information is contained in a series of medical articles published in the *New York Times* during the period from mid-1975 to 1987; unless the conditions have changed towards improvement since then, the condition is alarming. Complementary medicine crusades are significant signposts pointing towards the shifting nature of the changes yet to come. The current crisis in health care in Britain and America is ringing a bell towards the right direction. The direction of this bell is towards '*preventive medicine*'. In no distant future from now, practitioners who are not able to follow the new wind of change or at best embrace it will, as a matter of urgency, be swept aside by the public demand.

Just think of this: Considering the might and strength of the pharmaceutical multinationals, who could have thought or dreamt the possibility of the present-day swing of public demand towards the complementary medicine nearly ten years ago? It is important to remember that it is the same public who just a years ago cast 'all their votes into the pharmaceutical medical products' are today begging to share 'their' votes again between the pharmaceutical drugs/orthodoxy and complementary medicine. This wind of change came about as a result of public awareness and the effects of natural therapies. The efficiency and efficacy of our practices must be guided with the strongest efforts and professional standard. According to Dr Llaila Afrika, a naturopathic medical specialist, 'good health does not belong exclusively to any culture or race'. He said that this belongs to the entire humanity with their rights and demands for the appropriate products and effective services.

Chapter 2

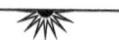

This chapter reviews the topic of preventive therapy—its aims, objectives, and importance in complementary health care. In this chapter, an attempt is made to outline the importance of various vitamins and minerals in complementary health care. Information on balanced diets and their problems is also reviewed. Suggestions of various means and methods of using dietary and supplementation therapy for the presentation of diseases are given. Reviewing the various methods of complementary medical practices presented in this book will enable the willing and able practitioners to select the best suitable line of prevention available.

2 Preventative Therapy

2.1 Description and Explanation

The topic of prevention is at the heart of this book. This idea can also be referred to as intermittent preventive therapy. These practices must be aimed at preparing and preventing diseases and illness. In our efforts to practice preventive therapy in complementary medicine, we must develop knowledge of what the human body requires in order for it to be free from diseases. For the physicians who are accustomed to illness diagnosis for treatment, this practice appears to be difficult at first, but once adopted, it will fall into the normal pattern of daily practice. It is important that we re-evaluate our understanding of natural medicine upon which the practice of complementary therapy is based. All the healing powers are inherent in the living organism (the human being). There is no curative 'virtue' in any drug or in anything outside the living organism. Nature has not provided remedies for disease. There is no such thing as a 'law of cure'; the only condition of recovery is obedience to physiological law. The so-called remedial agents do not act on the living human systems as it is generally believed but are rather acted upon by the vital force of the organism. By the term 'natural medicine' or 'natural therapy', people feel that it contains magical elements that remove diseases instantly. But that is not the case at all. There can be nothing wrong with the idea of setting up a complementary medicine preventive clinic. This will ensure that clients attend to this centre for counselling and advice on different methods of preventing illnesses.

Disease: This describes the state of a physiological and psychological imbalance. It is not, as commonly believed, an enemy at war with the powers of the living organism. It is a remedial effort, a process of purification and repair. It is not something to be destroyed, subdued, suppressed, killed, or cured but an action to be cooperated with. We must be very careful not be carried away by linguistic semantics. Once we understand the state of imbalance in human health this way, the understanding complementary practitioner is in a much better position to comprehend the behaviour of the unseen element causing the imbalance within his or her patients.

There is a whole school of thought built upon the idea that good health can be achieved as a result of successful 'prevention'. There are over 20,000 diseases catalogued and to be prevented, they say, by various vitamins, minerals, enzymes, herbs, massages, special types of baths, and special foods, etc. The problem is that those who practice preventing disease have so many diseases to prevent that they hardly get around to the actual job of preventing at all. The unfortunate result of this practice is that they cause more diseases to the human body with drugs used for the prevention than anything else. However, exuberant disease-free health is normal to the organism (human body) when it is supplied with the proper needs of life. The fact is that all diseases are caused. If we do not indulge in the behaviour and habits that causes disease, we will not have diseases: They are not bound to happen. In his quest for finding the causes of *diseases*, Dr Samuel Hahnemann (the founding father of homeopathic medicine) wondered whether God had created man and disease to live and work concurrently. Hahnemann did find an answer to the health problems of his day.

For us in the modern times, health crisis and the confusion that comes with it are the challenges staring us in the face. The term 'preventive therapy' in complementary medicine may lead some readers to believe that we are once again talking about or diving into the concept of prevention in its conventional meaning. Well, no, we are not digging into such an area at all. The preventive therapy in which we are called upon to dedicate our attention to is really simple and practical. Some complementary practitioners are doing this already, but it may not be as a deliberate programme or in a sufficient manner at all. It is not useful at all if we are engaged in complementary medicine bitterly but are critical of the orthodox medical practice and yet have no knowledge of the sources of the foods, the nutrients, and dietary supplementary therapy. We must therefore begin to re-evaluate the body of our professional knowledge in this field. It is critical that we go back to nature in an attempt to understand and start using the system, which are readily available and accessible and need minimum resources. Such a preventive approach must emphasise, as the essential factors of life and well-being, those influences and elements which, after many years of development, as a creature of nature, made mankind dependent upon the following: pure fresh air, free from impurities and free from pollution of any type, and pure fresh natural water. This means distilled water fresh from all impurities. The human body will not make use of anything in the form of chemicals or synthetic. Even when the water is pure, it can still be unhealthy for human consumption due to cross contamination during the handling. Both external cleanliness and internal cleanliness of human body are critical to a healthy living. The idea that frequent bathing will remove from human body all the oils on the body surface is primitive and an unhygienic belief to uphold. In modern times, the word 'hygiene' has grown weaker and weaker in meaning and in practice. The adage that cleanliness is godliness is now a thing of the past. Hospitals and clinics of every description including health centres concentrate mainly on diagnosis and examination of people armed with the view of finding sickness for treatment/the administration of drugs. While the treatment of illness is still a vital part of our health care concern, the changing times have called for more attention and more efforts towards preventive therapy.

In the past, complementary medicine was not considered worthy of any attention. But with time, both the general public and the mainstream medical profession have stated to soft-pedal. Therefore, we should have professional responsibility and accountability to both the public and our patients. 'To whom more is given, more will be expected.' We must learn about preventive therapy on eHow.com. Find information and videos including *Relapse Prevention Therapy, How to Prevent Suicide with Cognitive Therapy,* and *How to Use Fluoride Therapy.* We must familiarise ourselves with both the national government regulations on national health and the European regulations on health and the World Health Organisation. We must know and become aware of various private and state health centres responsible for laboratory tests and examinations. We must see ourselves as an integral part of the public health systems in any country we are residing. Above all, we must be aware of the need for constant updating of our professional knowledge and education.

The present-day public outcry demands that we devote more energy on counselling, advising, educating, communicating, examining, and carrying out frequent body alignment of our clients/patients, and above all, guiding them on their food choice and feeding behaviour rather than on 'medicine and medical treatment'. Practising complementary medicine with holistic principles at the forefront of our minds will carry with it the service of guidance and counselling of our patients towards total health care. This total care is implicit in maintaining a healthy lifestyle, healthy behaviour, and habits that will eventually lead to the prevention of illness. These being done, the condition resulting from these will assist the body's natural ability to resist the attack of disease and activate its defence mechanism against illness. Using those modalities which are compatible with the vital (force) curative activities of the body, complementary practitioners should rejoice and be proud to see that their patients are cutting down on many degenerative diseases. In preventive Therapy, practitioners must avoid from falling a victim to what Dr Hahnemann called 'alternative medical orthodoxy'.

Pursuing money income, we must never lose sight of the main professional responsibility summarised in the following words by Dr Hahnemann: 'The Physicians highest calling–his/her only calling, is to make sick people well'. And I add–to make them healthy and equip them towards the prevention of further illness. The so-called earlier detection of disease in people now being propounded by the orthodox medical practitioners suggests that diseases are within the human beings already and that the earlier detection will enable an earlier treatment and eventual eradication. But as complementary practitioners, our major concern must be constant and never-ending efforts towards prevention in the first instance. Once disease has invaded the human body, the distortion and imbalance created by such a foreign agent within the body, plus the most likely effects of the treatment, may set in motion a vicious cycle. The inherent ability of the human body to heal itself and its capacity to maintain a harmonious existence with itself and environment, all must form the cardinal basis upon which we should build.

2.2 The Principal Sources of Preventive Therapy

The Application of Nutrition and Dietary

Complementary practitioners must possess thorough knowledge and professional skill in nutrition and nutritive food resources. Without these skills and knowledge, the use of food and nutrition for the therapeutic prevention of diseases will not be achieved. Natural medicine recognises whole food to be nutritionally superior to the refined and processed foods as these contain more micronutrients, which the body needs. Yes, these micro-chemical elements in fruits and vegetables in their raw states are the chemicals to which the human body has been adapted to during the many years of co-evolution.

In her research at Dunn Clinical Nutrition Centre, in. Cambridge, Dr Shelia Brigham has stated as follows: 'Scientific Research on Soya Beans, has shown that eating Soya Bean based food can proactively prevent breast cancer (breast cancer affects one in twelve women in the United Kingdom) as well as the reduction of the symptom of menopause problem and combat heart disease in both men and women.' Organisations manufacturing nutritional supplements of vitamins and minerals have been trying to produce natural imitations of these products but their products remain synthetic. These synthetic products are not bio-available to the body. In natural foods of vegetable and fruits, there are no isolated nutrients. Ail the components of micro-nutrients work together synergistically.

For example, vitamin C, present in carrots with its bioflavoids when compared with the synthetic isolated vitamins, may look physically very attractive, but the body cannot utilise it since it goes into the body and comes out through the waste. With vitamin C present in the natural vegetables and fruits, you are sure to get the following nutri-chemicals:

- Ascorbic acid (the chemical name for vitamin C)
- Bioflavonoid, retina, quercitin, hesperidins, and flavones

- Proteins/amino acids, glycol–protein
- Lipo–protein
- Carbohydrate enzyme activators
- Isolated–flavour
- Glycosides and many other cofactors

On the other hand, synthetic vitamin C contains only ascorbic acid and nothing more. The life force which animates the biological structure of the human body is maintained and kept alive by foods in their bio-absorbable form. A larger percentage of these foods are vegetables and fruits.

Dietary Adjustment

Preventative therapy should be close to the hearts of every comple-mentary health care practitioner as a cardinal part of his/her profession. The concept that one is just practising homeopathy or Hebraism, with no regard to human nutrition and dietary, is now an outdated, old-fashioned approach. Both the therapeutic care treatment and early detection form of prevention are all well and good. But absolute prevention will always be better than cure. To understand the body's needs, frequent diagnosis, examinations, nutrition, and dietary therapy are paramount to enable the practitioner embark upon therapeutic guidance.

Complementary health care diagnostic approach, which assesses the body's constitution, vital reserve, and nutritional and structural integrity, will form a realistic foundation for the preventative health care measure. Complementary medicine practice must furthermore adhere to the prevention principle that commence generations need for the sake of the future ones. Patients who are properly informed during the consulting time will expect frequent health care checks, which should assess their structural integrity. Those patients who will not accept the whole person should be referred to the orthodox practitioners at once. Osteopathically, potential functioning weaknesses, thorough Irish and other clinical examinations, and evaluation of their nutritional biochemistry are all virtual. Deficiencies of essential physical stimulation such as deep breathing and moderate exercising including yogi therapy are all very important aids to circulation processes. These will also help the eliminative functions of the lung and skin.

Dietary Fibre and Disease Prevention

Dr C. Thomson, a naturopath, in his work, has outlined the far-reaching results of constipation which affects the process of regular squeezing action of the bowels, he emphasised the importance of a diet of unrefined grains, raw vegetables, and fruits to provide the body with roughage for the maintenance of the intestinal function, There are many evidences to suggest that most of the diseases prevalent in Western societies, compared to those in the developing nations of Africa, Asia, and the South America, may be linked with the diet of fibre in their diet. Conditions such as varicose veins, obesity, hypertension, heart diseases, thrombosis, gallstones, and other digestive diseases or disorders have all been linked with chronic bowel syndrome. The diet fibre is defined as the indigestible portion of grains and vegetable structure. These include cellulose and non-cellulose polysaccharides.

The Potentials of Raw Foods

In his pioneering work, the nutritionist Dr M. Bircher-Benner conceived the idea of 'sunlight theory of nutrition'. He believed that the second law of thermodynamic was applicable to nutrition. Thus, in a diet of raw vegetable food, we find the highest potentials, and these are degraded by health/sunrays. Dr Bircher-Benner based his advocacy of a diet containing a high proportion of fresh raw fruits and vegetables on this.

Another important fact was that Dr Pottenger and Simonson provided supporting evidence of the biological value of uncooked vegetables and fruits in nutritional studies, which were carried out over a period of twenty years on eight generations of cats. The animals were divided into two equal groups. After the period of a given time, the group which was fed on uncooked foods remained very healthy. But those fed on cooked foods ended up with bone and density deformities as well as other health problems. Although each nutrient must be proportionally represented to create a balanced diet in the human nutrition, in 1892, Prof. G. Bunge showed the importance of the proportion of bio-unavailable proteins and carbohydrates in vegetable foods to human health. Preventive therapy must ensure through advice, simulation discussion, counselling, and examinations that the diets of the patients do not lack woody fibre contained in bran, vegetables, and fruits. Foods in these classes contain the greatest proportion of vitamins: minerals and trace elements.

2.3 Agricultural Soil and Their Effects

The knowledge that the bio-quality of human nutrition is determined by the principle of wholeness throughout the food chain, from the soil upwards, is very important to complementary health care practitioners. Although they are not actually involved in the plant cultivation, plant nursery, the harvesting, and the processing, the use of chemicals as fertilisers and the nature of storage and handling of food materials calls for serious attention. All these are believed to impose an unnecessary burden by free compounds on the body of the consumer. This can gradually interfere with enzyme functions and undermine cellular integrity in the human body. In his scientific observation, Dr Robert Carrion expressed the view that human and animal health was dependent on the quality of the soil. In another note, he noticed significant differences in the health of communities in different parts of India. These differences he attributed in part to various soil qualities. One of the most inspiring advocates of organic farming movement, Sir Albert Howard made a similar observation with regard to the health of animals. In preventative therapy, we must build up in our daily practice the principle of counselling our patients to obtain foods that have been organically grown. This means foods that are fertilised only with natural manure/compost free from pesticides and not prepared with synthetic additives.

Antioxidants have been shown to reduce DNA (free radical) damage. This report includes the studies testing effects of Juice Plus (whole food concentrates of fruits and vegetables) supplementation on human cellular DNA. This highly regarded method was used to arrest DNA damage. Lymphocytes were analysed and treated with an alkaline reagent to unwind the DNA. The sample was then labelled with a fluorescent marker (for DNA and then electrophoreses). As the marked DNA migrated, a tail resembling a comet was saved in the media. Cells with no DNA abnormality had no tail, while abnormal DNA produced the tail with the appearance of a comet; the longer the tail, the more the DNA damage. These comet tail movements are quantified using a spectrophotometer: DNA damage was significantly reduced (66 per cent) in the peripheral blood lymphocytes of both male and female patients, with an average age of fifty years for over a period of eighty days. DNA damage was significantly peripheral blood Lymphocytes of both smokers.

The above scientific research findings were endorsed by Dr John F. Whitethorn, MD, in his prevention therapy profile in the use of juice and fruit—vegetable as whole food supplementation. The following information increases in plasma the anti-oxidant levels (building immune system) and decreases in serum lipid peroxides (toxins). Capsules for only 28 days.

- Beta Carotene + 510% could be the best sources such as kale, carrots, broccoli, oranges, and spinach. These reduce the risk of heart disease, cancer, and eye disorders.
- Alpha-carotene + 119%: These slow the growth of cells and boost the immune system. Best Sources: carrots, pumpkin, yellow corn, and seaweed.
- Lutelnizeaxanthin + 4.4%: These could reduce the risk of muscular degeneration (eye disorder) and lung, colon, and prostate cancer. Best sources: kale, spinach, beets, and sweet peppers.
- Limonene + 2046%: This could reduce the risk of cardiovascular disease, colon, pancreatic, and prostate cancer (appears to provide photo protection against ultraviolet (light greatest known photochemical). Best Sources: tomatoes and other red fruits and vegetables.
- Alpha-tocopherol + 58%: This is an active form of vitamin E. containing very strong anti-oxidant properties, which strengthen the white blood Cells that fight off disease. Normal nerve development depends on Vitamin E. Best sources: kale, spinach, and grains. Lipid peroxides are human precursors. Toxins are reduced by 75%. Serum, lipid per (body's toxins, they are free radical. Note: juice plus capsules contain apple, orange, pineapple, cranberry, peach, acerola cherries, papaya, carrots, barley, beets, kale, broccoli, cabbage, oats, spinach, tomato plus active enzymes, oxidants and phyto-chemical, or micronutrients.

CHAPTER 3

T his chapter evaluates various dietary therapies based on fruits and vegetables. The chapter goes on to explain how the bioavailability of these sources can cause the prevention of various diseases in human body. It looks at the skills and knowledge required of the practitioners for the uses of these resources.

Our discussions have been centred on nutrition and dietary therapy as an effective method of preventive measure in the practice of complementary medicine. In one of the Health and Well-being Seminars held recently in London by the manufacturers of the Juice Plus capsule supplementation products for the benefit of both conventional and complementary medicine, it was noticed that the majority of the doctors and the complementary practitioners had no knowledge of nutrition or dietary therapy. Although this book is not a text on the science of nutrition, it is important to briefly explain what are vitamins and minerals, what they do for the human body, and the consequences of their deficiencies. Although vitamins and minerals are not medicines in any sense of the word, lack of them or the inadequate (insufficient) supply or unavailability of their micronutrients in the body will certainly lead to serious diseases in the body. Conversely, their adequate and sufficient supply to the body will certainly prevent the attack of such diseases. But if the providers of these food supplements and the providers of herbal medicines are in competition with each, it is obvious that where two 'elephants are in a struggle, the grass will inevitably be the one to suffer'. In a situation where the practitioners and the providers of the products are driven solely by the profit motive, the safety of the patients will suffer. One hopes that the economic-motivated racketeering that brought down many other professions will not ravage the practice of complementary health care.

3.1 The Description of Food Supplements

The word 'vitamin' is usually misunderstood by many people including some health care practitioners. Once the word 'vitamin' is mentioned, people think of 'pill'. This is to confuse the image of medicine and drugs. Although vitamins can work as medicines and as drugs, they are certainly not drugs or medicines. Vitamins are organic substances very necessary for regulating and maintaining the body process. They are essential for the normal functioning of the body. Apart from being few, vitamins cannot be manufactured or synthesised by the human body. They are necessary for the growth, vitality, and general well-being. They are found in minute quantities in all organic foods. They are usually obtained from these foods or from the dietary supplement. These supplements are available in the form of tablets and capsules or pills. They are still food substances. Human life cannot be sustained without all the essential vitamins and minerals. Vitamins must never be seen as pep-pills or as a substitute for food. They cannot replace food at all. They cannot be assimilated without food in the body. They have no caloric or energy value on their own. Vitamins cannot act as a substitute for proteins or for other nutrients or even each other. In fact, they are not a component part of the human body structure. Those who take only vitamins and stop eating food may either die or never be healthy at all. Vitamins regulate the human metabolism (the set of chemical reactions that happen in living organisms to maintain life). These processes allow organisms to grow, reproduce, and maintain their structures. Metabolism keeps the body tuned up and functioning at a high performance level. Deficiency in even one vitamin will result in endangering the entire human body.

3.2 Vitamins' Deficiency, Their Symptoms and Common Diseases

The following summary table may help practitioners in the diagnosis and testing of patients for the possible deficiency in any of the vitamins.

Preventive Therapy in Complimentary Medicine

Affected Areas	Signs/Symptoms	Possible Vitamin Deficiencies
General	Fatigue, malaise, apathy, depression, and the loss of appetite	Usually 8 complex Vitamins B1 and B12
Nervous systems	Headache, tingling numbness, burning skin	Vitamin B6-Niacin Vitamins BI and B2 V
	Low back pain	Folic acid, vitamin B12
	Lack of muscular coordination	Vitamins B1, B12
	Personality changes	Niacin amide
	Loss of memory	Vitamins B1, B12
	Muscle wasting and weakness	Niacin amide and folic acid
	Loss of senses	Vitamin B1
	Dragging of the feet (foot drop)	Vitamin B6
	Reduced tendon jerks	Vitamin B1
	Sub-acute combined degeneration of the spinal cord.	Vitamin B1 Vitamin B12
	An increased stress	Vitamin B-complex Vitamins C, E
Skin	Haemorrhaging	Vitamins C, K
	Dry skin	Vitamin A
	Yellow colouration	Vitamin B12
	Hardening of the skin	Vitamin A
	Spiral and interrupted hair growth	Vitamin C Vitamin B2 Niacin amide
	General dermatitis	Antithetic acid
	Burning feet	Folic acid, vitamin B12
	Scar tissue	Vitamin E
	Pregnancy striate	Vitamin E

Affected Areas	Signs/Symptoms	Possible Vitamin Deficiencies
Eyes	Poor night vision	Vitamin A
	Dry eyes	Vitamins A, B2
	Blurred vision	Vitamin B1
	Bloodshot eyes	Vitamin B2
	Dim vision	Vitamin B1, Niacin amide
	Intraocular haemorrhage	Vitamins C, K
	Optic neuritis	Vitamins B1, B12
Lips, tongues, and mouth sores	Inflammation.	Vitamin B2
	Ulceration	Vitamin B2 v
	Fissures at corners of lips	Vitamins B2, B6, B1
	Lips that hurt	Vitamins B12, B2
	Sore tongue and inflamed tongue	
	Beefy red swollen tongue	
	Fissured tongue	
	Magenta-coloured tongue	
Gums	Bleeding and spongy	Vitamin C
	Gingivitis (inflamed).	Niacin amide
Face	Seborrhoea of nose and lips	Vitamins B2, B6
	Cheek pigmentation	Niacin amide
Skeletal system	Softening of the skin (babies)	Vitamin D
	Skeletal system	Vitamin D
	Swelling of the skull (babies)	Vitamin D
	Swelling of the joints (babies)	Vitamin C
	Painful bleeding of joints	
Gastrointestinal	Diarrhoea	Niacin amide
	Digestive disorders	Vitamin B1
	Paralytic ileums	Panthothenic acid
Blood	Anaemia	Folic acid, Vitamin B12
	Haemolytic anaemia	Vitamins C, B6
		Vitamin E

In a study carried out on the quality of agricultural products at the Federal Agricultural Research Centre in Geisenheim, Germany, the vitamin content of two varieties of apple, the spice of apples, which were otherwise identical in appearance, showed a wide discrepancy. These were attributable to the variations in the mineral contents of the soil in which they were grown. The variety of the apple grown in Ontario, Canada, was found to have more than six times the vitamin C content than in those grown in Germany. Therefore, the difference in the geographical soil is a major factor in considering the vitamins and mineral contents of the given food materials. Therefore, it is very important that the environment of the soils where food materials are grown is given attention. This factor can make much difference between the effectiveness and bioavailability of the products.

3.3 The Various Foods That Cause Illnesses

In some persons, once a certain age is reached, there is a reduction in the vitality of the cell. This reduced adaptation in energy makes them less tolerant to specific food items, for example, milk, refined carbohydrate, or meat. The cumulative effects of these may give rise to various health problems. This is prominent in cow milk protein caseinogen, which is very hard to digest. This substance can cause an increase in catarrh and some form of skin disorder. In some persons, the proteins Lacto albumin and Lacto globulin can give rise to allergic reaction. Some refined sources of carbohydrates, such as sugar, on frequent intake may contribute to various health disorders because of fibre and other essential constituents being removed during their processing. These may also result to be the cause of hyper-insulin in diabetics. Another example is that of the children born in Europe and America who may be used to the Western diets. If these children are suddenly exposed to highly spiced foods and some foods of high carbohydrate content, they may suffer from the problem of indigestion and stomach ulcer. There are many evidences of these occurrences.

In orthodox medical practice, protein intake is, generally, overemphasised in nutrition. It is important to know and bear in mind that excessive intake of animal protein can be harmful to health. Prof. Janssen of Tubingen in Germany demonstrated this in his experiment when he fed students on a diet of 1,500 g of meat, 31 g of white bread, and lemon water. After ten days, their capillaries became hardened. Some were dilated and broken. The gums developed scurry-like swelling and bled easily. They were on a strict meat-free diet for two months to restore normality. According to this experiment, protein combustion in the body produces excess acid which must be neutralised by vegetable foods rich in alkaline, such as fruits. The conclusion drawn from this research is that these are the principal causes of digestive changes leading to conditions such as arthritis and few other health disorders.

Diabetic Control

Planned regulation of dietary counselling as a basic therapeutic measure must form the cardinal principle of all of complementary natural medicine practice and not only for the naturopaths or the homoeopaths. The adjustment of each patient's diet should vary according to each individual anabolic or catabolic measure. In the elderly and chronically sick, anabolic steps may be required to improve the nutritional needs of the patients for their vitality and immunity. Although all the nutritional requirements should be obtained from the foods we eat, in modern times it is very hard to imagine how many people are there who can possibly meet the required daily allowance (RDA) due to several factors. These factors need the critical attention of each natural medicine practitioner if his professional principles of holistic health care are to be upheld.

3.4 Whole Food Mixed Diet and Vegetarian Diet

The principle of the wholeness of food to be eaten as near to its natural state as possible is important. Such foods must be balanced by containing all the nutrients required in the right quantity and quality that must be bio-available to the body.

The advocates of vegetarianism (the avoidance of all animal products including fish) maintain that this method of disease prevention can be very effective. The major advantage of this method is the higher ratio of alkaline to acid-forming foods. It has been found that neither the teeth nor the gastric enzymes of humans are adapted to a carnivorous diet. It has also been reported that there is an additional burden placed on the liver by such products and excess sodium contained in animal protein. Dr James Williamson maintains that animal meats are unsuitable for human beings because they contain the development of the animal soul forces, which is rather very hard to overcome spiritually. It is also believed that the full practice of vegetarianism will lead to vitamin B12 deficiency. This is because vitamin B12 is found only in animal products. However, in natural medicine, we must weigh the overall needs of the individual's spirituality and health and longevity needs.

However, folic acid present in vegetable foods may reduce the symptom of vitamin B12 deficiency. But after a few years, symptoms such as fatigue, weight loss, anaemia, and mild neurological disturbances may result. Attention is also drawn to the likely deficiency of zinc and calcium in these foods and to the large quantity of phytate-rich foods such as beans, legumes, and grains in the diet of vegetarians. Physic acid, which binds the zinc and calcium in these foods, renders them un-absorbable. But yeast, which is present in bread, destroys hydrate. A properly planned vegetarian diet can be a source of maintaining good health.

3.5 Fruits and Vegetables Only Diet

We are being reminded often every day that the fresh, raw fruits and vegetables are good for our health. Research has continued to find some vital elements in fruits and vegetables, such as vitamins, antioxidants, phytonutrients, minerals, enzymes, and fibres, which seem to strengthen the human immune system and contribute to health and longevity in various ways. It has been suggested that getting nutrients from whole food sources such as real fruits and vegetables is much healthier than supplementing the diet with specific, isolated nutrients. Both the US and UK departments of health have recommended that we eat two to four servings of fruits and three to six servings of fresh raw vegetables daily for normal functioning good health. The unfortunate thing is that growing evidence has shown that due to the fast pace of modern life, it is not possible or easy for the majority of people to meet this requirement in their daily lives. Furthermore, when these classes of foods are eaten at all, they are always in a state of being overprocessed, overstored, and overcooked. Most of all, they are never eaten in the right quantity and quality and in the right combination. Another limitation to the availability of these required food items is the buying and preparing of four to six servings of different food—fresh fruits and vegetables—every day. This task takes a tremendous amount of time and energy. The average individual does not have both the time and the means of doing this.

The tendency today is that people have developed great passion for constantly going for junk food. The usual excuses are as follows: We are too busy to be involved in the long processes of preparing food. Or it is that they do not have that amount of money required for the constant purchase of so many fruits and vegetables every day. Most people's eating behaviour is concentrated on buying fast and convenient foods than checking for their expiry date. But the health consequences of this behaviour are obvious.

Macrobiotics Dietary Therapy

Writing about the 'art of living', German Prof. Dr C. W. Hufeland, in the early nineteenth century, advocated whole grains food and plant foods indigenous to the locality of the *consumer*. With careful therapeutic planning for the needs of the individual patients, macrobiotic dietary therapy as an additional preventative system fulfils the requirements of a basic dietary therapy. For example, there exist many different stores throughout the modern cities of many nations, some of which cater for the indigenous food items of various kinds from all over the world. While the natural medicine practitioners are not expected to have knowledge of all the indigenous food items that exists, proper guidance and the direction of the patient towards the need for these commodities will be an aid to good macrobiotic dietary therapy.

3.6 Raw Fruits and Vegetables Juice Dietary Therapy

Raw fruits and vegetables have been recognised throughout the history of man as a natural source of the food substances needed to help protect the strength, vigour, and youthful appearance, which most mature humans desire. At the beginning of creation, God said, 'Behold; I have given you every plant yielding seeds; it shall be food for you' (Gen. 1:29). Fruits and vegetables were to be all that were eaten in the Garden of Eden. From the history of antiquity, it has been discovered that the ancient Egyptian Africans who lived around the Garden of Eden also ate raw fruits and raw vegetables as their native indigenous foods. History also says that these people lived much longer than modern man. The eating of animals as food we are told is of later development.

Fasting Dietary Therapy

This is the practice of voluntary abstention from food for a given period of time say from twelve hours to three months. Dr M Shelton in the United States has drawn a distinction between therapeutic fasting and starvation. He stated that during the period in question, if hunger is lacking, the patient is fasting, but once hunger returns, if the patient continue, fasting, he or she is only but starving. During such a period of the actual fasting the following health benefits may be achieved:

- A physiological rest of the digestive tract
- Mobilisation of detoxifying defence mechanisms
- Stimulus to subsequent recuperation

Fasting is particularly good for fibrite diseases such as influenza, tonsillitis, bronchitis, and some fevers in children. It is also vital for disorders such as gastroenteritis, asthma, sinusitis, and cholecysttis. It can provide the physiological stimulation essential for mobilising the healing mechanism of the body. Physical stimuli such as deep breathing and moderate exercises are all essential aid to fasting as they help in the circulation processes. These will also help to promote the eliminative functions of the lungs and the skin.

3.7 Mono-dietary Therapy

This is the practice of manipulating foods, that were performed to meet the low-fat and high-mono dietary.

This dietary therapy was the only treatment available in the era before insulin therapy. This is another form of dietetic stimulus. It is the restriction of the patients' intake of a given food item for some days. The effect of this therapy is the saturation of the system with the particular nutrients of which the food is composed. One of the best-known mono-diet fruit is that of grape cure. The patient may eat up to 6 lbs of the fruit a day. During the period in question, all liquid intakes should be just water and grape apple juice. This therapy is known to be effective for high blood pressure, cardiac problems, and general fluid retention. The benefits may be due to high potassium contents of the grapes.

Much of the nutritional substances in raw fruits and vegetables are usually concentrated in their natural juices. These juices are 'saturated in the cellulous fibres of the plants'. In order to extract the nutrients, the body must break down the fibrous cells. For the digestive system, especially in the elderly people, and sometimes dental problems for proper chewing, this can be a hard task. Properly controlled, the combined juice of raw fruits and vegetables with all their materials of minerals and vitamins will flood the body with the essential materials to build strong, healthy, and functioning cells. In this way, the body can be revitalised in an amazingly short period of time. This therapy is 'an age old Grand Mama method'. Although it has been taken for granted by man, the method is being accepted as vital for its role in complementary natural medicine preventative therapy. Only the juice of fresh, raw fruits and vegetables captures the whole synergistic complex of the healing ingredients contained within the living plant. These impressive therapeutic effects of the plant juice are not attributable to any single substance but to the complex effects of various elements contained only in raw, fresh plants. A message to the reader: If you are a devoted natural medicine practitioner, why not just experiment this by keeping a fridge full of some well-prepared raw fresh fruit and vegetable juice in your clinic. Depending on the diagnostic results of your patients, begin to administer some doses of the fruit juice. Carry out a weekly evaluation of the results of this experiment to see the effects and the improvement in the health of your patients. But please ensure that the juice is a representative of the sizable number of the combined raw fruits and raw vegetables.

As natural medicine therapists, we must resist the daily temptation of falling for 'that darling of the general health care, the pill'. Indeed, what makes the juice of raw fruits and raw vegetables a remedy is that you have chosen this method of disease prevention, but for heaven's sake, do not denigrate this. It is of almost no use if all that the practitioner is prepared to do is to advise the patient to obtain the fruit and vegetable juice from the nearest supermarket and live on the doses. All the health care precautions applicable to food items discussed above in the preventative therapy must also apply to raw fruit and vegetable juice dietary therapy. Those patients who cannot eat raw fruits and vegetables because of stomach disorders or ulcers can take fruit juice with no resultant problem at all. Walter Schoenenberger, a Swiss pharmacist, realised the healing and medicinal potential of plant juice early in the nineteenth century and became impressed by the efforts to encourage the spreading of this knowledge; the German government awarded him a gold medal for his contributions to public health. The most important factor to consider is to pay due attention to the hygienic conditions in the preparation and storage of the juice for consumption. Both the equipment, the utensils, and personal hygiene of the persons preparing and carrying out the processing of raw fruits and vegetable juices are all strictly important. Examples of effects of dank damage mutation, births defects, sterility, age related diseases chronic and overall ageing canc.

3.8 Dietary Supplementation and Mineral Deficiency

Osteoarthritis and the Meaning

In this book many authentic natural medical products from all over the world are subscribing to our recognition. Both their names and details are therefore shown here for the reader's perusal. There are no orthodox medical products shown here. Any reader interested in any of the products in this book can place an order through the details of address given.

The word 'arthritis' is taken from Greek words meaning 'inflamed joints' and is associated with a group of over 100 rheumatic diseases and conditions. These diseases may affect not only the joints but also the muscles, bones, tendons, and ligaments that support them. Osteoarthritis is the condition that results when the cartilage is slowly eroded, and bone begins grinding against bone. This is accompanied by bony outgrowths called osteophytes. Cysts may form, and the underlying bone thickens and becomes deformed. Other symptoms include knobby knuckles, grating and grinding sounds that emanate from arthritic joints, and muscle spasms, along with pain, stiffness, and loss of mobility. Osteoarthritis rarely spreads to other body parts but concentrates its erosive influence in one or just a few joints.

Who are at risk for osteoarthritis? While age alone does not cause osteoarthritis, the loss of joint cartilage is experienced more frequently with increasing age. Others at risk may include those who have some abnormality in the way their joint surfaces fit together or who have weak leg and thigh muscles, legs of unequal length, or a misalignment of the spine. Trauma to a joint caused either by an accident or by an occupation in which repetitive motions overuse a joint can also set the stage for osteoarthritis. Once deterioration begins, being overweight can exacerbate osteoarthritis.

Glucosamine Species

Glucosamine is a naturally occurring substance in the body, the purpose of which is to stimulate the manufacture of collagen (the protein portion of a fibrous substance that holds joints together). Collagen is also the main constituent of reticular cartilage. A large number of clinical studies have been conducted to quantify the effects of glucosamine on osteoarthritis. Results have been conflicting. A multi-centre clinical trial conducted by the National Institutes of Health in 2006 found that patients taking glucosamine HCl, chondroitin sulphate, or a combination of the two had no statistically significant improvement in their symptoms compared to patients taking a placebo. However, a secondary analysis suggested that supplementation with glucosamine may help to alleviate symptoms in patients with moderate to severe pain (Clegg, et al. 2006).

Although glucosamine's effect on joint damage is still debated, many medical experts believe this supplement reduces pain and it is safe. The usual dose is 500 mg three times a day.

Glucosamine is a modified sugar produced by the body. It is used to form larger molecules called glycosaminoglycans, which are involved in the formation and repair of cartilage. They are also used as lubricants and shock absorbers by our joints. Synthetically produced glucosamine is used to address the imbalance between production and destruction of naturally occurring glucosamine in osteoarthritis cartilage. The two chemical forms available are glucosamine sulphate (Arthro-Aid Direct, Bioglan, Blackmores, Arthrogen, Golden Glow, Healthstream, and Procosamine) and glucosamine hydrochloride (Arthro-Aid and Osteo-Eze).

Glucosamine can be administered as a topical cream, an oral tablet, an intra-muscular injection, and as an intra-articular injection (directly into the joint). There have been a number of studies that have reported an improvement in joint discomfort with the use of glucosamine (Houpt J. B., McMillan R., Wein C., and Paget-Dellio D., Effect of glucosamine hydrochloride in the treatment of pain of osteoarthritis of the knee, *Journal of Rheumatology*, 1999; 26 (11): 2423-30). There have also been reports comparing glucosamine to ibuprofen. Each of these studies showed a similar amount of relief in patients administered glucosamine and ibuprofen. In one study, glucosamine was shown to be more effective than ibuprofen (Muller-Fassbender H., Bach G. L., Haase W., Rovati L. C., and Setnikar L., Glucosamine sulfate compared to ibuprofen in osteoarthritis of the knee, *Osteoarthritis Cartilage*,1994; 2: 61-9). Glucosamine is a safe, natural product that has exhibited few side effects. Those that have been shown have been gastrointestinal in nature (Reginster J. Y., Deroisy R., Rovati L. C., Lee R. L., Lejeune E., Bruyere O.,

Giacovelli G., Henrotin Y., Dacre J. E., and Gossett C., Long-term effects of glucosamine sulphate on osteoarthritis progression: a randomised, placebo-controlled clinical trial, *Lancet,* 2001; 357 (9252): 251-6).

Chondroitin Sulphate

This is a naturally occurring molecule that is a component of cartilage. It helps keep the cartilage resilient by absorbing fluid into the connective tissue. Researchers also believe that chondroitin blocks the enzymes that break down cartilage as well as provide the building blocks for cartilage to repair itself. (Busci L. and Poor G., Efficacy and tolerability of oral chondroitin sulfate as a symptomatic slow-acting drug for osteoarthritis (SYSADOA) in the treatment of knee osteoarthritis, *Osteoarthritis Cartilage*). Chondroitin supplements are not known to exhibit any side effects. Chondroitin is commonly sold as chondroitin sulphate in capsule or tablet form. It is also available in combination with various forms of glucosamine and sometimes manganese as well. A dosage of 400 mg twice per day is recommended.

Hyaluronic acid is a fluid in the knee joint. A person with osteoarthritis of the knee has a reduced amount of hyaluronic acid in the joint. Injections are used to put more of the fluid into the joint and so provide more protection for it. The intended result for sufferers is that they experience relief from pain, which may last up to six months. However, the injections are very expensive, costing in the region of 0.

In a meta-analysis of eight hyaluronan trials involving 971 patients, the outcomes in patients treated with hyaluronan were superior to outcomes in patients treated with a placebo at the end of the treatment cycles and after six months (George E., Intra-articular hyaluronan treatment for osteoarthritis, *Ann Rheum Dis*, 1998; 57: 637-40). Other studies, however, have shown little or no benefit. If you feel that you could benefit from this treatment, consult your physician.

Ginger

For hundreds of years, ginger has been used as an anti-arthritis treatment. Ginger acts as an antagonist to prostaglandins. The dried rhizome of ginger contains approximately 1-4 per cent volatile oils. These are the medically active constituents of ginger and are also responsible for ginger's characteristic odour and taste. The aromatic constituents include zingiberene and bisabolene, while the pungent constituents are known as gingerols and shogaols. (Bliddal H., Rosetzsky A., Schlichting P., Weidner M. S., Andersen L. A., Ibfelt H. H., Christensen K., Jensen O. N. and Barslev J., A randomized, placebo-controlled, cross-over study of ginger extracts and ibuprofen in osteoarthritis, *Osteoarthritis Cartilage*, 2000; Jan; 8(1):9-12). Boswellia is an Ayurvedic plant that contains anti-inflammatory triterpenoids called boswellic acids. The aromatic gum resins from this tree have been used by practitioners of the avurvedic system of medicine to treat arthritis for centuries. An Ayurvedic herbal combination of ashwagandha, boswellia, and curcumin was evaluated in a randomised, double-blind, placebo controlled, crossover study in patients with osteoarthritis. Treatment with this formulation produced a significant drop in the severity of pain. ('Efficacy and tolerability of Boswellia serrata extract in treatment of osteoarthritis of knee-a randomized double blind placebo controlled trial' by Dr Kimmatkar N., Dr Thawani V., and Dr Hingorani L., Khiyani at MS Orthopedics, Indira Gandhi Medical College, Nagpur, India. *Phytomedicine*).

Glucosamine and Chondroitin

Glucosamine and chondroitin supplements are used to slow the progression of osteoarthritis and to lessen the pain associated with it. Glucosamine is sold in many forms, including glucosamine sulphate, glucosamine hydrochloride (HCl), and N-acetyl glucosamine (NAG), and may also contain a potassium chloride or sodium chloride salt. However, there appears to be no conclusive evidence that one form is better than another. Chondroitin is typically sold as chondroitin sulphate. The supplements appear to be more effective when taken together.

CHAPTER 4

African Traditional Medicine

This chapter looks at the definition and origin of African traditional medicine. It also presents information on various health degenerations of the modern African race resulting from the so-called modern civilisation. This chapter proceeds further into various aspects of preventive therapies demanding urgent attention in the present period. This chapter also sees how the modern African traditional medicine is linked to that of the ancient Khemetian Egyptians. It is here that the presentation of the programme outline of the new Federal College of Complementary and Alternative Medicine in Nigeria is explained. Here some useful information will be given about the danger of bowel infections and disease, diseases that affect male and female reproductive organs. A brief discussion on the African female's natural health therapy that affects both their internal and external beauty is given. A discussion on Dr Ssali's Mariandina nutritional food supplement products under the traditional African medicine is given. This chapter also deals with the importance of eating more of the African indigenous foods products as a means of continuing preventive therapy among the people of African origin. A brief outline of some psychosomatic and psychological health problems common among the Africans is also given.

4.1 The Nature and Origin of African Traditional Medicine

Although this section of the chapter does not deal with the ancient history of Africa, it is rather very interesting as information about one of the legends of the African founding father of medicine is given attention here. This man is called Imhotep. He was a priest and a high government official serving under the Egyptian Third Dynasty king, Djoser. Imhotep designed Djoser's tomb, a step pyramid in Saqqara that's considered the world's oldest stone building. Imhotep's work predates reliable records, but modern scholarship puts King Djoser's reign around 2640 BC, possibly ending around 2613 BC. Imhotep advised the king and supposedly produced journals (now lost) on medicine and healing, and he's credited with designing Djoser's tomb, a forty-acre complex near ancient Memphis, which required the mobilisation of thousands of labourers. Over the next 2000 years, Imhotep's legend grew. He was deified in Egypt, and the Greeks (who called him Imouthes) associated him with their God of medicine—Asclepius. Considered a semi-mythical figure until archaeological findings of the twentieth century, Imhotep is considered by many to be history's first scientist. Some people think the Joseph of the Bible and Imhotep are one and the same. Since 1990, Egypt's Saqqara Geophysical Survey Project has been working on what they believe is the site of Imhotep's tomb. 'Of the non royal population of Egypt, probably one man was known better than all others' (as given in the book *Imhotep, Doctor, Architect, High Priest, Scribe and Vizier to King Djoser* by Jimmy Dunn). Imhotep lived during the Old Kingdom and was born a commoner during the Third Dynasty. He was very skilled and was dedicated to the ideals of his nation. He was the manufacturer of products from plant seeds mixed with grapefruit seed extract and other alternative medicinal herbs which he used in healing. He was born *c.* 2700 BC, his birthplace was near Memphis, Egypt, he died *c.* 2600 BC, and is best known as the architect of the oldest Egyptian architecture.

Research into anthropology and archaeology shows that the origin of African traditional medicine is traced back to Dr Imhotep—the real father of medicine. This African of ancient Egypt (Kimit—the ancient indigenous Africans known as the mother of Western civilisation) was the originator of medicine and not Hippocrates who lived 2,000 years later. Imhotep Kanofer was born in Kimit, Egypt (Africa), on 21 May of the year 2980 BC. His mother was Khereduankh and his father was Kanofer. He was a distinguished architect and master builder. Imhotep spread the knowledge of medicine to Greece and Rome throughout the centuries. He was a scientist and most famous physician. He was a multi-genius who invented the sciences of architect, economics, engineering, psychosomatic healing, and astronomy. It was Imhotep who designed the step pyramid of Saqqara in Egypt. He was revered and called the great 'God of Medicine'. To say that we cannot trace and attribute the origin of medicine to the African race is madness! The Greeks renamed Imhotep 'Aeclepios', meaning the God of Healing. The symbol of medical profession—the caduceus—was the insignia found in his temples. His temple was, in fact, the first hospital known to the world at the time! From Egypt came the earliest medical books; the first observatory for human physiology; and the first experiment in surgery, pharmacy to anatomical and medical vocabulary. In the tribute to this African original father of medicine, the Institute of Traditional African Medicine has placed Imhotep's image in the centre of their official logo to commemorate his ancient ingenuity—the origin of natural medicine.

4.2 The Nature of the African Traditional Medicine

African traditional medicine, not just the plants science, the psychosomatic/psychotherapy and the approach to diagnoses. These include the very early knowledge of anaesthetics and antiseptic and the knowledge of vaccinations and surgical techniques in use. African herbal medicines are very effective. These had sustained lives very long before the coming of the white man. In fact, when the white Arabs and the white Europeans arrived, the ancient Africans believed that their 'August Visitors' had brought a faster and better medical system to improve upon their own existing system. But little did they know that their own medical system was being destroyed and replaced by that of the Europeans. In accordance with the theme of this book, *The Preventive Therapy*, my finding is that the natural health therapist must insist on advising Africans to begin to review their food and feeding habits. This approach will do much to prevent some of the modern diseases associated with their acquired Euro-centric lifestyle of food habits.

Research has shown that the people of African origin whose major sources of diets were indigenous commodities, free from chemical, derived their balance nutrients and protection from their foods. Usually, they had a high degree of resistance to disease, a high degree of immune system, and lived a healthier and longer life. These food commodities in their biochemistry possess therapeutic properties for maintaining good health with no side effects or addiction. Most natural remedies derive their ingredients from such food products.

4.3 The Typical Examples of African Health Food Commodities

Some of the typical examples of African health food commodities are as follows: yam and cocoyam; unripe plantains; unripe bananas); unripe pawpaw; cocoyam leaves; sweet potatoes and their leaves; green and red peppers; cassava and cassava leaves; tropical water melons and their seeds; egusi oil and its seeds; pumpkins and their seeds; tropical water leaves; Ugu and their seeds; Uha leaves; Ewedu, Okwuru, Ogbono and their oil; tropical chicken natural breed and their eggs and Gene fowl; tropical red ginger, tropical garlic, and tropical red onions; tropical snails and frogs; African/tropical fish both fresh and wood-dried, African wood-dried bushmeat; Okazi; Ngalangala, Ehuru, Achi, and ukpo; Nchuawa and Ugbogro; Adu; Nkwu; Eruru; Mbusu; Abuba-Eke (Piton oil); Akide, Odudu, Ukpara, and grasshoppers; grasscutter bushmeat; Nzu; and many more tropical African food commodities which I am not able to mention here. Anybody who tells you that any of the above listed items including the red oil from African palm tree is unhealthy, must substantiate this claim with independent, unbiased research evidence.

The following is one of the recent practices in the uses of African food products:

Soy Organic Garri and Poundo Yam

We are beginning to enter into the new age of awareness in the era of African health food commodities. This has come with our realisation that no one but ourselves will ever rediscover the potentialities inherent in our indigenous food commodities. We have now realised that the total health vitality and longevity are connected to every aspect of our lives and also that the quality of our lives is a matter of personal choice. We can ignore our connection to the natural balance of living or strive to create integrity, balance, and awareness in every aspect of our daily lives.

The envied physical energy and bio-longevity of the indigenous Africans are attributable to the types and organic nature of the food materials they eat. Both the animal and vegetable sources of their foods are basically organic. Organic food is a term that has acquired the meaning of foods grown under natural conditions (without the use of inorganic fertilisers, pesticides, or any other chemical process). For example, the animals feed on the tropical grassland and the green plant leaves full of natural bio-resources. These vegetables and the fruits grow naturally in rainforests where vitamin D is synthesised by the ultra rays of the sun.

The Natural Balance Brief Discussion About Yam

Yam is a native of tropical Africa. It is a stable food crop in much of the tropical world. It is not the same thing as the sweet potato. The two differ both in appearance and texture. Yam has almost 50 per cent more protein and three times more starch than sweet potatoes. It is a better source of energy. For example, 100 g of boiled yam will provide 133 calories compared to the sweet potato's eighty-four calories. Yam is also a good source of potassium, which is needed for muscle and nerve function. The yellow-flesh varieties are a useful source of beta carotene. Through laboratory research in various nations in Africa, especially in Ghana and Nigeria, careful refining and processing have produced yam powder of first-class quality. This poundo yam, as it is called, is usually exported to various nations of the world. Yam can be used for the production of cakes, biscuits, bread, and fufu. Yam can be prepared and eaten in various ways. For example, yam porridge, boiled yam, baked yam, roast yam, fried and sautéed yam, pounded yam, yam stew, and yam pepper soup.

Cassava

This is the basic raw material from which garri is produced. It is a tropical vegetable plant tuber of West African origin. Almost every nation in western Africa produces cassava in varying quantities. Cassava is made into garri, fufu, and other end products. The cassava flour powder is used in the production of bread and biscuits. The two principal species of cassava are the white spice family mainly used for making garri and the red spice family (ofume-Iwa in Efick Calabar River State of Nigeria). This type of cassava is used in various ways. They can be prepared and eaten exactly as yam unlike the white type. In whichever form the cassava is prepared, it is a major stable source of food in Nigeria and Ghana. In the southern part of Nigeria, mainly within the eastern states, cassava is predominantly the principal staple diet of the people.

The Cassava Stems

Being one of the most economic plants sources of food, the stems are planted in the months of March, July, and September and can be harvested after three to four months of planting depending on the nature of the soil. The unfortunate thing these days is that chemical fertilisers are now being used to induce faster and increased production of cassava in some parts of Africa. We are told that these types of fertilisers are substances that supply plant nutrients or amend soil fertility and that they are the most effective means of increasing crop production and improving the quality of food produced. We are also told that fertilisers enhance the natural fertility of the soil or replace the chemical elements taken from the soil by previous crops. The use of manure and composts as fertilisers is probably almost as old as agriculture. Modern chemical fertilisers include one or more of the three elements most important in plant nutrition: nitrogen, phosphorus, and potassium. Of secondary importance are the following elements: sulphur, magnesium, and calcium.

The Cassava Leaves

These are translucent, greenish, and also edible. The leaves are very rich in various vitamins and minerals such as vitamins A, B Complex, vitamin C, folic acid, calcium, magnesium, phosphorous, and vitamin D. The leaves can also be made into capsules in special preparation.

The Cassava Tuber

This part of the product is a major source of the starchy food of the indigenous people of the eras mentioned above. But starch is reduced by 80 per cent during the process of garri production, and this makes the garri diet a suitable lighter meal of fufu (or eba as the Nigerian nation calls it) for those people on a lower carbohydrate diet as opposed to the meal of fufu. During the processes of garri production, most of the water and heat soluble vitamins and mineral contents of the tuber such as vitamins C and B Complex are reduced. To replace these vitamin and mineral losses, the soya organic garri and the soya organic poundo yam products are fortified with natural phytonutrient blends. These contain the following ingredients.

Micro-nutrients present in the soya organic (organic soya bean) used in the process of fortification of isoflavones such as genistein and diazein are powerful phytoestrogen-protective agents against breast and prostate cancer. Each pack of the soya organic garri and soya organic poundo yam contains 30 mg of these soya organic micro-nutrients. One of the nutritional advantages of the soya organic garri is its higher content of the cellulous plant structure known as roughage. This substance is very important for the work of the small intestine in the absorption and assimilation of the micronutrients into the bloodstream. It can also protect against diverticulosis, spastic colon, haemorrhoids, cancer of the colon, and varicose veins.

It is high time that all the people of African origin begin to reverse back to their indigenous native foods. The Indians, the Chinese, the Japanese, and many other races of the world are relying on their native foods to survive. We must resist the temptation by anybody to bribe or use the law to deprive us from eating or dieting in accordance with our nature and indigenous tradition. We must begin to stop from being bamboozled into making the food of other cultures as our own. It is very foolish to depend on the foods of European origin and thereby promote their own economic well-being to our own detriment. In fact, even though they may live in our countries for many years they will still continue to buy their own type of food commodities. Wherever they live, they will always continue to reflect and support their indigenous economic and cultural affinity. If you are ever in any doubt of the bio-chemistry authenticity in any of the above listed African food items, feel free to take a sample to an unbiased food laboratory anywhere in the world. But please do not continue sending 'Coal to New Castle'. The world we in live is being controlled and influenced by the system of economic interest, and health matter is no exception at all!

We should never be afraid to claim that the origin of medicine in every land in the world is traceable to the African race. But the demon of imperialism and slavery did its best to set aside the African system of medicine to make way for the European system. They have trained many Africans to believe and accept that our medical practices are not systematic comparable to those of the Chinese and Indians. As we start to embark upon the redevelopment of African traditional medicine (ATM), we are not discovering a new field of science, but rather we are beginning to pick the bits and pieces of what has been left by the ravage of imperialism. Even at this, the African house 'niggers' will still find this very hard to accept. We must begin to rediscover our Ancient health care culture as our indigenous heritage. The African Egyptians and Ethiopians paid great attention to health, diseases, and sicknesses.

These were among the major facts of life in Ancient Egypt and Nubian. Diseases such as tuberculoses, leprosy, typhoid, and malaria fever were already flourishing. Much of the health imbalance was caused by poor water management, poor food control and management, and poor social hygiene and environment.

The rate of lifespan was very low. To eradicate the causes of disease and illnesses was the major concern of the African indigenous healers. These conditions set them to search in nature for an answer. In time, they discovered through natural instinct that both plants and animals were the sources of their foods. Consequently, they discovered too that the same products were also the sources of their health care and medicine. From this, it is clear that the ancient Africans were the originators of health care science. Their practice may have been at a rudimentary stage, but it was the system that sustained their lives. These food commodities will remain effective in the supply of natural nutrients as long as they are not grown with chemical fertilisers. Once these plants and animals means of their natural nutrients are replaced by chemicals, their lives will no longer subsist without a continuous never-ending supply of such fertilisers. This is one of the ways of creating negative agricultural dependence on the Western technology. Before the introduction of Western agricultural chemical fertilisers into the African communities, natural manure was the only sources of fertilisers throughout. The choice is now ours. Continue to be poisoned by the chemically produced foods or begin to research into our own natural sources of fertilisers for safety, protection, and survival. If we ignore these approaches, our death rate will increase, our birth rate will decrease, our life rate will decrease, and our infant mortality rate will increase. Has God destined us to perpetual subservience and dependence?

In the year 2980 BC, a child was born to the Ancient Africans of Egypt. He was called Imhotep or Imhotep Kaaofor (generally called Okafor by the Igbos of Nigeria.) In fact, the origin of this father of medicine can be traced to the Igbo nation—the origin of mankind. This extraordinary man became the lifesaver of the entire society of his land. Imhotep devoted most part of his ninety-nine years of existence on earth to discovering and developing the medical science of his kemetic nation now called Egypt. This unusual African man expanded and extended his genius into various fields such as the science of chemistry, mathematics, architecture, and engineering. In time, the knowledge we know today as psychotherapy, psychosomatic (healing without medicine (Dibia Afa), and the divination—healing through the divine power by tapping into the individual's psyche were used to treat people. This is today referred to as spiritual healing. Health research carried out in Asia, Europe, and America has shown that the people of African origin whose major sources of diets are of natural sources live longer and are also healthier. In natural medical practice, it is not the symptoms that must be cured, but the underlying cause for this symptom is only the body's call or warning that there are deficiencies to be supplied. For example, a man who goes without food for three days and nights, consequently, will be in pains, fever, headache, etc. Obviously, his sickness is not a disease but it is simply due to lack of food. If this condition ever continues, the symptoms or the body's process will not kill him. It is lack of food to provide for the body's processes that will kill him or her.

If the carers did not know how to cure the pains by providing the necessary food requirements, the ache arising from his lack of some of the resources will certainly lead to sickness. No medication of any kind will ever form a substitute for the body's calls for food and its nourishing phytonutrients. So it is the phytochemical present in various food items that may do the magic. Lack of any of them will set up certain symptoms, which is nature's method of indicating that certain types of the vital 'workers' of the body are absent and must be supplied. The thorough knowledge of these vital elements and the symptoms of their deficiency in the human body must form a major part of the practitioner's training and practice to ensure preventive therapy. This is the reason for my criticism of most of the complementary health care practitioners who go by the name of 'holistic medicine practitioners'. It is also the reason for my writing this book. Views of this nature, I am sure, are not new, but their emphasis is almost dying away slowly and needs to be replaced.

Natural medicine practitioners tend to behave in ways that seem to suggest that once people hear terms such as alternative medicine, they will rush with all confidence. In time this claim will be of no use at all, unless they are describing an operational functionality that goes to remedy the imbalance in the people's health condition. The fundamental basis of preventive therapy must be nutrition and dietary measure, which aims at application of wholeness. If we look around us, it is already evident that the orthodox approach to nutrition is based primarily on quantitative factors. In terms of calories, daily requirements of minerals and carbohydrates, and protein differentiation, complementary preventative therapy must, in addition to taking into account these, be concerned with the theory that food be eaten near to its natural state as possible given the correct quantity, the correct quality, and in the correct mix to arrive at the balanced meal for each person. Our understanding is that the refinement and processing of foods will always result in the loss of their essential vitamins, minerals, and trace elements; hence the balance and interaction cannot be satisfactorily replaced by any synthetic substitute.

Although an individual takes the greatest personal care over his or her daily food intake, as a matter of fact, the dietary habits, lifestyle, eating behaviour of people, and their social attitudes tend to place a barrier in the way towards a healthy level for their well-being. Preventive complementary therapy is for the practitioners to become skilful in the requirements of healthy dieting for maintaining the bio-availability. These were the natural medical and health care treatments used for many years before the arrival of the Arabs and Europeans. The system was found to be best suited to black-skinned African men and women, young and old. The system was based on our climate, temperature, temperament, spirit, body, mind, vegetations, and our total being. The black African system of health care ensured healthy life, peace of mind, vitality, and longevity. Although all human beings are biologically similar, some diseases and treatments suitable, for example, to some people of non-black skin may not be suitable for the Africans due to the differences in their indigenous soil, environment, food, vegetation, and ethno-spirituality.

4.4 The Traditional Medicine Preventive Measures

The principles of the African knowledge of illness and healing come from pre-ankh health and long life originated from our ancient heritage: natural sources of plants, animals, and minerals in the soil. Our ancestral Africans based their health care and well-being on these natural products for many centuries until the Europeans began to replace their system with chemical medicine. It is these chemical medicines which have reduced our natural resistance, hence resulting in countless diseases and early deaths. But thank God that we are now gradually rediscovering our African health care heritage. To rediscover the African health care heritage, a favourable environment free of corruption, adulteration, 'and monkey business magic' based on superstition must be checked in the prevailing stifling authoritarian regime dominated by Western-backed demagogues in some of the African nations. An effective practice of modern African traditional medicine must be based on the following principles:-

- Prevention and treatment
- Regeneration of the body defence mechanism
- The effective ejection of waste from the body
- The creation of harmony and balance within the body
- The prevention of low sperm counts in men and increase vitality
- The stabilisation of food intake and nutrients
- The prevention of fibroid in females

As naturopathic physicians, one of our major tasks must be to embark upon the body purification plan. The aim must be to clear the body of toxin that contributes to weight gain, fatigue, and chronic illnesses. Healing diet: 'Eating the right kind of foods is the major principle of detoxification therapy,' says Dr Elson M. Haas ND, director of the Preventive Medical Centre, Marin, San-Rafael, California, USA; the Late Prof. Charles Ssali, the director of Mariandina Natural Health Centre, UK and West Africa; and Dr Llaila Afrika, Naturopathic Health Centre, UK and USA.

In the modern African communities the disease of blood pressure is so common that its danger is hardly understood. Many of the complementary practitioners view it as a disease that should be treated or cured. Apart from the famous HIV disease as a killer, the next in the line of a killer disease is blood pressure (BP). It is therefore vital that we must establish, at least, a rudimentary knowledge of what BP actually means. In order to help us understand this, let us look at that 'natural pump' placed in the human body called 'heart'. The human heart is an engineering marvel—an elegant pump that receives oxygen rich in blood from the lungs and uses just the right amount of force to push it back through the arteries and out to the body's tissues.

Action: When all goes well during this activity of pumping, there is just enough pressure inside the arteries to maintain a steady flow of blood. But such pressure can be affected by exercise, stress, diet, and hormones, as well as by blood loss from menstruation or by severe injury. To keep the system working correctly in the face of constantly changing conditions, the heart makes continual adjustment. Its rate of beating speeds up or slows down and the strength of its contraction increases and decreases.

Blood Pressure: This measures how much the heart contracts (*systolic* pressure) and how much the arteries contract (*diastolic*) pressure. A reading of 140 systolic over 90 diastolic is considered as the upper limit of the normal level. Some sections of this book will give information on the appropriate procedure for the prevention and control of the problem of blood pressure. Actually, it can be referred to as a modern lifestyle health problem rather than as an infectious illness.

4.5 Bowel as the Major Source of Infection and Disease

Among the African communities both at home in Africa and within the Diaspora Africans, the malady of bowel infections due to the intestinal parasites is becoming rampant. This is because Africans no longer depend on their native indigenous food habits. With the increased enjoyment of Western lifestyle there are some heavy prices to be paid.

About 62 million people in the United States suffer from digestive illnesses. More than half the UK population suffer from a similar illness. A significant part of this epidemic is due to parasitic infections. It was believed before that parasitic infection was the syndrome of tropical climates attributable to the presence of dirty water, food, and unhygienic environmental conditions. But today, it has been discovered that parasitic infections are widespread in both Europe and America. They affect more than 150 million U.S. citizens and at least 40 per cent of the world population according to United Nations Health Organisation.

In the United Kingdom, laboratory evidence has proved that parasites are the missing diagnosis in the genesis of many chronic health problems, for example, the diseases of the gastrointestinal tract and endocrine system. For example, filarial worms, hookworms, whipworms, pinworms, and flatworms affect more than 4 million people around the world. These lead to illnesses such as elephantiasis, blindness, and serious intestinal diseases including haemorrhoids and dysentery. It will not matter at all whether a person is wealthy or poor; parasites have consciousness of equality and attack all socio-economic groups, including great scientists, statesmen, and women.

Significant Symptoms of Parasites Are as Follows

Abnormal pains and cramps; anaemia; arthritis; bloody stools; chronic fatigue syndrome; colitis; constipation/bloating; fever; flatulence; food allergy; foul-smelling stool; gastritis; headache; inflammatory bowel disease; intestinal permeability; irregular bowel movement; IBS: irritable bowel syndrome; joints and muscular aches and pains; low back pain; malabsorption of nutrients, hence bio-unviable; nervousness; rash and itching of the skin; abnormal weight loss; skin conditions; sleep disturbances; rectal bleeding; and vomiting. African people whose food brand loyalty is based on items such as pork and pork products, beef, chicken, and fish products not well done are all victims of major parasitic infections. Once the parasitic infection has occurred, they will colonise the large intestines, lay their eggs, and continue to extract their nutrients from your blood through the nutrients of the food you eat. In time, they will multiply and grow. The first-class food items they love most and feed upon are sugary foods, bananas, chocolates, ice creams, sweet potatoes, sweet drinks, under-done meats, and under-done eggs.

Intestinal parasites will not grow in the bowels of those whose daily diets contain the following food products:

> African bitter leaf; Uha; Okazi; Ewedu; Egusi; Ogbono; Utazi; Ehuru; Ugu; Nchuawu; Ose-Nsukka; red African pepper; garri, pounded yam; cassava; cocoyam, unripe plantains, unripe bananas; African dried bushmeat; African wood-dried fish; African red onions, garlic, ginger, and red cloves.

Those who must practice anal sex must use condoms otherwise they will become an agent for the cross-transmission of parasitic infection through the eggs. They can also transmit diseases such as anus cancer and ulcer of the rectum and that of the penis. Bisexual men and women must be aware that they can be infected or can carry any of these infections to their wives or from them. Those who practice oral sex must realise that whatever VD is present in the vagina, penis, or the anus, it will also infect the mouth directly. In fact, there is no way one can sock the vagina or anus without the mouth contact with excreta. If you are in doubt of this statement why not take a sample of excreta to a laboratory for a test. The colonies of bacterial contents of the waste will surprise you. Any doctor who told you that excreta contains no swarm of harmful bacteria must be suffering from professional duplicity.

4.6 Diseases of Male and Female Reproductive Systems

Problems of Male Reproductive System

They are as follows: weakness of virility; sex drive weakness; excretion with blood; lack of erection; defect during ejaculation; convulsion of the penis; swelling of the testicle; enlarged testicles; itching of the testicle skin; shrinking of the testicles; ascending of the testicle's skin; dropping of the testicles; slackness of the testicle skin; ulcer of the penis, testicles, and genital area; hard boils on the penis; obi-twitching of the penis; low sperm counts; premature ejaculation; excessive sex drive; constant erection of the penis; separation of the peritoneum; hernia of the abdomen and of the groin; and nymphomania.

Problems of Female Reproductive System

They are as follows: suppressed menses; excessive menstrual flow; excessive vaginal secretion; itching of the vagina; frigidity; low sexual drive; nymphomania; painful menstrual period; false pregnancy; inability to conceive; flatulence of womb; deviation of mouth of the womb; frequent miscarriage; abnormal vaginal odour; excessive vaginal wetting; insufficient breast milk; excessive breast milk; swelling and stretching of the breast; cessation of milk flow; bruising of the breasts; ulcer and wounds of the womb; haemorrhoids of the womb; boils of the womb; protrusion of the womb; inclination of the womb to one side; swelling of the womb; enlarged womb; cancer of the womb; and strangulation/twisting of the womb.

The above information about the common diseases in male and female is presented here to enable the complementary health care to begin to understand the health problems that may be faced by a large number of people. In fact, anyone who takes the matter of his or her health very seriously should go for regular health check-up from time to time. Nothing in the world must be seen to be more important than one's life, and good health is a crucial preamble of life.

4.7 African Femininity and Natural Health Therapy

The Beauty of African womanhood: 'Real women are made up of both biological and physiological qualities.' In the natural health care, the topic of African woman's body and physiognomy must be given special attention. In her physical body, the hair and the skin are the major and principal part of this discussion.

You should know it that hair being your crowning glory, it is the first thing that people notice about you. It is also the most immediate prospect of change that you possess. In its natural state, an African woman's hair is translucent, sparkling, woolly, and dark ebony. But it is most marvellous when it is well treated and conditioned with no chemical substance. Hair grows from a cluster of matrix cells beneath the skin. The cells divide rapidly and push the new hair up towards the scalp. To perform its functions, the hair follicles and matrix cells must be fed adequately enough. The hairs draw their food through the nutrients from the foods we eat. Therefore, your body, your skin, and your hairs are as good and rich as the foods you eat, the state of your environment, and the state of your mind!

The foods you eat, when you eat them, the condition of the foods, the state of your mind when you are eating them, the soap you use, the water you use for cleaning your hair, the cream and oil you use on your hair, the ingredients of their contents, and their quality and quantity—all these factors will affect and determine the life of your hair. Do remember that you are an African woman on whose shoulder all the problems of the African world are placed. You are the only source of our joy and inner spiritual tranquillity. It is implied therefore that you are the only source of the African man's composure, equanimity, calmness, level-headedness, coolness, self-possession, serenity, and peace of mind. Most men in other races of the world may derive these spiritual inner qualities from other sources, but for the people of African origin this is not the case. The reasons for this will be treated in my next book titled *The Graciousness of African Women in History*.

The way you wear your hair, its colour, condition, and your make-up all these not only reflect and indicate your outlook but also add up to a definitive physical statement about yourself. This is why due consideration must be given about the management of your hair. It is wrong to believe that the African woman's hair is the same as that of the Asian woman and the same as the European woman. Even among the African women, hair varies from individual to individual and must be seen and treated as such! You may not believe it but your inner feelings and mood reflect the shape and the life of your hair. You may think that your hair is an independent item just placed on your head. Well, it is not! It is not only your whole personality but your humanity as a woman! It is also definitive of your womanhood.

The following discussion is based on a hypothetical African woman who is a typical example of a naturally beautiful woman of African origin. She recognises what her body and her hair require to nourish and grow. Whatever style is introduced into your hair, it must project the whole African womanhood and your femininity. Never allow yourselves to be robbed of this natural quality—it is the only trump card you possess in life! If you are called upon to trade off your femininity for the so-called equality with any man—be he white or African—this must be resisted. Do remember that as an African woman, you have been and will remain the centre of attack by our oppressors. Once you are captured, the struggle between us—the African men and the oppressors—is over. During the years of our total oppression when our oppressors were at the apex—zenith—of their total control of our world, the image and natural beauty of the African women were relegated to the back. And she was downgraded. At our captivity in slavery and colonialism, the most demonic adjectives were used to describe the African women. But you see, that came to pass and the truth began to resurface. For example, go and research the backgrounds of most members of the world's leaders; the genes of an African woman will be traceable.

It is the resilience, the essence, and the natural quality of the specialness in you that had kept the African race going till today. Please do not let go. You have come a long way! Today you are more beautiful, more attractive, and more charming. In fact, when an African woman's lips curves upwards, you will see that her eyes become brighter and softer and may sparkle like diamonds. Besides a sincere and radiant smile, one of the most beautiful thing about you, which one sees on your face, is a pair of laughing eyes that are suggestive of peace and loving eyes! Your men may not know and value this creative energy in you. Please do pardon us, for we are all the products of the colonial/slavery imprint legacy! It is this psychological cloud that has not been allowing us to focus our attention on placing our female folk in their noble place. But whatever you do, you must avoid the excessive consumption of sugar, alcohol, and cigarettes.

There is no African family without African woman, and without families, there is no African society! But our men must begin to recognise these vital facts in our women! If we allow ourselves to treat our women in the ways that depreciate their true value, then they will be alienated from us, and these vibrant spiritual qualities in them will be allowed to lie dormant: latent, inactive, sleeping, resting, and undeveloped. They will remain hidden and quiescent. The potential negative effects of these on the entire African family will be discussed in my next book: *The Graciousness of the African Woman in History.*

A word of warning to those confused black men who believe that the hallmark of a female beauty should be a white woman as the role model. It is these men who are still under the thick cloud of the colonial/slavery imprint legacy that prevents them from seeing and appreciating the natural beauty bestowed upon the African womanhood. Like our rediscovery of natural medicine, there is something within the bodies of black women, which is therapeutically curative and which we must yet rediscover. But to enhance this quality, we, the African men, must aim at continuous pampering and nurturing of the growth and continuity of these spiritual essences present in our women. If we allow other people's technological advancements to erode and crush the spiritual essence inherent in the African womanhood, we will have ourselves to blame!

Do remember that the beauty of women, fashion, foods, oil, and medicine are the five most vital economic lifeblood of any group of people! Japanese or Chinese people will certainly go to war in order to prevent these resources escaping from their cultural control. We may even add that women are the most vital resource. Please do preserve your women, your oil, your foods, your fashion, and your medicine. You can include your religion to these resources. Those who control them will certainly control your physical and spiritual life! Those of us who sincerely believe that both Mohammed and Jesus Christ represented the Africans, please do think again. These two messiahs may have come from the African race, but religion as preached by them in their days have since been diluted, redefined, reprocessed, restructured, and reprogrammed to our own detriment! Those of us who sincerely believe that we should be much engaged in the preparation of ourselves to occupy the white man's place in heaven while the Europeans and the

Asians take charge of the physical world here on earth, including our resources, they must think again! We are proud of your femininity and wield the power of its full extent to become more pleasant, more raging, and more beautiful. You should never be pressurised into beginning to admire most of the Euro-centric African women with all the sweetness of the new womanhood who embody the mannish new women with all the qualities of femininity but crushed into lifelong loneliness and permanent singleness!

4.8 The Western Civilisation Diseases

This is a new focus to an otherwise old problem. The arrival of the Western system of life not only affected both the economic and social life of the Africans but also brought with it a profound change in the food and health care system of the people. The principal aim of this topic is to draw attention to various common illnesses affecting both females and males, old and young people of African origin. Among all other races of the world, Africans are found to be the only people who have 'swallowed' (especially the negative aspects) of the so-called modern Western civilisation with an accelerated high speed. But this blind high speed has brought with it an uncountable health care disaster to us. Indeed, it is very hard today to find any African community where heart attacks do not exist and where cancer is not known; an African community where there is no obesity, blood pressure, and male and female sex organ diseases; and an African community where a new killer disease such as HIV AIDS has not visited. The following are the old and new common illnesses so rampant among males and females of African origin:

- Blood pressure generally on the increase
- The diseases of unhealthy food brand loyalty
- Psychosomatic Illnesses on the increase
- Eczema disorder on the increase
- Hair loss disorder on the increase
- Parasitic infection of the colon on the increase
- Cross infection though bisexual syndrome on the increase
- An imperial imprint trauma increasingly reproducing
- Mental poisoning caused by racism and deprivation bitterness— all on the increase

- Acute Inner restlessness and depression on the increase
- Drunkenness and drug addiction on the increase
- An uncontrollable sexual urge/nymphomania syndrome on the increase

Western Illnesses Common Among African Males

- Weakness of vitality—low sexual drive
- Lack of erection and low sperm count
- Defection during ejaculation on the increase
- Swelling of the testicle
- The itching and shrinking of the testicle
- Ulcer and twitching of the penis
- Excessive sex drive and constant erection
- Nymphomania syndrome
- Sexual transmitted diseases including HIV AIDS
- Diseases transmitted through oral sex—parasitic worm and many more

Western Illnesses Common Among African Women

- Excessive menstrual flow on the increase
- Excessive vaginal secretion on the increase
- Vaginal itching and excessive vaginal wetting on the increase
- Low sexual drive and sexual frigidity on the increase
- Painful menstrual flow on the increase
- Abnormal vaginal odour on the increase
- Ulcer and wound of the womb on the increase
- Deviation on the mouth and protrusion of the womb on increase
- Haemorrhoid—piles and boils of the womb
- Inclination of the womb to one side on the increase
- Cancer and strangulation of the womb on the increase

4.9 Psychosomatic Syndrome/Traumatic Syndrome

This is behavioural-based body of acquired knowledge specifically common among the people of African origin. It is an invincible phenomenon militating over an individual and a group of people. The syndrome is a result of the African slavery and colonial imprint legacy.

Imprint legacy is the totality of acquired body of knowledge which had replaced and continues to re-shape the indigenous lifestyle of the modern Africans, for example, the displacement of the entire African communities through slavery raids; the capturing and shackling, brutal broad daylight raping of women and children in front of the public; tying up of legs and hands and gagging of mouths of the African males and females; and the destruction of their shrines, their temples, their religious altars, and the psychological pollution of their moral life. All have had dehumanising effects on what was left of the African humanity. This societal pillage gained momentum from the year AD 1458 and not until AD 1957. No African male or female was allowed to have a say in the governance and the control of their lives. For the past fifty years, the entire indigenous African societies have been wallowing in darkness trying to rediscover their humanity. But they have not paid any due attention to the effects of this syndrome in terms of their individual or collective health care.

Most of the time this syndrome causes serious illness and health imbalance, which the conventional medical profession is not able to detect or treat. Most people consider the material and physical world to be the only reality that exists. They see these as the only things that they can relate to their physical sense grasped by their rational minds. But on our viewing human beings with sanitised eyes, we can perceive numerous energy structures, energy movements, shapes, and colours within and around the physical body. This energy that we call the 'vital force' lends life to the physical body and provides it with sensations and means of expression. These are the powers at work behind the body's material appearance with all its functions and capabilities consisting of a complex network of energy system. This system finds expression within the individual and the collective attitude and behaviour.

Understanding the Syndrome

The understanding of the syndrome is vital in Afro-centric psycho-somatic disorder therapy. It is believed that the origin of our people's political, social, and economic behavioural inadequacies is connected with or to negative and destructive thoughts and belief patterns rooted deeply into their minds. Self-hatred and self-rejection are the typical examples of these problems. The thought or the feeling of abject poverty is one of the typical examples of such a mental attitude to life among the people of African origin. The totality of our individual and collective exposure and experiences of the imperial imprint legacy has produced in us an unauthentic perception of life and world view. This non-physical and mind-health-related problems are inter-connected.

The Effects of This Syndrome

The syndrome is an in-built negative feeling of inadequacy inherent in our people and finds expression in our daily activities, also in our individual and collective occupations. They also find expression in all our interactions with other people. This feeling leads to low self-esteem, low self-image, and self-hatred. It also generates endless questioning of self-worth. As a negative quality, it is responsible for the fratricidal behaviour inherent in all the people of African origin. They acquired this habit from the imperial contact with the Arabs and the Europeans. This was nurtured by our slavers and our colonists. It was also built into the Willie Lynch techniques for controlling slaves and Africans, which were used in the slave colonies. Having been internalised, this quality has continued to be part of our culture up to the present time. If it is true that the whites believe that the people of African origin are inferior to them, any display of inferiority complex is an acknowledgement of that claim! Often the very successful ones among us disagree that they possess any trace of this quality of mind at all.

But just look at an average healthy black man or woman you meet on the street, at the bank, or in a supermarket. Observe how they behave. Watch the frequent display of wealth or qualifications being expressed in their mood of dressing with a touch of obvious arrogance and showmanship! If you happen to know them, you dare not make the mistake of trying to greet them without adding their academic or traditional titles. With all other races of the world, the omission of such titles will not rock anger or provoke discord at all It is this inner discontentment that is responsible for our conspicuous consumption of goods and material at the dire expense of our national economy. Just look at the black children you meet on the street both in Africa and abroad; observe the quality of their dresses and the mobile phones in their hands. They always ensure that they possess the best. The cars they use, the shoes and the jewelleries they wear, all are very superior and expensive. Their consumption levels are their attempt to compensate for their individual and collective feeling of inadequacies.

Another example of this never-ending inner discontentment is that the 'madness' of the so-called technological catch up instead of the people putting all their efforts into building skills, capacities, and technical knowledge of the citizenry. Without a well-structured programme of re-orientation and liberation, this very quality of mind can never be erased from our individual and collective behaviour—psychosomatic syndrome and psychological imbalance in us—the Africans.

Examples of Psychosomatic and Psychological Health Imbalance Are as Follows:

- Mental torment
- Unknown fear of self and fear of others
- Weak will
- Subservience
- Easily discouraged
- Self-hatred and self-rejection
- Easily overwhelmed
- Sense of hopelessness
- Simplicity of heart
- Overzealous hospitality
- Lack of inner joy as the fruit of human spirit and creativity
- Evil and negative effects derived from human skin colour hatred
- Racial discrimination
- The negative effects of colonial-based education
- Evil danger of abject poverty
- The effects of chemical cosmetics
- The effects of fatigue and tension—stress
- The fear of being charmed by an enemy
- The effects of negative thoughts and feelings
- Negative memories of the past experiences
- The phobia of being hunted by demons of the forests and empty buildings
- The phobia of being possessed by invincible beings of a female spirit living in the sea called Mammy Water
- Bleached skin colour syndrome
- The feeling of inadequacy called inferiority complex
- The danger of superiority complex from reversed racism
- Cross-cultural racism syndrome
- Drug addiction syndrome

- The negative syndrome of loneliness and rejection
- The effects of negative words—lack of confidence in self
- The negative behaviour inherent from our imperial imprint legacy
- Multiple effects of skin colour discrimination
- Fratricidal syndrome

Once you are in the presence of people who expressly demonstrate that you are not accepted, you will unconsciously begin to represent their opinons and their actions against you. As you continue to exist alongside of these psychological enemies of yours, you will begin to not only hate yourself but also people of your own kind. The outcome of this self-hatred can be deep rooted and will take many years to be overcome. So you see, racial discrimination carries heavier 'negative loads' than is known. Self-bitterness, spiritual self-rejection, and fratricidal behaviour are generally part and parcel of the same evil. Why the effects of racial discrimination do not affect the Europeans in the same light as the people of African origin is because they are not at the receiving end of the economic ladder. Such respondent racism not backed with social and economic deprivation will be ineffective. Although colour discrimination is now unlawful in the UK, the traumatic effects are still present in the subconscious minds of the victims. When most of us get back to our homelands, we put up a pretence that all is well with us in Europe and America. But once the history of South Africa, Australia, and Alabama in the USA starts unfolding, the harsh facts can no longer be covered permanently. The issue of self-hatred and self-rejection 99 per cent of the time originates from personal struggles against economic and social deprivation. This is also the root cause of lower self-esteem. It is also the second root issue behind cardiovascular disease as a result of self-bitterness, self-rejection, and self-hatred. These produce coronary artery disease, otherwise known as congestive heart problem.

You may wonder why some of the above listed items should be included as causing ill health. It is important to recognise that any element capable of preventing a person from normal peaceful coexistence must be considered as illness. Each of the above listed has the ability of causing psychosomatic abnormality of physical health and behavioural imbalance. This is why complementary medical practitioners must see themselves as engaged in a holistic health care practice. The effects of any of these can be referred to as illness or sickness. Most of the time, the mainstream medical profession carries out various medical examinations of all sorts in order to identify the causes of such illness but to no avail! This means that the conventional medicine depending on its chemical medicine has no answer to these aspects of human health problems. The Eastern world, including African nations, in their indigenous communities has been using psychosomatic therapy for many years long before the arrival of the Western man.

One of the typical examples of psychosomatic behavioural syndrome is such as that found among the African rulers. They are usually voted into power to lead their nations for development and progress. But, instead, they engage themselves in amassing personal wealth and siphoning the wealth of their nations to other countries. Rulers such as Mubutu of Congo and Abacha of Nigeria are cases in point. Have you wondered the kind of inner spirit within these groups of Africans responsible for such abnormal behaviour? It can be called psychosomatic or cognitive dissonance. Cognitive dissonance is an uncomfortable feeling caused by holding conflicting ideas or interests simultaneously. These supposedly African leaders suffer from two conflicting needs: firstly, to lead their countries out of their neocolonial bondage, and secondly, the need to connive with the foreign franchisors to build their own personal wealth to the detriment of their citizenry. Cognition is the scientific term for the process of thought. In their inner self-value system, these rulers hardly perceive themselves as an integral part of the citizens they are called upon to lead. In normal circumstances, the resolving answer for this condition could have been a ghastly social revolution! But for the fear of a counter revolution by the foreign franchisors, the African citizens continue to endure the near slavery condition relentlessly. But will this condition ever continue indefinitely?

What Are the Preventive Measures?

Those who could have carried out such revolution are the products and the agents of the same malady that is rocking their societies. We have seen typical examples of such an inhuman-revolution through various military coups that have happened in Africa and other Third-World nations since their independence. However, the alternative sources of action open to us are the re-education of our people to start the process of self-re-orientation and re-adaptation.

Naturopathic Remedies

In this aspect of natural medicine, we apply purely natural methods of healing in accordance with the illness involved. Some health problems may not respond to any other approach of treatment. It is unfortunate that most people understand the application of medicine as the only method of treating, healing, and bringing about a healthy thorough assessment in the need for bio-alignment (complete overall); assessment of the body's need for adequate dietary requirement (ethnic food components); for balanced digestion, absorption, and assimilation; the evaluation for fresh air, pure clean water, adequate temperature, sufficient light, sufficient rest, sufficient sleep; regular cleanliness of both internal and external parts of the body; positive and orderly state of mind; clean environment; the correct synergy of colour scheme in house decoration; the correct music rhythm; and the correct aroma therapeutic effects of the surrounding. Naturopathic health care therapy in Africa must bear in mind the indigenous cultural ways of life in applying any principles of treatment. Whichever application of natural healing processes being applied, it must aim at the retrieval, revamping, rejuvenation, revitalisation, regeneration, reactivation, and restoration of human health: of body, mind, and spirit. It is the application of naturopathic principles that helps any other natural health treatment to be effective and successful.

Phytonutrients Herbal Health care Remedies

This is a system of natural health medicare best suited to black-skinned African men and women, old and young. This treatment is based on the tropical climate, temperament, temperature, spirit, body, mind, vegetation, the soil, bio-ecology, and our total being. Since our food and lifestyle vary from those of other races of the world, it follows therefore that we must begin to look for an alternative method of health care just like the Chinese and Indians. The application of African phytonutrient herbal medicine therapy will ensure healthy life, peace of mind, an increased vitality, and longevity. Although we are all human beings, some of the health care treatment on the non-black-skinned people may not be very suitable for the black Africans. This is due to the differences in the soil, environment, food habit, vegetations, and ethno-spirituality. Historically, there can be no doubt that the existence of medicine is traceable to the black African race. For example, the very first people, rulers, and the civilisation in India, Ethiopia, and Egypt were black Africans. Yoga and all other Eastern natural health therapy originated in Africa. Call it botanic or ethno-medicine, if you like, the system dates back to 7000 years BC. The African race had depended upon the herbal method of curing their illnesses long before the arrival of the European influence. We are gradually going back to the natural system! But we have no choice at all.

Some plants in ancient times were known for their colourful and aromatic properties. Egyptians used them for extracting perfumes from Ra's sweat and the divine essence. These are natural plants' essence derived from organic African forests. Before the arrival of the Arabs and Europeans in the African native lands and the subsequent corruption of their medicinal system, African indigenous healers made use of plant fragrances to heal. The great master healers knew and understood the essence of each plant and the effects they could have on human emotion and health. According the anthropological historians, the first medical healer long before Hippocrates (now called the father of medicine) was an African called Imhotep.

The African indigenous people had a highly developed sense of smell, and this enabled them to detect and classify the uses of each plant essence and oil. It is unfortunate that our pursuits of the Western imprint legacy have misdirected us to abandon most aspects of our lives that are indigenous African. The brainwashing of our people is so real that our developed sense of smell has gradually died away. But without the developed sense of smell, the Chinese medical system could not have progressed and the wine-brewing multimillion industries in France, Germany, Italy, Spain, South Africa, and Britain could hardly have ever developed. Even today, the European aromatherapy products depend on the application of the sense of smell of the specialists. Without the existence of the various aromatic fragrances, essences, and oils from the forest of Africa, the international business of body-shop cosmetics would not be flourishing. For those who want to know exactly how this essence works, please be informed that our sense of smell is very important and potent in every sense in making adjustments to our emotion and mental states. The olfactory nervous system which consists of many millions of nerve endings can pick up aroma via the nose. This, in turn, transmits a specific massage to the limbic system which is the emotional centre in the brain. It is here that the brain, through its central nervous system, commands the arteries to release and neutralise any congestion by the mucus. This action is instant. People who use this product describe it as 'magical'. It is not a magic at all but a scientific and natural principle.

Notwithstanding the African imprint legacy, we are beginning, through research and necessity, to accumulate a body of knowledge to constantly tell ourselves about certain fragrances/essences present in the African forest plants, which possess properties that can be extracted and used to relax, stimulate, uplift depression, help insomnia, give feelings of romance, and indeed have an effect on the vast array of emotional and mental states that one can possibly experience. These essences are free from any chemical mixture, and they are not another type of Vicks at all. They are purely natural and undiluted and must not be rubbed on the face. They are not recommended for pregnant women. *Instructions for use*: Take just a drop in your palm and rub your palms together until it is warm.–Slowly sniff through the nose deeply. The action is instant! Carry out this action any time you feel sad or depressed or cold. Put a few drops on your pillow before bedtime. A few drops also can be dropped in your hot bath to invigorate you. But please note that this is not a conventional perfume at all. *Functions*: uplifting, relaxing, refreshing, antidepressant, confidence-creating, stimulating and reducing and relieving headaches. It is also an analgesic, muscle-relieving and cold-relieving. It is also used for asthma and has a rejuvenating effect. Please look out for likely imitations. In his book titled *Nutricide*, Dr Lliala Afrika has advised us about the dangers of chemicalised food and their indiscriminate consumption by the Africans.

4.10 Mariandina Health Products by Prof. Charles Ssali

Mariandina is a natural formulation for the maintenance of good health in people of all ages. It provides the body with natural nutrients that are deficient in one's diet. These deficiencies include vitamins, minerals, enzymes, peptides, etc., which the body requires on a daily basis. *Mariandina A, B, and J* can provide those requirements because they are made of natural ingredients obtained from natural foods, vegetables, fruits, and plant hormones.

Those who are sick because of bacterial, fungal, and virus infections need additional nutrients because of their action to boost the immunity and the body's fighting power against diseases. To create *Mariandina* we went back to learn how Mother Nature puts together her medicinal herbs and fruits from which food comes. The fruits and vegetables spoken of in Genesis, chapter 3, are the way forward to good health. They provide nutrients and spare parts for our bodies. They are the source of healing and help in the prevention of degenerative processes of body cells, which if unchecked lead to ageing. This is the secret of the biblical Tree of Life. The damage to the body from pollution, poor nutrition, disease, stress, and injury can be repaired better by these natural food supplements than by the use of chemicals, which inflict further damage to the body because of their toxicity.

Mariandina A is an advanced unique natural composition consisting of twenty-eight natural herbs, vitamins, minerals, and rare elements such as vitamin C, vitamin A, vitamin E, vitamin B6, vitamin B12, folic acid, citrus bioflavanoids, iodine, niacin, biotin, calcium, zinc, iron, selenium, copper, manganese, and ginseng plus many more which boost the immune system, repair body cells and tissues, cleanse, provide stress relief, and energise the body.

Mariandina B is an advanced natural composition consisting of twenty-three natural herbs and vitamins such as Siberian Ginseng Powder, Alfalfa leaf, Golden seal root, vitamin E, Gotu Kola, Betacarotene, Kola nut, Bee pollen, Liquorice root, Hawthorn Berry, capsicum, Yellow Dock leaf, Echinacea, Purpurea, Ginkgo Biloba leaf, garlic, Co-enzyme Q-10, vitamin C, Di-basic calcium phosphate, and Guarana, which increase blood circulation in the brain, sexual organs, and heart to rejuvenate them to function more efficiently and overcome stress.

Mariandina J is a unique natural composition of twenty-nine powerful herbs such as Calendula, Echinacea, Astragalus, St. Johns wort, Bed Straw, mistletoe, thyme, camomile, Lecithin, Devil's claw, Spirulina, Dandelion, Codonopsis, Osha root, Berberis, Aquifolium, garlic, and Calmus root plus many more that detoxify and cleanse the body.

Marindina Herbal Syrup is a nutritional booster specially formulated to help maintain energy, health, and vitality in both adults and children. It contains a range of vitamins and minerals enriched with herbal extracts like Ginkgo Ginseng Sarsaparilla, etc., all in a base of honey and malt, balanced in a pleasant blackcurrant taste. It is suitable for vegetarians. *Recommended daily intake:* Children three to six years: one teaspoonful (5 ml) daily. Adults and children over six years: two teaspoonfuls (10 ml) daily.

How to take Mariandina:

When using the *Mariandina* products for general health, it is advisable to take one of each of *Mariandina range A, B, and J* in the morning and the same after the evening meal. This ensures detoxification while you sleep or during working hours. A midday course is useful for those desiring quicker results or if in a poor health status.

Higher doses are recommended for diseases where the user is also advised to drink one or two litres of water per day to wash out the impurities through the kidneys. In some mild conditions, one may use *Mariandina A* alone, but in severe illnesses, *Mariandina J and B* should be used in conjunction with *Mariandina A*. Adults should use two of each three times a day. In all cases, the addition of one formula B capsule three times a day helps to speed up benefits.

Children over the age of three may have one-fourth of the adult dosage of *Mariandina A, B, and J*. Those aged ten to fifteen years may take half the adult dose. Where tablets are available, they may be crushed and mixed with the child's food or a spoonful of honey.

One should continue with the usual treatment until it is no longer necessary.

For male disorders, *Mariandina A, B, and J* are used in dosages of two capsules of *Mariandina A*, two capsules of *Mariandina J*, and one capsule of *Mariandina B* twice a day. This course is recommended for at least three months before one can reduce it to once a day. This course may be taken three times a day in some cases.

In all cases smoking and use of habitual drugs routinely is discouraged.

For those using contraceptive pills, smokers, and alcoholics, the use of *Mariandina* is recommended in higher dosage because most of the nutrients are used to clear the backlog of impurities and toxins stored in the body fat.

In cases of high blood pressure, it is advisable to take *Mariandina A, B, and J* together with the anti-hypertension drugs from your own doctor until the blood pressure is controlled. This may take over six months. During this period, *Mariandina* helps the body to clear itself of cholesterol, open up coronary heart blood vessels, and improve brain circulation. This reduces the risk of stroke, heart attack, and kidney failure.

Patients diagnosed with multiple sclerosis should use *Mariandina A, B, and J* as indicated in the chart. Skin and intestinal disorders may be treated as recommended in the chart.

All users should increase their daily intake of fruits, vegetables, and water.

Natural Health Dosage Guide

Mariandina Is Not a Cure—Mariandina Helps the Body Fight the Natural Way

Dosage Guide information: 2 × 3 = Two capsules three times a day; 3 × 3 = three capsules three times a day

Diseases and Conditions	Adult dosage for Mariandina A	Adult dosage for Mariandina J	Adult/children's dosage for Mariandina B	Children's dosage for Mariandina A	Children's dosage for Mariandina J
Immune disorders	2 × 3	2 × 3	2 × 3	1/2 × 2	1/2 × 2
Arthritis	2 × 3	1 × 3	1 × 3	–	–
Asthma	2 × 3	1 × 3	1 × 3	1/2 × 2	1 × 3
Breast cancer	2 × 3	3 × 3	2 × 3	–	–
Bronchitis	2 × 3	1 × 3	1 × 2	–	–
Cancer	2 × 3	3 × 3	2 × 3	2 × 3	1 × 3
Colitis	2 × 3	1 × 3	1 × 3	–	–
Depression	2 × 3	2 × 3	2 × 3	–	–
Diabetes	2 × 3	1 × 3	2 × 3	2 × 3	1 × 3
Dizziness	2 × 3	1 × 3	1 × 3	–	–
Eczema	2 × 3	1 × 3	1 × 2	1 × 2	1 × 2
Gastroenteritis	2 × 3	1 × 2	1 × 3	1 × 2	–
General health	1 × 2	1 × 2	1 × 2	1 × 1	1 × 1
Genital herpes	2 × 3	2 × 3	1 × 3	–	–
Heart disease	2 × 3	1 × 3	1 × 2	1 × 2	1 × 2
Hepatitis B+C	2 × 3	2 × 3	2 × 3	1 × 2	1 × 2
Irritable bowels	2 × 3	1 × 3	1 × 3	1 × 2	1 × 3
Kidney diseases	2 × 3	1 × 1	1 × 3	1 × 2	1 × 2
Lupus	2 × 3	–	1 × 3	1 × 2	–
Loss of libido	2 × 2	2 × 2	1 × 2	–	–
Menopause	2 × 2	–	1 × 3	–	–

Measles	1×3	1×3	1×2	1×2	1×2
Multiple sclerosis	2×3	2×3	2×3	1×2	1×2
Period pain	2×3	2×3	1×2	1×2	1×2
Peptic ulcers	1×3	1×3	1×3	1×2	1×1
Pneumonia	2×3	1×3	1×3	1×2	1×1
Prostate cancer	2×3	3×3	2×3	–	–
Psoriasis	2×3	1×3	1×2	1×2	1×3
Rheumatic joints	2×3	1×3	1×3	$1/2 \times 2$	–
Sciatica	2×3	1×2	–	–	–
Sickle cells	$1 \times 2/1 \times 3$	1×1	1×2	1×3	1×1
Skin disorders	2×3	1×3	1×2	1×3	1×3
Strokes	2×3	1×3	2×3	–	–

4.11 Modern Traditional African Medicine

What do we mean by the word modern African medicine? It is improper to say that we are practising modern traditional medicine unless the following procedures are in place. A body should be set up to be responsible for such a practice. The following is an example.

The Federation of African Continental Traditional Medicine (FACTM) should be responsible for the following:

- Authentic and well-researched herbal resources must be established in all the nations of Africa to create central uniformity.
- Comparative studies must be made with reference to countries like China and India to learn their systems of control and validation.
- Standard of selection, procurement, storage, manufacture, and packaging of the products must be established.
- Scientific research laboratories must be set up in each of the member communities of the federation to be responsible and accountable to the FACTM.
- Educational standard of training, assessment, evaluation, and professional validation must be established.

Until the above-stated aims come to live, we will continue to take things as they are at the present time. The information at hand now sets about the prevailing African traditional medicine as follows:

In the modern times this is a holistic discipline involving indigenous herbalism and African spirituality, typically involving diviners, midwives, and herbalists. Practitioners of traditional African medicine claim to be able to cure various and diverse conditions such as cancers, psychiatric disorders, high blood pressure, cholera, most venereal diseases, epilepsy, asthma, eczema, fever, anxiety, depression, benign prostatic hyperplasia, urinary tract infections, gout, and healing of wounds and burns. Diagnosis is reached through spiritual means, and a treatment is prescribed, usually consisting of a herbal remedy that has not only healing abilities but also symbolic and spiritual significance. Traditional African medicine, with its belief that illness is not derived from chance occurrences but through spiritual or social imbalance, differs greatly from Western medicine, which is technically and analytically based. In the twenty-first century, modern pharmaceuticals and medical procedures remain inaccessible to large numbers of African people due to their relatively high cost and concentration of health centres in urban cosmopolitan cities. In recent years, the orthodox African medical practitioners have acknowledged that they have much to learn from traditional medical practice.

History—Colonial Era

Modern science has, in the past, considered methods of traditional knowledge as primitive. Under colonial rule, traditional diviners—healers were outlawed because they were considered by many nations to be practitioners of witchcraft and were declared illegal by the colonial authorities, creating a war against witchcraft and magic. During this time, attempts were also made to control the sale of herbal medicines. After Mozambique obtained independence in 1975, attempts to control traditional medicine went as far as sending diviners—healers to re-education camps. As colonialism and Christianity spread through Africa, colonialists built general hospitals and Christian missionaries built private ones with the hopes of making headway against widespread diseases. Little was done to investigate the legitimacy of these practices, as many foreigners believed that the native medical practices were pagan and superstitious and could only be suitably fixed by inheriting Western methods. During times of conflict, opposition has been particularly vehement as people are more likely to call on the supernatural realm.[1] Consequently, doctors and health practitioners have, in most cases, continued to shun traditional practitioners despite their contribution to meeting the basic health needs of the population.[2]

Modern Period

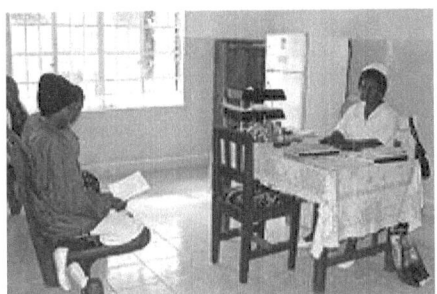

Nurse at Koidu Hospital in Sierra Leone
consulting with patients

In recent years, the treatments and remedies used in traditional African medicine have gained more appreciation from researchers in Western science. Developing countries have begun to realise the high costs of modern health care systems and the technologies that are required, thus proving Africa's dependence on it. Due to this, interest has recently been expressed in integrating traditional African medicine into the country within the continent's national health care systems. An African healer embraced this concept by making a forty-eight-bed hospital, the first of its kind, in Kwamhlanga, South Africa. This combines traditional methods with homeopathy Iridology and some Asian traditional approaches. However, the highly sophisticated technology involved in modern medicine, which is beginning to integrate into Africa's health care system, could possibly destroy Africa's deep-seated cultural values.

Why should this be the case? All other Eastern medical systems integrated in to the Western systems have not been destroyed by them. If the African traditional medical practitioners are properly trained, proficiently skilled, and well devoted, they can indeed compete with anybody in the world.

Diagnostics

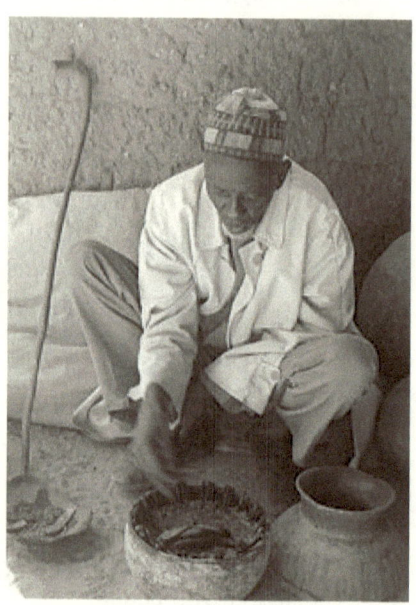

Will You Really Call the Above Practice a Modern
African Traditional Medicine, and How Can Anyone
Prevent Disease By This Approach and Method?

Looking at this man in this very particular practice and the so-called diagnosis, both require modernisation and more professionalism. We cannot continue to let people to continue practising African medicine in such unhygienic and degrading situations all in the name of Africa. I am very surprised that the African nations are not willing to set aside illiterate methods of handling an otherwise very important and delicate profession like medicine! I do hope that I am not going to be misconstrued as saying that you should abolish all the illiterate African medicine practitioners. No, what I am saying here is that each of the African national government ministries of health must as a matter of urgency begin to set up indigenous medical training centres. Consequently, in about five to ten years of time, African traditional medicine will have a crop of educated and professionally skilled men and women Africans who will advance this section of the national medical system. At the present time, African traditional medicine is not a system at all. But it will never become a system until such a time when the leadership in each of our nations in African is awake! In fact, the orthodox medical practitioners will never help you to set up and reorganise ATM. This is because the ATM men and women who emerge from various African 'swamps' are talking as if they are in competition with the mainstream medical system of their lands.

The man shown above is a Kapsiki crab sorcerer of Rhumsiki in the Extreme North Province of Cameroon. He is using a form of divination by interpreting the changes in the position of various objects as caused by a freshwater crab. The diagnoses and chosen methods of treatment in traditional African medicine rely heavily on spiritual aspects, oftentimes based on the belief that psycho-spiritual aspects should be addressed before medical aspects. In African culture, it is believed that 'nobody becomes sick without sufficient reason'. Traditional practitioners look at the ultimate 'who' rather than the 'what' when locating the cause and cure of an illness, and the answers given come from the cosmological beliefs of the people. Rather than looking to the medical or physical reasons behind an illness, traditional healers attempt to determine the root cause underlying it, which is believed to stem from a lack of balance between the patient and his or her social environment or the spiritual world, not by natural causes. Natural causes are, in fact, not seen as natural at all but manipulations of spirits or the gods. For example, sickness is sometimes said to be attributed to guilt by the person, family, or village for a sin or moral infringement. The illness, therefore, would stem from the displeasure of the gods or God due to an infraction of the universal moral law. According to the type of imbalance the individual is experiencing, an appropriate healing plant will be used, which is valued for its symbolic and spiritual significance as well as for its medicinal effect.

When a person falls ill, a traditional practitioner uses incantations to make a diagnosis. Incantations are thought to give the air of mystical and cosmic connections. Divination is typically used if the illness is not easily identified, otherwise the sickness may be quickly diagnosed and given a remedy. If divination is required, then the practitioner will advise the patient to consult a diviner who can further give a diagnosis and cure. Contact with the spirit world through divination often requires not only medication but also sacrifices.

4.12 Treatments

Traditional practitioners use a wide variety of treatments ranging from 'magic' to biomedical methods such as fasting and dieting, herbal therapies, bathing, massage, and surgical procedures. Migraines, coughs, abscesses, and pleurisy are often cured using the method of 'bleed-cupping' after which a herbal ointment is applied with follow-up herbal drugs. Animals are also sometimes used to transfer the illness to afterwards. Some cultures also adopt the method of rubbing hot herbal ointment across the patient's eyelids to cure headaches. Malaria is cured by both drinking and using the steam from a herbal mixture. Fevers are often cured using a steam bath. Also vomiting is induced or emetics are used to cure some diseases. For example, raw beef is soaked in the drink of an alcoholic person to induce vomiting and nausea and cure alcoholism. In Bight of Benin, the natives have been known to use the fat of a boa constrictor to cure gout and rheumatism; it is also thought to relieve chest pain when rubbed into the skin.

Medicinal Plants

Africa is endowed with many plants that can be used for medicinal purposes of which they have taken full advantage. In fact, out of the approximated 6,400 plant species used in tropical Africa, more than 4,000 are used as medicinal plants. Medicinal plants are used in the treatments of many diseases and illnesses, the uses and effects of which are of growing interest to Western societies. Not only are plants used and chosen for their healing abilities, but they also often have symbolic and spiritual significance. For example, leaves, seeds, and twigs that are white, black, and red are especially seen as symbolic or magical and possess special properties.[1] Examples of some medicinal plants include the following.

Prunus Africana with Stripped Bark of a Tree

- **Pygeum (*Prunus africana*)**: Pygeum is not only used in traditional African medicine but has also developed a following around the world as a cure for mild-to-moderate benign prostatic hyperplasia, claimed by its users to increase the ease of urination and reduce inflammation and cholesterol deposits. In traditional

African practice, the bark is made into tea, whereas elsewhere in the world it is found in powders, tinctures, and pills. Pygeum has been sold in Europe since the 1970s and is harvested in mass quantities in Cameroon and Madagascar each year.[1]

- **_Securidaca Longepedunculata_**: This is a tropical plant found almost everywhere across the continent with different uses in every part of Africa. In Tanzania, the dried bark and root are used as a laxative for nervous system disorders, with one cup of the mixture being taken daily for two weeks. In East Africa, dried leaves from the plant are used in the treatment of wounds and sores, coughs, venereal diseases, and snakebites. In Malawi, the leaves are also used for wounds, coughs, venereal diseases, and snakebites, as well as bilharzia, and the dried leaves are used to cure headaches. In other parts of the continent, parts of the plant are used to cure skin diseases, malaria, impotence, and epilepsy and are also used as an aphrodisiac.

A study entitled 'ACE Inhibitor Activity of Nutritive Plants in Kwa-Zulu Natal' was conducted by Irene Mackraj and S. Ramesar, both of the Department of Physiology and Physiological Chemistry; and H. Baijnath, Department of Biological and Conservation Sciences, University of Kwa-Zulu Natal, Durban, South Africa, to examine the effectiveness of sixteen plants growing in Africa's KwaZulu-Natal region, concluding that eight plant extracts may hold value for treating high blood pressure (hypertension).

The traditional African medicinal plants used by traditional healers that the team examined were as follows:

Plants	Description
Amaranthus dubius	A flowering plant, also known as spleen amaranth
Amaranthus hybridus	Commonly known as smooth pig-weed or slim amaranth
Amaranthus spinosus	Also known as spiny amaranth

Asystasia gangetica — An ornamental ground cover known as Chinese violet. Also used in Nigerian folk medicine for the management of asthma

Centella asiatica — A small herbaceous annual plant commonly referred to as Asiatic pennywort

Ceratotheca triloba — A tall annual plant that flowers in summer sometimes referred to as poppy sue

Chenopodium album — Also called lamb's quarters, this is a weedy annual plant

Emex australis — Commonly known as southern three corner jack

Galinsoga parviflora — Commonly referred to as gallant soldier

Justicia flava — Also known as yellow *justicia* and taken for coughs and treatment of fevers

Momordica balsamina — An African herbal traditional medicine also known as the balsam apple

Oxygonum sinuatum — An invasive weed with no common name

Physalis viscosa — Known as starhair ground cherry

Senna occidentalis — A very leafy tropical shrub whose seeds have been used in coffee and called septic weed

Solanum nodiflorum — Also known as white nightshade

Tulbaghia violacea — A bulbous plant with hairless leaves often referred to as society or wild garlic

Of the sixteen plants, *Amaranthus dubius, Amaranthus hybridus, Asystasia gangetica, Galinsoga parviflora, Justicia flava, Oxygonum sinuatum, Physalis viscosa,* and *Tulbaghia violacea* were found to have some positive effects, with the latter proving to be the most promising with the ability to lower one's blood pressure.

Spirituality

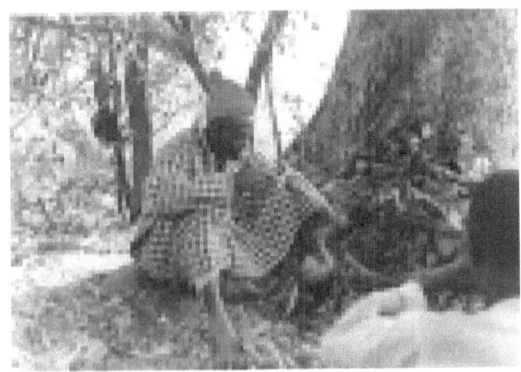

A famous Bedik diviner outside Iwol, Southeast Senegal
(West Africa). He predicted outcomes by examining
the colour of the organs of sacrificed chickens.

Some healers may employ the use of charms, incantations, and the casting of spells in their treatments. The dualistic nature of traditional African medicine between the body and soul, matter, and spirit and their interactions with one another are also seen as a form of magic. Richard Onwuanibe gives one form of magic the name 'extrasensory trojection'. This is the belief among the Igbos of Nigeria that medicine men can implant something into a person from a distance to inflict sickness on them. This is referred to by the Igbos as *egba ogwu*. To remove the malignant object, the intervention of a second medicine man is typically required, who then removes it by making an incision in the patient. *Egba ogwu* involves psychokinetic processes. Another form of magic used by these practitioners, which is more widely known, is sympathetic magic, in which a model is made of the victim. Actions performed on the model are transferred to the victim, in a manner similar to the familiar voodoo doll. 'In cases where spirits of deceased relatives trouble the living and cause illness, medicine men prescribe remedies, often in the form of propitiatory sacrifice, in order to put them to rest so that they will no longer trouble the living, especially children.'[5] Using charms and amulets to cure diseases and illnesses is an uncertain and clouded practice that requires more scientific investigation.

The Kalahari Desert (shown in red) and the surrounding Kalahari Basin (in orange).

In African cultures, the act of healing is considered a religious act. Therefore, the healing process often attempts to appeal to God because it is ultimately God who can not only inflict sickness but also provide a cure. Africans have a religious world view, which makes them aware of the feasibility of divine or spirit intervention in healing with many healers referring to the Supreme God as the source of their medical power. For example, the Kung people of the Kalahari Desert believe that the great God Hishe created all things and, therefore, controls all sickness and death. Hishe, however, bestows mystical powers for curing sickness on certain men. Hishe presents himself to these medicine men in dreams and hallucinations, giving them curative power. Because this god is generous enough to give this power to the medicine men, they are expected to practice healing freely. The Kung medicine men effect a cure by performing a tribal dance.[5] Loma Marshall, who took expeditions to South-west Africa with her family to study the Kung people, writing two books on their findings, describes the ceremonial curing dance as follows.

At the dances not only may the sick be cured, but pending evil and misfortune averted. The Kung believe that the great God may send *Gauwa* or the *gauwas* at any time with ill for someone and that these beings may be lurking awaiting their chance to inflict it. The medicine men in the dances combat them, drive them away, and protect the people. Usually there are several medicine men performing at the same time. To cure they go into trance, which varies in depth as the ceremony proceeds . . . When a man begins, he leaves the line of dancing men, and still singing, leans over the person he is going to cure, going eventually to every person present, even the infants. He places one hand on the person's chest, one on his or her back, and flutters his hands. The Kung believe that in this way he draws the sickness, real or potential, out of the person through his own arms into himself . . . Finally, the medicine man throws up his arms to cast the sickness out, hurling it into the darkness back to *Gauwa* or the *gauwasi*, who are there beyond the firelight, with a harp, yelping cry of 'Kai Kai Kai'.[8]

Loma Marshall does not give any information as to whether or not the dance is successful in curing the patient but says that it purges the people's emotions for their 'support and solace and hope'.

CHAPTER 5

T his chapter deals with various aspects of the so-called modern African traditional medicine. It also looks into the ratio of the orthodox doctors to the traditional practitioners in some African nations. This chapter surveys the relationship between the Western medical system and that of the traditional methods. The term 'African holistic health care' is explored. Attention is given to the establishment of a complementary medical college by the Federal Government of Nigeria. This chapter looks into the concept of naturopathic medicine and how it functions. Finally, the problem of coronary heart disease is explored.

5.1 Modern African Traditional Medicine

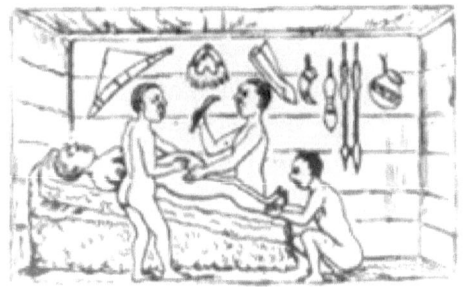

Successful Caesarean section performed by
indigenous healers in Kahura, Uganda. As
observed by R. W. Felkin in 1879

It is very shocking to see here in the above drawn photo that both the sick person and the native practitioners are all nude. May be this was what the culture and the practice at that stage in their history required. Whatever was the requirement, this is very disgraceful. However, a similar practice in Europe at that period in time is also very disgraceful and dehumanising.

Many traditional medicinal practitioners are people without education, who have rather received knowledge of medicinal plants and their effects on the human body from their forebears. They have a deep and personal involvement in the healing process and protect the therapeutic knowledge by keeping it a secret. In a manner similar to orthodox medicinal practice, the practitioners of traditional medicine specialise in particular areas of their profession. Some are experts in herbalism, whilst others are experts in spiritual healing (diviners), and some others specialise in a combination of both. There are also traditional bone setters and birth attendants. Herbalists are becoming more and more popular in Africa with an emerging herb trading market in Durban, which is said to attract between 700,000 and 900,000 traders per year from South Africa, Zimbabwe, and Mozambique. Smaller trade markets exist in virtually every community. Their knowledge of herbs has been invaluable in African communities, and they were the only ones who could gather them in most societies. Midwives also make extensive use of indigenous plants to aid childbirth. African healers commonly 'describe and explain illness in terms of social interaction and act on the belief that religion permeates every aspect of human existence'.

Payments

Traditional healers, like any other profession, are rewarded for their services. In African societies, the payment for a treatment depends on its efficacy. They do not request payment until after the treatment is given. This is another reason many prefer traditional healers to Western doctors who require payment before the patient has assessed the effectiveness of the treatment. The payment methods have changed over time with many practitioners now asking for monetary payment, especially in urban settings, rather than their receiving goods in exchange, as happening formerly. In fact, in the past, in my part of Africa, the healers did not ask for payment but rather requested that their clients pay them they have recovered from the illness. Today, such healers will not receive anything at all. This is because the so-called Western civilisation has removed from the African conscience the fear of God and moral duty.

Learning the Trade

Some healers learn the trade through personal experience while being treated as a patient who decides to become healers upon recovery. Others become traditional practitioners through a 'spiritual calling' and, therefore, their diagnoses and treatments are decided through the supernatural. In some cultures, a sign of calling can come from mental disarrangement said to be caused by *agwu Nshi,* the spirit of divining, through which the healer gains inspiration. Through this training, psychological stability is eventually attained. Another route is to receive the knowledge and skills passed down informally from a close family member such as a father or an uncle or even a mother or an aunt in the case of midwives. Apprenticeship to an established practitioner, who formally teaches the trade over a long period of time and is paid for his tutoring, is another route to becoming a healer. The training is complex, depending on the kind of medical practice that the aspiring practitioner wants to be a part of. Once the trainee is officially initiated as a healer, they are, in some societies, considered to be half man and half spirit, possessing the power to mediate between the human and supernatural world to invoke spiritual power in their healing processes.

Importance

In Africa, the importance of traditional healers and remedies made from indigenous plants plays a crucial role in the health of millions. According to the International Development Research Centre (IDRC), one estimate puts the number of Africans who routinely use these services for primary health care to be as high as 85 per cent in Sub-Saharan Africa. The relative ratios of traditional practitioners and university-trained doctors in relation to the whole population in African countries showcase this importance. For example, in Ghana, in Kwahu district, for every traditional practitioner there are 224 people against one university-trained doctor for nearly 21,000. In Swaziland, the same situation applies where for every healer there are 110 people, whereas for every university-trained doctor there are 10,000 people.[2] According to the Nairobi-based specialist in biodiversity and traditional medicine with the IDRC, Francois Gasengayire, there is one healer for every 200 people in the Southern Africa region, which is a much greater doctor-to-patient ratio than is found in North America.

5.2 Principles of Dietetic Control

The Ratio of Orthodox Doctors to Traditional Health Care Practitioners to Patients in East and Southern Africa:

Country	Doctor: Patient	TMP: Patient	References
Botswana	—	TMPs estimated at 2,000 in 1990	Moitsidi, 1993
Eritrea	Medical doctors estimated at 120 in 1995	—	Government of Eritrea, 1995
Ethiopia	1: 33,000	—	World Bank, 1993
Kenya	1: 7,142 (overall)	1: 987 (Urban-Mathare)	World Bank, 1993
	1: 833 (Urban-Mathare)	1: 378 (Rural-Kilungu)	Good, 1987
Lesotho		Licensed TMPs estimated at 8,579 in 1991	Scott, et al. 1996
Madagascar	1: 8,333		World Bank, 1993
Malawi	1: 50,000	1: 138	Msonthi and Seyani, 1986
Mozambique	1: 50,000	1:200	Green, et al. 1994
Namibia		1: 1,000 (Katutura) 1: 500 (Cuvelai) 1: 300 (Caprivi)	Lumpkin, 1994
Somalia	1: 14,285 (Overall) 1: 2,149 (Mogadishu), 1: 54,213 (Central region), 1: 216,539 (Sanag)		World Bank, 1993; Elmi, et al. 1983
South Africa	1: 1,639 (Overall)	1: 700–1,200 (Venda)	World Bank, 1993
	1: 17,400 (Homeland areas)		Savage, 1985*; Arnold and Gulumian, 1987*
Sudan	1: 11,000		World Bank, 1993

Country	Doctor: Patient	TMP: Patient	References
Swaziland	1: 10,000	1: 100	Green, 1985; Hoff and Maseko, 1986
Tanzania	1: 33,000	1: 350-450 in DSM	World Bank, 1993; Swantz, 1984
Uganda	1: 25,000	1: 708	World Bank, 1993; Amai, 1997
Zambia	1: 11,000		World Bank, 1993
Zimbabwe	1: 6,250	1: 234 (urban) 1: 956 (rural)	World Bank, 1993; Gelf and et al. 1985

* References with an asterisk are in Cunningham, 1993.

Note: TMP refers to a traditional medical practitioner.

This table, which displays the ratios of traditional medical practitioners to patients and Western practitioners to patients, shows that in many parts of Africa, practitioners trained in Western medicine are few and far between. Because of this, healers prove to be a large and influential group in primary health care and an integral part of the African culture and are required for the health of its people. Without them, many people would go untreated.

Medications and treatments that Western pharmaceutical companies manufacture are far too costly and not available widely enough for most Africans. Many rural African communities are not able to afford the high price of pharmaceuticals and cannot readily obtain them even if they were affordable; therefore, healers are their only means of medical help. According to Dr Sekagya Yahaya Hills, who is a university-trained dentist and a traditional healer in Uganda, there are promising signs that some of the plant-based remedies offered by medicine men are not just affordable but also effective, even in treating AIDS. Dr Hills read his 'Declaration of Traditional Healers' at the Thirteenth International Conference on AIDS and Sexually Transmitted Infections (STIs) in Africa, which summarised the important role of traditional medicine, stating: 'As traditional healers, we are the most trusted and accessible health care providers in our communities. We have varied and valuable experience in treating AIDS-related illness and accept the great responsibility of continuing to do so.' Because this form of medicine is 'the most affordable and accessible system of health care for the majority of the African rural population,' the African Union declared 2001-10 to be the decade for African traditional medicine with the goal of making 'safe, efficacious, quality, and affordable traditional medicines available to the vast majority of the people'.

5.3 Relationship with Western Medicine

Although Western medicine is successful in developed countries, it doesn't have the same positive impact in many of the underdeveloped African countries. Though Western practices can make an impact in health care practices, in certain areas such as in the spread of various diseases, it cannot integrate wholly into the culture and society. This makes the traditional African practitioners a vital part of their health care system. There are many reasons why the Western medical system does not work in Africa. Hospitals and medical facilities are difficult for many Africans to get to. With vast areas of land and poor road and transportation systems, many native Africans have to travel immense distances on foot to reach help. Once they arrive they are often required to wait in line for up to eight hours, especially in urban areas, as the lack of clinics and resources cause overcrowding. Patients are oftentimes not told the cause of their illness or much information about it all, so they have no way to prevent or prepare for it. The technology used is usually of poor quality, which affects the quality of treatment. Western medicine is also too expensive for the average African to afford, making it difficult for them to receive proper care. Finally, Western medicine removes native Africans from the culture and tradition and forces them into a setting that they are not comfortable with, away from their family and traditions which are of utmost importance to them. They do not get the proper spiritual healing that their culture seeks and traditional ideology requires.

However, there has been more interest expressed recently in the effects of some of the medicinal plants of Africa. 'The pharmaceutical industry has come to consider traditional medicine as a source for identification of bio-active agents that can be used in the preparation of synthetic medicine.' Pharmaceutical industries are looking into the medicinal effects of the most commonly and widely used plants to use in drugs. It's apparent that there are some things that can be learnt from traditional African practice. In comparing the techniques of African healers and Western techniques, Dr T. Adeoze Lambo, a Nigerian psychiatrist, stated, 'At about three years ago, we made an evaluation, a programme of their work, and compared this with our own, and we discovered that actually they were scoring almost 60 per cent success in their treatment of neurosis. And we were scoring 40 per cent-in fact, less than 40 per cent.'

Special Note:

Herbal medicine is an African tradition. For thousands of years, many people of the African continent had faithful and confident dependence on the use of various plants of the earth for the alleviation and avoidance of certain chronic and acute illnesses. Like healers in many cultures of the world, African herbalists have drawn on a large body of knowledge in the course of over 10,000 years, and yet the world has ignored and overlooked the African contribution to medicine and the healing arts. It is my hope that this small book will help to change that . . .

Traditionally, ancient African priests would orally transmit their herbal knowledge from one generation to the next. Not only was African medicine passed from generation to generation, starting in ancient Egypt (Kemet), but also from continent to continent . . . When Greek physicians took their oath to Aesculapius, they were really swearing into an African originally named Imhotep. During his lifetime, he was revered as the God of Medicine between 2780 and 2680 BC. Western societies have wrongly given credit to a Greek named Hippocrates, who had actually taken the Aesculapius (Imhotepian) oath and lived 2,000 years after the true "Father/God of Medicine" . . . The Dravidians (the black untouchables) of India who were the first inhabitants of that country migrated from Ethiopia via the Isthmus of Suez. They were the founders of Hinduism and Ayurveda medicine, which was a product of the esoteric philosophy of inner Africa . . . The only true African healing system which is still intact in its original language of African terminology is Yoruba medicine, which is widely practised on the African continent as well as in South America and the Caribbean . . . The principles of Yoruba medicine had been influenced by Egyptian holistic medicine about 4,000 years ago, developed by the mystic prophet Orunmile. Because of this root, Yoruba medicine shows the development of a distinctive African tradition, which in some ways has been carried out.

Anybody who possesses a smattering of appreciative knowledge of the Western world will know that there is no way a Euro-centric system of medicine will exist successfully alongside that of African traditional medicine. Their initial concept was to outwit our traditional approach to anything, and this domineering philosophy is deep-seated and cannot be wished away. For example, the Chinese and the Indians could not have developed their own systems of medicine by employing the Europeans or the American to do it for them. In fact, there is no African who is alive today, trained in the European system of medicine, and who will be capable or possess the willingness to work on such a revolutionary idea of developing the African indigenous medicine to a professional systematic standard. Here, I am not talking about the replacement of collectivises of few 'Botanic mixed Grill with a Euro-centric Baptismal Taggings'. The Chinese could not have achieved their own until 1948 when Chairman Maw said that enough was enough! Who is it in Africa to say what Chairman Maw said to the entire peasant farmers in China in 1948? In fact, if any European or any Euro-American ventures to encourage such a revolutionary development in the African medical system, you know that such an individual male or female will be banished or ostracised for life! Oh yes, anyone of them can speak in your favour and even can go to the extent of saying that African medicine is good, but to what avail is this statement?

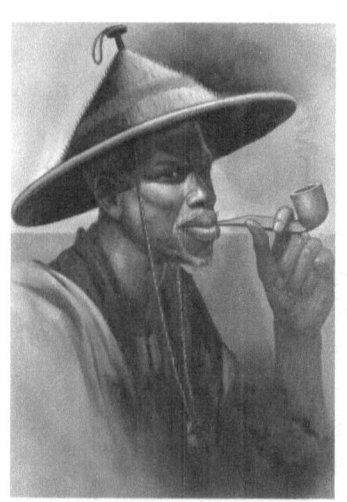

This picture is of a typical indigenous African elder in his late eighties still going strong and still grooving!

Indeed, his counterparts in Europe who have no relatives to care for them have long been forgotten. These types of elders are usually institutionalised. Among us Africans, our children, husbands, wives, in-laws, nieces, and uncles, all support us in our old age. It is these people who make up the African institution of family the lifeblood of our societies. This humanistic family system is seriously threatened by the Euro-African system of family life and the institution of marriage. For the African, the presence of family and its members has psycho-biological therapeutic effect in prevention of both physical and mental illnesses. Take away the existence of traditional family life from the African, his or her life loses its meaning! It is not the Europeans who are insisting that we should abandon the African system of family life but the so-called the African intellectuals. These modern African men and women who rush back to Africa after grabbing a few qualifications from the west and being propelled by the imperial imprint legacy are insistent on seeing to it that the African system of family life is flushed out totally. In addition to the family conducive life essential for the prolonged life of most African elders within the African communities in Africa, the next very important thing is their feeding habits and foods they eat. But since their foods are now under the control of chemical fertilisers, Africans will no longer enjoy the luxury of health and longevity they are used to.

This is a tragedy, and none of us know the answer at all.

During all my research tours in countries like Nigeria, Togo, Ivory Coast, Benin Republic, and Ghana, it was clear that the standard of herbal medical products was not receiving any attention of proper cultivation. It was clear that there is no law to regulate and control both the standard and procurement of the herbal leaves, roots, barks, seeds, flowers, and herbal fruits. One can see these herbal products littering all over the township market grounds along the gutters and stagnant waters, with colonies of blue bottle flies feasting and hibernating on them. In some of the occasions in these markets such as onyibo-markets near Lagos and Grand-Mche in Pobway in Ivory Coast, I have personally observed colonies and swarm of magus mixed with the herbs on the bear floor attracting passing dogs, birds, and vultures. In fact, most of the people who are called upon to govern African nations are very funny. How on earth could they be pressing for the efficacy and effectiveness of the so-called African herbs and sincerely refuse to see the need for any proper organisation of such a wonderful industry. Now we are told that some pharmacies and business investors from China have started to negotiate to take over the planting, organisation, harvesting, and production of herbals in various nations of Western Africa. What a joke! Looking at the pages of this book which describes African herbal medicine, what do you see? An industry in dying need of research and development! It may be that we are expecting the Europeans, the Americans, and the Asians to come and develop ours for us to their own detriment. You must be joking! The People's Republic of China has an enormous number of mouths to feed. For any one of us to believe that China will be there to develop us and not their own people, such a person's intelligence must be below that of a cow!

5.4 African Holistic Health

The concept of African holistic health means was put together by an African-American Dr Lliala Afrika who strongly believes that for the black people to be healthy in mind, body, and spirit, they must begin to reassess their consumption of the Western medicine and its threat to their bodies. You will find the tools of changes in his books, DVDs, and CDs to help you obtain and maintain optimum health and a productive life without harsh drugs or painful surgery. We are suffering and dying three times faster than all other cultures because we are being miseducated and deceived about health and nutrition! The reasons for African holistic health being so important are because the system treats the 'whole person'. Today more than ever, the need for grounded, self-aware holistic practitioners, skilled in the wisdom of the ages, is very crucial. Modern medical practices are unpredictable at best with very high failure rates. The use of synthetic drugs without consideration for the body, mind, and spirit as a whole has created very unhealthy populations around the world, says Dr Afrika. The need is evident, and people are ready for a change. Holistic health care does not deny the need for allopathic (drugs and surgery) medicine. It simply offers a safe, non-intrusive, organic approach to healing the person as opposed to medicating the symptoms of a disease.

children violence and learning It can reduce obesity and put people on diet that they can stay on for life. Traditional medicine cannot make these cl. Drug companies are making billions of dollars at our expense! We have well-documented facts that you can research yourself. Chemotherapy and radiation do not cure cancer . . . they cause it! Insulin is a salt. It does not cure diabetes! Sugar and junk foods make children violent! Conventional drugs ultimately make arthritis worse and destroy the body! High blood pressure can be eliminated with diet and natural herbs when carefully planned. Dieting to lose weight does not work.

The body will always make your food be your medicine and not medicine should be your food. All you are going to get from your doctor are expensive examinations and procedures, potent drug prescriptions, or surgery. They may help temporarily, but they don't give you a final cure. Prove us wrong! Holistic educational come with instructional booklets:

How to Overcome Cancer Without Drugs or Surgery Diabetes: How to Treat, Prevent and Overcome Diabetes Using Natural Holistic Remedies; diabetes: how You Get It, How You Get Rid of It; Overcoming Heart Disease Without Drugs or Surgery; Overcoming Heart Disease; Free Yourself from Arthritis Without Drugs or Surgery; Weight Loss and Obesity: How to Lose Weight Naturally and Permanently Without Diet or Exercise; Weight Loss and Obesity; Melanin: The Well-kept Secrets About Melanin and Race; Melanin: How Melanin Determines Your Race; Eating to Die: Why African Americans Are Dying Three Times Faster Than All Other Races; Eating to Die; The Best of Dr Afrika: Excerpts from Great Lectures; Things Your Doctor May Not be Telling You; Health in America; Myths About Health That Are Destroying Our Society; Health in America: Five Great Myths About Health That Are Destroying Our Society; Americans Are Dying Three Times Faster Than All Other Races; Growth and Development of the Black Child: How to Save Our Children; and How Sugar Destroys Your Heart and Other Vital Organs.

Coronary Heart Disease

This disease is caused by a thickening of the inside walls of the coronary arteries. This thickening called atherosclerosis narrows the space through which blood can flow, decreasing and sometimes completely cutting off the supply of oxygen and nutrients to the heart. It is usually caused by a combination of non-holistic practices such as poor nutrition, environmental pollution, destructive eating habits, and deterioration of the body. Many other factors can cause this disease reaction such as high and low blood pressure, acid ash, fat deposits, thermal glandular fatigue, and loss of vein and artery flexibility. The current fad, which suggests high cholesterol levels resulting in arteriosclerosis caused heart attacks, was started in 1913. It is founded upon giving high levels of cholesterol to rabbits (liver too small to break down fats). Further, the researcher never realised that the research was on disease damage and never gave disease damage any significance.

Atherosclerosis usually occurs when a person has high levels of cholesterol, a fat-like substance in the blood. Cholesterol and fat circulating in the blood build up on the walls of the arteries. This build-up narrows the arteries and can slow or block the flow of blood. When the level of cholesterol in the blood is high, there is a greater chance that it will be deposited onto the artery walls. This process begins in most people during childhood and the teenage years and worsens as they get older. In addition to high blood cholesterol, high blood pressure and smoking also contribute to CHD. On average, each of these doubles your chance of developing heart disease. Therefore, a person who has all three risk factors is eight times more likely to develop heart disease than someone who has none. Obesity and physical inactivity are other factors that can lead to CHD. Being overweight increases the likelihood of developing high blood cholesterol and high blood pressure while physical inactivity increases the risk of heart attack. Regular exercise, good nutrition, and smoking cessation are keys to controlling the risk factors for CHD.

Overweight/obesity: About 65 per cent of American adults are overweight or obese. Being overweight or obese increases the risk not only for heart disease but also for other conditions, including stroke, gallbladder disease, arthritis, breast, colon, and other cancers. Being overweight and obesity are determined by two key measures: body mass index or BMI and the waist circumference. BMI relates the height to weight.

Heart Attack Warning Signs

Heart attack happens; every minute counts. Know the warning signs. Smoking rates among African-American adults historically have been higher than among the general U.S. population. However, recent increases in teen smoking among African Americans document the need for continued prevention efforts. African Americans continue to suffer disproportionately from chronic and preventable diseases compared to white Americans. Of the three leading causes of death in African Americans—heart disease, cancer, and stroke—smoking and other tobacco use are major contributors to these illnesses. *Start! Walking Program*: The American Heart Association's Start! Walking Program helps your company encourage you and your co-workers to live healthier, happier lives.

5.5 Federal College of Complementary Medicine, Nigeria

The outpatient clinic of this college explains the importance of the institution. It seems that Nigeria among all other African countries is the only place where the government has shown interest in establishing a college of complementary medicine of this nature. The start of this body of training will definitely help to regularise the standard of this part of health care system in the country. In the following presentation given by FCCM, there are many preventive therapy techniques that we can learn.

The term *Alternative Medicine*, as used in the modern Western world, encompasses any healing practice 'that does not fall within the realm of Conventional Medicine'. Commonly cited examples include naturopathy, homeopathy, acupuncture, and osteopathy, in addition to a range of other practices. It is frequently grouped with *complementary medicine*, which generally refers to the same interventions when used in conjunction with mainstream techniques, under the umbrella term of *complementary and alternative medicine* or CAM. Some significant researchers in alternative medicine oppose this grouping, preferring to emphasise differences of approach but nevertheless use the term *CAM*, which has become standard.

Alternative medicine practices are as diverse in their foundations as in their methodologies. Practices may incorporate or base themselves on traditional medicine, spiritual beliefs, or newly conceived approaches to healing. Jurisdictions where alternative medical practices are sufficiently widespread may license and regulate them. The claims made by alternative medicine practitioners are generally not accepted by the medical community because it is believed that evidence-based assessment of safety and efficacy is either not available or has not been performed for many of these practices, but suffice it to say that complementary and alternative investigations are established on the safety and effectiveness of complementary and alternative medical practices; it will be adopted by conventional (orthodox) practitioners. Presently in the clinic at FEDCAM, the following sections are operational:

(i) Detoxification

Detoxification is one of the more widely used treatments and concepts in complementary and alternative medicine. It is based on the principle that illnesses can be caused by the accumulation of toxic substances (toxins) in the body. Eliminating existing toxins and avoiding new toxins are essential parts of the healing process. This is one of the main treatment procedures frequently recommended for our patients in the ICU.

Purpose of Detoxifying

Detoxification is helpful for those patients suffering from many chronic diseases and conditions, including allergies, anxiety, arthritis, asthma, chronic infections, depression, diabetes, headaches, heart disease, high cholesterol, digestive disorders, mental illness, and obesity. It is helpful for those with conditions that are influenced by environmental factors, such as cancer, as well as for those who have been exposed to high levels of toxic materials due to accident or occupation. Detoxification therapy is useful for those suffering from allergies or immune system problems that conventional medicine is unable to diagnose or treat, including chronic fatigue syndrome, environmental illness/multiple chemical sensitivity, and fibromyalgia. Symptoms for those suffering these conditions may include unexplained fatigue, increased allergies, hypersensitivity to common materials, intolerance to certain foods and indigestion, aches and pains, low grade fever, headaches, insomnia, depression, sore throats, sudden weight loss or gain, lowered resistance to infection, general malaise, and disability. Detoxification can be used as a beneficial preventative measure and as a tool to increase overall health, vitality, and resistance to disease.

Origin of Detoxification

Detoxification methods of healing have been used for thousands of years. Fasting is one of the oldest therapeutic practices in medicine. Hippocrates, the ancient Greek known as the 'Father of Western medicine', recommended fasting as a means. The problem of toxins in the environment is compounded because humans are at the top of these for improving health. Ayurvedic medicine, a traditional healing system that has developed over thousands of years, utilises detoxification methods to treat many chronic conditions and to prevent illness. Detoxification treatment has become one of the cornerstones of treating patients at the FEDCAM clinic. Conventional medicine notes that environmental factors can play a significant role in many illnesses. Environmental medicine is a field that studies exactly how those environmental factors influence disease. Conditions such as asthma, cancer, chronic fatigue syndrome, multiple chemical sensitivity, and many others are strongly influenced by exposure to toxic or allergenic substances in the environment and food chains and are more likely to be exposed to an accumulation of

toxic substances in the food supply. For instance, pesticides and herbicides are sprayed on grains that are then fed to farm animals. Toxic
substances are stored in the fatty tissue of those animals. In addition,
those animals are often injected with synthetic hormones, antibiotics, and other chemicals. When people eat meat products, they are
exposed to the full range of chemicals and additives used along the
entire agricultural chain. Detoxification specialists call this the build up
of toxin bioaccumulation. They assert that the bioaccumulation of toxic
substances over time is responsible for many physical and mental disorders, especially ones that are increasing rapidly (like asthma, cancer,
and mental illness). As a result, detoxification therapies are increasing
in importance and popularity.

Detoxification Therapies

Detoxification therapists use a variety of healing techniques after
a diagnosis is made. The first step is to eliminate a patient's exposure
to all toxic or allergenic substances. These include heavy metals,
chemicals, radiation (from X-rays, power lines, cell phones, computer
screens, and microwaves), smog, polluted water, foods, drugs, caffeine,
alcohol, perfume, excess noise, and stress. Specific treatments are
used to stimulate and assist the body's detoxification process. Dietary
change is immediately enacted, eliminating allergic and unhealthy
foods and emphasising foods that assist detoxification and support
healing. Detoxification diets are generally low in fat, high in fibre, and
vegetarian with an emphasis on raw food. Processed foods, alcohol, and
caffeine are avoided. Nutritional supplements such as vitamins, minerals,
antioxidants, amino acids, and essential fatty acids are often prescribed.
Spirulina is a sea algae that is frequently given to assist in eliminating
heavy metals. For toxic bowel syndrome and digestive tract disorders,
herbal laxatives and high fibre foods such as psyllium seeds may be
given to cleanse the digestive tract and promote elimination. Colonics are
used to cleanse the lower intestines. Digestive enzymes are prescribed
to improve digestion, and acidophilus and other friendly bacteria are
reintroduced into the system with nutritional supplements.

Fasting is another major therapy in detoxification. Fasting is one of
the quickest ways to promote the elimination of stored toxins in the body
and to prompt the healing process. People with severe toxic conditions
are supervised closely during fasting because the number of toxins in the

body temporarily increases as they are being released. Chelation therapy is used by detoxification specialists to rid the body of heavy metals. Chelates are particular substances that bind to heavy metals and speed up their elimination. Homeopathic remedies have also been shown to be effective for removing heavy metals. Sweating therapies can also detoxify the body because the skin is a major organ of elimination. Sweating helps release those toxins that are stored in the subcutaneous (under the skin) fat cells. Saunas, therapeutic baths, and exercise are some of these treatments. Body therapies may also be prescribed, including massage therapy, acupressure, shiatsu, manual lymph drainage, and polarity therapy. These body therapies seek to improve circulatory and structural problems, reduce stress, and promote healing responses in the body. In the preventive therapy, these applications are very useful and very important.

Detoxification Procedures

The detoxification procedure as carried out in the clinical services department of FEDCAM follows the principle of osmosis (drawing substances from a weaker solution to a stronger solution). It requires the patient dipping his/her feet inside a bowl containing clean water. The water is ionised by adding a small quantity of NaCl (table salt). The quantity of the NaCl needed will be determined by the detox machine. An array is dropped inside the ionised water. The array is to serve as a medium for extracting the toxins from different organs of the body. The whole procedure lasts for thirty minutes, and the colour of the eventual product depends on the organ of the body from where the toxins are being extracted as illustrated in the table below:

S No	Colour	Organ	End Product
1	Black (deep)	Liver	Toxin
2	Orange	Joints	Toxin
3	Green	Gallbladder	Toxin
4	Brown (slight)	Liver	Toxin
5	Suspended oil droplets cholesterol Whitish foam	Immune system	Toxin

S No	Colour	Organ	End Product
6	Suspended brown particles	Drug/food debris	A detoxifier Detoxification in progress (5 min) Detoxification ends (30 min)

(ii) General Rules and Regulations Governing the Treatment

Room

1. Every worker in the treatment room must put on his/her lab suit.
2. A noiseless environment must be maintained.
3. Eating is not allowed in the treatment room.
4. Anyone attending to a patient must put on his/her hand glove and nose mask.
5. Smoking is not allowed in the treatment room.
6. Cleanliness must be the order of the day.

(iii) Acupuncture Department

Acupuncture is a system of healing which has been practised in China and other Eastern countries for thousands of years. Today, countries such as America, Canada, Germany, and others have included acupuncture and other forms of complementary and alternative medicine into their health care delivery system. Although often described as a means of pain relief, acupuncture is in fact used to treat people with a wide range of illnesses. Its focus is on improving the overall well-being of the patient rather than the isolated treatment of specific symptoms. According to traditional Chinese philosophy, our health is dependent on the body's motivating energy known as 'Qi'—moving in a smooth and balanced way through a series of meridians (channels) beneath the skin. Chi consists of equal and opposite qualities—yin and yang, and when these become unbalanced, illness may result. By inserting fine needles into the channels of energy, an acupuncturist can stimulate the body's own healing response and help restore its natural balance. The flow of chi can be disturbed by a number of factors. These include emotional states such as anxiety, stress, anger, fear or grief, poor nutrition, weather conditions, hereditary factors, infections, poisons, and trauma. The principal aim of acupuncture in treating the whole person is to recover the equilibrium between the physical, emotional, and spiritual aspects of the individual. Most people's experience of needles is of those used in injections and blood tests. Acupuncture needles bear little resemblance to these. They are much finer and are solid rather than hollow. When the needle is inserted, the sensation is often described as a tingling or dull ache. Needles are inserted either for a second or two or may be left in place for thirty minutes or more, depending on the effect required. During treatment, patients commonly experience a heaviness in the limbs or a pleasant feeling of relaxation. Occasionally people may experience drowsiness after treatment, in which case it is advisable not to drive or do anything that can put you at risk. The benefits of acupuncture frequently include more than just relief from a particular condition. Many people find that it can also lead to increased energy levels, better appetite, and sleep as well as an enhanced sense of overall well-being.

Clinical Application of Acupuncture

In arthritis, migraine, insomnia, schizophrenia, waist/back pains, kidney disorders, Parkinson's disease, etc., which have been seen untreatable by Western medicine or traditional medicine have been successfully treated using acupuncture. Acupuncture generally involves several weekly or fortnightly treatments. Most courses consist of up to twelve sessions. A visit to an acupuncturist will involve an exam and an assessment of the patient's condition, the insertion of needles, and advice on self-care. Most sessions last about thirty minutes.

Acupuncture Procedures

The patient will be asked to lie down, either face-up, face-down, or on his/her side, depending on where the needless are inserted. The acupuncturist should use single-use disposable sterile needles. As each needle is inserted the patient should feel them, but initially without pain. However, when the needle reaches the right depth there should be a deep aching sensation. Sometimes the needles are heated or stimulated with electricity after insertion. Once inserted, the needles will remain there for fifteen to forty minutes.

A patient being treated for knee arthritis

(iv) Therapeutic Massage

Massage is the practice of soft tissue manipulation with physical (anatomical), functional (physiological), and psychological purposes and goals. The word comes from the French *massage* 'friction of kneading', or from Arabic *massa* meaning 'to touch, feel or handle' or from Latin *massa* meaning 'mass, dough'. In distinction the ancient Greek word for massage was *anatripsis*, and the Latin was *frictio*. Massage involves acting on and manipulating the body with pressure structured, unstructured, stationary, or moving—tension, motion, or vibration, done manually or with mechanical aids. Target tissues may include muscles, tendons, ligaments, skin joints, or other connective tissue, as well as lymphatic vessels or organs of the gasterointestinal system. Massage can be applied with the hands, fingers, elbows, knees, forearms, and feet. There are over eighty different recognised massage modalities. The most cited reasons for introducing massage as therapy have been client demand and perceived clinical effectiveness. In professional settings, massage involves the client being treated while lying on a massage table, sitting in a massage chair, or lying on a mat on the floor. The massage subject may be fully or partly unclothed. Parts of the body may be covered with towels or sheets. At FEDCAM, a bed called Migun therapeutic massage bed shown below is used for patients for the treatment of various diseases. It is an electrically operated device. A bed sheet is laid on it, and the patient is made to lie on his/her back. The power switch is turned on, and the ball-like objects move from the feet to the head. The treatment period for a session is usually forty minutes. The bed has an auto-stop facility. The diagram shown below explains the procedure.

A patient undergoing therapeutic massage on a Migun therapeutic massage bed.

(v) Shortwave Diathermy

Diathermy is the use of high-frequency electric current for deep heating of tissues in physical therapy. Shortwave, ultrasound, and microwave diathermy heat tissues at different depths for different purposes. Low heat warms tissue to ease muscle pain. Higher degrees of diathermy destroy tissue; this is useful in surgery, particularly on the eye or nerves, to coagulate, limit bleeding, and seal off traumatised tissues.

Shortwave diathermy is a form of heat treatment using high frequency electromagnetic currents. These cause molecules in deep tissue to vibrate, heating the tissues and increasing the blood flow to them. Diathermy is used to accelerate recovery and reduce pain in sports injuries such as bursitis, strains, and sprains. It is not used on acute injuries where there has been recent bleeding. Diathermy involves heating deep muscular tissues. When heat is applied to the painful area, cellular metabolism speeds up and the blood flow increases. The increased metabolism and circulation accelerates tissue repair. The heat helps the tissues relax and stretch, thus alleviating stiffness. Heat also reduces nerve fibre sensitivity, increasing the patient's pain threshold. The body part to be treated is placed between thick cloths. Heat is generated as the high-frequency waves travel through the body tissues between the plates. Shortwave diathermy is most often used to treat areas like the hip, which is covered with a dense tissue mass. It is also used to treat pelvic infections and sinusitis.

(vi) Homeopathy Department

Homeopathy is based on the idea that large doses of a substance cause a symptom while very small doses of that same substance will cure it. Homeopathy was developed by an eighteenth-century German doctor, Samuel Hahnemann, who founded a system based on the ancient concept of 'like cures like'. Substances that cause a certain symptom in a person are given to the person to relieve those symptoms. The 'law of proving' is the method used to test substances for their healing effect. Dr Hahnemann and his assistants conducted many provings, taking in plant, mineral, animal, and chemical material. They carefully wrote down the symptoms they felt with each substance. Later, when patients had those symptoms, they were treated with very dilute doses of that substance. This approach became the first law of homeopathy: the law of similars or 'like cures like.' Over time, volumes of information developed from Dr Hahnemann's years of 'provings'. These volumes are called the homeopathic pharmacopoeia, and they are still used as the source of homeopathic remedies. When a patient describes his symptoms, the symptoms are compared with this large collection of documented symptoms until a match is found. The patient is then treated with a highly diluted version of that substance. A person complaining of intense, throbbing headaches, for example, might be treated with a very diluted dose of belladonna (a poisonous herb used to make some medicines), because a tiny bite of that plant causes throbbing headaches.

Preparation of Homeopathic Remedies

After lengthy shaking, one drop of the new solution is mixed with another ninety-nine drops of water. This mixture is shaken vigorously, and then one drop is taken from it and added to another ninety-nine drops of liquid, and so on. This process is repeated as many as thirty, fifty, or more times. The end result can be a solution more dilute than one molecule of salt placed in an ocean. A molecule is the smallest possible amount of any substance. Most homeopathic remedies contain less than one molecule of the original plant or chemical extract.

Clinical Application of Homeopathy

Today, homeopathic remedies are used most often to treat problems such as arthritis, asthma, colds, flu, and allergies. These are some of the most common problems for which people seek medical advice. But some supporters believe that homeopathic remedies can cure many illnesses. Responsible practitioners do not use homeopathic remedies to treat diabetes, cancer, heart disease, or other major illnesses. Nor do they use it to treat surgical emergencies or serious infections or injuries. Some people believe that homeopathic medicine works by stimulating the body's own natural defences. Dr Hahnemann believed homeopathic remedies would replace the illness with a similar but weaker illness that the body's 'vital force' could more easily overcome. The reason most commonly offered today by homeopathic proponents is the remedy that water has a 'memory' of the original substance. What is this memory? Homeopaths say it is electromagnetic waves of the active ingredient it once contained. They say that vigorous shakings between each dilution make this memory possible. Another explanation, heard less often, is that all of the shaking and dilution activity releases the essence, or healing life force, of the original substance. Many advocates of homeopathy indicate that they do not know how it works and that later research will unlock that mystery. Homeopathic supporters have not been able to offer an explanation that scientists can reproduce or accept. How its remedies could work remains a perplexing problem for homeopathic proponents and is a major source of scientific scepticism. Clinical homeopathic research has produced varying results. Some studies indicate it is effective in the treatment of allergies, infant diarrhoea, and other problems; other studies do not. Researchers in Britain recently looked at the results from the most well-designed research projects about homeopathy. After a careful study, they decided that there was little reason to believe that homeopathic remedies work.

Most scientists say homeopathic remedies are basically water and can act only as placebos. A placebo is a 'sugar pill' which appears to reduce symptoms by means of mental suggestion. However, at the Federal College of Complementary and Alternative Medicine, homeopathic remedies involve using products that are safe and have no side effects. If only, through the power of the mind, they can be used to reduce the symptoms of self-limiting illnesses (aches and pains that will go away on their own in a week or so). Thus, homeopathic remedies help some people get through these problems with fewer symptoms and may shorten the length of these illnesses.

Radionic computer (MK 12/S/3/MA)

(vii) Radionic Computer

The instrument mentioned above used at FEDCAM is a radionic analysis/broadcasting instrument for use in electronic homeopathy. It is an ideal instrument for student training and is ideal for gaining experience in radionic testing, analysis, and broadcasting. This instrument makes it possible for you to copy a homeopathic remedy or, with the help of a rate, to produce (simulate) it yourself. The instrument is a compact, portable unit enclosed in a hand-built case with a detachable lid. This particular equipment is in use in our clinic at the Beckman Natmedics Health Centre in London.

5.6 Naturopathy Department

Naturopathy is a system of medicine based on the healing power of nature. Naturopathy is a holistic system, meaning that naturopathic doctors strive to find the cause of disease by understanding the body, mind, and spirit of the person. Most naturopathic practitioners use a variety of therapies and techniques such as nutrition, hydrotherapy, and herbal medicine. There are two areas of focus in naturopathy:

one is supporting the body's own healing abilities and the other is empowering people to make lifestyle changes necessary for the best possible health. While naturopathic practitioners treat both short-term illness and chronic conditions, theiremphasis is on preventing disease and educating patients. Complementary preventive therapy practitioners must pay due attention to this very approach.

A typical medicinal plant

The modern form of naturopathy can be traced to eighteenth- and nineteenth-century natural healing systems. Such systems include hydrotherapy (water therapy), which was popular in Germany, and nature cure, developed in Austria, based on the use of food, air, light, water, and herbs to treat illness. Benjamin Lust, a German immigrant, first introduced naturopathy to the United States in 1902 when he founded the American School of Naturopathy. The school emphasised the use of natural cures, proper bowel habits, and good hygiene as the tools for health. This was the first time that principles of a healthy diet, like increasing fibre intake and reducing saturated fats, became popular. In the mid-1920s to 1940, the use of naturopathic medicine declined. It was not until the 1960s that naturopathic-style holistic medicine became popular again. Today, naturopaths are licensed care providers in many American states. They offer a variety of natural therapies, including homeopathy, vitamin, and mineral supplements. Traditional Chinese medicine, relaxation techniques, and herbal remedies. A visit to a naturopathic doctor, or ND, will be similar to a visit to your family doctor. Your first visit may take more than an hour. The doctor will take a very thorough history, asking about your diet, lifestyle, stress, and environmental exposures. Next, the ND will do a physical examination, which may require laboratory tests. In addition to conventional tests, NDs may use unique laboratory techniques such as the comprehensive digestive stool analysis (CDSA). This test allows naturopaths to examine your digestive process as well as to see which nutrients your body is absorbing, among other things. Naturopathic NDs treat the whole person, which means that they consider a variety of factors before they diagnose an illness. An ND might look at your mental, emotional, and spiritual state; your diet; your family history; your environment; and your lifestyle before making a diagnosis. Some of the more common treatments used by naturopaths at the Beckman clinic and I am sure also at the FCM clinic will include

(1) nutritional counselling, (2) herbal medicine, (3) hydrotherapy (water therapy)—these therapies include drinking natural spring water, taking baths, alternating hot and cold applications, and water exercise, all of which are thought to stimulate healing and strengthen the immune system. (4) Electromagnetic therapy: Naturopaths consider patients to be participants in their health care, so you may be asked to make lifestyle changes (such as changing your sleeping, eating, and exercise habits). Which illnesses and conditions respond well to naturopathy? Because naturopaths combine so many therapies, it is difficult to single out specific illnesses that respond well to naturopathy. Naturopaths treat both acute and chronic conditions from arthritis to ear infections (otitis media), from HIV to asthma, from congestive heart failure to hepatitis. Naturopaths treat the whole person (rather than only treating a disease or its symptoms), aiming to help their patients maintain a balanced state of good health. Because of this holistic approach, naturopathy may be especially suited for treating chronic illnesses.

(viii) Hydrotherapy

Hydrotherapy is the use of water to revitalise, maintain, and restore health. Hydrotherapy treatments include saunas, steam baths, foot baths, sitz baths, and the application of cold and hot water compresses. Father Sebastian Kneipp, a nineteenth-century Bavarian monk, is said to be the father of hydrotherapy. Kneipp believed that disease could be cured by using water to eliminate waste from the body. Hydrotherapy is popular in Europe and Asia, where people 'take the waters' at hotsprings and mineral springs. In North America, it is often recommended as self-care by naturopathic doctors. There is a physiological basis to hydrotherapy. Cold is stimulating, and it causes superficial blood vessels to constrict, shunting the blood to internal organs. Hot water is relaxing, causes blood vessels to dilate, and removes wastes from body tissues. Alternating hot and cold water also improves elimination, decreases inflammation, and stimulates circulation. The human bodyis 65 per cent water and requires regular hydrating and replenishing of fluids. Most of us are familiar with the fatigue and malaise that can occur when we don't drink enough water. Macrobiotic theory has a very clear stance concerning water, whether it is used for drinking, bathing, or cooking. When we are helping our bodies to heal, or when we are focused on preventive care, the quality of the water we consume is critical. Environmental studies have revealed that much of the nation's public drinking water is contaminated by traces of hormones, toxins, and pharmaceutical drugs. Some cities have better water than others, but it's an issue that concerns all of us.

Macrobiotics recommends the use of high-quality spring, well, or filtered water, depending on where you live. Some practitioners recommend distilled water, because it is likely to be more pure than spring water and is a good carrier for healing protocols. There is conflicting information about consuming only distilled water, since all minerals and solid particles have been removed from it, but at FCAM, energised water is prescribed for the patients. It is prepared using a BioDisc: two parts hydrogen, one part oxygen. Also known as water, it's the most essential element next to air for our survival. The human body is a water machine running primarily on water and minerals. By weight, our body is about 72 per cent water. Naturally, the quality of water we consume affects our overall state of health. Every healing and life-giving process happens in our body through water. Our blood, the very substance of our existence, is more than 83 per cent water, flowing through our body distributing nutrients, oxygen, and antibodies on demand. The purity of the water we drink greatly impacts our strength and energy level. Any toxic chemical, chlorine included, that gets into our body, will use the body's strength and energy to repair and reduce the damage done by that contaminant. Consumption of water laced with contaminants will cause the properties of our blood to change and negatively affect virtually every aspect of our health. So enrich the drinking water you consume with energy from the BioDisc.

BioDisc/Energy Water (BDEW)

BioDisc is a natural energy-generating device. It's a wellness tool. When liquid is passed through the biofrequency created by the BioDisc, the molecular structure of the liquid is reformed to peak condition. The liquid turns into 'energised water' for consumption.

A BioDisc

It is a glass but guarded by a thick rubber to prevent it from breaking in case it hits the floor. Pour drinking water over the BioDisc. Collect and drink the energised water. It's energised instantly. Otherwise, stand the bottle of your drinking water on top of the disc for six hours or longer. If you poured chlorinated water, the taste and smell will disappear. Put in your refrigerator overnight, and everything in it will be energised.

FEDCAM has started a mass production of energy water called FEDCAM Energy Water.

Benefits of Energy Water (Bio-Energy Water)

By drinking the FEDCAM energy water, you will benefit in the following ways: (1) It helps to improve your sleep. (2) It will energise our body to be less fatigued. (3) It helps balance the 'ying' and 'yang' and boosts the 'chi' (life force). (4) The calming effects of the resonance increases mental cognition. (5) It helps to detoxify and hydrate all body cells. (6) It reduces stress levels. (7) It increases the intake of nutrients and food supplements. (8) It increases oxygenation of the blood. (9) It enhances the immune system of your body. (10) It will assist in pain relief.

(ix) Electromagnetic Therapy (EMT)

Electromagnetic therapy is a form of alternative medicine which treats diseases by applying electromagnetic radiation or pulsed electromagnetic fields (PEMF) to the body. These methods can treat a wide range of ailments, including ulcers, headaches, burns, chronic pain, nerve disorders, spinal cord injuries, diabetes, gum infections, asthma, bronchitis, arthritis, cerebral palsy, heart disease, and cancer. Equipment used at FEDCAM to achieve this is *Pyro-Energen*. Pyro-Energen (for the diagrams, refer to the college's prospectus) is the first electrotherapy or electro-medicine device in the world that uses *static electricity* to eradicate the origin and cause of viral diseases, cancer, and diseases of unknown cause.

The *Pyro-Energen* produces high-tension voltage of static electricity. It produces around 18,000 volts, depending on the climate or humidity and the insulation between the patient and the ground. However, the *Pyro-Energen's* static electricity does not induce any Joule heat to your body. It just simply surrounds your body. Thus, there are no side effects at all. Do you know that all of us are living under a certain electrified field of natural waves? When this kind of field is broken, then you get unhealthy. In today's modern world, there are now various kinds of pollutants; our planet is warming up, creating incurable diseases, and nature is losing a perfectly balanced electrical field of atmosphere. Aside from it, the individual's personal offence against humanity is also losing a certain electrical field (for your information simply, it can be considered something like that of human *aura*) that protects you from paranormal wave (origin of virus and diseases of unknown cause), which exists in fifth dimension.

Pyro-Energen (front view)

As seen in the illustration below, our body is surrounded by static electricity and the paranormal wave that creates diseases. *Pyro-Energen* does electrification outside the body (it does not pass through or penetrate the body), illustrated as negative electron (−), which discharge the paranormal wave, positive (+).

Operation Procedures of Pyro-Energen

The *Pyro-Energen* is used with a plate connected to the Output High Voltage. (1) Place the *Pyro-Energen* on a sturdy flat surface (e.g. on a plastic/wooden table or desk), away from nearby conductive materials. It may be in your bedroom or living room. Plug the output cable to the Output High Voltage. Connect the alligator clip to a metal sheet, foil, or screen. The cable from the *Pyro-Energen* to the metal screen should not be touching the ground. (2) Place the metal screen or sheet on a low plastic stool. Sit on a plastic or wooden chair. *Use only clean and dry plastic or wooden materials.* Don't use cane (bamboo or rattan) chairs as they could be poor insulators and could produce electrostatic leakage resulting in less effectiveness of the treatment. Place your feet (bare or with socks) on the metal sheet or screen. (3) Finally, have someone plug the power cord into the outlet.

If you need to use the *Pyro-Energen* alone, it is best to use it with a remote-controlled power outlet. If unavailable, one solution is to use a power extension bar that has a separate on and off switch, and use a plastic or wooden stick to turn on the switch. *Be sure not to bring the power cord near the Output High Voltage terminal and cable. Do not touch any appliance or anything or anyone that is grounded.* The two indicator lights should light up, then electrotherapy begins. (4) Children or pets may be held on the lap for treatment. (5) Treatment frequency of three to five times a day, at thirty minutes per session, is adequate. If you do not suffer from an illness or disease, once a day or twice a week of treatment is recommended to prevent disease and maintain health.

After Your Session

After you have completed, be sure to remove your feet first from the metal screen, then unplug the unit from the wall outlet or turn off the power extension bar if you're using one. Or have someone turn off the machine for you. One way to check if the *Pyro-Energen* is functioning properly, or if you are not grounded, and if you are well insulated, is to tear off thin bits of tissue paper or Kleenex and place it on a flat surface (made of wood or plastic), then bring your finger near it. The tissue paper will start to move or rise. This means that you are under electrostatic electrification. Poor insulation affects the intensity of static electricity surrounding your body. Under good insulation, the tissue paper should begin to move or rise when your fingers are three to four inches away from it.

Infrared Radiation Therapy

Radiant heat is simply a form of energy that heats objects directly through a process called conversion, without having to heat the air in between. Radiant heat is also called infrared energy (IR). Our sun is the principal source of radiant energy that we enjoy daily (some more so than others).

Have you ever been outside on a partly cloudy spring day of about fifty degrees Fahrenheit and felt quite comfortable until the sun was suddenly obscured by a cloud? Although the air temperature had not had time to drop, you felt chilled, as the cloud would not let the warming infrared rays through to reach you. Infrared light is an important energy force that promotes healing—a raising of the white blood cell count. Why is that good? Because more white blood cells mean greater immunity. Greater immunity means greater health and a better quality of life. Energy medicine is an ancient practice, and Chinese health practitioners would use healing touch therapies for improved cell growth, DNA synthesis, and protein synthesis in cells. Although these ancient practitioners did not know the technical terms as to why their therapy improved health, they were sure their patients got better. Over the past twenty-five years, Japanese and Chinese researchers and clinicians have done extensive research on infrared treatments and reported many provocative findings. Whole-body infrared therapy has been used for over eighty years by German physicians in an independently developed form. Among other benefits, whole-body infrared thermal systems make it possible for people in wheelchairs or those who are otherwise unable to exert themselves or those who won't follow through on an exercising and conditioning programme to achieve a cardiovascular training effect. This also allows for more variety in any ongoing exercise programme.

As for infrared's outstanding effect on caloric consumption and weight control, we find that burning from 600 to 2,400 calories in a thirty-minute session is quite routine. The infrared thermal system might then simulate the consumption of energy equal to that expended in a six-mile run during only a single session. This would be invaluable for those who don't exercise and those who can't exercise yet want an effective weight control and fitness maintenance programme.

Infrared radiation light

Evidently, the flushing of toxins from the lymph areas and from the largest organ of elimination, the skin, isthe source of many of these health improvements. Toxemia has been targeted as the number one reason so many of us are ill. With the elimination of these poisons from deep within the body, the organs can then do their job unhindered.

A patient receiving infrared radiation therapy

The list of health enhancements through the use of infrared therapy as used at FEDCAM is impressive, and it includes relief from all forms of arthritis; increase in the extensibility of collagen tissues; relief from muscle spasms and joint stiffness; increase in blood flow; assists in resolution of inflammatory infiltrates, oedema, and exudates; weight control; hypertension; arteriosclerosis; coronary artery disease; blood circulation; ear, nose, and throat conditions; skin conditions (including cellulite); and all-round beauty treatment.

Pharmacy

The clinical services department has a natural medical pharmacy where remedies for various ailments and diseases are made available to the patient. We are indeed very pleased to see that the Nigerian Federal Government has shown interest in complementary medicine by establishing a college of this nature. With this, it is now possible to regulate and control the standard of complementary medicine in Nigeria. One hopes that other nations in Africa will follow. I have no doubt in my mind that Nigerians will recognise the complementary inter-relationship between the orthodox medical system and complementary therapy. Once our attitude and the loudness of our mouth are under self-control, Nigeria public will live to benefit from the combined professionalism of an integrated medical system in the country.

5.7 Coronary Heart Disease

This disease is caused by a thickening of the inside walls of the coronary arteries. This thickening, called atherosclerosis narrows the space through which blood can flow, decreasing and sometimes completely cutting off the supply of oxygen and nutrients to the heart. It is usually caused by a combination of non-holistic practices such as poor nutrition, environmental pollution, destructive eating habits and deterioration of the body. Many other factors can cause this disease reaction such as high and low blood pressure, acid ash, fat deposits, thermal glandular fatigue and loss of vein and artery flexibility. The current fad, which suggests high cholesterol levels resulting in arteriosclerosis-caused heart attacks, was started in 1913. It is founded upon giving high levels of cholesterol to rabbits (liver too small to break down fats). Further, the researcher never realised that the research was on disease damage and never gave disease damage any significance.

Atherosclerosis usually occurs when a person has high levels of cholesterol, a fat-like substance in the blood. Cholesterol and fat circulating in the blood build up on the walls of the arteries. This buildup narrows the arteries and can slow or block the flow of blood. When the level of cholesterol in the blood is high, there is a greater chance that it will be deposited onto the artery walls. This process begins in most people during childhood and the teenage years and worsens as they get older.

In addition to high blood cholesterol, high blood pressure and smoking also contribute to CHD. On average, each of these doubles your chance of developing heart disease. Therefore, a person who has all three risk factors is eight times more likely to develop heart disease than someone who has none. Obesity and physical inactivity are other factors that can lead to CHD. Being overweight increases the likelihood of developing high blood cholesterol and high blood pressure while physical inactivity increases the risk of heart attack. Regular exercise, good nutrition, and smoking cessation are keys to controlling the risk factors for CHD.

Overweight/obesity

About 65 per cent of American adults are overweight or obese. Being overweight or obese increases the risk not only for heart disease but also for other conditions, including stroke, gallbladder disease, arthritis, breast, colon, and other cancers. Being overweight and obesity are determined by two key measures: body mass index or BMI and the waist circumference. BMI relates the height to weight.

Heart Attack Warning Signs When a heart attack happens, every minute counts. Know the warning signs. Smoking rates among African-American adults historically have been higher than among the general U.S. population. However, recent increases in teen smoking among African Americans document the need for continued prevention efforts. African Americans continue to suffer disproportionately from chronic and preventable disease compared to white Americans. Of the three leading causes of death in African Americans—heart disease, cancer, and stroke—smoking and other tobacco use are major contributors to these illnesses.

CHAPTER 6

This chapter deals with various research findings in the garlic compound. Here the book gives tips on various health matters that can be remedied using garlic herbal medication. Complementary health care practitioners must be very careful in the application of the recommended dose of the products. This chapter explains the principles of dietetic control therapy based on various forms of dietary supplementation. It also elucidates the importance of the new vegetable and fruit whole food capsules scientifically approved for better and healthy living and prevention of diseases. This chapter gives an illustration of the various scientific research works done on the matters of dietary therapy. This chapter also gives the presentation of the elaborate research findings on the importance of garlic for preventive therapy and treatment.

6.1 Research Findings in Garlic Compounds

The following research findings have been included in this book to enable natural health practitioners to have the knowledge and the basis of using garlic as one of the major herbal resources in natural medicine. But the principal purpose of my presenting the details of the research findings is to demonstrate the various uses of this herb. There are many types of potential diseases which can be prevented by the uses of garlic in the dietary programme. Such diseases are shown in this book. For all information given in this book, the potential practitioners should ask and enquire the about the following: (1) What does this information mean in terms of my practice and preventive therapy? (2) Are there any scientific and proven evidence that shows the efficacy of this product (s)? (3) How would/should we apply the given product(s) to my practice? (4) Where would/should we obtain any or all of these product(s)? (5) Do we have the knowledge and the professional skills in the usage of these products?

(6) The fact that the named products have worked for the patience or clients in other societies or communities or any individuals in any given countries dose that mean that as a practitioner I will obtain the same result in using the same product under my own given local condition? (7) These questions that must apply to the entire book are primarily about preventive therapy in complementary medicine. It is neither a text book nor an instruction book on complementary medicine and should not be seen as such. (8) Such unguided assumptions of 'street wisdom' which are often expressed by people about the uses of herbs for treatment must be considered in relation to the consequence. The same legal requirements of professional duties and responsibilities of all health practitioners must also apply to the complementary practitioners.

The healthy properties of garlic are legend and have been identified and validated by hard empirical science in over a thousand scientific reports in this last decade. Areas of beneficial activity include anti-AIDS, anti-cancer, anti-cardiovascular disease, and anti-infectious properties, among others. Garlic is furthermore uniquely the richest dietary source of many otherwise rare healthy sulphur compounds, plus organic selenium, as well as being one of the best sources of organic germanium (after ginseng and green tea, the latter is the richest food source known), besides an impressive array of other essential nutrients and active health-promoting phytochemicals. Various forms of garlic are available, the most effective being fresh, powdered, distilled, and especially aged garlic; the latter lacks the irritant effect of fresh garlic, yet possesses equal or greater bioactive range and potency.

Pharmacologic Activities of Aged Garlic Extraction
Comparison with Other Garlic Preparations

We investigated the pharmacologic activities of four garlic preparations: raw garlic juice (RGJ), heated garlic juice (HGJ), dehydrated garlic powder (DGP), and aged garlic extract (AGE). The study used three animal models, i.e. testicular hypogonadism (hypospermatogensis and impotence) induced by warm water treatment, intoxication of acetaldehyde, and growth of inoculated tumour cells. RGJ was found to be effective only in the recovery of testicular function. The efficacy of HGJ was observed in three models; however, it did not improve impotence. DGP was effective in recovery of spermatogenesis and stimulated acetaldehyde detoxification. Significant beneficial effects of AGE were found in all three models. Although all four garlic preparations significantly enhanced natural killer (NK) and killer cell activities of the spleen cells of tumour-bearing mice, only AGE and HGJ inhibited the growth of inoculated tumour cells. These results suggest that different types of garlic preparations have different pharmacologic properties, and among the four garlic preparations studied, AGE could be the most useful garlic preparation (Kasuga S., et al., *J. Nutr.*, 131(3): 1080S, 2001).

Antioxidant Healing: The Effects of Aged Garlic Extract

Oxidative modification of DNA, proteins, and lipids by reactive oxygen species (ROS) plays a role in ageing and disease, including cardiovascular, neurodegenerative, and inflammatory diseases and cancer. Extracts of fresh garlic that are aged over a prolonged period to produce aged garlic extract (AGE) contain antioxidant phytochemicals that prevent oxidant damage. These include unique water-soluble organosulphur compounds, lipid-soluble organosulphur components, and flavonoids, notably allixin and selenium. Long-term extraction of garlic (up to 20 mo) ages the extract, creating antioxidant properties by modifying unstable molecules with antioxidant activity, such as allicin, and increasing stable and highly bioavailable water-soluble organ sulphur compounds, such as S:-allylcysteine and S:-allylmercaptocysteine. AGE exerts antioxidant action by scavenging ROS, enhancing the cellular antioxidant enzymes, superoxide dismutase, catalase, and glutathione peroxidase, and increasing glutathione in the cells. AGE inhibits lipid peroxidation, reducing ischemic/reperfusion damage and inhibiting oxidative modification of LDL, thus protecting endothelial cells from the injury by the oxidised molecules, which contributes to atherosclerosis. AGE inhibits the activation of the oxidant-induced transcription factor, nuclear factor (NF)-kappaB, which has clinical significance in human immunodeficiency virus gene expression and parthenogenesis. AGE protects DNA against free radical-mediated damage and mutations, inhibits multiuse carcinogenesis, and defends against ionising radiation and UV-induced damage, including protection against some forms of UV-induced immunosuppressant. AGE may have a role in protecting against loss of brain function in ageing and possesses other anti-ageing effects, as suggested by its ability to increase cognitive functions, memory, and longevity in a senescence-accelerated mouse model. AGE has been shown to protect against the cardiotoxic effects of doxorubicin, an antineoplastic agent used in cancer therapy and against liver toxicity caused by carbon tetrachloride (an industrial chemical) and acetaminophen, an analgesic. Substantial experimental evidence shows the ability of AGE to protect against oxidant-induced disease, acute damage from ageing, radiation and chemical exposure, and long-term toxic damage. Although additional observations are warranted in humans, compelling evidence supports the beneficial health effects attributed to AGE, i.e. reducing the risk of cardiovascular disease, stroke, cancer, and ageing, including the oxidant-mediated brain cell damage that is implicated in Alzheimer's disease.

6.2 Scientific Abstracts

Allyl sulphur compounds are the major active constituents found in crushed garlic. Research has revealed that garlic and its lipid- or water-soluble components have many pharmacologic properties; however, studies also demonstrate that heating has a negative influence on these beneficial effects. Our studies showed that as little as 60 s of microwave heating or forty-five minutes of oven heating can block garlic's ability to inhibit *in vivo* binding of mammary carcinogen DMBA metabolites. Allowing crushed garlic to 'stand' for ten minutes before microwave heating for 60 s prevented the total loss of anti-carcinogenic activity, which relates to its anticancer properties (Song K. and Milner J., *J. Nutr.*, 131(3): 1054S, 2001).

Garlic exhibits a broad antibiotic spectrum against both gram-positive and gram-negative bacteria. Noteworthy results published include the following: (1) raw juice of garlic was found to be effective against many common pathogenic bacteria—intestinal bacteria, which are responsible for diarrhoea in humans and animals; (2) garlic is effective even against those strains that have become resistant to antibiotics; (3) the combination of garlic with antibiotics leads to partial or total synergism; (4) complete lack of resistance has been observed repeatedly; (5) even toxin production by microorganisms is prevented by garlic. Helicobacter pylori (*H. pylori*) is a bacterium implicated in the aetiology of stomach cancer and ulcers. The incidence of stomach cancer is lower in populations with a high intake of allium vegetables. We have demonstrated *in vitro* that H. pylori is susceptible to garlic extract at a fairly moderate concentration. Even some antibiotic-resistant *H. pylori* strains are susceptible to garlic (Sivam G., *J. Nutr.*, 131(3): 1106S, 2001).

The antimicrobial effects of aqueous garlic extracts are well established but those of garlic oil (GO) are little known. GO sulphide constituents and garlic powder (GP) were compared in tests against human enteric bacteria. All bacteria tested, which included both gram-negative and positive bacteria and pathogenic forms, were susceptible to garlic materials. Based upon its thiosulphinate content, GP was more active than GO against most bacteria, although some properties of GO are identified as offering greater therapeutic potential (Ross Z., *Apple Environ. Microbiol.*, 67(1): 475, 2001). The effects of garlic preparations, including dehydrated raw garlic powder (RGP), dehydrated boiled garlic powder (BGP), and aged garlic extract (AGE), on the gastric mucosa were determined. Among the three preparations, RGP caused severe damage, including erosion. BGP also caused reddening of the mucosa, whereas AGE did not cause any undesirable effects. These results suggest that caution be used with regard to safety and effectiveness when choosing a garlic preparation because some preparations may have undesirable effects, including gastrointestinal problems (Hoshino T., *J. Nutr.*, 131(3): 1109S, 2001).

Epidemiological and laboratory studies provide insight into the anti-carcinogenic potential of garlic and its constituent compounds. Part of the protection from these compounds probably relates to a block in nitrosamine formation and metabolism. However, blockage in the initiation and promotion phases of the carcinogenicity of various compounds, including polycyclic hydrocarbons, provides evidence that garlic and its constituents can alter several phase I and II enzymes. Their ability to block tumours in a variety of sites, including skin, mammary, and colon, suggests a general mechanism of action. Changes in DNA repair and in immunocompetence may also account for some of this protection. Some, but not all, allyl sulphur compounds can also effectively retard tumour proliferation and induce apoptosis. Changes in cellular thinly and phosphorylation stains may account for some of these anti-tumorigenic properties. The anti-carcinogenic potential of garlic can be influenced by several dietary components including specific fatty acids, selenium, and vitamin A. Garlic and its constituents can suppress carcinogen formation, carcinogen bio-activation, and tumour proliferation (Milner J., *J. Nutr.*, 131(3): 1027S, 2001) In the past decade, the cancer-protective effects of garlic have been well established by epidemiologic studies and animal experiments. However, the cardiovascular-protective properties of garlic are less well understood, in particular, the reported hypercholesterolemia effect. In a recent randomised, double-blind, placebo-controlled intervention study, we showed that aged garlic extract (AGE) supplementation was effective in lowering the plasma concentration of the total cholesterol by 7 per cent and the LDL cholesterol by 10 per cent in hypercholesterolemia men compared with subjects consuming a placebo 2001).

Aged garlic protects the small intestine from anti-tumour drug-induced damage (Horie T., et al., *J. Nutr.* 131(3s): 1071, 2001).

Most chemical and biological studies about garlic have been conducted using organ sulphur compounds. However, a variety of steroid spooning from garlic are being increasingly recognised for their importance in biological processes. This report demonstrates *in vitro* antifungal anti-tumour cytotoxicity and blood coagulability as well as cholesterol-lowering effects of steroid spooning from garlic and aged garlic extract (Matsuura H., *J. Nutr.*, 131(3): 1000S, 2001).

Animal and *in vitro* studies provide evidence of an anti-carcinogenic effect of active ingredients in garlic. This study reviewed the epidemiologic literature on garlic consumption. Site-specific case–control studies of stomach and colorectal cancer, in which multiple reports were available, suggest a protective effect of high intake of raw and/or cooked garlic. Evidence from available studies suggests a preventive effect of garlic consumption in stomach and colorectal cancers (Fleischauer A., *J. Nutr.*, 131(3): 1032S, 2001).

There is increasing evidence that allium derivatives from garlic have significant anti-proliferative actions on human cancers. Both hormone-responsive and hormone-unresponsive cells lines respond to these derivatives. The effects shown by allium derivatives include induction of apoptosis, regulation of cell cycle progression, and modification of pathways of signal transduction. Allium derivatives appear to regulate nuclear factors involved in immune function and inflammation, as well as in cellular proliferation. Our own studies indicate that allium derivatives inhibit proliferation of the human prostate cancer cell line and the human breast cancer cell line.

Oxidative modification of LDL has been recognised as playing an impor-tant role in the initiation and progression of atherosclerosis. In this study, we determined that aged garlic extract (AGE) may be useful for prevention of atherosclerosis (Ide N. and Lau B., *J. Nutr.*, 131(3): 1020S, 2001).

Garlic is known for its pharmacologic and nutritional properties. In previous studies, garlic elicited a reduction in plasma levels of lipids by inhibiting hepatic cholesterol synthesis. The aim of this study was to investigate in an *in vivo* model the effects of garlic extract and some fractions on cholesterol levels and vascular reactivity in cholesterol-fed rats. The plasma concentration of cholesterol was 58 mg/dL (100 per cent) at the beginning of the study and increased to 102 mg/dL (153 per cent; hypercholesterolemia group) at the end of the treatment. Plasma total cholesterol decreased in all groups treated with garlic; moreover, this effect was higher in rats fed with raw garlic fractions and extracts. LDL decreased significantly with respect to the hypercholesterolemia group in all groups treated with garlic fractions and extracts (P: < 0.01). These data suggest that garlic fractions could prevent diet-induced hypercholesterolemia and vascular alterations in the endothelium-dependent relaxation associated with atherosclerosis.

Using various kinds of models, we examined the effects of aged garlic extract (AGE) on immune functions. These studies strongly suggest that AGE could be a promising candidate as an immune modifier, which maintains the homeostasis of immune functions. These studies strongly suggest that AGE could be a promising candidate as an immune modifier, which maintains the homeostasis of immune functions (Kyo E., et al. *J. Nutr.*, 131(3): 1075S, 2001). The health benefits of garlic likely arise from a wide variety of components, possibly working synergistically. The complex chemistry of garlic makes it plausible that variations in processing can yield quite different preparations. Highly unstable thiosulphinates, such as allicin, disappear during processing and are quickly transformed into a variety of organ sulphur components. The efficacy and safety of these preparations in preparing dietary supplements based on garlic are also contingent on the processing methods employed. Although there are many garlic supplements commercially available, they fall into one of four categories, i.e. dehydrated garlic powder, garlic oil, garlic oil macerate, and aged garlic extract (AGE). Garlic and garlic supplements are consumed in many cultures for their hyperlipidemia, anti-platelet, and procirculatory effects. In addition to these proclaimed beneficial effects, some garlic preparations also appear to possess hepatoprotective, immune-enhancing, anticancer, and chemo preventive activities (Imagoes H., et al. *J. Nutr.*, 131(3): 955S, 2001).

It has been known for several decades that hypercholesterolemia is a major risk factor for atherosclerosis and that lowering of cholesterol can significantly reduce the risk for cardiovascular diseases. More recently, oxidation of LDL has been recognised as playing an important role in the initiation and progression of atherosclerosis. Short-term supplementation of garlic in human subjects has demonstrated an increased resistance of LDL to oxidation. These data suggest that suppressed LDL oxidation may be one of the powerful mechanisms accounting for the anti-atherosclerotic properties of garlic (Lau B., *J. Nutr.*, 131(3): 985S, 2001).

Of the many beneficial actions of garlic, inhibition of the growth of cancer is perhaps the most remarkable. Our previous animal studies demonstrated that aged garlic extract was highly effective, and unlike the approved immunotherapy for human bladder cancer, bacillus Chalmette-Guerin (BCG), garlic was effective when added to the diet. Garlic can detoxify carcinogens by stimulation of cytochrome P (450) enzymes or by its antioxidant activity or sulphur compound binding. Studies demonstrate a direct toxic effect of garlic on sarcoma and gastric, colon, bladder, and prostate cancer cells in tissue culture. The most likely explanation of this effect is immune stimulation. Comparison of the effects of garlic on BCG immunotherapy reveals many similarities. Both stimulate proliferation of lymphocytes and macrophage phagocytes, induce the infiltration of macrophages and lymphocytes in transplanted, induce splendid hypertrophy, stimulate release of interleukin-2, tumour necrosis factor-alpha, and interferon-gamma, and enhance natural killer cell, killer cell, and lymphocyte-activated killer cell activity. These activities represent effective stimulation of the immune response. Studies suggest that garlic may be useful in preventing the suppression of immune response that is associated with increased risk of malignancy. Data suggest that maintenance of immune stimulation can significantly reduce the risk of cancer (Lamm D. and Riggs D., *J. Nutr.*, 131(3): 1067S, 2001).

Aged garlic extract (AGE) has been shown previously to have moderate cholesterol-lowering and blood pressure-reducing effects. We investigated whether platelet function, a potential risk factor for cardiovascular disease, can be inhibited by AGE administration. AGE exerts selective inhibition on platelet aggregation and adhesion, platelet functions that may be important for the development of cardiovascular events such as myocardial infarction and ischemic stroke (Steiner M., *J. Nutr.*, 131(3): 980S, 2001).

Garlic detoxifies chemical carcinogens, prevents carcinogenesis, and can also directly inhibit the growth of cancer cells. Garlic stimulates immunity, including macrophage activity, natural killer and killer cells, and LAK cells, and increases the production of IL-2, TNF, and interferon-gamma. These cytokines are associated with the beneficial Th1 anti-tumour response, which is characteristic of effective cancer immunotherapy. Garlic stimulates the proliferation of macrophages and lymphocytes and protects against the suppression of immunity by chemotherapy and ultraviolet radiation. Garlic is not a panacea for cancer, but its broad range of beneficial effects is worthy of serious consideration for the prevention and treatment of cancer.

Nephritic syndrome (NS) is characterised by proteinuria, oxidative stress, and endogenous, an excessive amount of fat and fatty substances in the blood (hyperlipidemia). Hyperlipidemia and oxidative stress may be involved in coronary heart disease and the progression of renal damage in these patients. Garlic has been suggested to be beneficial in various disease states. Some of the beneficial effects of garlic may be secondary to its hypolipidemic and antioxidant properties. Garlic treatment diminishes significantly total-cholesterol, LDL-cholesterol, and triglycerides, but not HDL-cholesterol in chronic NS. These data indicate that garlic treatment ameliorates hyperlipidemia and renal damage in chronic NS, which is unrelated to proteinuria or antioxidant enzymes (Pedraza-Chaverri J., *Mol. Cell Biochem.*, 211(1-2): 69, 2000).

The immuno-dulatory effects of naturally occurring sculpture compounds in garlic include the total white blood cell (WBC) count being enhanced significantly and bone-marrow cellular also being increased significantly in treated animals, suggesting an immunostimulating effect for garlic sculpture compounds. (Kuttan G, *J. Ethno-pharmacology*) In the rates that were fed with a high cholesterol diet mixed with garlic powder, there was a significant reduction in their serum cholesterol levels compared with the group which were on a diet containing high cholesterol without garlic powder. The blood pressure of the animals receiving garlic powder and high cholesterol diet was significantly lower as compared to the high cholesterol and control diet group. These results show that garlic is beneficial in reducing blood cholesterol, triglycerides levels, and systolic blood pressure in hypercholesterolemia rats. Our experimental results show that garlic may beneficially affect two risk factors for atherosclerosis—hyperlipidemia and hypertension (Ali M., et al. *Prostaglandins Leukot Essent Fatty Acids*).

To find a better contact solvent to dissolve gallstones, we studied *in vitro* use of garlic oil and compared it with monooctanoin. Garlic oil dissolved the cholesterol gallstones in proportion to the concentration used. The gallstone fragmentation was faster (six hours versus thirty-six hours) and more (88.30 per cent versus 71.01 per cent) by garlic oil in comparison to monooctanoin in test tubes and even in artificial gallbladder and common bile duct models. Garlic oil is a better contact dissolving agent of gallstones than monooctanoin (Nijhawan S., et al. *Trop. Gastroenterol.*, 21(4): 177, 2000). Chronic Helicobacter pylori disease is reduced with allium vegetable intake. This study was designed to assess the *in vivo* anti-*H. pylori* potential of a variety of garlic substances. The MICs (range 8-32 mg/ml) and minimum bactericidal concentrations (MBCs) (range 16–32 mg/ml) of undiluted garlic oil (GO) were smaller than those of garlic powder (GP) (MIC range 250-500 mog/ml; MBC range 250-500 mg/ml) but greater than the MIC of allicin (4. 0 mg/ml) present in GP. Substantial *in vitro* anti-H. pylori effects of pure GO and GP and their dually sulphur components exist, suggesting their potential for *in vivo* clinical use against H. pylori infections.

Reactive oxygen species are involved in gentamicin (GM) nephrotoxicity, and garlic is effective in preventing or ameliorating oxidative stress. The protective effect of garlic is associated with the prevention of the decrease of Mn-SOD and GPx activities and with the rise of lipoperoxidation in renal cortex (Pedraza-Chaverri J., et al. *Free Radix Biol-Med.*, 1; 29(7): 602, 2000). Garlic has been widely reported to protect against cardiovascular disease by reducing serum cholesterol concentrations and blood pressure and by inhibiting platelet aggregation. However, most of these studies have been performed in hypercholesterolemia subjects or in animal models. We performed a thirteen-week study in normolipidemic subjects who ingested 5 mL of aged garlic extract per day. Dietary supplementation significantly inhibited both the total percentage and initial rate of platelet aggregation. We conclude that AGE, when taken as a dietary supplement by normolipidemic subjects, may be beneficial in protecting against cardiovascular disease as a result of inhibiting platelet aggregation (Rahman K. and Billington D., *J. Nutr.*, 130(11): 2662, 2000). Due to the high incidence of atherosclerosis in diabetes, this study investigated the effect of garlic extract on the coronary vascular ultra-structural changes. At present, garlic extract may open a new era in the medicinal use of garlic to prevent diabetic cardiovascular complications (Peterman S., et al. *Drug Deliv.*, 7(2): 91, 2000).

Garlic has been shown to have applications as an antimicrobial, antitumour, hypolipidaemic, antiarthritic, and hypoglycemic agent. In particular, the use of garlic in the treatment and prevention of cardiovascular disease and cancer is an area of considerable investigation and interest (Ali M., *Prostaglandins Leukot Essent Fatty Acids*, 62(2): 55, 2000). Extensive evidence points to the ability of allyl sulphides from garlic to suppress tumour proliferation both *in vitro* and *in vivo*. Both concentration and duration of exposure can increase the antiproliferative effects of lipid- and water-soluble allyl sulphides. Part of their antiproliferative effects may relate to an increase in membrane fluidity and a suppression of integrand glycoprotein IIb–IIIa-mediated adhesion. Allyl sulphides are also recognised for their ability to suppress cellular proliferation by blocking cells in the G2/M phase and by the induction of apoptosis. This increase in the G2/M and apoptotic cell populations correlates with elevated cellular peroxide production. The composition of the entire diet and genetic/epigenetic factors will likely determine the true benefits that might arise from allyl sulphur compounds from garlic (Knowles L. and Milner J., *Drug Metabolic Drug Interact.* 17(1–4): 81, 2000).

Six different mixtures of garlic distilled oils have been assayed against a number of yeasts (*C. albicans, C. tropicalis,* and *B. capitatus*), gram-positive bacteria (*S. aurous* and *B. subtitles*) and gram-negative bacteria (*P. aeruginosa* and *E. coli*). Results support a specific antifungal more than an antibacterial activity (Avato P., *Phytomedicine*, 7(3): 239, 2000).

The anti-platelet activity of methyl allyltrisulphide (MATS), a component commonly present in steam-distilled garlic oil, has been demonstrated by the authors. In addition, our recent findings that to a promyelocytic leukaemia cell HL60, Allium oils shows marked anti-euplastic effects representing both growth suppression and differentiation activities. (Ariga T, Bio factors.) In the circulation of sickle cell anaemia patients, a certain population of erythrocytes has an elevated density. These abnormally dense cells are believed to be at the root of the painful crisis and anaemia of the patients. We have found that aged garlic extract (AGE) as well as its components with antioxidant activity inhibited the formation of dense cells *in vitro*. The degree of inhibition *in vitro* by antioxidants taken orally may be related to their efficacy in inhibiting dense cell formation in the patients (Ohnishi S. and Ohnishi T., *J. Nutr.*, 131(3): 1085S, 2001) The antibacterial activity of garlic powder was tested by using garlic bulbs post-harvested one year. The use of powder from fresh garlic was more effective for antibacterial activity than that from old garlic. The antibacterial activity was resistant to heat treatment of 100 degrees Celsius for twenty minutes. The antibacterial activity was shown against pathogenic bacteria such as methicillin-resistant Staphylococcus aurous (MRSA), Salmonella enteritidis, and Candida albicans. Thus, the practical use of garlic powder is expected to prevent bacteria-caused food poisoning (Sasaki J., et al. *J. Nutr. Sci.*

Vitamin (Tokyo), 45(6): 785, 1999) Allicin, one of the active principles of freshly crushed garlic homogenates, has a variety of antimicrobial activities. Allicin in its pure form exhibits (i) antibacterial activity against a wide range of gram-negative and gram-positive bacteria, including multidrug-resistant enterotoxicogenic strains of Escherichia coli; (ii) antifungal activity, particularly against Candida albicans; (iii) antiparasitic activity, including some major human intestinal protozoan parasites such as Entamoeba histolytica; and (iv) antiviral activity.

6.3 Garlic and Candidiasis: Cause or Cure

Thomson, Director, Gaia Research Institutive of Natural Health Diet Guru Mary-Anne Shearer, in a newsletter recently linked Candida overgrowth to the use of antibiotics, even natural ones like garlic, causing confusion among readers and enthusiasts along the grapevine. Sure, synthetic antibiotics and even natural antibiotics like garlic (and colloidal silver) can cause or contribute to the problem, but not necessarily so, unless colon ecology is seriously deranged prior to or because of inappropriate use of these substances. With correct usage, in the case of higher doses, involving a 'viable' robotic at the appropriate time after an intensive antimicrobial intervention and a cessation thereof, at least temporarily with garlic (or colloidal silver) whilst the beneficial organisms are established in a non-competitive milieu, colon ecology can be effectively corrected and maintained, in spite of, if not because of, the (correct) use of these useful substances.

Arthritis, virginities, and oral thrush are caused by a yeast-like fungus of the Candida group. Because of solid scientific research, garlic is the number one natural treatment for Candida infections, used by thousands of holistic physicians in America (Stephen Fulder, PhD, *Garlic: Nature's Original Remedy*, Healing Arts Press, 1991) and is often recommended as a nutritional supplement and as a primary food by natural health professionals in rational dietary programmes for Candidiasis (Benjamin Lau, MD, PhD, *Garlic for Health*; Candida albicans following earlier garlic antibiotic experiments, researchers expressed the opinion that garlic extracts possessed the potent ability to kill dangerous organisms without destroying those vitally necessary to body health (Klosa J., *German Medical Monthly*, Mar 1950). Whilst it is not quite true to say that garlic selects only the unfriendly organisms for attack, it does tend to attack foes rather than friends, but nevertheless knocks out some of each. However, the beneficial bacteria that live naturally in the gut soon recover, whilst the invaders do not. At lower doses, garlic does not kill invaders but simply stops their multiplication, affording the body an opportunity to marshal its own defences. Garlic is the only antibiotic which at the same time as fighting microbial invaders also protects the body against poisons produced by infection (Stephen Fuller, PhD, *Garlic: Nature's Original Remedy*, Healing Arts Press).

Garlic is a unique antibiotic because it also nourishes beneficial bacteria, since oligosaccharides found in foods such as garlic and onions are robotics which selectively stimulate the growth activities of both good lactobacilli, Acidophilus and Bifid bacteria, in the colon, thereby improving health (Gibson G., et al. Aspects of health and disease involving the human colonic macrobiotic, Summary Report of a First Plenary Meeting on Functional Food Science in Europe, *Intl Life Sci. Inst.*, 2-4 Apr, 1996); (Macfarlane G. and Cummings J., *BMJ*, 318(999), 1999); (Roberfroid M., *Am. J. Clin. Nutr.*, 71(6), 2000). Fungal growth is inhibited by low concentrations of garlic, and lactic acid bacteria are the least sensitive microorganisms to the inhibitory effects of garlic, requiring higher concentrations (Rees L., et al., *World J Microbial Biotechnology*, 9: 303, 1993). See for online literature reviews.

The Herxheimer effect is pronounced in the use of garlic, but the duration appears to be less than with antibiotics (*Novus Research Report No* A-66013, Novus Research Archive, August, 1995). The maximum tolerable dose of a fresh extract of garlic administered orally to human volunteers was determined to be 25 ml of garlic extract. Larger amounts caused severe burning sensations in the oesophagus and the stomach and vomiting. After oral ingestion of 25 ml of the extract, anticandidal and anti-ryptococcal activities were detected in undiluted serum 0.5 and 1 h after ingestion. After high doses, even the blood can kill the infecting fungi (Caporaso N., et al., *Antimicrob. Agents Chemotherapy*, 23(5), 1983) Current therapeutic dose recommendations are 4 gms of fresh garlic or 1-2 cloves per day (Murray J., *Literature Review*, Univ. Med. Dent., New Jersey, 1999).

Out of fifty medicinal plants belonging to twenty-six families studied for their antimicrobial activity, only nine showed antifungal activity. Garlic exhibited activity against both filamentous and non-filamentous fungi (Srinivasan D., et al., *J. Ethnopharmacol.*, 74 (3), 2001). Garlic has a variety of antimicrobial activities: antibacterial, antifungal (particularly against *Candida albicans*), antiparasitic (including protozoa), and antiviral. Beneficial effects against Candida and candidacies have been demonstrated in several diverse scientific studies: (Kabelík J., *Pharmazie*, 25(4), 1970); (Tynecka Z. and Goś Z., *Acta Microbiol*. Pol B, 5(1), 1973); (Tynecka Z. and Goś Z). Allicin is a compound found in garlic and responsible for much of the therapeutic properties of garlic. It has never been found in the blood of people who have consumed garlic, indicating that it is rapidly converted to other compounds (Reuter H., *Phototherapy*, 12: 83, 1991). Allicin is the product of an enzymatic reaction. When fresh garlic is crushed, allinase acts upon the compound alliins to produce allicin. This natural compound loses much of its beneficial properties within hours because it begins to react with garlic's other compounds as soon as the clove is crushed. However, the end product is ajoene, which possesses antifungal qualities (Yamada Y. and Azuma K., *Anti-microbe Agents Chemother*., 1977 11(4), 1977). The antifungal activity of six fractions derived from garlic was investigated in an *in vitro* system. Ajoene had the strongest activity. The growth of Candida albicans was inhibited by ajoene at less than 20 mg/ml (Yoshida S., et al. *Appl. Environ. Microbiol*., 53 (3), 1987).

The mode of anti-Candida action of garlic was studied in Candida albicans. Protein and nucleic acid syntheses were inhibited to the same extent as growth, but lipid synthesis was completely arrested. Blockage of lipid synthesis is likely an important component of the anticandidal activity of garlic. (Adetumbi M., et al. *Antimicrob Agents Chemother*., 30(3), 1986) Garlic treatment affected the structure and integrity of the outer surface of the yeast cells. Growth of *C. albicans* in the presence of garlic suggests that it exerts its effect by oxidation, causing inactivation of enzymes and subsequent microbial growth inhibition (Ghannoum M. J. *Gen. Microbiol*., 134 (Pt 11), 1988). Researchers have confirmed that the phagocytic-enhancing activity of garlic can be attributed to the control of Candida albicans in a living model to this effect (Tadi P., et al. *Intl Clin. Nutr. Rev.*, 10(4), 1990). Garlic strongly enhances phagocytosis of peritoneal macrophages (the ability of immune cells to engulf foreign agents) and increases natural killer cell activity both *in vitro* and *in vivo* (Kyo E., et al. *Phytomed*, 4(4), 1997).

Although Candida organisms are primarily inhabitants of the lower alimentary canal, it is often also genital and even cutaneous. Candidiasis may actually presage progression to AIDS, where Candida overgrowth can be a major opportunistic complication, causing invasive oral infections, even in the oesophagus, upper respiratory tract, and lungs. In addition to controlling this, garlic has furthermore been found to enhance natural killer cell activity and to improve helper/suppressor T-cell ratios in AIDS patients after only six weeks of intake to within the normal range for all subjects. Patients in these studies noted significant improvements in their candidiasis (Abdullah T., et al. *J. Nat. Med. Assoc.*, 80(4), 1988); (Abdullah T., et al., *Deutsche Zeitschrift Fur Onkologie*, 21:52, 1989). Garlic has especially potent antifungal activity toward growing Candida albicans cells, clearly superior to all established appropriate antibiotics tested (Moore G. and Atkins R., *Mycologia*, 69:341, 1977) (most of which are still in use today in some form or another), and with microbicidal concentrations 10-100 times higher than inhibitory concentrations (Naganawa R., et al., *Appl. Environ. Microbiol.*, 62:11, 1996), the control potential far exceeds any negative potential.

Closer to home, Prof. Sid Cywes, at the University of Cape Town, and Peter de Wet, Chief Paediatric Surgery Research Technologist at the Red Cross Children's Hospital, tried garlic out on the culture medium for burn infections and other organisms and were astonished that it could also combat serious candida yeast infections (*MRC News*, Med. Res. Council SA, 31(5), 2000). Since then, about thirty very sick infants, where broad-spectrum antibiotics failed to bring improvement, have been given fresh allicin enterally. The allicin treatment brought about a significant success. One of the active ingredients in garlic is a compound called allicin. On crushing fresh garlic, an enzyme called alliinase is released which rapidly converts the odourless compound alliin into allicin bearing the typical odour of garlic. Allicin is highly unstable and rapidly converts to other sulphur compounds such as ajoene. It is however allicin and agene which have been the main subjects of research. These compounds block the enzymes that are necessary for metabolism of the micro-organisms. They have also been shown to inhibit the growth of more than twenty-three organisms, and a very interesting point is that no resistance has been found up to date (Limson J., Feature: The science behind the legendary healing properties of garlic, *Science in Africa* (Online), Saturday 24 November 21:17:10, 2001). The safe, diverse microbicidal potential of garlic obviously still delights researchers, in spite of its non-patentability:

6.4 The Problem of Treating AIDS

AIDS secondary to HIV infection is currently characterised by immune deficiency that is refractory to immune-enhancing interventions. Once the number of CD4+ T-cells drops to the level of about 200 CD4+/mm3 in the peripheral blood, the action of antiretroviral drugs in various combinations, immune-modulating herbs, antioxidants, and/or immune stimulant therapies (e.g. levamisole, IL-2, topical DNCB, vaccine products) on the CD4+ levels is negligible (there may be a modest, temporary rise). Whereas substantial increases in peripheral blood CD4+ levels can be observed in most HIV+ individuals treated by such therapies when the initial CD4+ count is above about 300, the same treatments fail to positively affect CD4+ levels once AIDS occurs, even in the same individuals who previously responded quite favourably. In virtually all published reports and in personal communications regarding unpublished observations of treatment results, the current evidence is that patients with a CD4+ count substantially below 200 have not been able to achieve a CD4+ count that is substantially above 200 (not reaching even 300), which is sustainable for more than a few months. Although peripheral blood CD4+ counts are not in themselves considered accurate measures of the full effect of therapeutic interventions, CD4+ levels and CD4+ percentage of total lymphocytes remain satisfactory predictors of survival (as do incidence of certain opportunistic infections, such as CMV, measures of cell mass and cell membrane integrity, and nutritional stress indicators such as low albumin). Since mortality is usually the result of the impact of secondary infections and/or cancers that arise in the immune-compromised situation, coupled with the side effects of drug therapies aimed at controlling the infections and cancers, the CD4+ and percent CD4+ serve as indicators of overall immune competence in relation to fighting fatal infections and cancers. A modest prolongation in the median lifespan for those infected by AIDS observed over the past decade has been attributed largely to effective prophylaxis and treatment of PCP, the first of the many potentially fatal infections to arise as the CD4+ levels approach and decline below 200. Other potentially fatal infections that arise when the CD4+ count falls below about fifty, such as MAC and CMV, have not been as easy to control, with progress measured in weeks rather than months. Another portion of the prolonged lifespan is attributed to a brief delay in decline of CD4+ counts when antiretroviral drugs are used before the CD4+ level reaches 200. Together, these account for about one to two years of extended longevity compared to the experience during the first decade of viral transmission and disease development.

Recently, it was revealed that the production of CD4+ T-cells is maintained at a high rate throughout most of the course of the HIV disease and that HIV replication is also maintained at a high rate (on the order of 109 visions daily). The maintenance of some balance between these two is accomplished both by competition (HIV results in destruction of CD4+ T-cells, and the CD4+ T-cells are part of the immune attack against HIV) and by symbiotic relationship (the presence of HIV stimulates production of CD4+ T-cells, and the T-cells in turn provide a replication base for HIV). In most cases, HIV gains the upper hand slowly over a period of years (giving the appearance that HIV is a slow virus), until AIDS is developed (possibly initiated by the activation of other viruses), and then, in many cases, the failure of the immune system proceeds more rapidly, probably because of the influence of chronic and acquired secondary infectious agents and perhaps because of fatigue of the bone marrow cells (accelerated by suppressive drugs) or the immune cells themselves.

Why Therapies May Fail

It is possible that some of the therapies attempted in the treatment of AIDS fail to affect CD4+ levels because of improper use. For example, we may find that antiretroviral drugs should be used only for short periods of time (e.g. a few days to a few weeks) to rapidly inhibit HIV but not allow for either drug toxicity (often marked by declining RBC and increasing MCV, initiation and progression of neuropathy, and, for some drugs, development of pancreatitis) or a high proportion of resistant strain virions to develop. This short application might be best applied when the individual is to be treated for a second condition (aside from HIV itself) to enhance the body's ability to fight the infection by relieving it of the heavy burden of HIV for a few days. An eruption of herpes might best be treated by a short course of zidovudine plus acyclovir, or PCP might be treated by a short course of sulpha drugs plus ddI so that the immune system has a chance to assist the drug therapy in overcoming the infectious episode. In contrast, continued use of the drugs leads to accumulating toxicity problems, with HIV drug resistance as well, even with some of the new combination therapies. By more quickly eliminating secondary infections and giving the body a short break from the HIV fight, it might be possible, especially when applying other methods as well, to produce better clinical results.

It has been suggested—by the current author and others—that natural therapies for HIV infection, including ingestion of antioxidants that reduce the stimuli for HIV replication, are likely to fail because of inadequate dosage. Too little material may be ingested orally (because of the dosage form or improper instructions or compliance with instructions), and only a fraction of the material may be absorbed, especially in those with AIDS. It is possible that the natural therapies succeed in bolstering some portions of the immune system that may help delay morbidity and mortality for several months, but they may not affect certain aspects of the immune system, as reflected in the CD4+ counts, critical to preventing catastrophic events (e.g. wasting accompanying an infectious disease or cancer).

The focus of most immune-based herbal therapies for HIV infection has been the ingestion of mixtures of Chinese tonic herbs, such as astragalus, ganoderma, ligustrum, ginseng, cordyceps, epimedium, lycium, and deer antler, or the ingestion of nutrients or metabolic substances, such as vitamin C, zinc, selenium, l-carnitine, coenzyme Q10, and beta carotene. Investigations in China show that the herbs increase immune functions in laboratory animals and human subjects that suffer from immune suppression due to cancer drugs, corticosteroids, and unknown causes that may include viruses other than HIV. In the USA and China, the tonic herbs are often administered along with broad-spectrum antiviral herbs (e.g. isatis, hu-chang, viola, phellodendron, sophora, dandelion, andrographis) that inhibit a wide range of micro-organisms *in vitro*, inhibit infections and tumours in laboratory animals, and have been applied in complex formulas to treat infections and tumours in clinical trials of non-HIV infected persons with success.

The antiviral herbs are given to those with HIV in the United States in relatively low dosage, partly because it is believed that high dosage will cause digestive system disturbances, partly because of the expense of high dosage approaches (not covered by insurance and not afforded by most patients), and partly because of the unwillingness or inability of patients to consume higher dosages. HIV begins to interfere with digestive processes early in its pathogenesis, and this interference worsens as the disease progresses, causing significant malabsorption, contributing to symptoms of abdominal bloating and diarrhoea, and limiting the use of drugs, herbs, or other ingested therapeutic materials. It is not known whether higher dosages would be effective if they could be administered. Long-term administration of low-to-moderate dosages of tonic and antiviral herbs has not caused apparent adverse effects but has not halted CD4+ T-cell declines in those with AIDS and appears to provide only a temporary stabilisation (about one year) in those with relatively high initial CD4+ levels.

Anti-infection Natural Therapies

Until a means is found to reverse the continuing immunological decline observed in those with AIDS, it is necessary to identify and apply the best therapies available, which are aimed specifically at preventing and treating opportunistic infections and cancers. The current drug therapies are not entirely satisfactory because, as examples, the sulpha drugs often cause allergy reactions, the MAC drugs frequently cause digestive system disturbances, and antiviral drugs easily cause bone marrow inhibition. A number of broad-spectrum anti-infection herbs have been identified by Chinese researchers, including garlic, licorice, stemona, phellodendron, scute, and sophora. Licorice is utilised primarily as a virus inhibitor, is clinically effective for hepatitis B, and shows laboratory inhibition of HIV, both retroviruses (one active component, glycyrrhizin, has been developed as a drug therapy in Japan by Minophagen and is being tried in the United States for AIDS). A dosage of about 15 g per day of the dried licorice roots from China, extracted by hot water and consumed either as a liquid or a dried extract, is approximately the effective dosage for hepatitis B and rarely causes side effects. Higher doses may cause side effects due to stimulation of aldosterone production (alters sodium/potassium balance), though some of this effect may be countered by consuming certain amino acids (cysteine and glycine) at the same time.

Scute contains the flavonoid baicalin (as well as several related flavonoids) which has been shown by Japanese research to inhibit both retorviruses and cancer. It is an ingredient in a basic seven-herb formula, Sho-Saiko-To (Minor Bupleurum Combination), which is given to patients with hepatitis B or HIV infection; the formula was developed about 1,800 years ago to treat malaria or a similar infectious disease that produced alternating fever and chills. Sophora and phellodendron are common ingredients in Chinese herb formulas for treating infections of the skin, lungs, and intestines. Both contain alkaloids that have anti-cancer potential (e.g. matrine in sophora and berberine in phellodendron). Stemona is mainly used to treat lung infections, including tuberculosis and whooping cough, and it has been shown to have a broad spectrum of antipathogenic actions, inhibiting viruses, bacteria, and fungi. No obvious side effects have been observed from using these herbs in the daily dosages applied at the Institute's clinics (equal to about 10-2 g of each crude herb, extracted by hot water and dried to powder).

Garlic is the most extensively studied herb for inhibiting infections, and its application to AIDS has been repeatedly suggested as a result of laboratory and clinical investigations, based on its apparent or implied efficacy and known safety. Nonetheless, it is not common practice for health professionals to recommend ingestion of garlic to AIDS patients. This is an unfortunate situation as garlic has the advantages of being easily accessible, inexpensive, and generally free of side effects—other than producing an obvious odour, which apparently deters a substantial number of potential users.

In China, garlic is utilised in the treatment of intestinal tuberculosis, a condition equivalent to MAC. Purple-skinned garlic, a variety which is considered 'stronger' than ordinary white-skinned garlic, is given in a daily dosage of 50 g until the condition is resolved. If this type of garlic is indeed stronger than the one which is more widely available, then a higher daily dosage of the white-skinned garlic may be required. One to two ounces of white-skinned garlic bulb (28-56 g; 56 g is about one whole garlic head) daily is currently suggested at ITM's clinics for treatment of infection in those with AIDS. For the purpose of contributing to preventing infection, a lower dosage of about three cloves per day is suggested. The garlic can be consumed with the evening meal to avoid having a lingering garlic odour throughout the day or prepared as a blender drink in the morning (a recipe developed with ginger, garlic, water, lemon juice, sweetened with sugar and/or honey has proven generally acceptable).

Consuming large amounts of raw garlic may cause gastric irritation in some individuals, though this can be minimised by consuming, at the same time, vitamin B1 which complexes with the active sulphur compounds to reduce their irritant effect. One can also consume, at the same time or just prior to ingesting the raw garlic, a small amount of oil (e.g. olive oil or butter), which can coat the stomach lining and disperse the irritant compounds. In most persons, garlic is not irritating, and in fact, it is used as a treatment for gastric ulcer in China. For those who object to ingesting raw garlic because of its taste or characteristic odour, there are a number of garlic preparations that have been made as 'odourless garlic.' Unfortunately, the anti-infection and immune-modulating activity of these preparations is not known; their ability to lower cholesterol and triglycerides and to reduce platelet sticking is often well established but may involve different active components. The number of capsules or tablets equivalent to two ounces of raw garlic is quite high. Garlic extracts (aged, odour reduced) are also available in liquid form. There is a small number of published documentation suggesting that the aged garlic extract (Kyolic) does have anti-infection properties, but these are probably retained only in the original liquid form, not the dried liquid that is prepared in tablets or capsules, according to informal clinical observations.

6.5 Active Constituents and Pharmacology

The primary antiseptic ingredients of garlic are sulphur compounds (thiols), of which aliens (S-allylcysteine S-oxide) is considered especially important. Alien is odourless but is converted by an enzyme in garlic, called alliance, to allicin, one of the highly odoriferous compounds. The odourless garlic products usually contain alien or similar compounds which either retain the same activity or are converted to allicin and other active substances after ingestion. MAC isolates from AIDS patients have been shown to be inhibited by garlic extract, indicating that at least a portion of the *in vivo* activity noted in Chinese treatments for tuberculosis may be attributed to direct inhibition of Mycobacterium species. Isolates of Mycobacterium tuberculosis are inhibited by garlic extract *in vitro*.

Anti-CMV activity of garlic was demonstrated *in vitro* at the Institute of Hematology in Beijing (results published in 1990 and 1993). Antiviral activity had been proposed earlier as a basis for the apparent ability of garlic to treat influenza and common cold; *in vitro* tests reveal that garlic extract inhibits influenza B and herpes simplex 1 (herpes viruses are cofactors in stimulating HIV replication). Antifungal activity of garlic has also been demonstrated *in vitro*, notably with Candida, Cryptococcus, and Aspergillis, pathogens that affect those with AIDS; it has been used successfully in Chinese clinical treatment of 'fungal pneumonia'. Trichomonos is killed by garlic juice. The 'antibiotic' activity of garlic is not limited to direct inhibition or killing of micro-organisms. In AIDS patients treated with an aged garlic extract, natural killer cell activity increased dramatically in just six weeks, and that effect was maintained for at least an additional six weeks, with continued ingestion of garlic.

In twelve weeks' time, CD4+/CD8+ ratios, which are abnormally low in those with AIDS, increased substantially in nine out of ten patients treated by the garlic extract. A protein fraction from aged garlic extracts has been shown to enhance cytotoxicity and proliferation of lymphocytes from the blood of HIV-individuals when stimulated by IL-2.

If tumour cells are treated with garlic extract before injection into animals, tumours do not develop. If garlic is injected into tumours, the level of immune cells (neutrophils and macrophages) within the tumours increases. Garlic extract also reduces free radicals (cysteine and other sulphur compounds are well known as free-radical scavengers), inhibits tumorogenesis by chemical induction (aflatoxin and others), and aids elimination of lead (the latter effect is achieved by ingesting just 1.2 g of raw garlic each time, three times daily for one month). Garlic inhibits formation of carcinogenic n-nitroso compounds from dietary components and protects the stomach from HCl-induced lesions. Garlic also inhibits the immune suppression caused by exposure to UVB light. Further, antidiabetic activity of garlic has been revealed with laboratory animals; for example, rabbits experience a dose-dependent hypoglycemia in response to garlic extract. It also improves glucose tolerance (sugar metabolism disorders arise in many persons with AIDS).

Although the cardiovascular effects of garlic are not of major concern to those with HIV infection, it is worthwhile to note the dosage that is necessary to produce an observable effect. When given to HIV-humans, garlic at a dosage of just 5 g per day lowers triglycerides, and at 10 g per day it also decreases cholesterol levels and increases fibrinolytic activity and clotting time. Since CMV and free radicals have been implicated in the development of atheromas, regular ingestion of raw garlic at a dosage of 10 per day appears to be a reasonable preventive for atherosclerosis by reducing blood fats, platelet sticking, free radicals, and CMV activity. Garlic is also reported to reduce blood pressure in hypertensive patients.

Pharmacokinetics

Oral ingestion of garlic is often effective for obtaining the desired clinical effects. Absorption studies in rats, mice, and dogs indicate nearly 100 per cent bioavailability of monitored components, such as S-allylcysteine. Distribution is to the plasma, liver, and kidneys. Oral pharmacokinetics of alliin, allicin, and vinyldithiine in rats showed varying times to peak blood levels from 10 to 120 minutes for the different compounds. Gastric juice activates some garlic ingredients, including some with antiprotozoal activity. Antibacterial components begin to appear in the blood about thirty minutes after intake but may take some time to accumulate in the organs. Most of the oily components, such as allicin, are eliminated in six to eight hours. For clinical application in treatment of infectious diseases, Chinese physicians prescribe garlic extracts to be taken every two to four hours. In China, pertussis has been treated successfully in children by administering garlic extract sweetened with sugar orally. The extract was administered every two hours, at the rate of about 20 g raw garlic per day for children over age five (it is common practice for children aged six to twelve to receive about one-third the adult dose).

In pharmacokinetic studies of garlic extract given by enema or IV injection to rabbits, it was shown that allicin had a half life of 2.3 hours by IV but only 1.5 hours by enema. Accumulation after daily administration was not noted. The main target organs appear to be the lung and heart, suggesting that garlic may be particularly valuable in the treatment of PCP and other lung infections as well as the rarer condition of myocarditis. Radioactively labelled allicin given through IV to mice showed the highest concentration in the lungs, followed by the heart, intestines, blood, fat, and brain, with little in the muscles, spleen, or liver. Allicin, which is oily, is converted within ten minutes to water-soluble metabolites, and it is rapidly distributed to the organs.

A Unique Allicin Preparation

A garlic extract rich in allicin has been prepared in Shanghai for intravenous administration. The vials of liquid (containing 30 mg of allicin from about 15 g of raw garlic) have been used in the United States at three research centres. Dr Qingcai Zhang, who arranged the import of this material, has been prescribing it to about 200 AIDS patients in New York City; a small number of patients treated at the Search Alliance clinic in Los Angeles have used it in a successful attempt to duplicate claimed results, and the Institute for Traditional Medicine has been recommending it to patients in Portland for the past two years.

The main method of use for the liquid extract thus far has been by retention enema. This is a means of delivering the garlic extract to the lower bowel for treatment of cryptosporidiosis, and it is also a method of delivering it rapidly to the bloodstream for those who do not have an IV line. According to preliminary and unpublished reports, cryptosporidium-caused diarrhoea can be resolved within five to ten days using two vials of the allicin preparation each time (usually once per day). In one case, electron microscope analysis of biopsied intestinal tissue demonstrated complete elimination of cryptosporidium. Elimination of this organism is not expected by the use of current drug therapies, such as oral humatin. In China, bacillary and amoebic dysentery are treated by retention enema using a 10 per cent garlic liquid at a dose of 30-100 ml per day for about one week.

Another method of administration being used in New York and in Portland is inhalation of garlic vapours. The liquid extract is combined with sterile water (or sterile saline) and used alone or with solubilised n-acetyl-cysteine (Mucomyst) and applied by a nebuliser to treat respiratory infections (lung and/or sinus). Dr Zhang reports effectiveness for treating bronchitis and sinus infections; adverse response has not been observed. In Portland, one case of asthmatic response in a patient being treated for sinus infection who had a long history of severe asthma was noted; otherwise, the patient reports have been favourable.

A mucokinetic drug, S-carboxymethylcysteine (Mucodyne) differs only slightly from alliin. This compound is also found in radish seeds, used extensively in China for mucous disorders. According to Dr Irwin Ziment, a specialist in respiratory drugs, 'one would expect that people who are habitual eaters of garlic and radishes maintain optimal muckiness, thereby reducing their susceptibility to chronic bronchitis'. The action of both the garlic and n-acetyl-cytokine is to restore movement of mucus so that infections are less likely to occur and anti-infection herbs, drugs, and immune components can reach the infecting organisms that end up being protected by the thick mucus coat. Garlic also directly inhibits the pathogens involved. In China, garlic liquid prepared with sesame oil, zanthoxylum (Szechwan hot pepper), and apricot seeds instilled into the sinus with an applicator successfully treated tuberculosis sinus. The average course of therapy was three months.

IV administration has also been applied in New York and in Portland. One individual in Portland has administered one-half vial of IV garlic preparation (diluted with sterile saline) each day for several weeks via a Hickman line without adverse effect (this was administered with gancyclovir in the treatment of CMV retinitis). Application of this extract to the central line without dilution (not the recommended method) produced a temporary dizziness, but no other adverse effect. Several other individuals have applied the garlic via an IV drip to peripheral veins (one method is to include it in the high volume drip used for administration of fascine). No adverse reactions have been noted, but this method is inconvenient for daily administration if one is not already using regular IVs, as the duration of the drip is long and one needs to establish an open line each day. The effectiveness of IV administration for AIDS-related infections has not yet been determined. In China, injection of the garlic extract into non–HIV-infected patients was reported to cure Cryptococcus meningitis, one of the deadly opportunistic infections encountered with AIDS.

Current limitations with using the liquid allicin preparation include difficulties related to packaging (sealed glass vials that must be broken open), uncertainties about sterility and purity (no problems have been noted, but because the manufacturing is foreign, there is no U.S. oversight), cost (about $3/vial, with recommended daily use of 1/2 to 2 vials per day, not covered by insurance), and limited access (there are currently few distribution points in the United States). Because garlic is readily absorbed with oral administration in many different forms of preparation, the liquid allicin probably only needs to be used for the retention enema, nebulae, and IV. While it can be ingested orally, it is unlikely to have any specific advantage over eating 15 g of raw garlic except for the small volume of liquid involved. The use of IV garlic compared to other methods of delivery is recommended based on the pharmacokinetics; IV garlic yields a longer allicin half life and better distribution to organs that are affected by certain infections.

6.6 Potential Adverse Effects

In the Western medical literature, only one case of serious reaction to oral garlic ingestion has been noted, and this was a haemorrhage suggested to have resulted from ingestion of large quantities of garlic. It is reported in the Chinese literature that prolonged IV infusion could induce phlebitis. A possible explanation for these occurrences is irritation of the venous walls by very high levels of the garlic compounds. Since those with AIDS often have a low level of platelets, a precaution should be taken to avoid spontaneous bleeding. One simple method is by ingesting substantial amounts of balconied. Balconied improve the integrity of blood vessel walls and are applied to prevent spontaneous bleeding, yet they counter the pathological tendency to form clots. Sauté contains anti-haemorrhage falconoid, including bacilli.

AIDS sometimes results in elevated triglycerides (secondary to elevated tumour necrosis factor levels) and frequently results in lowered cholesterol (probably due to cytokine effects as well). The low levels of cholesterol (in the range 100–150) may have pathological consequences. It is not known if chronic ingestion of high levels of garlic will worsen this condition, and therefore cholesterol levels should be monitored in those with AIDS undertaking garlic therapy; however, it is likely that the cholesterol-lowering effects of garlic in non-infected individuals will not have much implication for those with HIV-induced low cholesterol levels. The mechanism of cholesterol lowering with garlic is revealed in two types of studies. Subjects fed a large amount of butter along with garlic show lower serum cholesterol levels soon after eating than those who consume butter without garlic, suggesting inhibition of cholesterol uptake and/or speeding of cholesterol clearing. *In vitro* studies of rat hepatocytes suggest that garlic can reduce choleste-rogenesis by the liver. Long-term administration of garlic causes an average decline of about 9 per cent in the cholesterol levels of patients with hypercholesterolemia, but studies have not been done to determine if it would cause such a decline in those with normal or subnormal cholesterol levels.

Garlic is applied topically in China for the treatment of fungal infection of the skin. Contact dermatitis has been reported as the result of applying fresh-cut garlic bulb to the skin, but prepared garlic extracts appear to be free of this allergic potential.

Unlike several other anti-infection Chinese herbs, garlic does not appear to cause digestive disturbance in large doses as long as irritant effects are countered by vitamin B1 or oils. Garlic can be eaten with certain oily foods, such as pine nuts or walnuts, which are suggested as potentially useful for those with HIV infection. According to traditional Chinese medical texts, garlic is listed as an antiparasitic herb, which is said to 'strengthen the stomach' and to resolve phlegm accumulation. It is commonly prescribed in a dosage of 6–15 g per day (one to three large cloves). No toxicity or caution is mentioned for this dosage range. Dr Zhang reports only one case of apparent adverse effect of allicin therapy, which was an individual who was suffering from kidney failure at the time of administration of the garlic extract. The patient's condition worsened rather than improved. At the Eppley Institute in Omaha, sixteen volunteers were provided garlic extract from six to seven cloves of garlic (i.e. about 20 g) daily for three months to evaluate its effect on the metabolism of acetaminophen. Although there was little effect of garlic on the metabolism of this drug, there were no reported problems with administering this level of garlic.

Garlic in the Context of Natural Therapies for HIV

A protocol relying on antioxidant and anti-infection strategies is being evaluated at ITM's HIV clinic. The protocol includes ingestion of vitamins (e.g. beta carotene, vitamin C, and vitamin E), minerals (e.g. calcium, magnesium, zinc, and selenium), metabolic factors (e.g. coenzyme Q10 and 1-carnation), flavonoids, extracts of certain Chinese herbs, including licorice, and immune-modulating polysaccharides from mushrooms, seaweed, and sea cucumber. For those with AIDS, ingestion of garlic is also recommended, in the form of either raw garlic or the aged garlic extract (Kyolic). When no obvious opportunistic infection is present, the daily dosage of garlic to be ingested is 10 g raw garlic (daily) or one-half teaspoon liquid of aged garlic extract each time, three times daily. When an infection is present, the dosage is increased to 28 g of raw garlic or up to twice the usual dose of the garlic extract. This protocol is intended to replace (or, as necessary, complement) the continual—but not the occasional—utilisation of nucleosides, anti-MAC drugs, and other drugs currently in use in standard medical practice, especially those used for controlling thrush. For those who are experiencing lung infection, ingestion of tablets made from stemona, sophora, and phellodendron is recommended along with inhalation of aerosolised garlic (to complement oral ingestion of garlic). For intestinal infections, the same tablets are utilised, along with oral ingestion of garlic plus garlic extract used by retention enema.

CHAPTER 7

In this chapter, the topics of nutrition and health are dealt with. This chapter shows that most of the health care problems emerge from lack of proper care for the appropriate nutrients in the food intake. The issues of vegetables, nuts and fruits are discussed in full. Information about the appropriate sources of the nutrients is given.

7.1 Health and Nutrition

Let food be thy medicine and let medicine be thy food. (Imhotep)

It is important to start this very chapter with avocado pear to demonstrate its impact in diet.

Avocado Pears—a Very Healthy Vegetable and Fruit

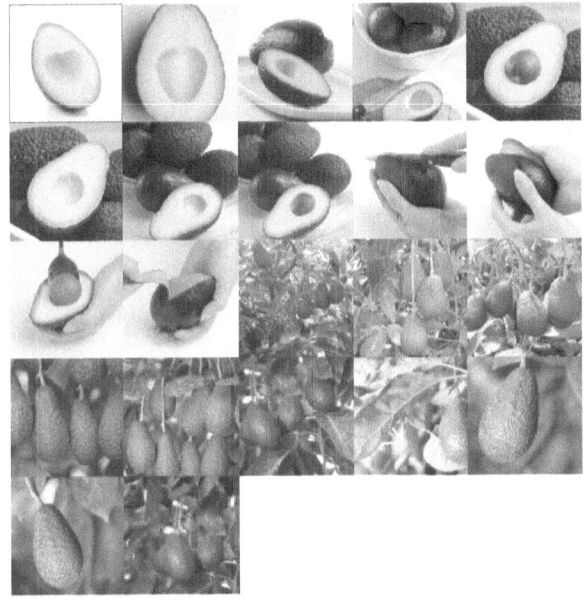

Avocados contain twelve of the thirteen known vitamins and several minerals. Half a medium avocado (72 g) contains just 137 calories, 50 per cent less than a plain bagel. Gram for gram, an avocado contains almost twice the amount of cholesterol-lowering monounsaturated (or 'good') fat as salmon avocados contain 12.5 per cent more potassium than the sportsperson's favourite—bananas. They're not only delicious but also contain eleven out of the thirteen known vitamins, including vitamins E, B6, and B5. In fact, in the vegetable and fruit world, avocado is the only one item that might be described as containing almost all the vitamins and minerals. Since the product is not traditionally subjected to heat in cooking, it means that the nutritive contents are consumed directly natural. It is therefore a better source of preventive nutritional therapy. This item of food can be prepared and eaten at any time of day and can accompany any dish. Because it is not to be subjected to any cooking process, care must be taken to ensure that it is served under a strict condition of hygiene.

The constant attention given to the topic of nutrition and dietary therapy in this book is a serious indication of the preventive value of the subject. I wonder whether a complementary health practitioner will ever think that any form of drug possesses an inherent power to prevent diseases than our knowledge of what the human body requires to equip and protect itself. Daily discoveries are being made around the world, which prove that vitamins, minerals, and food compounds have the ability to both prevent prostate disease and actually target and kill cancer cells. Many of these nutrients are needed in therapeutic doses, amounts which make it necessary to isolate these compounds and take in supplement form. This said however, we simply don't know enough about all the properties of a particular plant to isolate one or two compounds and get the synergistic effect of the whole plant. There are over 20,000 known bioflavonoids and 800 arytenoids, of which only a handful have been studied. This makes it very important not to rely on supplementing alone as the answer to your nutritional needs. Please use organically grown produce and beef that has been grass-fed whenever possible. Having said that, however, you can utilise your local grocery for this programme. Any complementary medicine practitioner who does not understand or does not possess the thorough knowledge of food and nutrition must, as a matter of fact, resign and resort to the sale of local newspapers, instead.

Amino Acids

Amino acids are the building blocks our bodies rely on. The body uses twenty-two amino acids that it gets from the protein we eat to construct over 50,000 protein structures. More than 5,000 amino acid complexes are used by the immune system. Glutathione, for instance, is composed of three amino acids and is one of the bodies' primary means of controlling free radicals which damage the cells of the body. Why, protein taken as one tablespoon of cottage cheese will increase the glutathione levels in the prostate by 60 per cent, and this is only one of the 5,000 protein structures the body utilises in the immune response. It is extremely important to completely break down the protein we ingest into individual amino acids; this can happen only if adequate protease enzymes are present in the digestive tract. Partially digested protein is known as peptides. Peptides severely limit the body's ability to fully utilise protein. Ensure that you advise your clients to get enough enzymes in their diet. Protein does have a downside in the fact that it is acidic; sugar, simple carbohydrates, alcohol, and soft drinks are also acidic. Ideally, our diets should be 20 per cent acid-forming foods and 80 per cent alkali-forming foods. Just one soft drink per day or a meal with little vegetables and a large piece of meat can cause our bodies to become so acidic that it creates an ideal environment for cancer and other degenerative diseases. Therefore you are cautioned that you guide your clients on adequate protein content in their diet, but excessive amounts are to be avoided, as are the use of other foods which are acid-forming too.

Recommended protein foods: Lean cuts of beef (preferably grass-fed), chicken and turkey (limit any fat from meat fed with grains such as corn and wheat), wild game, cold water fish, beans (any plant-based protein), eggs (especially omega 3 enriched), soy milk (all soy products), goat's milk, cottage cheese, plain yogurt, nuts, and protein supplements/amino acids. Limit meat to the size of a deck of cards with each meal.

Protein foods to avoid: Pork, fatty cuts of domestic livestock, dairy, most cheese, and peanuts (alpha toxin mould). Do not burn or cook meat at high temperatures.

Fats

A shift that is taking place is the recognition that fats are essential for us; every cell uses fat for the structure of the cell wall. The body utilises fat for many other purposes and should be furnished from a number of sources in order to ensure that the many and varied needs for fats are being met. Cod liver oil and flaxseed oil are excellent sources of omega 3 fatty acids which are absolutely essential for good health. Other sources of omega 3 are wild game, grass-fed cattle, and cold water fish. Due to the pollution of all bodies of water, all fish have some degree of contamination. Mercury is at the head of the list, and large ocean-dwelling fish have toxins such as mercury; the larger the fish, the more it is contaminated. Be careful that you don't consume fish without taking selenium, a mineral shown to chelate mercury and other heavy metals. Many contaminants we consume act as xenoestrogens and should be removed regularly. An excellent way of getting omega 3 fatty acids without getting the contaminants is to take quality cod liver oil. I would also refer you to the research of Dr Joanna Budwig; she used flaxseed oil and cottage cheese with great results in treating cancer. Another reason for consuming omega 3's with EPA's and DHA's is they help inhibit the cox 2 enzyme, which causes inflammation, a contributing factor in prostate cancer. Omega 6 fatty acid is essential as well and can be obtained from borage oil, evening primrose oil, corn oil, soybean oil, and any meat which has been grain-fed. Unlike omega 3 oil that most people are deficient in, the average person gets too much omega 6 fattyacid, and this causes unpleasant reactions in the body. Too much omega 6 has also been linked to cancer, as it is metabolised into 5-hete acid. Many researchers feel 5-hete is a primary fuel used for tumour growth. As with most nutrition, the body needs the correct ratio of omega 3 and omega 6 to function best. This ratio should be no more than 4 g of omega 6 to 1 g of omega 3.

The average American has a ratio of forty to one. To further add insult to injury, there are several sources of omega 6 that we are not getting, such as evening primrose oil; these sources provide components of omega 6 which are beneficial but not found in grains. Almost all omega 6 that we get comes from corn, wheat, or soybean. One component of omega 6 we get from grains is metabolised into archidonic acid. An enzyme called 5-lipoxygenase (5-lo) is used to metabolise arachidonic acid into the aforementioned 5-hete. Other oils such as olive and canola for example are very nutritious and should be incorporated into the diet. Many of these are Omega 9. We will not take the time here to get into the debate about the saturation of oils, but we do believe that if you limit your intake of omega 6 and use olive oil for cooking and salad dressings, you will be much healthier. The Mediterranean diet is recognised as being very healthy; it uses fish, vegetables, and olive oil as the main staples. Caution should also be taken to keep fats from going rancid. Just as precaution should be taken prior to consumption, taking antioxidants to protect fats in the cells and fats found in the bloodstream is just as important. This can be accomplished with colourful fruits, berries, and vegetables as well as antioxidants in the supplement form. One last caution about fat and that is heterocyclic amines. When you superheat any oil (frying) or when you char meat on the grill, you alter the composition of the fat into these compounds (heterocyclic amines), which are known carcinogens.

Recommended oils: Cod liver oil—Since 1987, laboratory studies have repeatedly illustrated that DHA and EPA slow or arrest the growth of human prostate cancer cells. Researchers showed that this growth arrest is associated with decreased conversion of arachidonic acid to its potentially damaging metabolite 5-hete. The other oils are flaxseed oil, olive oil, Smart Balance Spread, butter (use sparingly), grape seed oil, and virgin coconut oil.

Oils to avoid: Any oil with hydrogenated or partially hydrogenated oil, corn oil, soybean oil, lard, any oil which has been used for frying, and margarine.

7.2 Vegetables, Fruits, and Nuts

Vegetables, grains, and sugars are our source of carbohydrates; the body utilises carbohydrates primarily for energy. The main problem with carbohydrates is that we have abused them. Processing of grains, refining of sugars, and juicing of fruits cause the rapid absorption and conversion of carbohydrates into glucose. This elevated glucose enters the bloodstream and causes the body to release insulin in order to either drive the glucose into the cells to be used for ATP (energy) or to be stored for later use as fat. Sugar and insulin are closely linked to prostate cancer, and problems only occur when excess is involved. When the modern American diet is consumed, excess is inevitable. This makes the elimination of sugar, high glycemic fruits, and fruit juices essential, as is elimination of other simple carbohydrates such as flour, white rice, white potatoes, and most breads. Another problem with carbohydrates is that when they are heated to high temperatures in the cooking process, they form a carcinogen known as acryl amides. When eating fruits, vegetables, or grains, it is a good idea to eat them with as little processing and cooking as possible. This helps preserve nutrients and enzymes. There are exceptions; vegetables can often be juiced to remove fibre and increase the available nutrients, and tomatoes which have been cooked will have more available lycopene content than fresh tomatoes. A good salad dressing to use is flaxseed oil and cottage cheese; noni juice might also be added to the mixture. Soy should be incorporated into your diet; a study done at the Moffitt Cancer Centre in Tampa, Florida, is just one which shows that consumption of soy fights prostate cancer. Their study shows that in 69 per cent of the men taking soy PSA levels either dropped or remained stable. Twenty per cent had a three-point reduction in just three months. It is also a good idea to eat some olive oil or flaxseed oil with each meal or supplement. A recent study conducted by Wendy White, Associate Professor of Food Science and Nutrition at Iowa State University, shows that eating salad vegetables with some added fat promotes the absorption of lycopene, alpha-, and beta-carotenes, all of which aid in the fight against cancer and heart disease.

On the flipside, eating a salad completely devoid of fat deprives your body of these beneficial substances. Likewise, you can eat a handful of carrot sticks, but without the accompanying Ranch dressing or dip, your body can kiss the beta-carotene goodbye. Another wonderful benefit of vegetables is their synergistic value. Simply put, they work better together than they do in isolation. In a study, published in the December 2004 issue of the *Journal of Nutrition*, rats fed a combination of tomatoes and broccoli had markedly less prostate tumour growth than rats that ate diets containing either food alone and also less tumour growth than rats that ate diets containing specific cancer-fighting substances isolated from tomatoes and broccoli. This also creates a problem for researchers who have been taught to isolate a substance to test its efficacy. Studies that examine individual substances in isolation are simply not designed to tell us anything about the interactions that occur between those substances, much less between foods that each contains their own anti-cancer arsenals. Our recommendation is to incorporate those foods that have been shown to fight prostate cancer, but do not neglect to maintain other fruits and vegetables which might also add to and support vegetables such as carrots, cabbage, and tomatoes.

Recommended vegetables: Eat all with exceptions listed below, Especially important are cabbage and cabbage juice (especially cabbage juice), all cruciferous vegetables as well as sprouted broccoli seeds, garlic, tomatoes (paste and sauce especially), millet (millet has vitamin B17), and brown rice. Lightly steaming vegetables is better than cooking at high temperatures. Much more of the nutrients are made available by steaming and eating raw. One recent review paper (Craig W. J., Photochemical: guardians of our health, *J. Am. Diet Assoc.* 1997 October 97 (10 Suppl 2): S199–204) says, 'The foods and herbs with the highest anticancer activity include garlic, soybeans, cabbage, ginger, licorice, and the unbelliferous vegetables (caraway, carrots, celery, dill, parsley). Citrus, in addition to providing an ample supply of vitamin C, folic acid, potassium, and pectin, contains a host of active phytochemicals. The phytochemicals in whole grains reduce the risk of cardiovascular disease and cancer.'

Vegetables to avoid: Corn (especially corn meal), wheat (especially white flour), white rice, and white potatoes. Limit carrots to three per eight ounce glass of juice. Eat all the carrots you desire. The sugar content of the carrot juice is the only concern. Do not use microwave to cook vegetables as tests show that almost all of the nutrients are destroyed by this cooking method. Herbs and Spices: Eat any herb or spice you want. Try to get three cloves of garlic per day and pungent onions raw and cooked. Ginger root is very important as are hot peppers. Research shows that curry powder or turmeric has curcumin which is a potent flavinoid against prostate cancer. Use this whenever you can on wild rice or in soups.

Recommended fruits: All berries; red raspberries have been shown to be very effective against PC. You can get the same benefit from them fresh, frozen, or cooked. Research shows that one cup per week stops prostate cancer growth. Blue and black berries are a close second to red raspberries, lemons, whole oranges (one per day max), grapefruit, apples (one per meal), and any other high-fibre low-glycolic fruit; make sure to eat them whole in order to retain the fibre and slow absorption of sugar. Most of the nutrients that come from fruits are found in the skin and the seeds. Do not peel an apple unless you are eating the peel and throwing the pulp away.

Fruits to avoid: All fruit juices, high glycemic fruits (peaches and tropical fruits, for example), and melons (cantaloupes are fine to eat). Cancer cells metabolise energy almost exclusively from glucose; unlike a normal cell, it does not need oxygen and utilises anaerobic metabolism. Since it is so inefficient compared to aerobic metabolism, cancers have a voracious appetite for glucose to sustain themselves. This is why excess consumption of sugars tends to promote cancer growth. Avoid simple sugar as table sugar or fructose found in fruit juices. *Recommended nuts:* Bitter almonds and apricot seeds are a great source of vitamin B17 or laetrile which has been purported to be anti-tumour; sweet almonds (this type is found in most stores), walnuts, and Brazil nuts are most recommended. With the exception of peanuts, all others are permissible. Don't skin almonds. Eat lots of almonds with their brown skins intact. When almonds are blanched to remove their skins, they lose up to 80 per cent of their antioxidants. Nut power is concentrated in the skins; people who ate almond skins showed higher blood levels of antioxidants and increased protection against 'oxidation', a factor that promotes heart disease (Jeffrey Blumberg, PhD, Tufts University).

7.3 The Phytonutrients

Nuts to avoid: peanuts; they have Alfa toxin moulds. *Recommended breads:* Ezekiel (sprouted grain), soy bread (research showed that it cut down some diseases). *Breads to avoid:* all breads (especially those made with white flour), crackers, and chips.

Beverages

The body is estimated to be 70 per cent water, and staying properly hydrated is extremely important. If you are not consuming adequate amounts of pure water, you must start immediately. Tap water is most definitely not pure; it has more chemicals, heavy metals, and bacteria than is safe for a healthy person, much less someone with a health challenge. Many researchers feel that chlorinated water is unsafe to drink, bathe in, or even to breathe (steam). We recommend that you get a whole house water filter and a reverse osmosis filter for your drinking and cooking water. There is some controversy as to whether distilled water is good for you over the long term. This is due to the fact that water is a very strong natural solvent. This means that it will try to absorb anything it comes in contact with; if you add sugar to it, it becomes sweet, or add tea leaves and you get tea. When water comes into contact with even minute traces of a chemical compound such as a pesticide or herbicide, you get water with the ability to give you cancer. Distilling water can remove any suspended particulates from water to make it pure, but it then becomes what is termed as hungry water, and it also becomes acidic, around 5.5 ph. We would highly recommend you to add a liquid mineral complex such as Agape Living Water or add enough baking soda to neutralise the ph and lessen the water's likelihood of leaching vital minerals from the body. *Recommended beverages:* Water that has been through a reverse osmosis filter, distilled water (distilled water is especially good for cleansing), black tea, green tea, ginger tea, essiac tea, soy milk, goat's milk, raw organic cow milk, and vegetable juice (especially cabbage). If you are habituated to coffee, one cup per day is allowed, provided you add enough baking soda to neutralise the acid.

Beverages to avoid: All alcohols, all soft drinks, fruit juices, milk, spring water, and tap water.

In fact, most of what goes by the name of fruit juices are nothing but water, colour, flavour, and sugar. If the manufacturers ever venture into producing purely natural fruit juice, the addictives and preservatives added will certainly render the products unprofitable business and a health hazard. Whether you have a health challenge, or you want to maintain your health, diet is a critical component in your overall strategy. Eating the right foods, properly prepared, can be a tremendous ally or the wrong foods can actually make you sick. Clean water is just as important. Digestive enzymes are another factor to consider. Until a food has been properly digested it will not aid your health. One last nutrient you need to be concerned about is salt. You are an electrical being; when electricity stops you die. Your bodily fluids have the same salinity as the ocean, and it is vital you get enough salt (sodium chloride) to maintain this salinity. The problem arises with what is sold to us for salt. It has been stripped of all nutrients except sodium chloride, and additives are added to allow it to flow. We recommend your return to a more natural salt to meet your requirements for this vital nutrient. Books have been written on each of the topics I discussed here, and this information should be only a rudimentary understanding of what you need to do in order to be and stay healthy. It is more than a little coincidental that the foods listed in the Bible are being confirmed today by new scientific methods as being healthy. Many herbs and oils that the Bible mentions are also being proven to have medicinal value. In closing, do not forget the words of Hippocrates, the acknowledged father of modern medicine: "That your food should be your medicine and your medicine be your food." The words came from an African Egyptian, Imhotep, who lived between 2985 and 290 BC.

7.4 Juicing

We recommend detoxification drinks utilising a variety of vegetables, which have a powerful effect on the body's recuperative powers because of the rich array of easily absorbed nutrients. Fresh juices contain proteins, carbohydrates, chlorophyll, mineral electrolytes, and healing aromatic oils. But most importantly, fresh juice therapy makes available to every cell in our bodies large amounts of plant enzymes and phytonutrients, which are an integral part of the healing and restoration process.

Green Drinks, Vegetable Juices, and Blood Tonics: Green drinks are a vital component to the success of every cleansing programme. The molecular composition of chlorophyll is so close to that of human haemoglobin that these drinks can act as 'mini transfusions' for the blood and tonics for the brain and immune system. They are an excellent nutrient source of vitamins, minerals, proteins, and enzymes. They contain large amounts of vitamins C, B1, B2, B3, antithetic acid, folic acid, carotene, and choline. They are high in minerals, like potassium, calcium, magnesium, iron, copper, phosphorus, and manganese. They are full of enzymes for digestion and assimilation, some containing over 1,000 of the known enzymes necessary for human cell response and growth. Green drinks also have anti-infective properties, carry off acid wastes, and neutralise body pH and are excellent for mucous cleansing. They can help clear the skin, cleanse the kidneys, and purify and build the blood.

Green drinks and vegetable juices are potent fuel in maintaining good health, yet don't come burdened by the fats that accompany animal products. Incorporate cabbage, kale, or broccoli into your juices.

Tips On Juicing Programme: You get about 30 per cent of available nutrients from eating a fresh vegetable and much less if you don't chew your food well; as much as 90 per cent of enzymes, vitamins, minerals, and phyto-compounds are available when you juice.

a) I highly recommend cruciferous vegetables such as cabbage and broccoli. The goal is to drink three glasses per day. Even one will be of tremendous benefit.

b) Use carrots, except in very moderate amounts as it is high in sugar content and will trigger insulin release. Use no more than three per eight ounce glass of juice.

c) Do not use fruits to juice with, the same reason as is given for carrots. A few grapes or one-fourth of an apple may be used if you cannot tolerate the taste of vegetable juice alone. Remember that cancer is a sugar feeder, and fructose found in fruits is as bad as table sugar and *sugar feeds cancer*!

d) Broccoli sprouts are up to 100 times more potent in key nutrients than mature broccoli or cabbage. Use broccoli sprouts in salads and juice them after they are a few days old. Mix them with whatever vegetable you are juicing. You can get broccoli sprouts from the store, or better yet, sprout your own. Make sure to use only organic seeds certified for sprouting. You might go to the library or purchase a book on sprouting.

e) To enhance the taste of cabbage, you can add some kale leaves. Kale is as beneficial as cabbage, and you will probably enjoy the taste better than cabbage alone.

f) You might add vegetables such as cucumber, celery, turnips, spinach, green onion, peppers (hot or sweet), alfalfa sprouts, or wheat grass to your cabbage juice. Don't add more that 1/2 of any one or combination of these other vegetables to the cruciferous (cabbage or broccoli) juice.

g) To enhance the juices' detoxifying effect for heavy metals, add some cilantro or parsley (preferably cilantro).

h) Try not to juice more than you will drink in a twenty-four-hour period. Store any juice that you do not intend to consume immediately in an air-tight container, preferably a glass jar. By putting it in the freezer until it has almost frozen and then putting it in the refrigerator, you will slow down the degradation of the juice.

i) If you use cabbage juice for thirty days, it is a good idea to switch vegetables for a week or two. The long-term use of any one vegetable can cause you to become allergic to it. This is not likely, but is something to consider.

j) Juicing is messy and time consuming; it may not taste as well as we would like, but there is nothing you can do that will have a greater impact on your health. You get vitamins, essential fatty acids, minerals, chlorophyll, and most importantly you get phytonutrients and enzymes in large enough amounts as to be therapeutic. When you juice with cruciferous vegetables, you get nutrients such as sulphorafane and indole compounds that have been proven to be deadly prostate cancer fighters. If pharmaceutical companies could patent these compounds and sell them, they would be hailed as modern marvels, and they would charge you $100 per capsule.

k) If you don't have a juicer (go and get one), but in the meantime you can get some of the nutrients by boiling the vegetables in water and then drinking the water after the vegetable has been brought to a boil for at least five minutes. In fact, it has been shown that the water-soluble nutrients such as the phyto-compounds are leached out into the water by as much as 95 per cent. You will kill the enzymes, and you will not get nearly all the other nutrients in this manner.

Sprouts

Sprouting seeds neutralises acids and enzyme inhibitors which make seeds and grains hard to digest. Sprouting also increases vitamin and protein levels in the seed. Broccoli, for example, has many times more sulphor-apane in sprouts than that in the mature stalk, and broccoli sprouts have high levels of the cancer-fighting compound IP6 (Inositol Hexa Phosphate).

Tips for Sprouting:

a) Start with clean seeds and/or raw nuts.
b) Place seeds in a glass jar and fill no more than one-third with seeds. There are sprouting trays that you can purchase as well.

c) Cover seeds with filtered water (fill jar half full).
d) Cover the mouth of jar with a clean piece of nylon panty hose.
e) Let seeds set for twenty-four hours. Drain water and rinse and invert the jar so that it drains.
f) At least once a day, you should cover seeds with water. Let it stand for five minutes and drain.
g) The seeds should sprout in three to five days.
h) Use sprouts and start a new jar in a couple of days so that you have sprouts coming off as you need them. After sprouts are four days old, you can juice what you have left for a very nutritious drink.

Flaxseed Oil Recipes

Some research has shown flaxseed oil to be harmful when taken alone; this is due to the fact that lipids are only water-soluble and free-flowing when bound to protein, thus the importance of protein-rich cottage cheese. When high-quality, electron-rich fats are combined with proteins, the electrons are protected until the body requires energy. This energy source is then fully and immediately available to the body on demand, as nature intended.

Dr Johanna Budwig Mix/Breakfast Drink

Put the following in your blender: One cup organic cottage cheese (low fat, not the too hard one, best make your own) or plain yogurt; 2–5 tbsp of flaxseed oil; 1–3 tbsp of freshly ground flaxseed (coffee grinder ($15) works fine; 1 scoop of indentured whey protein; 1/2 cup of red raspberries fresh or frozen; and enough soy milk to make a glassful.

How to Prepare 'The Spread':

Put 8.5 ounce flax oil into a mixer bowl. Add 1 lb of 1 per cent cottage cheese (organic if available) and add Stevita to taste. Turn on the mixer, and add just enough unsweetened soy milk or water to get the contents of the bowl to blend in together. In five minutes, a preparation of custard consistency results that has *no* taste of the oil (and no oily 'ring' should be seen when you rinse out the bowl).

Note: When flax oil is blended like this, it does not cause diarrhoea even when given in large amounts. It reacts chemically with the (sulphur) proteins of the cottage cheese, yoghurt, etc.

How to prepare 'The Mayo' (mayonnaise): Mix together two tablespoons flax oil, two tablespoons of soy milk, and two tablespoons of yoghurt. Then add two tablespoons of lemon juice (or apple cider vinegar) and add one teaspoon of mustard plus some herbs such as marjoram or dill.

Ginger Tea: Grind about half an inch of fresh ginger root into a paste and place in a mug. Add boiling water and 'steep' for several minutes. Strain the clear liquid.

7.5 Fruits and Vegetables Dietary Therapy

In a recent article adapted from Dr Patrick Hollyford's *Optimum Nutrition Bible* in the *Institute of Optimum Nutrition Magazine*, 1998, New Year's issue, a comprehensive menu guideline containing 65 per cent fruits and vegetables was given as a typical example of the twenty-first century diet aimed at the prevention of diseases. Dr Hollyford's *Optimum Nutrition Bible* is a breath of fresh air on the latest research in health promotion effects of the so-called super foods. This marvellous current research finding is another authentic endorsement that the correct quality, quantity, and appropriate combination for the provision of adequate nutrients bioavailable to the body are better preventive therapy than medicine in certain diseases in natural complementary medicine therapy. Surely, this article has touched at the base of the matter. Once the practice is generally accepted, it will form a central meeting point between the orthodox and complementary health care systems. In that article, Dr Hollyford went further to suggest that doctors' prescription in the twenty-first century will be based on a diet which should direct the patient to eat two cloves of garlic, a serving of broccoli, Shiitake mushroom, and tofu every day in addition to other meals. It is maintained that these food items and many others contain nutricells, naturally occurring chemicals, or phytonutrients, which have the power to keep diseases at bay. It is from this standpoint that the writer of that article devised a diet menu with the above food items included for the new millennium designed to actively promote longevity and prevent diseases.

However, it is one thing to prescribe an adequate list of food items in a recommended menu but another thing to achieve the end result. Apart from the financial limitations involved in the people's affordability of the food items, there are many other factors, which may create limitations to the achievement of the desired objectives. These include the patient's individual lifestyle, dining behaviour, purchasing, storage preparation, and cooking and eating habits. Even at a dietetics ward of a hospital, patients on special dietary prescription would virtually have to be guided before they could eat up the required amount of food, especially the fruits and vegetable items. Children and women are the worst group in avoiding these menu items. My personal experience as a food production technician in the dietetics department at Harmasrsmith Hospital, South London, bears witness to these facts.

7.6 Fruits and Vegetables 1-1 Capsules

For many years now, dieticians and catering practitioners in health care centres have wondered whether the day will come when some of the items in the menu, especially fruits and vegetables, will be available in the form of tablets or capsules for easy consumption and assimilation into the body. Well, thank the good Lord; that day is now with us. Dr Santillo, a naturopath at Memphis in Tennessee in the United States, not long ago, came up with an invention of such fruit and vegetable capsules as a very convenient dietary supplementation. Dr Santillo named this wonderful natural whole food capsule, as Juice Plus. The cardinal objective of this capsule invention is to help solve the problems of the shortage in the essential phytonutrients in the daily dietary required allowance (DRA). Although Juice Plus capsules are not an alternative to the required daily intake of fruits and vegetables, they are a whole food supplementation that will surely take care of any shortage of the cell building and body system cleansers of the human organism.

The Juice Plus and Its Advantages

- Its bio-availability to the body without waste.
- Its storage durability-less perishable over the given period of time unlike the fresh fruits and vegetables.
- Its easy availability with less effort.
- Convenient to take just two daily.

- Hygienic and safe—no fear of contamination.
- Economic both in terms of time and money.
- Comprehensive whole food supplementation.
- Proven effectiveness with scientific support.
- Portable to carry, to store, and to use.
- Free from any adulteration or cross infection since the seventeen raw fruits and vegetables are organically produced and prepared with the greatest care.

Each bottle of the Juice Plus contains 120 capsules, and on average, this works out to be £1.26 per day. This demonstrates how cheap the products work out to be. Where on earth can anyone obtain five to six servings of fresh fruits and vegetables of this nutritional value at this cost?

7.7 Professional Research Supports

In his article titled 'Prevention Plus', a proof in the *American Health and Wellness Newsletter* of November 1997, Dr John F. Whitehorn, MD, believes that 'nutrition is the cornerstone of good health'. Recommending the prescription of fruits and vegetables in the form of capsules, Dr Whitethorn maintains that in the next several years, people will start going to their various health care centres like they are going presently for blood tests or to check their cholesterol levels and to check their levels of photo-chemicals and antioxidants. 'Doctors will be testing to see how, properly protected the patients are and not how sick they are,' he stated. There is no substitute for fresh, raw fruits and vegetables; this is why the manufacturers of Juice Plus say that their product is the next best thing to actually eating them. But the 15,000 and more members of the Federation of American Societies in Experimental Biology recently held that Juice Plus may even be more effective than fresh fruits and vegetables in protecting against disease like heart disease and cancer.

Another professional support is from Dr John Wise, the Vice President of Research and Development at National Alternative International of America, who was invited to present to this body the results of two studies on Juice Plus. The research works are as follows:

a) From the original bio-availability research work published, he concluded that 'it appeared that antioxidants are more readily absorbed through Juice Plus that are the same micro-nutrient in the raw fruits and vegetable's. We know that a diet high in consumption of various fruits and vegetables is linked to reduced risk of coronary heart disease, stroke and certain types of cancer. Dr Wise explained that they were largely because of the antioxidants they deliver.

b) In the studies conducted at King's College Medical School, University of London, it was found that everyone who took Juice Plus twice every day showed a dramatic increase in the levels of antioxidants beta carotene, vitamin E, and vitamin C in their blood much higher than could be obtained from the average consumption of fruits and vegetable. As stated by Dr Wise, parts of this explanation are that Juice Plus provides nutrients from seventeen different fruits and vegetables and grains every day in a readily bio-availability form. Also, the participants in both studies used Juice Plus to supplement their intake of fruits and vegetable just as recommended.

Although Dr Patrick Gilford's typical dietary therapy for a new millennium is a demonstration by several research findings, the most comprehensive programming of independent scientific research ever undertaken in the history of nutrition according to the current therapeutic bio-availability research in June 1996 is published in the *Reviewed Medicine Journal* in the UK.

The Effects of Juice Plus on the Human Immune System

Research from the University of Arizona Cancer Centre presented to the American Society of Cell Biology at the annual meeting of the Society in December 1998 was highly significant. In it, elderly patients of over sixty-five were recognised to have decreased immune functions (weak immune systems), which rendered them more susceptible to infections, cancer, allergies, and auto-immune diseases. This weakness is characterised by overactive B-cells and weak T-cells. The weak T-cells (the generals) allow the B-cells (the foot soldiers) to become overactive, lose focus, and become wasteful of effort resulting in counter-productive energy expenditure. It is as if they are shooting at random in all directions including 'friendly fire' at self.

Examples of Clinical Immune Dysfunction

Some of the examples are as follows: auto-immune disease, allergies, hernolytic anaemia, asthma, rheumatoid arthritis, chronic fatigue syndrome, multiple scleroses, AIDS, lupus erythematous cancer, diabetes mellitus, types of thyroids, and myasthenia gravis.

Scientific research evidence is mounting that nutrition plays an important role in immune physiology in humans. The report shows the effects of eighty days of Juice Plus consumption on individuals taking two fruit capsules each morning and two vegetable capsules each evening. Patients aged sixty to eighty-six were studied at baseline, forty days, and eighty days with the following result findings:

a) Supplementation increased T-cells proliferation. Catatonic T-cells kill infected cells, viruses, and some bacteria. Augmented T-cell response allows for an increase in the number (size of the army) to fight infection.

b) Supplementation enhanced the activity of natural killer (NK) cells. This increases the ability to fight cancer cells and some specific infection.

c) Supplementation enhanced the production of regulatory hormones of communication between immune cells known as cytokines IL-2 and IL-6. This enhances the entire response to infection.

Effects of Juice in DNA

In the same research findings, it was proved that failure to protect or repair the DNA subjects each patient's cell to numerous opportunities for mutation and cellular death. DNA is the blueprint used in cell duplication. The DNA must not be disrupted or changed in any fashion in order for normal healthy cells to be made. Free radical (oxidative) damage to DNA is cumulative and is felt to be associated with ageing, disease, cancer, and death of patients.

Cellular DNA takes an average of 10,000 oxidative hits per day. These oxidative hits continue and require a great deal of energy for repair. Examples of the effects are radiation, smoke, pollution, drugs, and many chemicals.

CHAPTER 8

The European Complementary Medicine

T his chapter gives detailed explanation and information on various complementary health care practices common in the European nations. Sometimes the information presents similar practices; this is understandable. This chapter moves from practices such as homeopathy, naturopathy, herbal medicines and aromatherapies to hydrotherapy. There is a discussion on the types of herbal medicine and the system in various European countries.

8.1 Homeopathic Medicine

The practice of homeopathic medicine in the United Kingdom is very advanced and widely spread throughout the kingdom. Sometimes the homeopaths are also placed at various health centres according to the necessary requirements. The principal reasons for presenting these various practices here is to enable us see what is available and to know what possible applications we can use for the purpose of preventive therapy in a given case. Among all the complementary health care practices available, homeopathy is widely popular, and it is next to herbal therapy.

The highest ideal of cure is rapid, gentle and permanent restoration of the health or removal and annihilation of the disease in its whole extent, in the shortest, most reliable and most harmless way on easily comprehensible principles. (Samuel Hahnemann, founder of homeopathy)

The long-term benefit of homeopathy to the patient is that it not only alleviates the presenting symptoms but it re-establishes internal order at the deepest levels and thereby provides a lasting cure. (George Vithoulkas, Director, Athenian School of Homoeopathic Medicine.)

Discovered in the late 1700s, homeopathy is a low-cost, non-toxic system of medicine. The system of homoeopathic healing assists the natural tendency of the body to heal itself. It recognises that all symptoms of ill health are expressions of disharmony within the whole person and that it is the patient who needs treatment not the disease. There are three principles on which homeopathy is formulated:

- *Like cures like (law of similars)*: Any substance that can produce the symptoms of an illness in a healthy human being can cure those same symptoms in a sick human being.
- *The more dilute the remedy, the greater its potency (law of the infinitesimal dose):* Homoeopathic remedies are usually prepared through a process of diluting with pure water or alcohol and successions (vigorous shaking) such that the more diluted a substance gets, the more potent it becomes.
- *An illness is specific to the individual (a holistic medical model):* Homoeopaths consult compendiums called repertories to determine the remedy which will most closely match the patient's symptoms. Homoeopathic medicines are drug components made by homoeopathic pharmacies consisting of plants, minerals, and animal extracts. Remedies (usually in liquid, tablet, or powder form) are prescribed in accordance with a patient's symptoms and health conditions while individual characteristics such as emotions and physical condition are also taken into account. Conditions benefited by homeopathy include diabetes, arthritis, bronchial asthma, epilepsy, skin eruptions, allergic conditions, and mental or emotional disorders. At the outset of homoeopathic treatment, your homoeopath will need to know all about you in order to find the right remedy for you as an individual. This will include past medical history, lifestyle, and any general complaints. This initial consultation may last an hour or more and will be treated in the strictest confidence.

Homeopathy: What It Is

Homeopathy is a system of medicine that is made from traces of plant, mineral, and organic ingredients. These medicines are prepared by a pharmacological process called potentisation. This process involves consecutive dilutions of a natural ingredient in some medium, usually water. The strength of the potency is inversely proportional to the number of dilutions (Ullman 1995). There is no physical trace of the original ingredient after the process is completed. A single remedy has the name of the original ingredient. The remedy can be taken orally in a liquid base or as a sugar pill. Modern homeopathic companies also produce remedies as ointments, lotions, eye drops, syrups, and sprays.

Origins

A German physician named Samuel Hahnemann (1755-1843) founded homeopathy. He derived the term from the Greek words 'homoios' and 'pathos'. Homoios is Greek for similar and pathos is Greek for suffering. The principle theory of homeopathy was previously described by Hippocrates in ancient Greece. Mayans, Chinese, Greeks, Native American Indians, and Asian Indians used this method of healing well before Hahnemann coined the phrase—homeopathy. Hahnemann was credited with making this principle theory into a systematic medical science (Ullman 1997).

Principle Beliefs

The principle belief of homeopathy is that like cures like, also known as the law of similars. This means that the same substances that cause illness and disease are used to cure it. The systematic provings of natural substances as homeopathic remedies are found in the *Materia Medica*. This literature is a detailed collection of reactions to substances in a healthy person. Therefore, homeopaths can prescribe remedies based on your symptoms.

Homeopathy is a highly individualised form of treatment. The homeopathic perspective is that there are no diseases, only diseased people. The basis of this perspective stems from the idea that we all experience diseases in different ways. It is too limiting to diagnose a person with a specific disease and expect one form of treatment to work on everyone. Therefore, homeopaths prescribe medicines that take into account both physical and psychological symptoms each person experiences. Homeopathy individualises treatment to a person's unique pattern of symptoms.

'Homeopathy has a highly systematic, rigorous method of investigating its medicine, using human subjects as the sounding board to understand the healing direction of various plant, mineral and animal substances' (Hershoff 2000). It is not known what the precise mechanism of healing is. It is difficult to prove its effectiveness through contemporary scientific methods. Researchers in the *Lancet* and *British Medical Journal* conducted studies that prove the effectiveness of homeopathy; however, they cannot explain them through the views of current biology (Hershoff 2000). Researchers at CalTech have discovered magnetic particles throughout the human brain. They speculate that dilutions create a higher level of the electromagnetic field, thus triggering the defence mechanisms of the body (Ullman 1995). There is no direct scientific evidence to prove, or disprove, why homeopathy is effective.

'First, do no harm' was Hippocrates famous passage for medical practitioners. Homeopathy, as a system of medicine, is considered highly safe. Homeopathic theory states that taking random remedies will not cause any harm. It is hypothesised that only the correct remedy will interact with the brain to trigger the healing response. Modern medicine fails in this aspect with upwards of 200,000 deaths caused by prescription drugs according to the *Journal of the American Medical Association* in the early 1990s.

Who Is Using It and Why?

Great Britain

Homeopathy is popular in Great Britain. It has been used to treat the royal family since the 1830s. Studies from the *New York Times* show that the number of visits to homeopathic physicians is increasing 39 per cent per year. A questionnaire of 268 patients in England reported some insight into why they use homeopathy. One of the responses included 'positive valuation of complimentary treatment' (Furnham 1996). The general attitude towards homeopathy is evident in their classification of homeopathy. They use the term 'complementary medicine', instead of alternative medicine (Hershoff 2000). Therefore, the terminology implies that it is accepted as a growing part of mainstream health care. On the other hand, alternative medicine implies that it is a separate entity from mainstream health care. Further homeopathy receives positive attention in the media. The royal family has been under its treatment for over a hundred years. Also, British Olympic teams claimed that a homeopathic (Arnica) ointment was their secret weapon.

The attitude of British health care professionals towards homeopathy is more positive than in the United States. A British consumer organisation survey concluded that 70 per cent who had tried homeopathy were cured or improved by it. A study in the *London Times* showed that 42 per cent of surveyed physicians refer patients to homeopaths. A survey published in the *British Medical Journal* noted that out of 100 recently graduated British physicians, 80 per cent expressed an interest in being trained in homeopathy, acupuncture, or hypnosis. This attitude may in part be due to the changes in organisation of homeopathic doctors in Great Britain. They wanted to gain credibility in the general population, government, and orthodox medical professionals. They acquired a number of professional properties in the process enhancing their legitimacy (Cant 1995).

Another study reported some motivations for using homeopathy. They included control over treatment, lack of personal care, and waiting lists for treatment (Ernst 2000). The British National Health Service (NHS) has some features that correspond to the motivations for using homeopathy. The NHS suffered from underfunding and a lack of resources. This leads to limitations on treatments, and patients turn to homeopathy for a sense of control. Also the limited resources lead to the waiting lists for treatment. Many seek homeopathy as an alternative to be treated at once. Also, studies reported regional inequalities and class differences in treatment. General practitioners spend more time with upper class patients (Gabe 2001). Therefore, much of the population does not receive adequate attention. They may then seek homeopathic doctors for the individualised care that homeopathy requires.

Attacks against the Practice

United States

Homeopathy was introduced in the United States in the late 1820s by German immigrants. It flourished for about a hundred years, and by the turn of the century there were over 100 hospitals, 143 societies, and over 15,000 practitioners (Rogers 1997). After this period, the popularity of homeopathy began to decline. Its decline was partly due to the American Medical Association. The theories of modern medicine and Western views were contrary to the principles of homeopathy. The rise of scientific medicine eventually led to a single model of medical practice. 'Medicine focused solely on the internal environment (the body), largely ignoring the external environment' (Conrad). The AMA successfully secured a monopoly and had an unrivaled professional dominance.

The attitudes of the United States government also reflect doubts in homeopathic treatments. The Food and Drug Administration (FDA) refused to acknowledge homeopathic remedies as effective drugs. Instead, they created standards listed in the Homeopathic Pharmacopoeia of the United States (HPUS). This was not a sign of acceptance by the government. It was instead a method to take action against possibly dangerous products masquerading as homeopathic medicines (Rogers 1997). The government passed licensing concerns to the states. There are only three states with homeopathic licensing boards. Therefore, there is no national standard for homeopathic practitioners. The ultimate decision is left up to the state, which is not always good for homeopaths. North Carolina Board of Medical Examiners revoked the license of a homeopath concluding that he was 'failing to conform to the standards of acceptable and prevailing medical practice' (NCAHF 1994).

The National Council Against Health Fraud in the United States issued a recommendation for consumers to avoid purchasing homeopathic products and avoid consultations with homeopathic doctors (NCAHF 1994). Similar organisations are sceptical because there is no scientific evidence of how homeopathy works. Studies from the British Medical Journal have proved rates of effectiveness through randomised, double-blind placebo-controlled studies (Taylor 2000).

The attitudes of American doctors are vastly different from British doctors. American doctors lead attacks against homeopathy. They have published several critical works on the practice of homeopathy. They attribute the alleged effectiveness of homeopathy to several reasons. They claim that they would have been cured anyway as diseases are cyclical and because of the placebo effect and false psychological perceptions (Barrett 2000). It is hard for consumers of medical care to ignore the attitudes of the highest regarded profession in the United States—doctors.

8.2 Herbal Medicine

The history of herbal medicine is so wide and extensive. The nature and the origin of herbal products into the Europeans nations is certainly connected with the Romans and the Greeks who made close contact with the ancient Kametian Egyptian Africans. As time moved on and human progress and advancement improved upon what they gathered from others. Today, no nation can categorically say that its own medicinal herbs are purely indigenous. In fact, the concept of multi-nationalism has affected every aspect of people's lives globally. Literally speaking, we are interdependent of each other. Although an extensive in formation are given here, I have by no means exhausted the entire body of knowledge in Herbal medicine world.

Herbalism is a traditional medicinal or folk medicine practice based on the use of plants and plant extracts. Herbalism is also known as *botanical medicine, medical herbalism, herbal medicine, herbology*, and *phytotherapy*. The scope of herbal medicine is sometimes extended to include fungal and bee products, as well as minerals, shells, and certain animal parts. Pharmacognosy is the study of medicines derived from natural sources. Traditional use of medicines is recognised as a way to learn about potential future medicines. In 2001, researchers identified 122 compounds used in mainstream medicine, which were derived from 'ethnomedical' plant sources; 80 per cent of these compounds were used in the same or related manner as the traditional ethnomedical use.

Many plants synthesise substances that are useful to the maintenance of health in humans and other animals. These include aromatic substances, most of which are phenols or their oxygen-substituted derivatives such as tannins. Many are secondary metabolites, of which at least 12,000 have been isolated—a number estimated to be less than 10 per cent of the total. In many cases, substances such as alkaloids serve as plant defence mechanisms against predation by micro-organisms, insects, and herbivores. Many of the herbs and spices used by humans to season food yield useful medicinal compounds. Similarly to prescription drugs, a number of herbs are thought to be likely to cause adverse effects. Furthermore, 'adulteration', inappropriate formulation, or lack of understanding of plant and drug interactions have led to adverse reactions that are sometimes life-threatening or lethal.

8.3 Anthropology of Herbalism

Further information: Zoo-pharmacognosy

People on all continents have used hundreds to thousands of indigenous plants for treatment of ailments since prehistoric times. Medicinal herbs were found in the personal effects of *Ötzi the Iceman*, whose body was frozen in the Ötztal Alps for more than 5,300 years. These herbs appear to have been used to treat the parasites found in his intestines. Anthropologists theorise that animals evolved a tendency to seek out bitter plant parts in response to illness.

Indigenous healers often claim to have learnt by observing that sick animals change their food preferences to nibble at bitter herbs they would normally reject. Field biologists have provided corroborating evidence based on observation of diverse species, such as chimpanzees, chickens, sheep, and butterflies. Lowland gorillas take 90 per cent of their diet from the fruits of *Aframomum melegueta*, a relative of the ginger plant, which is a potent antimicrobial and apparently keeps shigellosis and similar infections at bay. Researchers from Ohio Wesleyan University found that some birds select nesting material rich in antimicrobial agents which protect their young from harmful bacteria. Sick animals tend to forage plants rich in secondary metabolites, such as tannins and alkaloids.[10] Since these phytochemicals often have antiviral, antibacterial, antifungal, and antihelminthic properties, a plausible case can be made for self-medication by animals in the wild.

Some animals have digestive systems especially adapted to cope with certain plant toxins. For example, the koala can live on the leaves and shoots of the eucalyptus, a plant that is dangerous to most animals. A plant that is harmless to a particular animal may not be safe for humans to ingest. A reasonable conjecture is that these discoveries were traditionally collected by the medicine people of indigenous tribes, who then passed on safety information and cautions. The use of herbs and spices in cuisine was developed in part as a response to the threat of food-borne pathogens. Studies show that in tropical climates where pathogens are the most abundant, recipes are the most highly spiced. Further, the spices with the most potent antimicrobial activity tend to be selected. In all cultures, vegetables are less spiced than meat, presumably because they are more resistant to spoilage.

History of Borage for Its Cultivation—Harvesting, Curative, and Uses

In the written record, the study of herbs dates back over 5,000 years to the Sumerians, who described well-established medicinal uses for plants such as laurel, caraway, and thyme. Ancient Egyptian medicine of 1000 BC is known to have used garlic, opium, castor oil, coriander, mint, indigo, and other herbs for medicine, and the Old Testament also mentions herb use and cultivation, including mandrake, vetch, caraway, wheat, barley, and rye. Indian Ayurveda medicine has used herbs such as turmeric possibly as early as 1900 BC. Many other herbs and minerals used in Ayurveda were later described by ancient Indian herbalists such as Charaka and Sushruta during the first millennium BC. The *Sushruta Samhita* attributed to Sushruta in the sixth century BC describes 700 medicinal plants, sixty-four preparations from mineral sources, and fifty-seven preparations based on animal sources. The first Chinese herbal book, the Shennong Bencao Jing, compiled during the Han Dynasty but dating back to a much earlier date, possibly 2700 BC[citation needed], lists 365 medicinal plants and their uses—including ma-Huang, the shrub that introduced the drug ephedrine to modern medicine. Succeeding generations augmented on the *Shennong Bencao Jing*, as in the Yaoxing Lun (*Treatise on the Nature of Medicinal Herbs*), a seventh-century Tang Dynasty treatise on herbal medicine.

The ancient Greeks and Romans made medicinal use of plants. Greek and Roman medicinal practices, as preserved in the writings of Hippocrates and—especially—Galen, provided the pattern for later Western medicine. Hippocrates advocated the use of a few simple herbal drugs—along with fresh air, rest, and proper diet. Galen, on the other hand, recommended large doses of drug mixtures—including plant, animal, and mineral ingredients. The Greek physician compiled the first European treatise on the properties and uses of medicinal plants, *De Materia Medica*. In the first century AD, Dioscorides wrote a compendium of more than 500 plants that remained an authoritative reference into the seventeenth century. Similarly important for herbalists and botanists of later centuries was the Greek book that founded the science of botany, Theophrastus' *Historia Plantarum*, written in the fourth century BC.

8.4 Their Cultivation: Harvesting, Curing, and Uses

Middle Ages

The uses of plants for medicine and other purposes changed little in early medieval Europe. Many Greek and Roman writings on medicine, as on other subjects, were preserved by hand-copying of manuscripts in monasteries. The monasteries thus tended to become local centres of medical knowledge, and their herb gardens provided the raw materials for simple treatment of common disorders.

Modern Era

The fifteenth, sixteenth, and seventeenth centuries were the great age of herbals, many of them available for the first time in English and other languages rather than Latin or Greek. The first herbal to be published in English was the anonymous *Grete Herball* of 1526. The two best-known herbals in English were *The Herball or General History of Plants* (1597) by John Gerard and *The English Physician Enlarged* (1653) by Nicholas Culpeper. Gerard's text was basically a pirated translation of a book by the Belgian herbalist Dodoens and his illustrations came from a German botanical work. The original edition contained many errors due to faulty matching of the two parts. Culpeper's blend of traditional medicine with astrology, magic, and folklore was ridiculed by the physicians of his day, yet his book—like Gerard's and other herbals—enjoyed phenomenal popularity. The age of exploration and the Columbian exchange introduced new medicinal plants to Europe. The *Badianus Manuscript* was an illustrated Aztec herbal translated into Latin in the sixteenth century. The second millennium, however, also saw the beginning of a slow erosion of the pre-eminent position held by plants as sources of therapeutic effects. This began with the Black Death, which the then dominant four element medical system proved powerless to stop. A century later, Paracelsus introduced the use of active chemical drugs (like arsenic, copper sulphate, iron, mercury, and sulphur). These were accepted even though they had toxic effects because of the urgent need to treat Syphilis. The rapid development of chemistry and the other physical sciences led increasingly to the dominance of chemotherapy—chemical medicine—as the orthodox system of the twentieth century.

Role of in modern human society

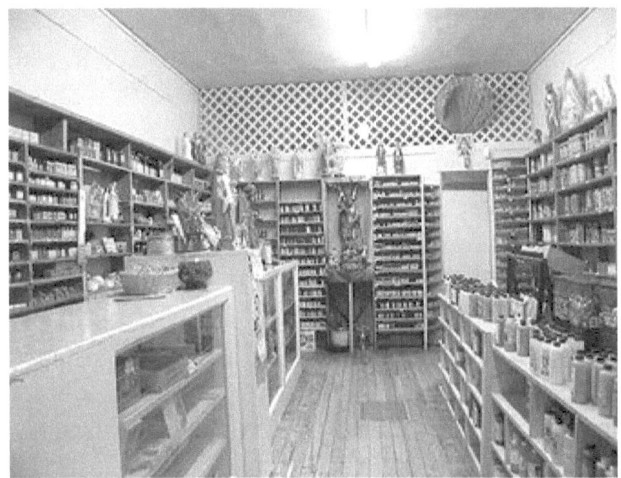

Botánicas, such as this one in Jamaica Plain, Massachusetts, cater to the Latino community and sell herbal cures and folk medicine alongside statues of saints, candles decorated with prayers, lucky bamboo, and other items.

The use of herbs to treat disease is almost universal among non-industrialised societies. A number of traditions came to dominate the practice of herbal medicine at the end of the twentieth century:

- The 'classical' herbal medicine system, based on Greek and Roman sources
- The Siddha and Ayurvedic medicine systems from various South Asian Countries
- Chinese herbal medicine (Chinese herbology)
- Traditional African medicine: Indigenous—Ethno-medic sources
- Unani—Tibb medicine
- Shamanic herbalism: a catch-all phrase for information mostly supplied from South America and the Himalayas
- Native American medicine

Many of the pharmaceuticals currently available to physicians have a long history of use as herbal remedies, including opium, aspirin, digitalis, and quinine. The World Health Organisation (WHO) estimates that 80 per cent of the world's population presently uses herbal medicine for some aspects of primary health care. Pharmaceuticals are prohibitively expensive for most of the world's population, half of which lives on less than U.S. $2 per day. In comparison, herbal medicines can be grown from seeds or gathered from nature for little or no cost. In addition to the use in the developing world, herbal medicine is used in industrialised nations by alternative medicine practitioners such as naturopaths. A 1998 survey of herbalists in the UK found that many of the herbs recommended by them were used traditionally but had not been evaluated in clinical trials. In Australia, a 2007 survey found that these Western herbalists tend to prescribe liquid herbal combinations of herbs rather than tablets of single herbs.

The use of, and search for, drugs and dietary supplements derived from plants have accelerated in recent years. Pharmacologists, microbiologists, botanists, and natural-product chemists are combing the Earth for phytochemicals and leads that could be developed for treatment of various diseases. In fact, according to the World Health Organisation, approximately 25 per cent of modern drugs used in the United States have been derived from plants. Among the 120 active compounds currently isolated from the higher plants and widely used in modern medicine today, 80 per cent show a positive correlation between their modern therapeutic use and the traditional use of the plants from which they are derived. More than two-thirds of the world's plant species—at least 35,000 of which are estimated to have medicinal value—come from the developing countries. At least 7,000 medical compounds in the modern pharmacopoeia are derived from plants]

Biological background

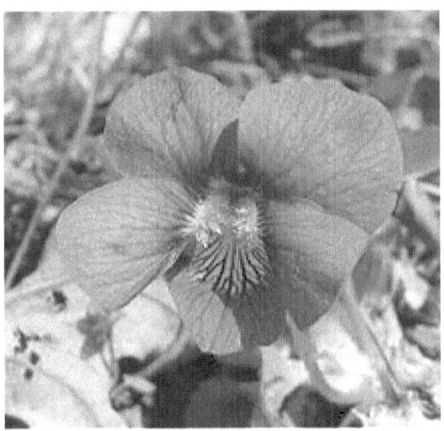

The Anthocyanins in sweet violets produce deep red shades.

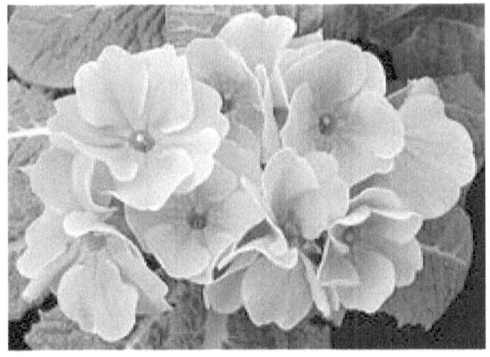

The arytenoids in primroses produce bright
red, yellow, and orange shades.

All plants produce chemical compounds as part of their normal metabolic activities. These are arbitrarily divided into primary metabolites, such as sugars and fats found in all plants, and secondary metabolites, compounds not essential for basic function found in a smaller range of plants, some useful ones found only in a particular genus or species. Pigments harvest light, protect the organism from radiation, and display colours to attract pollinators. Many common weeds, such as nettle, dandelion, and chickweed, have medicinal properties. The functions of secondary metabolites are varied. For example, some secondary metabolites are toxins used to deter predation, and others are pheromones used to attract insects for pollination. Phytoalexins protect against bacterial and fungal attacks. Allelochemicals inhibit rival plants that are competing for soil and light. Plants upregulate and downregulate their biochemical paths in response to the local mix of herbivores, pollinators, and micro-organisms. The chemical profile of a single plant may vary over time as it reacts to changing conditions. It is the secondary metabolites and pigments that can have therapeutic actions in humans and which can be refined to produce drugs. Plants synthesise a bewildering variety of phytochemicals, but most are derivatives of a few biochemical motifs. Alkaloids contain a ring with nitrogen. Many alkaloids have dramatic effects on the central nervous system. Caffeine is an alkaloid that provides a mild lift, but the alkaloids in datura cause severe intoxication and even death. Phenolics contain phenol rings. The anthocyanins that give grapes their purple colour, the isoflavones, the phytoestrogens from soy, and the tannins that give tea its astringency are phenolics. Terpenoids are built up from terpene-building blocks. Each terpene consists of two paired isoprenes. The names monoterpenes, sesquiterpenes, diterpenes, and triterpenes are based on the number of isoprene units. The fragrance of rose and lavender is due to monoterpenes. The carotenoids produce the reds, yellows, and oranges of pumpkins, corns, and tomatoes. Glycosides consist of a glucose moiety attached to an aglycone. The aglycone is a molecule that is bioactive in its free form but inert until the glycoside bond is broken by water or enzymes. This mechanism allows the plant to defer the availability of the molecule to an appropriate time, similar to a safety lock on a gun. An example is the cyanoglycosides in cherry pits that release toxins only when bitten by a herbivore.

The word 'drug' itself comes from the Dutch word 'droog' (via the French word 'Drogue'), which means 'dried plant'. Some examples are inulin from the roots of dahlias, quinine from the cinchona, morphine and codeine from the poppy, and digoxin from the foxglove. The active ingredient in willow bark, once prescribed by Hippocrates, is salicin, which is converted in the body into salicylic acid. The discovery of salicylic acid would eventually lead to the development of the acetylated form acetylsalicylic acid, also known as 'aspirin', when it was isolated from a plant known as meadowsweet. The word *aspirin* comes from an abbreviation of meadowsweet's Latin genus *Spiraea*, with an additional 'A' at the beginning to acknowledge acetylation, and 'in' was added at the end for easier pronunciation. 'Aspirin' was originally a brand name and is still a protected trademark in some countries. This medication was patented by Bayer AG.

8.5 Herbal Philosophy

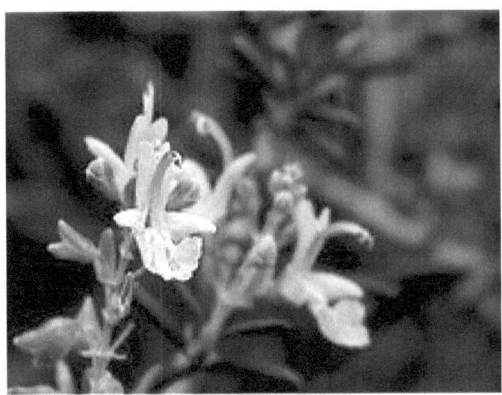

Rosemary

Four approaches to the use of plants as medicine include the following:

1) The magical/shamanic: Almost all non-modern societies recognise this kind of use. The practitioner is regarded as endowed with gifts or powers that allow him/her to use herbs in a way that is hidden from the average person, and the herbs are said to affect the spirit or soul of the person.

2) The energetic: This approach includes the major systems of TCM, Ayurveda, and unani. Herbs are regarded as having actions in terms of their energies and affecting the energies of the body. The practitioner may have extensive training and ideally be sensitive to energy, but need not have supernatural powers.

3) The functional dynamic: This approach was used by early physiomedical practitioners, whose doctrine forms the basis of contemporary practice in the UK. Herbs have a functional action, which is not necessarily linked to a physical compound, although often to a physiological function, but there is no explicit recourse to concepts involving energy.

4) The chemical modern practitioners—called phytotherapists—attempt to explain herb actions in terms of their chemical con-

stituents. It is generally assumed that the specific combination of secondary metabolites in the plant is responsible for the activity claimed or demonstrated—a concept called synergy. Most modern herbalists concede that pharmaceuticals are more effective in emergency situations where time is of the essence. An example would be where a patient had an acute heart attack that posed imminent danger. However they claim that over the long term herbs can help the patient resist disease, and that in addition, they provide nutritional and immunological support that pharmaceuticals lack. They view their goal as prevention as well as cure.

Herbalists tend to use extracts from parts of plants, such as the roots or leaves, but not isolate particular phytochemicals. Pharmaceutical medicine prefers single ingredients on the grounds that dosage can be more easily quantified. It is also possible to patent single compounds and therefore generate income. Herbalists often reject the notion of a single active ingredient, arguing that the different phytochemicals present in many herbs will interact to enhance the therapeutic effects of the herb and dilute toxicity. Furthermore, they argue that a single ingredient may contribute to multiple effects. Herbalists deny that herbal synergism can be duplicated with synthetic chemicals. They argue that phytochemical interactions and trace components may alter the drug response in ways that cannot currently be replicated with a combination of a few putative active ingredients. Pharmaceutical researchers recognise the concept of drug synergism, but note that clinical trials may be used to investigate the efficacy of a particular herbal preparation, provided the formulation of that herb is consistent.

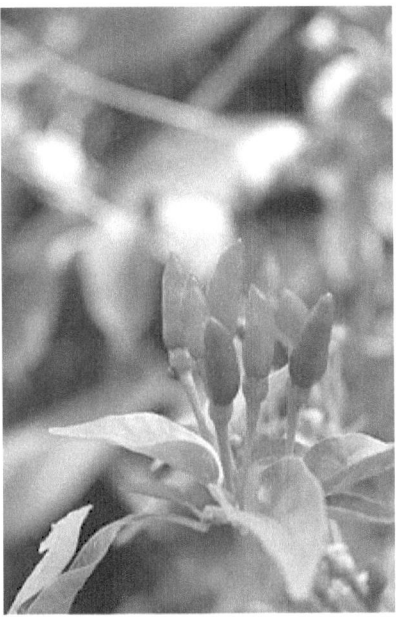

Thai chili peppers contain capsaicin.

In specific cases the claims of synergy and multifunctionality have been supported by science. The open question is how widely both can be generalised. Herbalists would argue that cases of synergy can be widely generalised, on the basis of their interpretation of evolutionary history, not necessarily shared by the pharmaceutical community. Plants are subject to similar selection pressures as humans, and therefore they must develop resistance to threats such as radiation, reactive oxygen species, and microbial attack in order to survive. Optimal chemical defences have been selected for and have thus developed over millions of years. Human diseases are multifactorial and may be treated by consuming the chemical defences that they believe to be present in herbs. Bacteria, inflammation, nutrition, and ROS (reactive oxygen species) may all play a role in arterial disease.[50] Herbalists claim a single herb may simultaneously address several of these factors. Likewise a factor such as ROS may underlie more than one condition.[51] In short, herbalists view their field as the study of a web of relationships rather than a quest for a single cause and a single cure for a single condition. In selecting herbal treatments, herbalists may use forms of information that are not applicable to pharmacists. Because herbs can moonlight as vegetables, teas, or spices they have a huge consumer base, and large-scale epidemiological studies become feasible. Ethnobotanical studies are another source of information. For example, when indigenous peoples from geographically dispersed areas use closely related herbs for the same purpose that is taken as supporting evidence for its efficacy Herbalists contend that historical medical records and herbals are underutilised resources. They favour the use of convergent information in assessing the medical value of plants. An example would be when *in vitro* activity is consistent with traditional use.

Popularity

A survey released in May 2004 by the National Center for Complementary and Alternative Medicine focused on who used complementary and alternative medicines (CAM), what was used, and why it was used. The survey was limited to adults, aged eighteen years and over during 2002, living in the United States. According to this survey, herbal therapy, or use of natural products other than vitamins and minerals, was the most commonly used CAM therapy (18.9 per cent) when all use of prayer was excluded. Herbal remedies are very common in Europe. In Germany, herbal medications are dispensed by apothecaries (e.g. Apotheke). Prescription drugs are sold alongside essential oils, herbal extracts, or herbal teas. Herbal remedies are seen by some as a treatment to be preferred to pure medical compounds which have been industrially produced.

In the United Kingdom, the training of medical herbalists is done by state-funded universities. For example, bachelor of science degrees in herbal medicine are offered at Universities such as University of East London, Middlesex University, University of Central Lancashire, University of Westminster, University of Lincoln, and Napier University in Edinburgh at the present. In the United States, a bachelor of science degree in herbal sciences is offered at Bastyr University, and a master of science degree in herbal medicine is offered at Tai Sophia Institute. There are also many smaller organisations and teachers offering certifications. A 2004 Cochrane Collaboration review found that herbal therapies are supported by strong evidence but are not widely used in all clinical settings.

Types of Herbal Medicine Systems

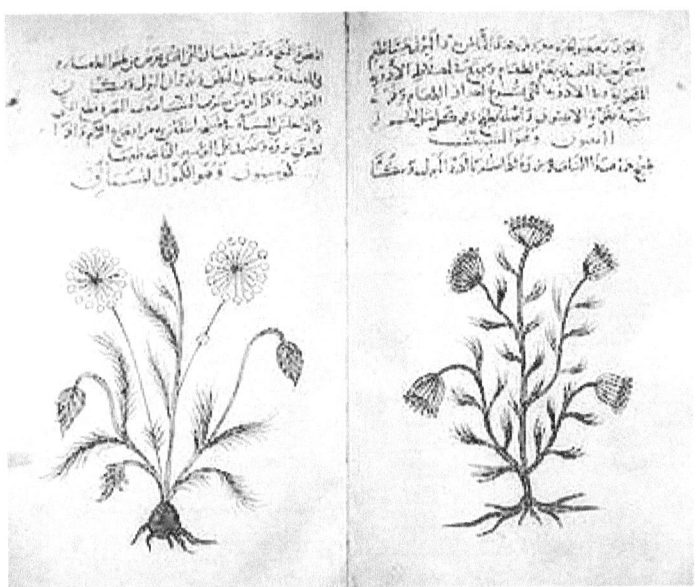

Dioscorides' Materia Medica, *c.* 1334 copy in Arabic,
describes medicinal features of cumin and dill.

Use of medicinal plants can be as informal as, for example, culinary use or consumption of herbal tea or supplement, although the sale of some herbs considered dangerous is often restricted to the public. Sometimes such herbs are provided to professional herbalists by specialist companies. Many herbalists, both professional and amateur, often grow or 'wildcraft' their own herbs. Some researchers trained in both Western and traditional Chinese medicine have attempted to deconstruct ancient medical texts in the light of modern science. One idea is that the yin–yang balance, at least with regard to herbs, corresponds to the pro-oxidant and anti-oxidant balance. This interpretation is supported by several investigations of the ORAC ratings of various yin and yang herbs.

In America, early settlers relied on plants imported from Europe and also from local Indian knowledge. One particularly successful practitioner, Samuel Thomson, developed a hugely popular system of medicine. This approach was subsequently broadened to include concepts introduced from modern physiology, a discipline called physiomedicalism. Another group, the eclectics, were a later offshoot from the orthodox medical profession, who were looking to avoid the then current medical treatments of mercury and bleeding and introduced herbal medicine into their practices. Both groups were eventually overcome by the actions of the American Medical Association, which was formed for this purpose. Cherokee medicine tends to divide herbs into foods, medicines, and toxins and to use seven plants in the treatment of disease, which is defined from both spiritual and physiological aspects, according to Cherokee herbalist David Winston. In India, Ayurvedic medicine has quite complex formulas with thirty or more ingredients, including a sizable number of ingredients that have undergone 'alchemical processing', chosen to balance 'Vata', 'Pitta', or 'Kapha'. In Tamil Nadu, Tamils have their own medicinal system now popularly called the Siddha medicinal system. The Siddha system is entirely in the Tamil language. It contains roughly 300,000 verses covering diverse aspects of medicine such as anatomy, sex ('kokokam' is the sexual treatise of par excellence), herbal, mineral, and metallic compositions to cure many diseases that are relevant even today. Ayurveda is in Sanskrit, but Sanskrit was not generally used as a mother tongue, and hence its medicines are mostly taken from Siddha and other local traditions.

In addition, there are more modern theories of herbal combination like William LeSassier's triune formula which combined Pythagorean imagery with Chinese medicine ideas and resulted in nine herb formulas which supplemented, drained, or neutrally nourished the main organ systems affected and three associated systems[citation needed]. His system has been taught to thousands of influential American herbalists through his own apprenticeship programmes during his lifetime, the William LeSassier Archive and the David Winston Center for Herbal Studies. Different chemicals in herbs are more abundant than in a single drug. Some chemicals in herbs may work as growth hormones or antibiotics, nutrients, and toxin neutralisers.

Many traditional African remedies have performed well in initial laboratory tests to ensure they are not toxic and in tests on animals. Gawo, a herb used in traditional treatments, has been tested in rats by researchers from Nigeria's University of Jos and the National Institute for Pharmaceutical Research and Development. According to research in the African Journal of Biotechnology, Gawo passed tests for toxicity and reduced induced fevers, diarrhoea, and inflammation. Phytotherapy is the study and use of extracts from natural origin as medicines or in promoting good health. Ethno-medical is the comparative study of how different cultures view disease and how they treat or prevent it, *also* the medical beliefs and practices of indigenous cultures, for example, the medical knowledge among Igbo traditional healers in Nigeria. The summary conclusion to be drawn from here is that herbalism is the principal foundation of the entire medical world whatever system that exists. Even the so-called chemical medicine must have their own bio-availability to the soil contents of their origin.

8.6 Anthroposophical Complementary Medicine

This is a combination of both the orthodox conventional medicine and the natural treatment approach to medicine. It focuses on strengthening the patient's organism and individuality. In fact, this approach is nearest to the application of homeopathy and herbal health care. *Anthroposophical* medicine is a holistic and salutogenetic approach to medicine focusing on strengthening the patient's organism and individuality. The self-determination, autonomy, and dignity of patients are central theme therapies intended to enhance a patient's capacities to heal. The medical system was founded in the 1920s by Rudolf Steiner in conjunction with Dr Ita Wegman as an extension to conventional medicine. It is based on the spiritual philosophy of anthroposophy. Conventional medical treatments, including surgery and medications, are employed as necessary, and anthroposophical physicians must have a conventional medical education, including a degree from an established and certified medical school, as well as extensive postgraduate study. There are currently anthroposophical medical practices in eighty countries worldwide.

Ita Wegeman was the co-founder of *anthroposophical medicine* before 1900 in Berlin, Germany. The first steps towards an anthroposophical approach to medicine were made before 1920, when homeopathic physicians and pharmacists began working with Rudolf Steiner, who recommended new medicinal substances as well as specific methods for preparing these. In 1921, Dr Ita Wegman opened the first anthroposophic medical clinic, now known as the Ita Wegman Clinic in Arlesheim, Switzerland. Dr Wegman was soon joined by a number of other doctors. They began to train the first anthroposophic nurses for the clinic. At Wegman's request, Steiner regularly visited the clinic and suggested treatment regimes for particular patients. Between 1921 and 1925, he also gave several series of lectures on medicine. In 1925, Wegman and Steiner wrote the first book on the anthroposophical approach to medicine named *Fundamentals of Therapy*. The clinic expanded and soon opened a branch in Ascona. Dr Wegman lectured widely, visiting Holland and England particularly frequently, and an increasing number of doctors began to include the anthroposophical approach in their practices. A cancer clinic, the Lukas clinic, opened in Arlesheim in 1963.

Methodology

Anthroposophical medicine approaches disease as an imbalance in the biological organism and employs treatment strategies intended to restore this balance. Anthroposophical approaches include anthroposophical medicines based upon modified homeopathic principles, physical therapies including massage therapy, and artistic therapies. Many of these are intended to support the patient's capacity for self-healing. Anthroposophical medicine is based upon the anthroposophical view of the human being, which considers the patient's: physical constitution in the following order:

- Life or Etheric body, seen as the organising principle directing growth and regeneration; Astral body, understood as the bearer of affect and consciousness; and Ego, seen as the capacity for self-reflection and free will. Anthroposophical doctors generally restrict the use of antibiotics and antipyretics and have a differentiated individual approach to vaccinations. Some children treated by anthroposophist doctors are vaccinated only against tetanus and polio, and some vaccinations are given later than recommended by health authorities.

Distribution of Anthroposophical Medicine

There are about twenty-eight anthroposophic hospitals, departments of hospitals, rehabilitation centres, and sanatoria located in Germany, Switzerland, Sweden, the Netherlands, Great Britain, Italy, the USA, and Brazil, as well as over 140 outpatient clinics worldwide. Four of the German and Swiss anthroposophic hospitals are state-sponsored, three are academic teaching hospitals under the coordination of nearby universities. Three European universities (Bern, Hamburg and Witten/ Herdecke) have professorships in anthroposophic medicine, and other universities offer courses on the field. Anthroposophic medicine is recognised in Germany as a 'special therapy system', along with homeopathy and herbal medicine under the Medicines Act, and has its own committee at the Federal Institute for Drugs and Medical Devices. Anthroposophical medical treatment has been a recognised specialty within Swiss governmental health policy since 1999. The International Federation of Anthroposophical Medical Associations estimates that there are currently approximately 2,000 anthroposophical doctors worldwide. Based on the number of prescriptions it has been estimated that anthroposophic medicinal products are prescribed by more than 30,000 physicians.

Studies of Efficacy

Out of 195 studies of anthroposophic medicine published through 2006, 186 found positive outcomes, defined as comparable or better results than with conventional treatment with respect to at least one clinically relevant outcome measure or a clinically relevant improvement resulting from the treatment. Eight studies found no advantage and one study showed a negative trend. The criteria used in the studies range from subjective judgements of quality-of-life improvements to objectively measured reductions in symptoms. A number of the studies were found to have clear methodological weaknesses, but a significant number of well-designed studies remain. A study of the effectiveness of anthroposophical medicine found long-standing improvements of disease symptoms and quality of life in patients with mental, respiratory, and musculoskeletal diseases and other chronic conditions; the study did not compare results with other treatment regimens, and the participants also received conventional medical treatment as conventional medical treatments such as surgery and medications are taken alongside this complementary therapy according to most practitioners' recommendations. A study of anthroposophic treatment of chronic illness found that 'anthroposophic therapies were associated with long-term reduction of chronic disease symptoms, improvement of health-related quality of life, and health cost reduction'.

- A comparison of the effectiveness of treatments of chronic lower back pain found that anthroposophically treated patients showed at least comparable improvements to conventionally treated patients and significantly more pronounced improvement on three scales: mental health, general health, and vitality. As with other forms of alternative medicine, for many treatments used in anthroposophical medicine, proofs of efficacy have not been made through strictly controlled medical testing.

Parsifal Study of Anthroposophical Lifestyle

An analysis of some of the data from the multicentre PARSIFAL study, involving 6,630 children aged five to thirteen in five European countries, concluded that certain factors in the anthroposophic lifestyle, such as restrictive use of vaccinations, antibiotics, and antipyretics, were associated with a reduced risk of allergic disease. Measles was more common in the anthroposophic group children, likely because of the reduced use of vaccinations in that group.

Mistletoe Treatment for Cancer

The use of mistletoe extracts in the treatment of cancer was first proposed by Rudolf Steiner and developed by anthroposophical researchers; it is now probably the best-known anthroposophic therapy. Various forms of the medication are widely available in Central Europe, where the treatment regimen of up to two-thirds of all oncology patients includes mistletoe. The extracts are generally no longer used to reduce or inhibit tumour growth, but to improve the patients' quality of life and to reduce tumour-induced symptoms and the side effects of chemotherapy and radiotherapy; a wide array of clinical studies support the efficacy of the treatment regimen for the latter purposes. There are also phytotherapeutic preparations using non-homeopathic doses of mistletoe; these should not be confused with the anthroposophical preparations.

In the United States, mistletoe 'holds interest as a potential anticancer agent because extracts derived from it have been shown to kill cancer cells *in vitro*,' but no forms of the extract have been approved by the FDA for any indications. Mistletoe extracts may not be distributed in or imported into the United States except for the purpose of clinical research. Although preclinical (animal) studies suggested a potential role for mistletoe extracts in cancer therapies, no such effects have been convincingly reported. Evidence for the efficacy of mistletoe as an anticancer drug from human studies is weak. Though numerous cohort studies and case series have reported tumour remission and regression, double blinded studies have tended not to support this effect, and the cohort and case studies have been criticised as biased due to their small size and lack of double-blinding. Mistletoe extracts are also frequently used to treat cancer patients in Holland and in Great Britain. The treatment has been approved as palliative therapy for malignant tumours in Germany. In the United States it is approved for clinical trial only, and numerous clinical trials have evaluated its effectiveness. Approximately thirty types of mistletoe extracts are used clinically; the most commonly used is known as Iscador. Though no serious side effects are normally found from mistletoe treatments, in one case a patient allergic to mistletoe went into anaphylactic shock. Minor side effects of injections reported include redness, pain, or, in a few cases, subcutaneous inflammation. The National Cancer Institute (U.S.) position on mistletoe is as follows: 'At this time, there is not enough evidence to recommend the use of mistletoe as a treatment for cancer except in carefully designed clinical trials. These trials will give more information about whether mistletoe can be useful in treating certain types of cancer.'

Reviews

- One review of studies of mistletoe concludes that Iscador (mistletoe) has been shown to be effective against cancers in animals, inhibiting metastasis, reducing the size of and causing necrosis of induced tumours, that there is evidence that mistletoe stimulates the immune system, but that there is no evidence of its efficacy in treating humans.
- In a survey of 105 clinical studies, one study concludes that 'the best evidence is for a reduction of side effects from conventional oncological therapies (chemotherapy, radiation therapy, surgical removal). An improvement in quality of life is also very probable. That remission of tumours can be induced through injection of mistletoe extracts is well-demonstrated, which accords with preclinical research into cytotoxicity and into the use for animal tumours, but this effect appears to be dependent upon the dose

and method of application, and is only present in exceptional cases with the usual small doses.' One review concluded: 'Although there is laboratory evidence of biological activity that may be beneficial to cancer patients, the evidence of clinical benefit from human studies remains weak and inconclusive. Because of the absence of serious side effects and the limited evidence that mistletoe products may offer some therapeutic advantages, further research is warranted.' The National Cancer Institute has concluded that mistletoe extract has been shown to kill cancer cells in the laboratory and to boost the immune system in animals, that there is evidence that mistletoe can boost the immune system in human beings, but that almost all of the studies done on human beings have major weaknesses that raise doubts about the reliability of their findings. According to the American Cancer Society, 'A number of laboratory experiments suggest mistletoe may have the potential to treat cancer, but these results have not yet been reflected in clinical trials. Available evidence from well-designed clinical trials that have studied mistletoe did not support claims that mistletoe could improve length or quality of life. Review of evidence from carefully conducted controlled human clinical studies indicates that mistletoe does not have any significant anti-tumour activity. Most of the studies that have found positive results from mistletoe extract in the treatment or prevention of cancer are not considered scientifically dependable . . . Researchers are working to identify the most important components, which are thought to be the lectins (proteins). Laboratory experiments also hint that mistletoe increases the activity of lymphocytes, which are cells that attack invading organisms.'

The principal points of conclusions to be drawn from this particular research finding are many. Before we can begin to claim efficacy and effectiveness of any remedy—be they herbal, homeopathic, or any others, such claim must be supported by evidence. It is professionally myopic to say that scientific research evidence is only open to the conventional medical system and not to the complementary therapy.

8.7 Osteopathic Medicine and Arthritis

This practice is a distinctive branch of mainstream medical profession. In the UK, It is a complementary medical practice founded by Andrew Taylor Still, doctor of osteopathic medicine in U.S. Medical School. Osteopathy or osteopathic medicine is an approach to health care that emphasises the role of the musculoskeletal system in health and disease. Doctors of osteopathic medicine (DOs) receive similar training as medical doctors (MDs) with additional training in osteopathic and holistic medicine. In this book many authentic natural medical products from all over the world are subscribing to our recognition. Both their names and details are therefore shown here for the reader's perusal. There are no orthodox medical products shown here. Any reader interested in any of the products in this book can place an order directly to the company or the clinic in charge. Neither the author nor the publishers can be held responsible for any of the products mentioned in this book if at all.

Arthritis as a Degenerative Disease

The information about arthritis given here is very necessary because it relates to the osteopathic health problem. The word 'arthritis' is taken from Greek words meaning 'inflamed joints' and is associated with a group of well over 100 rheumatic diseases and conditions. These diseases may affect not only the joints but also the muscles, bones, tendons, and ligaments that support them. Osteoarthritis is the condition that results when cartilage is slowly eroded, and bone begins grinding against bone. This is accompanied by bony outgrowths called osteophytes. Cysts may form, and the underlying bone thickens and becomes deformed. Other symptoms include knobby knuckles, grating and grinding sounds that emanate from arthritic joints, and muscle spasms, along with pain, stiffness, and loss of mobility. Osteoarthritis rarely spreads to other body parts but concentrates its erosive influence in one or just a few joints. Who are at risk for osteoarthritis? While age alone does not cause osteoarthritis, the loss of joint cartilage is experienced more frequently with increasing age. Others at risk may include those who have some abnormality in the way their joint surfaces fit together or who have weak leg and thigh muscles, legs of unequal length, or a misalignment of the spine. Trauma to a joint caused either by an accident or by an occupation in which repetitive motions overuse a joint can also set the stage for osteoarthritis. Once deterioration begins, being overweight can exacerbate osteoarthritis. These health conditions are more predominant within the cold temperate region of the world and may become worse during the winter period of the year. It is unfortunate that some people believe that painkiller substance can be used to cure the arthritic pains. Complementary health care practitioners seeking preventive therapy must be very careful. It may be true that the orthodox pharmaceutical products can ameliorate many health imbalances, but the concept of know-all and care-all is a myopic way of looking life in the present day.

Glucosamine Sulphate: Natural Treatment

Glucosamine is a naturally occurring substance in the body, the purpose of which is to stimulate the manufacture of collagen (the protein portion of a fibrous substance that holds joints together). Collagen is also the main constituent of articular cartilage. A large number of clinical studies have been conducted to quantify the effects of glucosamine on osteoarthritis. Results have been conflicting. A multi-centre clinical trial conducted by the National Institutes of Health in 2006 found that patients taking glucosamine HCl, chondroitin sulphate, or a combination of the two had no statistically significant improvement in their symptoms compared to patients taking a placebo. However, a secondary analysis suggested that supplementation with glucosamine may help to alleviate symptoms in patients with moderate-to-severe pain (Cleg, et al. 2006). Although glucosamine's effect on joint damage is still debated, many medical experts believe this supplement reduces pain and is safe. The usual dose is 500 mg three times a day. This information must be used very carefully taking into account the patient's given condition, age, and other related illnesses.

Glucosamine is a modified sugar produced by the body. It is used to form larger molecules called glycosaminoglycans, which are involved in the formation and repair of cartilage. They are also used as lubricants and shock absorbers by our joints. Synthetically produced, glucosamine is used to address the imbalance between production and destruction of naturally occurring glucosamine in osteoarthritis cartilage. The two chemical forms available are glucosamine sulphate (Arthro-Aid Direct, Bioglan, Blackmores, Arthrogen, GoldenGlow, Healthstream, and Procosamine); and glucosamine hydrochloride (Arthro-Aid and Osteo-Eze).

Glucosamine can be administered as a topical cream, an oral tablet, an intra-muscular injection, and as an intra-articular injection (directly into the joint). There have been a number of studies that have reported an improvement in joint discomfort with the use of glucosamine (Houpt J. B., McMillan R., Wein C., and Paget-Dellio D., Effect of glucosamine hydrochloride in the treatment of pain of osteoarthritis of the knee, *Journal of Rheumatology* 1999; 26 (11): 2423-30). There have also been reports comparing glucosamine to ibuprofen. Each of these studies showed a similar amount of relief in patients administered glucosamine and ibuprofen. In one study, glucosamine was shown to be more effective than ibuprofen (Muller-Fassbender H., Bach G. L., Haase W., Rovati L. C. and Setnikar L., Glucosamine sulfate compared to ibuprofen in osteoarthritis of the knee, *Osteoarthritis Cartilage*1994; 2: 61-9). Glucosamine is a safe, natural product that has exhibited few side effects. Those that have been shown have been gastrointestinal in nature (Reginster J. Y., Deroisy R., Rovati L. C., Lee R. L., Lejeune E., Bruyere O., Giacovelli G., Henrotin Y., Dacre J. E. and Gossett C., Long-term effects of glucosamine sulphate on osteoarthrits progression: a randomised, placebo-controlled clinical trial, *Lancet* 2001; 357 (9252): 251-6).

Chondroitin Sulphate

This is a naturally occurring molecule that is a component of cartilage. It helps keep the cartilage resilient by absorbing fluid into the connective tissue. Researchers also believe that chondroitin blocks the enzymes that break down cartilage as well as provide the building blocks for cartilage to repair itself in ageing or otherwise (Busci L. and Poor G., Efficacy and tolerability of oral chondroitin sulfate as a symptomatic slow-acting drug for osteoarthritis (SYSADOA) in the treatment of knee osteoarthritis, *Osteoarthritis Cartilage*). Chondroitin supplements are not known to exhibit any side effects. Chondroitin is commonly sold as chondroitin sulphate in capsule or tablet form. It is also available in combination with various forms of glucosamine and sometimes manganese as well. A dosage of 400 mg twice per day is recommended.

Hyaluronic acid is a fluid in the knee joint. A person with osteoarthritis of the knee has a reduced amount of hyaluronic acid in the joint. Injections are used to put more of the fluid into the joint and so provide more protection for it. The intended result for sufferers is that they experience relief from pain, which may last up to six months. However, the injections are very expensive, costing in the region of O. In a meta-analysis of eight hyaluronan trials involving 971 patients, outcomes in patients treated with hyaluronan were superior to outcomes in patients treated with a placebo at the end of the treatment cycles and after six months (George E., Intra-articular hyaluronan treatment for osteoarthritis, *Ann. Rheum. Dis.* 1998; 57: 637-40). Other studies, however, have shown little or no benefit. If you feel that you could benefit from this treatment, consult your physician.

Ginger

For hundreds of years, ginger has been used as an anti-arthritis treatment. Ginger acts as an antagonist to prostaglandins. The dried rhizome of ginger contains approximately 1-4 per cent volatile oils. These are the medically active constituents of ginger and are also responsible for ginger's characteristic odour and taste. The aromatic constituents include zingiberene and bisabolene, while the pungent constituents are known as gingerols and shogaols (Bliddal H., Rosetzsky A., Schlichting P., Weidner M. S., Andersen L. A., Ibfelt H. H., Christensen K., Jensen O. N. and Barslev J., A randomized, placebo-controlled, cross-over study of ginger extracts and ibuprofen in osteoarthritis, *Osteoarthritis Cartilage,* 2000, Jan; 8(1):9-12).

Boswellia is an Ayurvedic plant that contains anti-inflammatory triterpinoids called boswellic acids. The aromatic gum resins from this tree have been used by practitioners of the Ayurvedic system of medicine to treat arthritis for centuries. An Ayurvedic herbal combination of ashwagandha, boswellia, and curcumin was evaluated in a randomised, double-blind, placebo-controlled, crossover study in patients with osteoarthritis. Treatment with this formulation produced a significant drop in severity of pain (Kimmatkar N., Thawani V., Hingorani L. and Khiyani., Efficacy and tolerability of Boswellia serrata extract in treatment of osteoarthritis of knee—a randomized double blind placebo controlled trial at MS Orthopedics, Indira Gandhi Medical College, Nagpur, India, *Phytomedicine* 2003).

Glucosamine and Chondroitin

Glucosamine and chondroitin supplements are used to slow the progression of osteoarthritis and to lessen the pain associated with it. Glucosamine is sold in many forms, including glucosamine sulphate, glucosamine hydrochloride (HCl), and N-acetyl glucosamine (NAG), and may also contain a potassium chloride or sodium chloride salt. However, there appears to be no conclusive evidence that one form is better than another. Chondroitin is typically sold as chondroitin sulphate. The supplements appear to be more effective when taken together.

8.8 Aromatherapy—European

Aromatherapy is the use of essential oils from plants for healing. Although the word 'aroma' makes it sound as if the oils would be inhaled, they can also be massaged into the skin or—rarely—taken by mouth. Essential oils should never be taken by mouth without specific instruction from a trained and qualified specialist. Whether inhaled or applied on the skin, essential oils are gaining new attention as an alternative treatment for infections, stress, and other health problems. However, in most cases scientific evidence is still lacking.

The Meaning of Essential Oils

Essential oils are concentrated extracts taken from the roots, leaves, seeds, or blossoms of plants. Each contains its own mix of active ingredients, and this mix determines what the oil is used for. Some oils are used to promote physical healing—for example, to treat swelling or fungal infections. Others are used for their emotional value—they may enhance relaxation or make a room smell pleasant. Orange blossom oil, for example, contains a large amount of an active ingredient that is thought to be calming.

The History of Aromatherapy

Essential oils have been used for therapeutic purposes for nearly 6,000 years. The ancient Chinese, Indians, Egyptians, Greeks, and Romans used them in cosmetics, perfumes, and drugs. Essential oils were also commonly used for spiritual, therapeutic, hygienic, and ritualistic purposes.

More recently, René-Maurice Gattefossé, a French chemist, discovered the healing properties of lavender oil when he applied it to a burn on his hand caused by an explosion in his laboratory. He then started to analyse the chemical properties of essential oils and how they were used to treat burns, skin infections, gangrene, and wounds in soldiers during World War I. In 1928, Gattefossé founded the science of aromatherapy. By the 1950s, massage therapists, beauticians, nurses, physiotherapists, doctors, and other health care providers began using aromatherapy.

Aromatherapy did not become popular in the United States until the 1980s. Today, many lotions, candles, and beauty products are sold as 'aromatherapy'. However, many of these products contain synthetic fragrances that do not have the same properties as essential oils.

The Way Aromatherapy Works

Researchers are not entirely clear how aromatherapy may work. Some experts believe our sense of smell may play a role. The 'smell' receptors in your nose communicate with parts of your brain (the amygdala and hippocampus) that serve as storehouses for emotions and memories. When you breathe in essential oil molecules, some researchers believe that they stimulate these parts of your brain and influence physical, emotional, and mental health. For example, lavender is believed to stimulate the activity of brain cells in the amygdala similar to the way some sedative medications work. Other researchers think that some molecules from essential oils may interact in the blood with hormones or enzymes.

Aromatherapy massage is a popular way of using essential oils because it works in several ways at the same time. Your skin absorbs essential oils, and you also breathe them in. Plus, you experience the physical therapy of the massage itself.

During an Aromatherapy Session

Professional aromatherapists, nurses, physical therapists, pharmacists, and massage therapists can provide topical or inhaled aromatherapy treatment. Only specially trained professionals can provide treatment that involves taking essential oils by mouth.

During an aromatherapy session, the practitioner will ask about your medical history and symptoms, as well any scents you may like. You may be directed to breathe in essential oils directly from a piece of cloth or indirectly through steam inhalations, vaporisers, or sprays. The practitioner may also apply diluted essential oils to your skin during a massage. In most cases, the practitioner will tell you how to use aromatherapy at home, by mixing essential oils into your bath, for example.

Aromatherapy Good in Many Ways

Aromatherapy is used in a wide range of settings—from health spas to hospitals—to treat a variety of conditions. In general, it seems to relieve pain, improve mood, and promote a sense of relaxation.

Several clinical studies suggest that when essential oils (particularly rose, lavender, and frankincense) were used by qualified midwives, pregnant women felt less anxiety and fear, had a stronger sense of well-being, and had less need for pain medications during delivery. Many women also report that peppermint oil relieves nausea and vomiting during labour.

Massage therapy with essential oils (combined with medications or therapy) may benefit people with depression. The scents are thought by some to stimulate positive emotions in the area of the brain responsible for memories and emotions, but the benefits seem to be related to relaxation caused by the scents and the massage. A person's belief that the treatment will help also influences whether it works.

In test tubes, chemical compounds from some essential oils have shown antibacterial and anti-fungal properties. Some evidence also suggests that citrus oils may strengthen the immune system and that peppermint oil may help with digestion. Fennel, aniseed, sage, and clary-sage have estrogen-like compounds, which may help relieve symptoms of premenstrual syndrome and menopause. However, human studies are lacking.

Other conditions for which aromatherapy may be helpful include the following:

1) Alopecia areata (hair loss).
2) Agitation, possibly including agitation related to dementia.

3) Anxiety.
4) Constipation (with abdominal massage using aromatherapy).
5) Insomnia.
6) Pain: Studies have found that people with rheumatoid arthritis, cancer (using topical chamomile), and headaches (using topical peppermint) require fewer pain medications when they use aromatherapy.
7) Itching, a common side effect for those receiving dialysis.
8) Psoriasis.

Those Who Should Avoid Aromatherapy

1) Pregnant women, people with severe asthma, and people with a history of allergies should avoid all essential oils.
2) Pregnant women and people with a history of seizures should avoid hyssop oil.
3) People with high blood pressure should avoid stimulating essential oils such as rosemary and spike lavender.
4) People with estrogen-dependent tumours (such as breast or ovarian cancer) should not use oils with estrogen-like compounds such as fennel, aniseed, sage, and clay-sage.

Things You Should Watch Out For

Most topical and inhaled essential oils are generally considered safe. You should never take essential oils by mouth unless you are under the supervision of a trained professional. Some oils are toxic, and taking them by mouth could be fatal. Rarely, aromatherapy can induce side effects, such as rash, headache, liver and nerve damage, as well as harm to a fetus. Oils that are high in phenols, such as cinnamon, can irritate the skin. Add water or base massage oil (such as almond or sesame oil) to the essential oil before applying to your skin. Avoid using near your eyes. Essential oils are highly volatile and flammable, so they should never be used near an open flame. Animal studies suggest that active ingredients in certain essential oils may interact with some medications. Researchers don't know if they have the same effect in humans. Eucalyptus, for example, may cause certain medications, including pentobarbital (used for seizures) and amphetamine (used for narcolepsy and attention-deficit hyperactivity disorder) to be less effective.

The Future of Aromatherapy

Although essential oils have been used for centuries, few studies have looked into the safety and effectiveness of aromatherapy in people. Scientific evidence is lacking. And there are some concerns about the safety and quality of certain essential oils. More research is needed before aromatherapy becomes a widely accepted alternative remedy.

8.9 Ancient Egyptian Traditional Medicine

The primary purpose of presenting the research findings on ancient Egyptian medicine in this book is to know the historical background of modern African herbal therapy. The second aim is to show the origin of the modern African medical cosmology. These details will enable us to understand the nature and any possible preventive modality of modern diseases. The Egyptians believed that disease and death were caused by a god, a spirit, or some other supernatural force. They had shamans–physicians, who would discover the particular entity causing the disease and then drive it out with magic rituals or talismans as well as medicines. The duties of Egyptian physicians included creating medications, providing magic spells and prayers to provide healing, mending broken bones, dentistry, embalming, surgery, and autopsy. Physicians were often very specialised. From the tombstone of Iry, chief physician to a pharaoh of the Sixth Dynasty, we learn that he was also the 'palace eye physician' and the 'palace stomach bowel physician' and bore the titles 'One understanding the internal fluids' and 'Guardian of the anus' (Ead).

A common disease among the Egyptians was the parasitic disease Schistosomiasis, an infection by the larval worm of a snail. Humans are infected when they come into contact with the free swimming worm, which is released by the snail into water. The worm burrows into the skin and enters the veins of the human host and causes anaemia, loss of appetite, urinary infection, and loss of resistance to other diseases. The commoners also suffered from the injuries and deformities caused by hard labour to which they were exposed. They suffered from insect-borne diseases such as malaria and trachoma, an eye disease, small pox, measles, tuberculosis, and cholera. It is believed that there were occasional outbreaks of the bubonic plague spread along trade routes from the east. They contracted diseases such as trichinae, parasitic worms, and tuberculosis from their livestock. Leprosy, which had originated in Egypt, was relatively rare, possibly because of the immunity that tuberculosis sufferers have. Silicosis of the lungs, caused by breathing in sand particles, was a common cause of pneumonia for the ancient Egyptians. The ancient Egyptians also suffered from diet-related ailments such as malnutrition, vitamin and mineral deficiencies, dental abrasion, and ailments normal to all humans such as arthritis.

A great deal of our knowledge of ancient Egyptian medicine comes from the Edwin Smith Papyrus, the Ebers Papyrus, and the Kahun Papyrus. The Edwin Smith Papyrus and the Ebers Papyrus date from the seventeenth and sixteenth centuries BCE. These manuscripts are believed to be derived from earlier sources. They contain recipes and spells for the treatment of a great variety of diseases or symptoms. They discuss the diagnosis of diseases and provide information of an anatomy. They detail the ancient Egyptian concept of medicine, anatomy, and physiology. The Kahun Papyrus is a gynaecological text that deals with topics such as the reproductive organs, conception, testing for pregnancy, birth, and contraception. Among those materials prescribed for contraception are crocodile dung, honey, and sour milk.

Thanks to the medical papyri, we know of many of the ancient Egyptian treatments and prescriptions for diseases. They call for the treatment of many disorders and the use of a variety of substances, plant, animal, mineral, as well as the droppings and urine of a number of animals. They knew how to use suppositories, herbal dressings, and enemas and widely used castor oil. Honey and milk were used for the respiratory system as well as throat irritations. Honey, a natural antibiotic, was also widely used to dress wounds. Aloe vera was used to treat worms, relieve headaches, soothe chest pains, burns, ulcers, and for skin diseases. Frankincense was used to treat throat and larynx infections, stop bleeding, as well as treat asthma. Dill was used to sooth flatulence, also for its laxative and diuretic properties. Caraway was used to treat flatulence and as a breath freshener. Balsam apple or Apple of Jerusalem was used as a laxative. Garlic was believed to provide vitality, soothe flatulence, aid digestion, shrink haemorrhoids, and rid body of spirits. Camphor tree was used to reduce fevers, soothe gums, and treat epilepsy. Juniper tree was utilised to treat digestive ailments, soothe chest pains, and soothe stomach cramps. Mustard seeds were used to induce vomiting and relieve chest pains. Onions could be used to induce perspiration, prevent colds, and used as a diuretic. Parsley was used as a diuretic. Mint was used to soothe flatulence, aid digestion, stop vomiting, and as a breath freshener. Sandalwood was used to aid digestion, stop diarrhoea, and to treat gout. Sesame was used to soothe asthma. Poppy seeds were used to relieve insomnia, headaches, and as an anaesthetic. Thyme was also used as a pain reliever. *Resources:* Majno, Guido, *The Healing Hand,* Harvard University Press, Cambridge, 1975; Silverburg, Robert, *The Dawn of Medicine,* Putnam Publishing, New York, 1966; Dawson, Warren R, *The Beginnings, Egypt & Assyria,* Hafner Publishing Company, New York, 1964; Sanders, J. B, *Transitions from Ancient Egyptian to Greek medicine,* University of Kansas Press, Lawrence, 1963.

CHAPTER 9

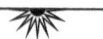

Asian Traditional Medicine System

This chapter gives a full discussion on various traditional medicines that some Asian countries follow.

The chapter looks at the Chines traditional medicines and shows how this has influenced traditional healing systems in various Asian countries.

9.1 Tibetan Healing

Two thousand years ago the indigenous people of Tibet had a traditional medical system, and like the medical systems of most indigenous people, it was connected to the native spiritual system; in the case of Tibet this was the Bön religion. Over several centuries, medical knowledge was incorporated from the Indian Ayurvedic system, the Chinese system, and the medical systems of Hellenic Greece and Persia. In addition, this system incorporated the Buddhist thought that was also introduced during that time. Tibetan medicine has existed in its present form for over one thousand years. In Buddhist thought, all suffering and hence all illness is caused by the three poisons: attachment, anger, and ignorance. Dr Yeshi Donden remarked that 'the root (of illness) is beginningless ignorance' and that 'ignorance is with us like our own shadow . . . even if we think that we are in very good health, actually we have had the basic cause of illness since beginningless time.' The basic theory of Tibetan medicine is to keep in balance the humours which are rLung (pronounced loong), mKhris-pa, and Bad-kan. In English, these are generally translated as wind, bile, and phlegm.

Diagnosis is done by observation and with an interview of the patient, taking of pulses, examination of urine and faeces, and examination of the tongue. Treatment can include consultations on lifestyle and diet, recommendations of mantras and meditation, moxabustion (burning of the herb mugwort), the use of supplements, massage with specially formulated herbal oil, and occasionally acupuncture. The Tibetan physician focuses her attention on spiritual factors even in the treatment of the simplest illnesses. Every Tibetan physician vows to 'regard medicine as an offering to the Medicine Buddha and all other medicine deities' and considers her 'medical instruments as holy objects'. Even the pharmaceuticals, which are mixtures of vegetable, animal, and mineral compounds, are prepared with meticulous attention to religious ritual.

9.2 Chinese Medicine

Traditional Chinese medicine, also known as *TCM*, includes a range of traditional medicine practices originating in China. Although well accepted in the mainstream of medical care throughout East Asia [citation needed], it is considered an alternative medical system in much of the Western world. TCM practices include treatments such as Chinese herbal medicine, acupuncture, dietary therapy, and Tui na massage. Qigong and Taijiquan are also closely associated with TCM [citation needed]. Major theories include yin yang, the five phases, the human body meridian/channel system, Zang Fu organ theory, six-channel pattern identification, four aspect pattern identification, etc. Modern TCM was systematised in the 1950s under the People's Republic of China and Mao Zedong[citation needed]. Prior to this, Chinese medicine was mainly practised within family lineage systems [citation needed].

History: Ancient (Classical) History

The same philosophy that informs about Taoist and Buddhist thought informs the philosophy of traditional Chinese medicine, which reflects the classical Chinese belief that the life and activity of individual human beings have an intimate relationship with the environment on all levels. In legend, as a result of a dialogue with his minister, Qibo the Yellow Emperor (2698–2596 BCE) is supposed by Chinese tradition to have composed his *Neijing: Suwen* or *Inner Canon: Basic Questions* (the book by Huangdi Neijing *Yellow Emperor's Inner Canon* title is often mistranslated as *Yellow Emperor's Classic of Internal Medicine*). Modern scholarly opinion holds that the extant text of this title was compiled by an anonymous scholar no earlier than the Han dynasty, just over two thousand years ago. During the Han Dynasty (202 BC–AD 220), Zhang Zhongjing China's Hippocrates, who was mayor of Chang-sha towards the end of the second century AD, wrote a *Treatise on Cold Damage*, which contains the earliest known reference to *Neijing Suwen*. Another prominent Eastern Han physician was Hua Tuo (c. AD 140-208), who anaesthetised patients during surgery with a formula of wine and powdered cannabis. Hua's physical, surgical, and herbal treatments were also used to cure headaches, dizziness, worms, fevers, coughing, blocked throat, and even a diagnosis for one lady that she had a dead fetus within her that needed to be taken out. The Jin dynasty practitioner and advocate of acupuncture and moxibustion, Huang-fu Mi (AD 215-82), also quoted the Yellow Emperor in his *Jia Yi Jing c.* AD 265. During the Tang dynasty, Wang Bing claimed to have located a copy of the originals of the *Neijing Suwen*, which he expanded and edited substantially. This work was revisited by an imperial commission during the eleventh century AD.

There were noted advances in Chinese medicine during the Middle Ages. Emperor Gaozong (r. 649-83) of the Tang Dynasty (618-907) commissioned the scholarly compilation of a *materia medica* in 657 that documented 833 medicinal substances taken from stones, minerals, metals, plants, herbs, animals, vegetables, fruits, and cereal crops.[2] In his *Bencao Tujing* (*Illustrated Pharmacopoeia*), the scholar-official Su Song (1020-1101) not only systematically categorised herbs and minerals according to their pharmaceutical uses but he also took an interest in zoology.[3][4][5][6] For example, Su made systematic descriptions of animal species and the environmental regions they could be found, such as the freshwater crab species *Eriocheir sinensis* found in the Huai River running through Anhui, in waterways near the capital city, as well as reservoirs and marshes of Hebei.

Some sinologists see TCM of the last few centuries as part of the evolution of a culture, from shamans blaming illnesses on evil spirits to 'proto-scientific' systems of correspondence. Any reference to supernatural forces is usually the result of romantic translations or poor understanding and will not be found in the Taoist-inspired classics of acupuncture such as the Huang Di Nei Jing. The system's development has, over its history, been analysed both sceptically and extensively, and the practice and development of it has waxed and waned over the centuries and cultures through which it has travelled, and yet the system has still survived thus far. It is true that the focus from the beginning has been on pragmatism—not necessarily understanding of the mechanisms of the actions—and that this has hindered its modern acceptance in the West. This despite that there were times such as the early eighteenth century when 'acupuncture and moxa were a matter of course in polite European society'. TCM describes the modern practice of Chinese medicine as a result of sweeping reforms that took place after 1950 in the People's Republic of China. The term 'Classical Chinese medicine' (CCM) often refers to medical practices that rely on theories and methods dating from before the fall of the Qing Dynasty.

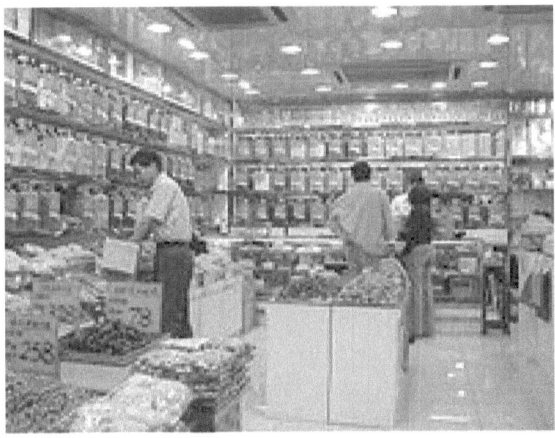

A Typical Tam Shop in Hong Kong

Ancient (Classical) History

The same philosophy that informs Taoist and Buddhist thought informs the philosophy of traditional Chinese medicine, which reflects the classical Chinese belief that the life and activity of individual human beings have an intimate relationship with the environment on all levels.

In legend, as a result of a dialogue with his minister Qibo the Yellow Emperor (2698–2596 BCE) is supposed by Chinese tradition to have composed his Neijing: Suwen or Inner Canon: Basic Questions (The book Huangdi Neijing, Yellow Emperor's Inner Canon's title is often mistranslated as Yellow Emperor's Classic of Internal Medicine. Modern scholarly opinion holds that the extant text of this title was compiled by an anonymous scholar no earlier than the Han dynasty, just over two-thousand years ago. During the Han Dynasty (202 BC–AD 220), Zhang Zhongjing China's Hippocrates, who was mayor of Chang-sha toward the end of the second century AD, wrote a Treatise on Cold Damage, which contains the earliest known reference to Neijing Suwen. Another prominent Eastern Han physician was Hua Tuo (c. AD 140–208), who anaesthetised patients during surgery with a formula of wine and powdered cannabis. Hua's physical, surgical, and herbal treatments were also used to cure headaches, dizziness, worms, fevers, coughing, blocked throat, and even a diagnosis for one lady that she had a dead fetus within her that needed to be taken out. The Jin dynasty practi-tioner and advocate of acupuncture and moxibustion, Huang-fu Mi (AD 215–282), also quoted the Yellow Emperor in his Jia Yi Jing c. AD 265. During the Tang dynasty, Wang Bing claimed to have located a copy of the originals of the Neijing Suwen, which he expanded and edited substantially. This work was revisited by an imperial commission during the eleventh century AD.

There were noted advances in Chinese medicine during the Middle Ages. Emperor Gaozong (r. 649–683) of the Tang Dynasty (618–907) commissioned the scholarly compilation of a materia medica in 657 that documented 833 medicinal substances taken from stones, minerals, metals, plants, herbs, animals, vegetables, fruits, and cereal crops.[2] In his Bencao Tujing (Illustrated Pharmacopoeia), the scholar-official Su Song (1020–1101) not only systematically categorised herbs and minerals according to their pharmaceutical uses, but he also took an interest in zoology.[3][4][5][6] For example, Su made systematic descriptions of animal species and the environmental regions they could be found, such as the freshwater crab species Eriocheir sinensis found in the Huai River running through Anhui, in waterways near the capital city, as well as reservoirs and marshes of Hebei. Some sinologists see TCM of the last few centuries as part of the evolution of a culture, from shamans blaming illnesses on evil spirits to 'proto-scientific' systems of correspondence.[8] Any reference to supernatural forces is usually the result of romantic translations or poor understanding and will not be found in the Taoist-inspired classics of acupuncture such as the Huang Di Nei Jing. The system's development has, over its history, been analysed both sceptically and extensively, and the practice and development of it has waxed and waned over the centuries and cultures through which it has travelled[9]–yet the system has still survived thus far. It is true that the focus from the beginning has been on pragmatism-not necessarily understanding of the mechanisms of the actions-and that this has hindered its modern

Timeline

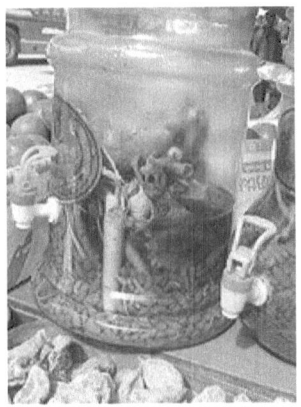

Macerated medicinal liquor with wolfberry, tokay gecko, and ginseng, for sale at a traditional medicine market in Xi'an, China. The history of TCM can be summarised by a list of important doctors and books.

- Unknown, *Huángdì nèijīng* (Yellow Emperor's Inner Canon)-Sùwèn and Língshū. The earliest classic of TCM passed on to the present.
- Warring States Period (fifth century BC to 221 BC): Silk manuscripts recording channels and collaterals, *Zubi shiyi mai jiu jin* (Moxibustion Classic of the Eleven Channels of Legs and Arms), and *Yinyang shiyi mai jiu jing* (Moxibustion Classic on the Eleven Yin and Yang Channels). The latter was part of a cache of texts found in Mawangdui in the 1970s.

9.3 Japanese Traditional Medicine—Kampo

Kampo medicine is the Japanese study and adaptation of traditional Chinese medicine. The basic works of Chinese medicine came to Japan between the seventh and ninth centuries. Since then, the Japanese have created their own unique herbal medical system and diagnosis. Kampo uses most of the Chinese medical system including acupuncture and moxibustion but is primarily concerned with the study of herbs.

Herbal medicines in Japan are regulated as pharmaceutical preparations, unlike other places such as the USA, Europe, etc., where most herbal preparations are regulated as dietary supplements (technically foods, not medicines). Both the industry and the government conduct extensive monitoring of agricultural and manufacturing processes as well as post-marketing surveillance to guarantee the safety of these preparations. Furthermore, access to Kampo herbal medicines is guaranteed as part of Japan's national health plan for each of its citizens. In the West, however, Kampo still remains a secret to all but a few. Kampo, like the traditional medicines of modern China, Vietnam, and Korea, has roots that extend back to ancient China's Han Dynasty (200 BC to AD 220). The term *Kampo* itself incorporates two characters: (kan) an adjectival modifier for things Chinese and (po) denoting 'way' or 'method'. Thus, Kampo means 'the way of the Chinese'. Although Kampo has developed within Japan's borders and within Japan's culture over the past 1,400 years, only recently have Kampo practitioners expressed interest in sharing Kampo's unique insights with the world. Approved kampo medicinesMain article: Kampo list

Today in Japan, Kampo is integrated into the national health care system. In 1967, the Ministry of Health, Labour and Welfare approved four kampo medicines for reimbursement under the National Health Insurance (NHI) program. In 1976, eighty-two kampo medicines were approved by the Ministry of Health, Labour and Welfare. Currently, 148 kampo medicines are approved for reimbursement. Rather than modifying formulas as in traditional Chinese medicine, the Japanese kampo tradition uses fixed combinations of herbs in standardised proportions according to the classical literature of Chinese medicine. Kampo medicines are produced by various manufacturers. However, each medicine is composed of exactly the same ingredients under the ministry's standardisation methodology. The medicines are therefore prepared under strict manufacturing conditions that rival pharmaceutical companies. In October 2000, a nationwide study reported that 72 per cent of registered physicians prescribe kampo medicine regulations, and therefore safety is much stronger and tighter for Japanese Kampo than Chinese traditional medicine due to strict enforcement of laws and standardisation.

Herbs Used in Kampo Medicines

Main article: Kampong herb list

The fourteenth edition of the *Japanese Pharmacopoeia* (JP) Nihon yakkyokuhō) lists 165 herbal ingredients that are used in kampo medicines. Lots of the Kampo products are routinely tested for heavy metals, purity, and microbial content to eliminate any contaminant. Kampo medicines are tested for the levels of key chemical constituents as markers for quality control on every formula. This is carried out from the blending of the raw herbs to the end product according to the ministry's pharmaceutical standards. Medicinal mushrooms like Reishi and Shiitake are herbal products with a long history of use. In Japan, the *Agaricus blazei* mushroom is a highly popular herb, which is used by close to 500,000 people.[1] In Japan, *Agaricus blazei* is also the most popular herb used by cancer patients.[2] The second-most used herb is an isolate from the Shiitake mushroom, known as active hexose correlated compound.

Kampo Outside Japan

In the United States, kampo is practised mostly by acupuncturists, Chinese medicine practitioners, naturopath physicians, and other alternative medicine professionals. The only available brand of the products in the United States is under Honso distributed by Honso USA, Inc. out of Phoenix, Arizona. In year 2002, Honso USA revealed its professional Kampo herbal formulas to licensed health care professionals in the United State. These products have been used by Japanese physicians under prescription for many decades. Kampo herbal formulas are studied under clinical trials, such as the clinical study of Honso Shosaikoto (HO9) for treatment of hepatitis C at New York Memorial Sloan-Kettering Cancer Center and liver cirrhosis caused by hepatitis C at UCSD Liver Center. Both clinical trials are sponsored by Honso USA, Inc., a branch of Honso Pharmaceutical Co., Ltd., Nagoya, Japan. The Kampo herbal combination Shosaikoto (SST) has been used extensively in China and Japan to treat chronic liver disease and other inflammatory diseases. Over 200 research papers have demonstrated SST's therapeutic roles of anti-inflammatory, anti-fibrotic, and chemopreventive properties that both preclinical and clinical research suggest are effective for various forms of liver diseases, including chronic hepatitis.

References

1. Wen Dan, Sho-saiko-to, a Clinically Documented Herbal Preparation for Treating Chronic Liver Disease, *HerbalGram: The Journal of the American Botanical Council*, Issue: 73 Pages: 34-43, 2007.
2. Rister Robert, *Japanese Herbal Medicine: The Healing Art of Kampo*. Avery, 1999. (ISBN 0-89529-836-8)
3. Tsumura Akira, Kampo: How the Japanese Updated Traditional Herbal Medicine, *Japan Publications*, 1991. (ISBN 0-87040-792-9).
4. Shibata Yoshiharu and Jean Wu, Kampo Treatment for Climacteric Disorders: A Handbook for Practitioners, *Paradigm Publications*, 1997. (ISBN 0-912111).

9.4 Indian Traditional Medicine—Ayurveda

Sanskrit *Āyurveda*, the 'science of life', or *Ayurvedic medicine* is a system of traditional medicine native to the Indian subcontinent and practised in other parts of the world as a form of alternative medicine. In Sanskrit, the word *Ayurveda* consists of the words *āyus*, meaning 'longevity', and *veda*, meaning 'related to knowledge' or 'science'. Evolving throughout its history, Ayurveda remains an influential system of medicine in South Asia. The earliest literature on Indian medical practice appeared during the Vedic period in India. The *Suśruta Saṃhitā* and the *Charaka Saṃhitā* were influential works on traditional medicine during this era. Over the following centuries, Ayurvedic practitioners developed a number of medicinal preparations and surgical procedures for the treatment of various ailments and diseases.

In Western medicine, Ayurveda is classified as a system of complementary and alternative medicine (CAM) that is used to complement, rather than replace, the treatment regimen and relationship that exists between a patient and their existing physician.[5]

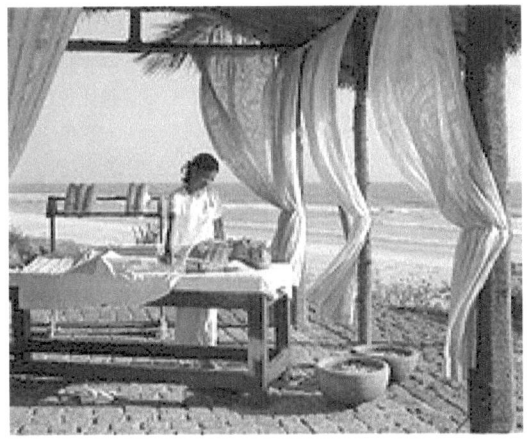

Traditional Indian Ayurvedic Spa in Goa

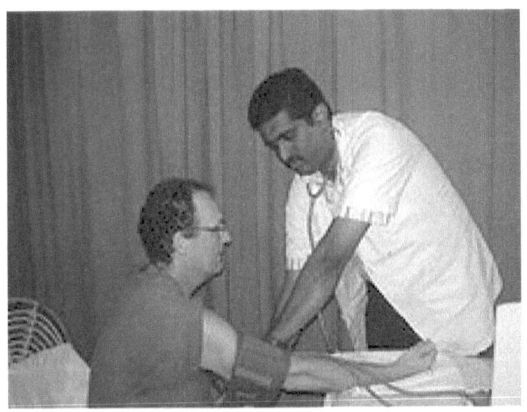

Ayurveda Doctor with Patient

Ayurveda is grounded in a metaphysics of the 'five great elements' (Devanāgarī: Prithvi—earth, Aap—water, Tej—fire, Vaayu—air, and Akash—ether)—all of which compose the Universe, including the human body.[1] Chyle or plasma (called *rasa dhatu*), blood (*rakta dhatu*), flesh (*mamsa dhatu*), fat (*medha dhatu*), bone (*asthi dhatu*), marrow (*majja dhatu*), and semen or female reproductive tissue (*shukra dhatu*) are held to be the seven primary constituent elements—saptadhatu (Devanāgarī: of the body.[6] Ayurveda deals elaborately with measures of healthful living during the entire span of life and its various phases. Ayurveda stresses a balance of three elemental energies or humours: *vata* (air and space—'wind'), *pitta* (fire and water—'bile'), and *kapha* (water and earth—'phlegm'). According to Ayurveda, these three regulatory principles—*Doshas* (literally that which deteriorates) are important for health, because when they are in a more balanced state, the body will function to its fullest, and when imbalanced, the body will be affected negatively in certain ways. Ayurveda holds that each human possesses a unique combination of *Doshas*. In Ayurveda, the human body perceives attributes of experiences as 20 *Guna* (meaning qualities).[7] Surgery and surgical instruments are employed.[7] It is believed that building a healthy metabolic system, attaining good digestion and proper excretion leads to vitality.[7] Ayurveda also focuses on exercise, yoga, meditation, and massage.[8] Thus, body, mind, and spirit/consciousness need to be addressed both individually and in unison for health to ensue. Several philosophers in India combined religion and traditional medicine—notable examples being that of Hinduism and Ayurveda. Shown in the image is the philosopher Nagarjuna—known chiefly for his doctrine of the *Mādhyamaka* (middle path)—who wrote medical works *The Hundred Prescriptions* and *The Precious Collection*, among others.[12]

Balance

Buddhism has been an influence on the development of many of Ayurveda's central ideas—particularly its fascination with balance, known in Buddhism as *Mādhyamaka*. Balance is emphasised; suppressing natural urges is seen to be unhealthy, and doing so may almost certainly lead to illness.[13] However, people are cautioned to stay within the limits of reasonable balance and measure.[13] For example, emphasis is placed on moderation of food intake[1], sleep, sexual intercourse, and the intake of medicine.[13]

Diagnosis

The Charaka Samhita recommends a tenfold examination of the patient. The qualities to be judged are as follows:

- Constitution
- Abnormality
- Essence
- Stability

- Body measurements
- Diet suitability
- Psychic strength
- Digestive capacity
- Physical fitness
- Age

In addition, Chopra (2003) identifies five influential criteria for diagnosis:

- Origin of the disease
- Prodrominal (precursory) symptoms
- Typical symptoms of the fully developed disease
- Observing the effect of therapeutic procedures
- The pathological process

Ayurvedic practitioners approach diagnosis by using all five senses. Hearing is used to observe the condition of breathing and speech. The study of the vital pressure points or marma is of special importance.

Hygiene

Hygiene is an Indian cultural value and a central practice of Ayurvedic medicine. Hygienic living involves regular bathing, cleansing of teeth, skin care, and eye washing.[6] Occasional anointing of the body with oil is also prescribed.

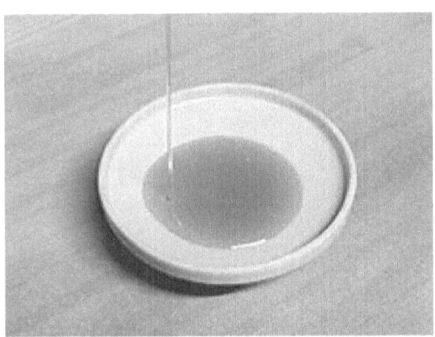

Oils such as sesame and sunflower oil are extensively used in Ayurvedic medicine. Studies show that both these oils contain substantial amount of linoleate in triglyceride form. Oils rich in linoleic acid may have antineoplastic properties.

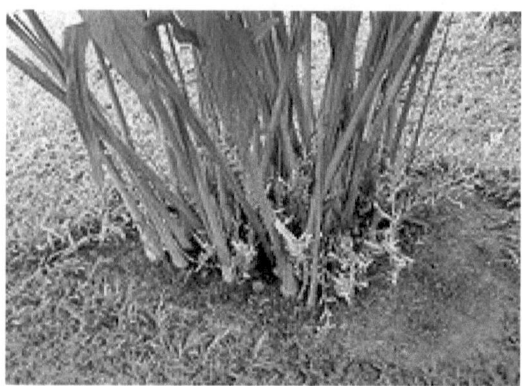

Hundreds of plant-based medicines are used in Ayurvedic medicine—including cardamom and cinnamon.

Treatments

Ayurveda stresses the use of plant-based medicines and treatments. [6] Hundreds of plant-based medicines are employed, including cardamom and cinnamon.[6] Some animal products may also be used, for example, milk, bones, and gallstones. In addition, fats are used both for consumption and for external use.[6] Minerals, including sulphur, arsenic, lead, copper sulphate, and gold, are also consumed as prescribed. This practice of adding minerals to herbal medicine is known as *rasa shastra*. In some cases, alcohol is used as a narcotic for the patient undergoing an operation. The advent of Islam introduced opium as a narcotic.[10] Both oil and tar are used to stop bleeding.[6] Traumatic bleeding is said to be stopped by four different methods: ligation of the blood vessel; cauterisation by heat; using different herbal or animal preparations locally which facilitate clotting; and different medical preparations which constrict the bleeding or oozing vessels. Different oils may be used in a number of ways including regular consumption as a part of food, anointing, smearing, *head massage*, and prescribed application to infected areas.

Shrotas

Ensuring the proper functions of channels (shrotas) that transport fluids from one point to another is a vital goal of Ayurvedic medicine, because the lack of healthy shrotas is thought to cause rheumatism, epilepsy, paralysis, convulsions, and insanity. Practitioners induce sweating and prescribe steam-based treatments as a means to open up the channels and dilute the Doshas that cause the blockages and lead to disease.

History

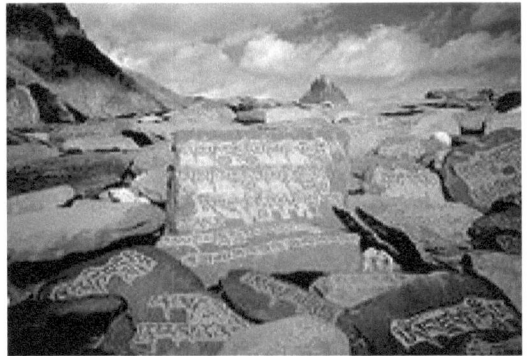

The mantra written on rocks.

Chanting mantras has been a feature of Ayurveda since the *Atharvaveda*, a largely religious text, was compiled. Around 1500 BC, Ayurveda's fundamental and applied principles got organised and enunciated. Ayurveda traces its origins to the Vedas, *Atharvaveda* in particular, and is connected to Hindu religion. *Atharvaveda* (one of the four most ancient books of Indian knowledge, wisdom, and culture) contains 114 hymns or formulations for the treatment of diseases. Ayurveda originated in and developed from these hymns. In this sense, Ayurveda is considered by some to have divine origin. Indian medicine has a long history and is one of the oldest organised systems of medicine. Its earliest concepts are set out in the sacred writings called the Vedas, especially in the metrical passages of the Atharvaveda, which may possibly date as far back as the second millennium BC. According to a later writer, the system of medicine was received by Dhanvantari from Brahma, and Dhanvantari was deified as the God of Medicine. In later times his status was gradually reduced, until he was credited with having been an earthly king.[6] The *Sushruta Samhita* of Sushruta appeared during the first millennium BC. Dwivedi and Dwivedi (2007)—on the work of the surgeon Sushruta—write:

The main vehicle of the transmission of knowledge during that period was by oral method. The language used was Sanskrit—the vedic language of that period (2000-500 BC). The most authentic compilation of his teachings and work is presently available in a treatise called *Sushruta Samhita*. This contains 184 chapters and description of 1,120 illnesses, 700 medicinal plants, 64 preparations from mineral sources and 57 preparations based on animal sources.

Underwood and Rhodes (2008) hold that this early phase of traditional Indian medicine identified 'fever (takman), cough, consumption, diarrhoea, dropsy, abscesses, seizures, tumours, and skin diseases (including leprosy)'. Treatment of complex ailments, including angina pectoris, diabetes, hypertension, and stones, also ensued during this period.[4][20] Plastic surgery, cataract surgery, puncturing to release fluids in the abdomen, extraction of foreign elements, treatment of anal fistulas, treating fractures, amputations, cesarean sections, and stitching of wounds were known. The use of herbs and surgical instruments became widespread The *Charaka Samhita* text is arguably the principal classic reference. It gives emphasis to the triune nature of each person: body care, mental regulation, and spiritual/consciousness refinement.

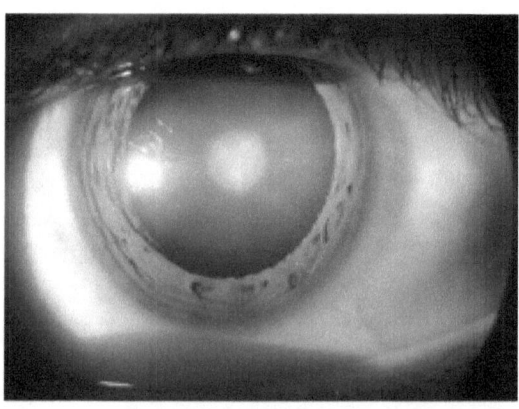

Cataract in human eye—magnified view
seen on examination with a slit lamp.

Cataract surgery was known to the physician Sushruta in the first millennium BC[21] and was performed with a special tool called the *jabamukhi salaka*, a curved needle used to loosen the lens and push the cataract out of the field of vision.[21] The eye would later be soaked with warm butter and then bandaged. Other early works of Ayurveda include the *Charaka Samhita*, attributed to Charaka The earliest surviving excavated written material which contains the works of Sushruta is the *Bower Manuscript*, dated to the fourth century AD . The Bower manuscript quotes directly from Sushruta and is of special interest to historians due to the presence of Indian medicine and its concepts in Central Asia.[23] Vagbhata, the son of a senior doctor by the name of Simhagupta,[24] also compiled his works on traditional medicine. Early Ayurveda had a school of physicians and a school of surgeons.[2] Tradition holds that the text *Agnivesh tantra*, written by the sage Agnivesh, a student of the sage Bharadwaja, influenced the writings of Ayurveda. The Chinese pilgrim Fa Hsien (*c.* AD 337–422) wrote about the health care system of the Gupta empire (320–550) and described the institutional approach of Indian medicine, also visible in the works of Charaka, who mentions a clinic and how it should be equipped.[26] Madhava (fl. 700), Sarngadhara (fl. 1300), and Bhavamisra (fl. 1500) compiled works on Indian medicine. [23] The medical works of both Sushruta and Charaka were translated into the Arabic language during the Abbasid Caliphate (*c.* 750).[27] These Arabic works made their way into Europe via intermediaries.[27] In Italy, the Branca family of Sicily and Gaspare Tagliacozzi (Bologna) became familiar with the techniques of Sushruta. British physicians travelled to India to see rhinoplasty being performed by native methods. Reports on Indian rhinoplasty were published in the *Gentleman's Magazine* in 1794.[28] Joseph Constantine Carpue spent twenty years in India studying local plastic surgery methods.[28] Carpue was able to perform the first major surgery in the Western world in 1815. Instruments described in the *Sushruta Samhita* were further modified in the Western World.

Current Status Within India:

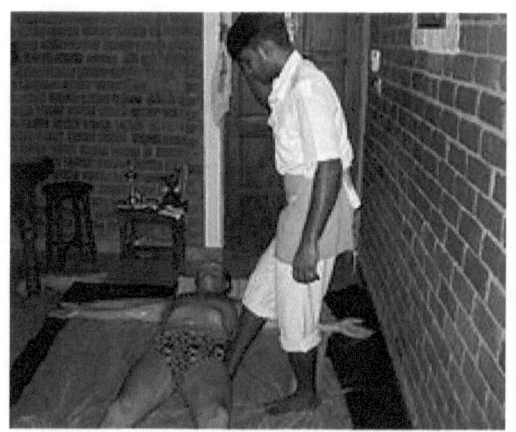

Foot Massage

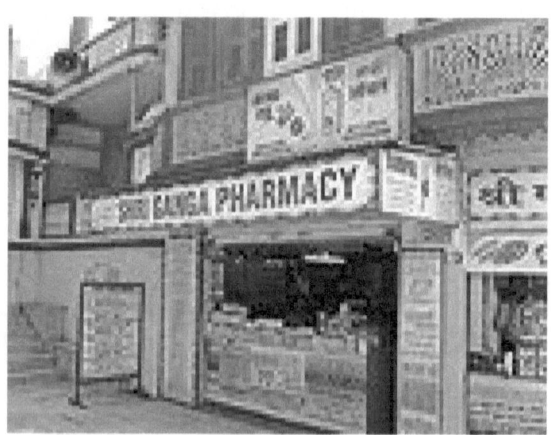

A Typical Ayurvedic Pharmacy, Rishikesh

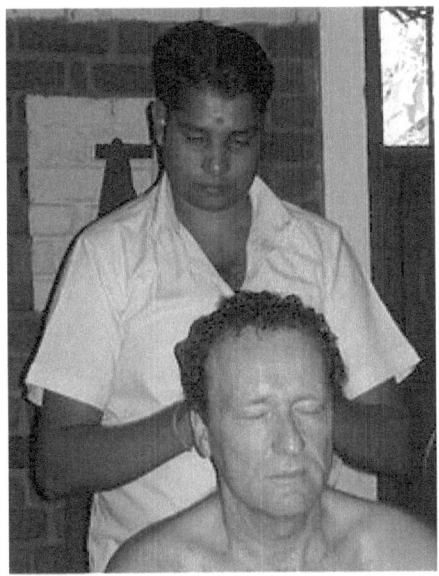

Head Massage

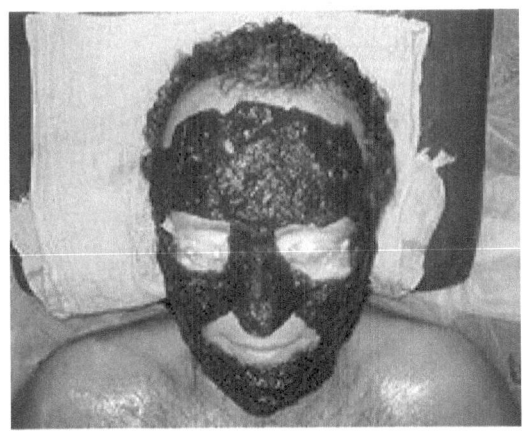

Facemask

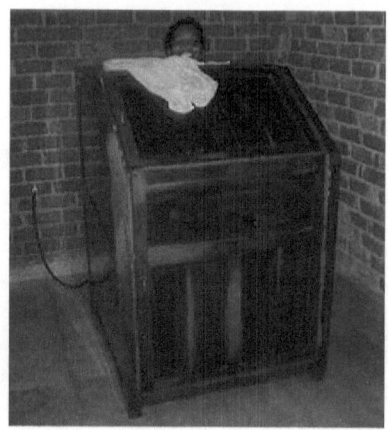

Steambox

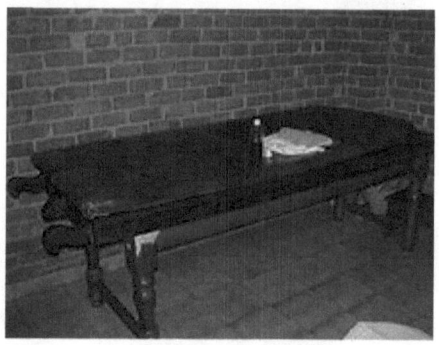

Massage Table

In 1970, the Indian Medical Central Council Act which aims to stand-ardise qualifications for Ayurveda and provide accredited institutions for its study and research was passed by the parliament of India. In India, over 100 colleges offer degrees in traditional Ayurvedic medicine. [8] The Indian government supports research and teaching in Ayurveda through many channels at both the national and state levels and helps institutionalise traditional medicine so that it can be studied in major towns and cities.[31] The state-sponsored Central Council for Research in Ayurveda and Siddha (CCRAS) is the premier institution for promotion of traditional medicine in India.[32] The studies conducted by this institution encompass clinical, drug, literary, and family welfare research. To fight biopiracy and unethical patents, the Government of India, in 2001, set up the Traditional Knowledge Digital Library as a repository of 1,200 formulations of various systems of Indian medicine, such as Ayurveda, Unani, and Siddha. The library also has fifty traditional Ayurveda books digitised and available online. Central Council of Indian Medicine (CCIM) a statutory body established in 1971, under Department of Ayurveda, Yoga and Naturopathy, Unani, Siddha and Homoeopathy (AYUSH), Ministry of Health and Family Welfare, Government of India, monitors higher education in Ayurveda.[36] The Bachelor of Ayurveda, Medicine and Surgery (BAMS) degree is the basic five-and-a-half year course of graduation. It includes eighteen different subjects comprising courses on anatomy with cadaver dissections, physiology, pharmacology, pathology, modern clinical medicine and clinical surgery, and paediatrics, along with subjects on Ayurveda like *Charaka Samhita*, history and evolution of Ayurveda, identification and usage of herbs (*dravyaguna*), and Ayurvedic philosophy in diagnostics and treatment. Many clinics in urban and rural areas are run by professionals who qualify from these institutes. Mukherjee and Wahile cite World Health Organisation statistics to demonstrate the popularity of traditional medicine as the primary system of health care.

Outside India

Academic institutions related to traditional medicine in India have contributed to Ayurveda's international visibility.[38] Kurup (2003) comments on the role of Gujarat Ayurved University:[38]

Several international and national initiatives have been formed to legitimise the practice of Ayurvedic medicine as CAM in countries outside India:

1. WHO policy of traditional medicine practice
2. The U.S. National Center for Complementary and Alternative Medicine
3. The National Institute of Ayurvedic Medicine
4. The National Ayurvedic Medical Association
5. The European Federation for Complementary and Alternative Medicine
6. The European Ayurveda Association

In 2009, the United States of America National Center for Complementary and Alternative Medicine (NCCAM) of the National Institutes of Health expended $1.2 million[45] of its $123 million annual budget on Ayurvedic medicine-related research. Due to different laws and medical regulations in the rest of the world, the unregulated practice and commercialisation of Ayurvedic medicine has raised ethical and legal issues; in some cases, this damages the reputation of Ayurvedic medicine outside India.[46][47][48]

Journals

A variety of peer reviewed journals focus on the topic of Ayurvedic medicine:

1. Ancient Science of Life
2. Theoretical and Experimental Journal of Ayurveda and Siddha
3. Journal of Research and Education in Indian Medicine (*JREIM*), AYU
4. The International Journal for Ayurveda Research

None of the journals except IJAR are PubMed indexed. The first subspeciality journal for the field of Ayurvedic medicine was launched in July 2010. It's focus is rheumatology and it is titled the *Journal of Clinical Rheumatology* in Ayurveda.

Patents

In December 1993, the University of Mississippi Medical Center had a patent issued to them by United States Patent and Trademark Office on the use of turmeric for healing. The patent was contested by India's industrial research organisation, Council for Scientific and Industrial Research (CSIR), on the grounds that traditional Ayurvedic practitioners were already aware of the healing properties of the substance for centuries and that this prior art made the patent a case of bio-piracy.[58] The Government of India had become involved in promoting traditional medicine by 1997.[3] R A Mashelkar, director-general of the Indian Council of Scientific and Industrial Research, made the following observation: 'This is a significant development of far-reaching consequences for the protection of the traditional knowledge base in the public domain, which has been an emotional issue for not only the people of India but also for the other third world countries.'

Scientific Evidence

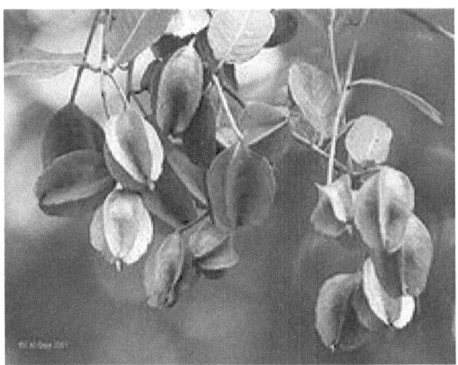

Chemical structure of curcumin used in Ayurvedic
medicine, shown here in its ketone form.

Research suggests that *Terminalia arjuna* is useful in alleviating the
pain of angina pectoris and in treating heart failure and coronary artery
disease. *T. arjuna* may also be useful in treating hypercholesterolemia.
As a traditional medicine, many Ayurveda products have not been
tested in rigorous scientific studies and clinical trials. In India, research
in Ayurveda is largely undertaken by the statutory body of the Central
Government, the Central Council for Research in Ayurveda and Siddha
(CCRAS), through a national network of research institutes. A systematic
review of Ayurveda treatments for rheumatoid arthritis concluded that
there was insufficient evidence, as most of the trials were not done
properly, and the one high-quality trial showed no benefits. A review
of Ayurveda and cardiovascular disease concluded that while the herbal
evidence is not yet convincing, the spices are appropriate, some herbs
are promising, and yoga is also a promising complementary treatment.
Some Ayurvedic products, mainly herbs used for phytotherapy, have
been tested with promising results. Studies suggest that turmeric and
its derivative curcumin are antioxidants.[64][65] *Tinspora cordifolia* has
been tested. Among the medhya *rasayanas* (intellect rejuvenation), two

varieties of *Salvia* have been tested in small trials; one trial provided evidence that *Salvia lavandulifolia* (Spanish sage) may improve word recall in young adults, and another provided evidence that *Salvia officinalis* (Common sage) may improve symptoms in Alzheimer's patients. In some cases, Ayurvedic medicine may provide clues to therapeutic compounds. For example, derivatives of snake venom have various therapeutic properties. Many plants used as *rasayana* (rejuvenation) medications are potent antioxidants. Neem appears to have beneficial pharmacological properties.

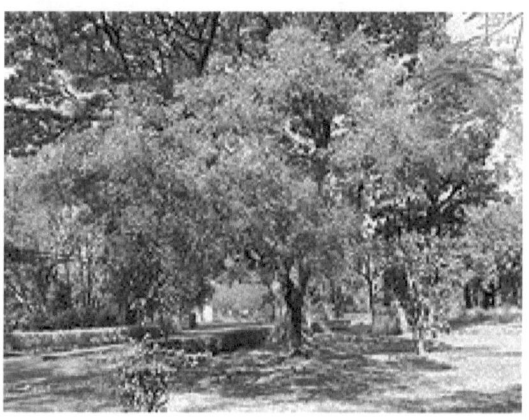

Azadirachta indica—believed to have immunopotentiating abilities and used often as an anti-infective—has been found to enhance the production of IL-2 and increase immunity in human volunteers by boosting lymphocyte and T-cell count in three weeks.

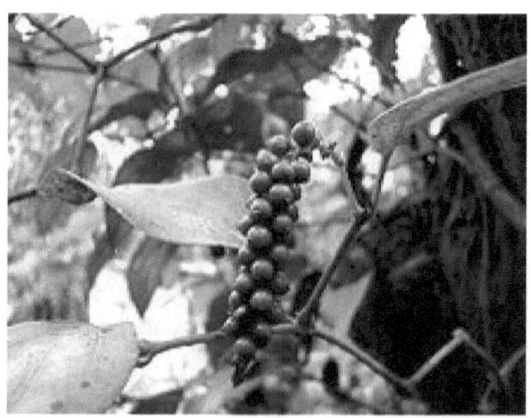

Black pepper and long pepper are combined with ginger to form the traditional *trikatu* mixture in Ayurveda. This mixture increases appetite, promotes the secretion of digestive juices, and cures certain gastric disorders, particularly achlorhydria and hypochlorhydria. Mitra and Rangesh (2003) hold that cardamom and cinnamon stimulate digestive enzymes that break down polymeric macromolecules in the human body.[16] Research suggests that *T. arjuna* is useful in alleviating the pain of angina pectoris and in treating heart failure and coronary artery disease.[60] *T. arjuna* may also be useful in treating hypercholesterolemia.

Safety

Rasa shastra, the practice of adding metals, minerals, or gems to herbs, is a source of toxic heavy metals such as *lead, mercury*, and *arsenic*. Adverse reactions to herbs due to their pharmacology are described in traditional Ayurvedic texts, but Ayurvedic practitioners are reluctant to admit that herbs could be toxic, and reliable information on herbal toxicity is not readily available. A 2004 study found such toxic metals in 20 per cent of Ayurvedic preparations that were made in South Asia for sale around Boston and extrapolated the data to the United States more broadly. It concluded that excess consumption of these products could cause health risks.[76] A 2008 study of more than 230 products found that approximately 20 per cent of remedies (and 40 per cent of rasa shastra medicines) purchased over the Internet from both U.S. and Indian suppliers contained lead, mercury, or arsenic. Traditionally the toxicity of these materials is believed to be reduced through purification processes such as *samskaras* or shodhanas (for metals), which is similar to the Chinese pao zhi, although the Ayurvedic technique is more complex and may involve prayers as well as physical pharmacy techniques. One medical journal reported: 'Crude aconite is an extremely lethal substance, yet Ayurveda looks upon it as a therapeutic entity.' Crude aconite is always processed, i.e. it undergoes 'samskaras' before being utilised in the Ayurvedic formulations. This study was undertaken in mice to ascertain whether 'processed' aconite is less toxic as compared to the crude or unprocessed one. It was seen that crude aconite was significantly toxic to mice (100 per cent mortality at a dose of 2.6 mg/mouse) whereas the fully processed aconite was absolutely non-toxic (no mortality at a dose even eight times as high as that of crude aconite). Further, all the steps in the processing were essential for complete detoxification. Following concerns about metal toxicity, the government of India ruled that Ayurvedic products must specify their metallic content directly on the labels of the product. The harmful effects of the samples are attributed in part to the adulterated raw material and lack of workers trained in traditional medicine.[82] In a letter to the Indian Academy of Sciences, director of the Interdisciplinary School of Health Sciences, University of Pune, Patwardhan Bhushan stated that metal adulteration is due to contamination and carelessness during the much faster modern manufacturing processes and does not occur with traditional methods of preparation.

9.5 Ancient Egyptian Traditional Medicine

This chapter surveys the traditional medicine as existed in the ancient Egypt and trace the journey to the modern times. The chapter also presents some information as how the early Egytian system of traditional medicine has influenced the development of the Chinese traditional medicine and all other societies.

We are being told that Paracelsus who lived in AD 1493-1541 was regarded as the founder of alternative medicine. This statement and claim can only be true as far as the German nation is concerned. As back as 2700-2600 BC Imhotep in Memphis, Egypt, was already practising traditional alternative medicine. It is held that his ancient medicine practice was the beginning of what is today known as modern medicine. Before this period in time, every other traditional medicine was learnt from the Greeks who learnt from Imhotep in ancient Egypt. It is very important that we acknowledge the real origin of medicine dating back to that period in time. The purpose of this section of the book is to expose the traditional medicine that existed during the ancient Egyptian periods. The second purpose is to show they applied preventive therapy within their practice. The third purpose is to trace the origin of medicine (herbal medicine) to them. It is known that most of the modern medical practices can find their origin in the ancient Egypt. Let us therefore see from the following information how this relates to that fact.

Until the nineteenth century, the main sources of information about ancient Egyptian medicine were writings from later in antiquity. Homer c. 800 BC remarked in the Ebers Papyrus treatment for cancer: recounting a 'tumor against the god Xenus'; it recommends 'do thou nothing there against'. Odyssey: 'In Egypt, the men are more skilled in medicine than any of human kind' and 'the Egyptians were skilled in medicine more than any other art.' The Greek historian Herodotus visited Egypt around 440 BC and wrote extensively of his observations of their medicinal practices. Pliny the Elder also wrote favourably of them in historical review. Hippocrates (the 'father of medicine'), Herophilos, Erasistratus, and later Galen studied at the temple of Amenhotep and acknowledged *the contribution of ancient Egyptian medicine to Greek medicine.*

In 1822, the translation of the Rosetta stone finally allowed the translation of ancient Egyptian hieroglyphic inscriptions and papyri, including many related to medical matters. The resultant interest in Egyptology in the nineteenth century led to the discovery of several sets of extensive ancient medical documents, including the Ebers papyrus, the Edwin Smith Papyrus, the Hearst Papyrus, and others dating back as far as 3000 BC. The Edwin Smith Papyrus is a textbook on surgery and details anatomical observations and the 'examination, diagnosis, treatment, and prognosis' of numerous ailments. It was probably written around 1600 BC but is regarded as a copy of several earlier texts. Medical information in it dates from as early as 3000 BC. Imhotep in the Third Dynasty is credited as the original author of the papyrus text and the founder of ancient Egyptian medicine. The earliest known surgery was performed in Egypt around 2750 BC. The Ebers papyrus *c.* 1550 BC is full of incantations and foul applications meant to turn away disease-causing demons and also includes 877 prescriptions.[5] It may also contain the earliest documented awareness of tumours, if the poorly understood ancient medical terminology has been correctly interpreted. Other information comes from the images that often adorn the walls of Egyptian tombs and the translation of the accompanying inscriptions. Advances in modern medical technology also contributed to the understanding of ancient Egyptian medicine. Paleopathologists were able to use X-rays and later CAT scans to view the bones and organs of mummies. Electron microscopes, mass spectrometry, and various forensic techniques allowed scientists unique glimpses of the state of health in Egypt 4,000 years ago.

9.6 Practices

Ancient Egyptian medical instruments depicted in a Ptolemaic period inscription on the Temple of Kom Ombo. Medical knowledge in ancient Egypt had an excellent reputation, and rulers of other empires would ask the Egyptian pharaoh to send them their best physician to treat their loved ones. Egyptians had some knowledge of human anatomy. For example, in the classic mummification process, mummifiers knew how to insert a long, hooked implement through a nostril, breaking the thin bone of the brain case to remove the brain. They also must have had a general idea of the location in the body cavity of the inner organs, which they removed through a small incision in the left groin. But whether this knowledge was passed on to the practitioners of medicine is unknown and does not seem to have had any impact on their medical theories. Egyptian physicians were aware of the existence of the pulse and of a connection between pulse and heart. The author of the Smith Papyrus even had a vague idea of a cardiac system, although not of blood circulation, and he was unable, or deemed it unimportant, to distinguish between blood vessels, tendons, and nerves. They developed their theory of 'channels' that carried air, water, and blood to the body by analogies with the River Nile; if it became blocked, crops became unhealthy, and they applied this principle to the body: If a person was unwell, they would use laxatives to unblock the 'channels'.[7]

Quite a few medical practices were effective, such as many of the surgical procedures given in the Edwin Smith papyrus. Mostly, the physicians' advice for staying healthy was to wash and shave the body, including under the arms, and this may have prevented infections. They also advised patients to look after their diet and avoid foods such as raw fish or other animals considered to be unclean.

Many practices were ineffective or harmful. Michael D. Parkins says that 72 per cent of 260 medical prescriptions in the Hearst Papyrus had no known curative elements,[8] and many contained animal dung which contains products of fermentation and moulds, some of them having curative properties,[9] but also bacteria posed a grave threat of infection. Being unable to distinguish between the original infection and the unwholesome effects of the faeces treatment, they may have been impressed by the few cases when the patient's condition improved.

Magic and Religion

Magic and religion were an integral part of everyday life in ancient Egypt. Evil gods and demons were thought to be responsible for many ailments, so often the treatments involved a supernatural element, such as beginning treatment with an appeal to a deity. There does not appear to have existed a clear distinction between what nowadays one would consider the very distinct callings of priests and physicians. The healers, many of them priests of Sekhmet, often used incantations and magic as part of treatment. The widespread belief in magic and religion may have resulted in a powerful placebo effect; that is, the perceived validity of the cure may have contributed to its effectiveness. The impact of the emphasis on magic is seen in the selection of remedies or ingredients for them. Ingredients were sometimes selected seemingly because they were derived from a substance, plant, or animal that had characteristics which in some way corresponded to the symptoms of the patient. This is known as the principle of *simila similibus* (similar with simila') and is found throughout the history of medicine up to the modern practice of homeopathy. Thus, an ostrich egg is included in the treatment of a broken skull, and an amulet portraying a hedgehog might be used against baldness.

Amulets in general were very popular, being worn for many magical purposes. Health-related amulets are classified as homeopoetic, phylactic, and theophoric. Homeopoetic amulets portray an animal or part of an animal, from which the wearer hopes to gain positive attributes like strength or speed. Phylactic amulets protected against harmful gods and demons. The famous Eye of Horus was often used on a phylactic amulet. Theophoric amulets represented Egyptian gods; one represented the girdle of Isis and was intended to stem the flow of blood at miscarriage. They were often made of bone, hanging from a leather strap.

9.7 Doctors and Other Healers

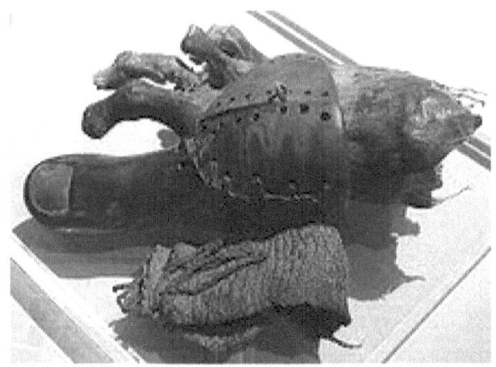

This wood and leather prosthetic toe was used
by an amputee to facilitate walking

The ancient Egyptian word for doctor is 'wabau'. This title has a long history. The earliest recorded physician in the world, Hesy-Ra, practised in ancient Egypt. He was 'Chief of Dentists and Physicians' to King Djoser, who ruled in the twenty-seventh century BC.[10] The lady Peseshet (2400 BC) may be the first recorded female doctor: She was possibly the mother of Akhethotep, and on a stela dedicated to her in his tomb she is referred to as *imy-r swnwt*, which has been translated as 'Lady overseer of the lady physicians' (*swnwt* is the feminine of *swnw*). There were many ranks and specialisations in the field of medicine. Royalty employed their own *SWNW*, even their own specialists. There were inspectors of doctors, overseers, and chief doctors. Known ancient Egyptian specialists are ophthalmologist, gastroenterologist, proctologist, dentist, 'doctor who supervises butchers', and an unspecified 'inspector of liquids'. The ancient Egyptian term for proctologist, *neru phuyt*, literally translates as 'shepherd of the anus'. Institutions, so-called *Houses of Life*, are known to have been established in ancient Egypt since the First Dynasty and may have had medical functions, being at times associated in inscriptions with physicians, such as Peftauawyneit and Wedjahorresnet living in the middle of the first millennium BCE.[11] By the time of the Nineteenthth Dynasty, their employees enjoyed benefits such as medical insurance, pensions, and sick leave.

The Egyptian Concept of Disease, Death, and Life

The Egyptians believed that disease and death were caused by a god, a spirit, or some other supernatural force. They had shamans—physicians, who would discover the particular entity causing the disease and then drive it out with magic rituals or talismans, as well as medicines. The duties of Egyptian physicians included creating medications, providing magic spells and prayers to provide healing, mending broken bones, dentistry, embalming, surgery, and autopsy. Physicians were often very specialised. From the tombstone of Iry, chief physician to a pharaoh of the Sixth Dynasty, we learn that he was also 'palace eye physician' and 'palace stomach bowel physician' and bore the titles 'one understanding the internal fluids' and 'guardian of the anus'.

A common disease among the Egyptians was the parasitic disease Schistosomiasis, an infection by the larval worm of a snail. Humans are infected when they come into contact with the free swimming worm, which is released by the snail into water. The worm burrows into the skin and enters the veins of the human host and causes anaemia, loss of appetite, urinary infection, and loss of resistance to other diseases. The commoners also suffered from the injuries and deformities caused by hard labour. They suffered from insect-borne diseases such as malaria and trachoma, an eye disease, small pox, measles, tuberculosis, and cholera. It is believed that there were occasional outbreaks of the bubonic plague spread along trade routes from the east. They contracted diseases such as trichinae, parasitic worms, and tuberculosis from their livestock. Leprosy, which had originated in Egypt, was relatively rare, possibly because of the immunity that tuberculosis sufferers have. Silicosis of the lungs, caused by breathing in sand particles, was a common cause of pneumonia for the ancient Egyptians. The ancient Egyptians also suffered from diet-related ailments such as malnutrition, vitamin and mineral deficiencies, dental abrasion, and ailments normal to all humans such as arthritis.

A great deal of our knowledge of ancient Egyptian medicine comes from the Edwin Smith Papyrus, the Ebers Papyrus, and the Kahun Papyrus. The Edwin Smith Papyrus and the Ebers Papyrus date from the seventeenth and sixteenth centuries BCE. These manuscripts are believed to be derived from earlier sources. They contain recipes and spells for the treatment of a great variety of diseases or symptoms. They discuss the diagnosis of diseases and provide information of an anatomy. They detail the ancient Egyptian concept of medicine, anatomy, and physiology. The Kahun Papyrus is a gynaecological text that deals with topics such as the reproductive organs, conception, testing for pregnancy, birth, and contraception. Among those materials prescribed for contraception are crocodile dung, honey, and sour milk. Thanks to the medical papyri, we know of many of the ancient Egyptian treatments and prescriptions for diseases. They call for the treatment of many disorders and the use of a variety of substances, plant, animal, mineral, as well as the droppings and urine of a number of animals. They knew how to use suppositories, herbal dressings and enemas, and widely used castor oil.

Honey and milk were used for the respiratory system as well as throat irritations. Honey, a natural antibiotic, was also widely used to dress wounds. Aloe vera was used to treat worms, relieve headaches, soothe chest pains, burns, ulcers, and for skin diseases. Frankincense was used to treat throat and larynx infections, stop bleeding, as well as treating asthma. Dill was used to soothe flatulence, also for its laxative and diuretic properties. Caraway was used to treat flatulence and as a breath freshener. Balsam apple or Apple of Jerusalem was used as a laxative. Garlic was believed to provide vitality, soothe flatulence, aid digestion, shrink haemorrhoids, and rid body of spirits. Camphor tree was used to reduce fevers, soothe gums, and treat epilepsy. Juniper tree was utilised to treat digestive ailments, soothe chest pains, and soothe stomach cramps. Mustard seeds were used to induce vomiting and relieve chest pains. Onions could be used to induce perspiration, prevent colds, and used as a diuretic. Parsley was used as a diuretic. Mint was used to soothe flatulence, aid digestion, stop vomiting, and as a breath freshener. Sandalwood was used to aid digestion, stop diarrhoea, and to treat gout. Sesame was used to soothe asthma. Poppy seeds were used to relieve insomnia, headaches, and as an anaesthetic. Thyme was also used as a pain reliever. *Resources:* Majno, Guido, *The Healing Hand*, Harvard University Press, Cambridge, 1975; Silverburg, Robert, *The Dawn of Medicine*, Putnam Publishing, New York, 1966; Dawson, Warren R, *The Beginnings, Egypt & Assyria*, Hafner Publishing Company, New York, 1964; Sanders, J B, *Transitions from Ancient Egyptian to Greek Medicine*, University of Kansas Press, Lawrence, 1963.

Ancient Egyptian Sanitation

Proper sanitation is an important factor in any city in order to address problems of health and sanitation. These issues were also important in the ancient world. The ancient Egyptians practised sanitation but in the widest sense of the word as modern technologies were not available to them. The degree of sanitation available to certain individuals varied according to their social status. Where did ancient Egyptians relieve themselves? If they had the means, bathrooms were built right in their homes. There is evidence that in the New Kingdom the gentry had small bathrooms in their homes. In the larger homes next to the master bedroom, there was a bathroom that consisted of a shallow stone tub that the person stood in and had water poured over him. There is no evidence that the common people had bathrooms in their homes. In modern society a sanitation company picks up our weekly refuse. In ancient Egyptian, it was the responsibility of each household to dispose of their garbage at the communal dump—the irrigation canals. As a result, these dump canals were breeding grounds for vermin and disease. Some homes in the cities may have had trays of earth for drainage and disposal of waste. For the most part, however, ancient Egyptians simply dumped their waste in canals or open fields. Water is an important part of any sanitation process, and the ancient Egyptians had plenty of water from the mighty Nile River and the irrigation systems built from it. Gathering water for individual homes was done by groups of women. The women went to the river or canal to get the water while the men actually worked in groups doing the laundry. The canals and river were also used by the common people for bathing purposes. The sanitation methods of the ancient Egyptians may seem crude when compared to the modern conveniences available in the twenty-first century. They did have what appears to have been a workable, viable sanitation system.

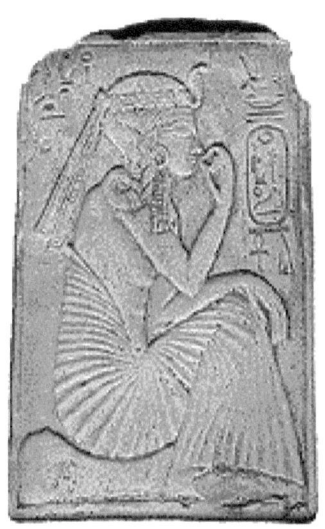

CHAPTER 10

T his chapter explores the Native American traditional medicine in existence long before the arrival of the Europeans in North America. This chapter also explains the historical development of

10.1 The Native American Traditional Medicine

The populations of the people who are now referred to as the Native Americans used to be called the Red Indians. These people are the indigenous original humans of what came to be known as modern America. Like the most parts of African continent, their culture and the major parts of their lives have been eroded by the European settlers and their descendants. In this presentation, we will see whether their practice of traditional medicine has any bearing with what is obtainable in Europe or African, and if so, what can we learn from them in terms of preventive therapy?

Native American medicine is a term that refers to the historical collection of information and treatment modalities of many different North American tribes, over thousands of years.

Many about the practices of these various peoples have been passed down through strictly oral traditions, a factor that makes documentation of its origin and initial use a relative mystery. What is known to date is that much of their existing medicinal knowledge was in use when the Europeans first visited this land more than 500 years ago. Some estimates suggest the first medical practices of the North American Indians some 40,000 years ago.

In a manner similar to that of TCM and Ayurveda, the approach of Native American medicine is one that takes all aspects of one's inner self, lifestyle, emotions, social setting, as well as their natural surroundings into consideration when recommending treatment.

The philosophy is one that strives to bridge the unseen relationships that exist between man and the natural world that surrounds him. At the core of the approach is a respect for the impact each has upon the other. The overall balance, and through it health, is a target that is achieved by taking into full consideration the forces that flow within, and without one's body, and in the growth of his/her understanding of the apparently simple truth that all life relies inherently upon all other life.

Native American medicine is a tradition that is rich in subtlety and difficult to document and communicate fully outside of its varied traditions and ceremonies. With a body of knowledge spread across hundreds of tribes, thousands of miles, and many years of unrecorded use, there is little that can be said to be standardised about its practice.

Although similarities in approach can be seen across the various tribes, the differences are also clear, often relative to the lifestyles and needs of each specific region, as well as the medicinal properties of those plants native to that region.

It has also been noted that even the approach of various practitioners within one tribe could differ significantly, based on the individualised and intuitive grasp each had on the world around him.

This lack of 'standardisation' was not seen as an indication of weakness surrounding the varied treatments but as an added strength, respecting each individual's connection with the natural world, and from that connection, their ability to offer a fuller and more all-encompassing approach to the treatment of those in need of healing.

The preferences of the patient are always respected within this cultural tradition. Its focus on a reverence for all things naturally designates the patient with a complete freedom to utilise their understanding and connections to enable a determination of their own path towards balance and ultimately towards healing.

Although many of the ceremonial practices of Native American medicine have survived centuries of tribal extermination and integration, one must presume that knowledge of profound value has been lost.

As a medical tradition never recorded in writing, the death of individuals designated to carry forward these practices to the generations that followed would immediately end a path of communication stretching back thousands of years, one ripe with information that can never be reclaimed.

In spite of this tragedy, what has survived intact to this day is a body of knowledge that continues to impact the health of both Native Americans and non-natives alike. Many common natural and pharmaceutical remedies make use of plants and herbs discovered and utilised by these peoples, for hundreds, if not thousands of years.

As the tide of medical theory begins to swing back towards an approach that recognises and respects every aspect of the individual, science and those in need search out the knowledge behind this highly regarded tradition, with the intent of an improved well-being for all.

10.2 The Historical Aspects of the Native American Traditional Medicine

The term *native American* suggests that the people who are now occupying the geo-economic land mass of America are neither native nor the original indigenous people of the place. These indigenous people are sometimes referred to as the American Indians. In fact, this is the appropriate term which could have been used to describe the indigenous people of South Africa instead of referring to them 'the Black Africans'.

Native American medicine refers to the combined health practices of over 500 distinct nations that inhabited the Americas before the arrival of Europeans at the end of the fifteenth century. Specific practices varied among tribes, but all of native medicine is based on the understanding that man is part of nature and health is a matter of balance. The natural world thrives when its complex web of interrelationships is honoured, nurtured, and kept in harmony. Native American philosophy recognises aspects of the natural world that cannot be seen by the eye or by technology but which can be experienced directly and intuitively. Just as each human has an immeasurable inner life which powerfully influences the well-being, so nature includes unseen but compelling forces which must be addressed and integrated for true balance to be achieved.

Native medicine may be as old as 40,000 years. The culture never developed the written language, so there was no documentation of Native American medicine until the Europeans arrived 500 years ago. Until recently, documentation has been limited to the observations of those outside the culture. Such writing describes the outward appearances of Native American medicine but cannot capture its rich subtlety and is therefore incomplete documentation. Native medicine must be embodied in a lifestyle that honours all creation and cannot be reduced to an academic body of knowledge and technique. Native American elders generally decline opportunities to share knowledge for fear that their sacred knowledge would be exploited.

Those Who Carry the Teachings Outside the Culture Risk Excommunication

Intrinsically holistic to a degree, conventional medicine is only beginning to conceptualise. Native American medicine addresses imbalance on every level of life, from the most personal inner life to the most overt behaviour. Disease is not defined by physical pathology, but viewed from an expanded context that includes body, mind, spirit, emotions, social group, and lifestyle. Without written language, native medicine never crystallised as a formal body of knowledge with standard practices. Native Americans understand that there are endless ways to achieve balance and that effective treatment is a marriage of a skilled, compassionate practitioner and committed patient. The uniqueness of each healer's approach is not simply tolerated, it is prized. Of equal importance is the patient's choice to heal. Patients' preferences are always honoured. To disregard them, or to use even subtle force, could never effectively establish harmony.

Native American medicine historically included many sophisticated interventions that have been lost in whole or in part, such as various forms of bodywork, bone setting, midwifery, naturopathy, hydrotherapy, and botanical and nutritional medicine. Ceremonial and ritual medicine is the largest surviving piece of Native American medicine. But it is still only a small part of what was available 500 years ago. An undocumented living tradition can only survive through living practitioners. As whole tribes died out, much traditional knowledge was lost. And as the number of indigenous Americans drastically decreased, so did native pride. More Native Americans took up European ways, especially the Christian religion. Fewer people took interest in keeping the traditions alive. There is evidence that some of this decline may be reversing. Native Americans are increasingly interested in preserving their culture, and healers from other perspectives are keen to learn ancient native wisdom traditions. Elder healers view interest from outside their culture with scepticism. Although some elders feel that sharing native medicine across cultures might help preserve it, most do not trust non-native cultures to honour the integrity of the teachings. Perhaps the power of Native American medicine is seen most dramatically in the fact that despite 500 years of tragic decline, it remains as fluid today as ever, a constantly evolving, living response to the needs of its people and the times.

Native American medicine is a complete system that addresses both healing and cure. Health requires balance in every sphere of one's life, from the most personal inner world to lifestyle and social connections. Native medicine places the roots of any imbalance in the world of spirit. Spiritual interventions are thus seen as critical to the success of any treatment plan. There are many ways to restore balance, and it is understood that each healer will have her own perspective drawn from her unique set of skills and life experience. Someone in need of healing looks for a practitioner who has been successful in similar situations. Native American understanding of harmonious balance is highly sophisticated. It demands that a unique treatment plan be designed to match the uniqueness of each case. From the Native American perspective, standardised practices, including even standardised fees, do not address the individual's needs and therefore compromise the integrity and power of the treatment. Although it is understood that the healing process is an exchange and involves a fee, native healers are proscribed from ever setting prices for their work. Native healers are aware that treatments are most effective when the patient is a deeply engaged participant. The process of negotiating a fee is often the beginning of the healing process.

The healing elder is the culture's primary access to healing power. In a system without technology and standardised practice, the responsibility for treatment failure falls squarely on the practitioner. There is simply no one else to blame. A practitioner who has too many failures loses the reputation as a powerful healer. Thus the medicine person is careful to evaluate each situation carefully; only on accepting those cases does he feel confident that he can help. He makes subtle assessments of the patient, knowing that subjective factors such as readiness to heal, value placed on treatment, and strength of will are powerful determiners of outcome. The client assesses his situation, makes an offer to the medicine practitioner, and waits to see if it is accepted. Negotiations are never carried out face to face. The client might leave an offering outside the healer's door. If it is still there in the morning, the healer has not accepted the case. The patient can go elsewhere or make another offering. Once the healer and patient come to an agreement, treatment may start with a behavioural prescription to strengthen the client's commitment, such as performing a selfless act, making amends with an estranged family member, or climbing a sacred mountain. The hierarchy of interventions chosen depends on the healer, the family, and the situation. Native healers choose the simplest interventions judged effective for a specific situation. Techniques commonly recommended include self-inquiry to identify what needs to be changed, lifestyle modification, herbs (echinacea, goldenseal, burdock root, sage, among others), prayer, various types of massage, and ceremonies such as sweat lodge and vision quest.

How It Works and When to Use It:
Different Theories on How It Works

Native American medicine works by returning the individual to a state of harmonious balance both within himself and in relationship to the outer world. This holistic approach seeks to create a change not only in pathology but also in the patient's understanding, a change towards healthier self-concept and greater appreciation of the world around him. Such growth supports the patient in necessary behaviour modifications. The healer's intention is that the person should not be simply cured of a disease, but transformed through the experience of disease.

Conditions It Works Best For

Native medicine recognises that true healing often requires technology as well as spirit. Although the spirit of native medicine survives, most of its healing technology has been lost with the decimation of the tribal culture over the last 500 years, the same period in which modern science was created. In recent history, conventional medicine has made astounding technical strides. Since Native medicine engages and prepares the patient for healing and the maintenance of health, it is useful in all situations, even when it alone may not be sufficient. Although herbal interventions must be used conservatively when pharmaceuticals are part of the treatment, spiritual interventions are never contraindicated. The following two patient stories illustrate a traditional Native American medicine approach to healing and the impact this type of intervention can have in shifting experience and opening up new possibilities of thought.

We sat in the hot, steamy darkness of the sweat lodge—Barb, her husband, the medicine man, and his helpers. Barb had come to explore why her breast cancer continued to spread, despite 'doing everything right'. On surface examination, she was. She attended yoga; fellow church members prayed for her regularly. She had the most famous oncologist in her region and the newest therapies. She had regular acupuncture, received intravenous vitamins, had healing massages, and ate a vegan diet. Nevertheless, her cancer continued to spread. We had travelled to South Dakota to visit a Native American healer. I was making my regular pilgrimage, and Barb had asked to join me. She thought a traditional healer might be able to turn things around for her.

We were at the point in the sweat lodge where the door opened, and the steam poured out. We cooled off while water made its slow passage, dipper by dipper full, around the assembled circle. Sonny, the medicine man, spoke quietly enough so that everyone listened. 'Big nose says to ask you what hasn't changed,' he said. 'He doesn't care what you have been doing. He wants me to ask you what hasn't changed.' Barb began to sob, spilling water from the battered, aluminum dipper that had just reached her.

'I'm still a failure,' she said. 'Not only am I a failure as a wife, a mother, and a lawyer,' she said, 'but I'm now a failure at healing myself as well.' Big Nose was Sonny's main spirit helper. In life, Big Nose had been Sonny's grandfather. Now Sonny relied upon him for instructions on how to heal. Sonny liked to kid us that he was a slow learner, saying that it had taken him thirteen years of vision quests before Big Nose had finally come to him to teach him about how he was to heal. For thirteen years, Sonny made the journey to the top of Bear Butte to sit for four days and nights, 'crying for a vision'. Finally Big Nose came. Through Sonny, Big Nose told Barbara that she was not a failure. Her problem lay in the bad things that she said to herself in a continual dialogue. Barbara agreed. Later we talked about what psychologists call 'negative self-talk'. Big Nose wanted that to stop. He said he didn't know if Barbara could get well or not, though he would ask. Nevertheless, he said, she was not a failure.

As a result of the sweat lodge, Barbara stopped many of her healing activities that kept her busy all day long and actually distracted from her need to feel good about herself. Sonny collected herbs that Big Nose told him might help. We prayed that Barb would be present with us in the sweat lodge in South Dakota at this same time next year. Sonny explained to her that it would be arrogant to pray for complete healing. That was up to God. We little people should consent ourselves with asking for another year of life. Later, Sonny took Barb to see Joe, who helped Sonny during times of trouble. Joe did a shaking tent ceremony for Barb and told her that she needed to live the next year as if it were her last. If you do that, he said, the spirits might give you another year. What were the herbs? Burdock root, golden seal, echinacea, bear root, and sage. All collected in the wild where they naturally grew. Joe did the sucking cure, where he symbolically sucked the cancer out of her body. He knew he didn't get it all, but thought that he had given her a head start in living fully for that next year. Considering these words, Barb decided to take her kids out of school and take a trip around the world. 'Live or die,' she said; her kids would have something they would always remember. 'We'll visit every great beach in the world.'

Or consider another woman who came to Arizona to work with a medicine man for healing. We went into the sweat lodge, and the medicine man asked her why she didn't like bakers. She was clueless about what he meant. 'Haven't you been to 20 different healers?' he asked her. Sure she said. This lodge was constructed of twisted palo-verde branches, smaller than could be built with the willow that grow naturally in South Dakota. We sat on desert sand, so different from the rich, black earth of South Dakota. The ceremony remained consistent, however, and we sat with the door open, taking a break from the heat and the nasal singing. 'It's like going to bakers and throwing away their bread because it's not what you want,' the medicine man said. 'Each of those bakers has made something wonderful for you,' he said. 'All of it is good, all of it is different. Some bake whole wheat, others sour dough, yet others pumpernickel,' he said. 'Any one of those breads could sustain you. Yet you throw their bread in the sand. You keep looking for the perfect bread, and you'll never find it. Just insult a lot of bakers.'

This conversation led the woman, who suffered from serious arthritis, to an understanding of the futility of her search. Ed, the medicine man, asked her to pick a healer and stick with him. Then he went into the desert and collected herbs for her. He asked her to bring her whole family, which she did. He performed a kind of intense massage, natural to his desert ancestors. He suggested foods she should eat, including corn, bean, and squash. He brought her special teas to drink. Medicine men understand that dramatic change is sometimes necessary to facilitate healing. In both cases, treatment was individualised to what was needed to facilitate that change. The change is considered primary. The herbs, the massage, and the prayers are secondary to support that change. Right relationships is a frequent Cherokee slogan for healing—correcting relationships to self, family, community members, and the spiritual world. Illness is seen as a consequence of relationship disturbance.

Training

Native American healers are traditionally trained as apprentices over an indeterminate, extended period of time. Students align themselves with a healing elder whom they trust to supervise their overall growth. The bond between elder and apprentice is profound, and elders do not readily accept students. There may be years of testing the student's intention and commitment before the dynamic stage of training begins. This preparation period is considered essential, a time in which the prospective apprentice learns patience, respect, and perhaps most importantly, how to receive knowledge.

Although Native Americans have adopted written language, native medicine continues to be an oral tradition. The wisdom of the elders is shared through stories and cannot be learnt in an academic setting. That technical knowledge which has survived the last 500 years is never separated from its natural context. Skills such as herbalism require finely tuned senses and the ability to commune with nature. Only through experience can students learn the intuitional skills that are necessary for successful treatment in this system. The chosen elder teacher judges the readiness of an apprentice to begin the practice of medicine.

Ethno-medicine

The field of ethno-medicine is a subsection of medical anthropology dealing with the common theme of disease treatment in all societies. All cultures have a system of knowledge and related practices that are passed down several generations. These practices pertain to the biological, social, and psychological aspects of every individual. It is a complex system of organising various illnesses and injuries relating to the body and the spirit. Ethnomedical practices are linked to environmental, biological, and cultural factors, which affect the pattern of disease recognition and the behaviour associated with certain illnesses (Levinson 1996: 436). According to the Encyclopedia of Anthropology (1996), ethno-medicine is defined as information specific to a given culture that allows its members to diagnose and categorise illness and trauma, explains their onset or cause, and seeks appropriate therapies for restoration or maintenance of patient (Levinson 1996: 436).

Western medicine is an exception to traditional ethno-cultural practices because it encompasses all cultural factors, while ethno-medicine refers particularly to practices which are culturally and geographically constrained. Systems of ethno-medicine emphasise that all things in life are interconnected, especially by a person's actions within the society (Levinson 1996: 437). Inappropriate social behaviour is often linked to the influence of spirits, dietices, witches, sorcerors, etc. who inflict disease or injury upon an individual as punishment. Depending upon the degree of knowledge, cultures differ in the reasoning of effective treatments for certain illnesses. Less-developed cultures tend to refer to religious taboos as the cause for the degree of bad luck in a person's health and well-being. Causes of disease are often related to the presence of a foreign object in a person's body or the disapproval of a spirit who has witnessed the patient's past behaviour. This provides a functional role for social behaviour within a society (Levinson 1996: 437). The knowledge accumulated by generations of indigenous sources provides a wide range of plant-based vocabulary and develops specific human-plant interactions. Specific plants with therapeutic benefits are categorised by smell, taste, texture, shape, and so forth (Levinson 1996: 438).

10.3 Japanese Traditional Medicine

The basic works of Chinese medicine came to Japan between the seventh and ninth centuries. Since then, the Japanese have created their own unique herbal medical system and diagnosis. Kampo uses most of the Chinese medical system including acupuncture and moxibustion but is primarily concerned with the study of herbs. Since the Chinese medicine originated from the Egyptian Africans, it follows therefore that even the Japanese medicine has the African origin.

Herbal medicines in Japan are regulated as pharmaceutical preparations, unlike other places such as the USA, Europe, etc., where most herbal preparations are regulated as dietary supplements (technically foods, not medicines). Both the industry and the government conduct extensive monitoring of agricultural and manufacturing processes as well as post-marketing surveillance to guarantee the safety of these preparations. Furthermore, access to Kampo herbal medicines is guaranteed as part of Japan's national health plan for each of its citizens. In the West, however, Kampo still remains a secret to all but a few. Kampo, like the traditional medicines of modern China, Vietnam, and Korea, has roots that extend back to ancient China's Han Dynasty (200 BC to AD 220). The term *Kampo* itself incorporates two characters: (kan) an adjectival modifier for things Chinese and (po) denoting 'way' or 'method'. Thus, Kampo means 'the way of the Chinese'. Although Kampo has developed within Japan's borders and within Japan's culture over the past 1,400 years, only recently have Kampo practitioners expressed interest in sharing Kampo's unique insights with the world. Approved kampo medicinesMain article: Kampo list

Today in Japan, Kampo is integrated into the national health care system. In 1967, the Ministry of Health, Labour and Welfare approved four kampo medicines for reimbursement under the National Health Insurance (NHI) programme. In 1976, eighty-two kampo medicines were approved by the Ministry of Health, Labour and Welfare. Currently, 148 kampo medicines are approved for reimbursement. Rather than modifying formulas as in traditional Chinese medicine, the Japanese kampo tradition uses fixed combinations of herbs in standardised proportions according to the classical literature of Chinese medicine. Kampo medicines are produced by various manufacturers. However, each medicine is composed of exactly the same ingredients under the Ministry's standardisation methodology. The medicines are therefore prepared under strict manufacturing conditions that rival pharmaceutical companies. In October 2000, a nationwide study reported that 72 per cent of registered physicians prescribe kampo medicines. Regulations, and therefore safety, are much stronger and tighter for Japanese kampo than Chinese traditional medicine due to strict enforcement of laws and standardisation.

Herbs Used in Kampo Medicines

Main article: Kampo herb list

The fourteenth edition of the *Japanese Pharmacopoeia* (JP) Nihon yakkyokuhō) lists 165 herbal ingredients that are used in kampong medicines. Lots of the Kampo products are routinely tested for heavy metals, purity, and microbial content to eliminate any contaminant. Kampo medicines are tested for the levels of key chemical constituents as markers for quality control on every formula. This is carried out from the blending of the raw herbs to the end product according to the ministry's pharmaceutical standards. Medicinal mushrooms like Reishi and Shiitake are herbal products with a long history of use. In Japan, the *Agaricus blazei* mushroom is a highly popular herb, which is used by close to 500,000 people.[1] In Japan, *Agaricus blazei* is also the most popular herb used by cancer patients.[2] The secondmost used herb, is an isolate from the Shiitake mushroom, known as active hexose correlated compound.

Kampo Outside Japan

In the United States, kampo is practised mostly by acupuncturists, Chinese medicine practitioners, naturopath physicians, and other alternative medicine professionals. The only available brand of the products in the United States is under Honso distributed by Honso USA, Inc. out of Phoenix, Arizona. In year 2002, Honso USA revealed its professional Kampo herbal formulas to licensed health care professionals in the United States. These products have been used by Japanese physicians under prescription for many decades. Kampo herbal formulas are studied under clinical trials, such as the clinical study of Honso Shosaikoto (HO9) for treatment of hepatitis C at New York Memorial Sloan-Kettering Cancer Center and liver cirrhosis caused by hepatitis C at UCSD Liver Center. Both clinical trials are sponsored by Honso USA, Inc., a branch of Honso Pharmaceutical Co., Ltd., Nagoya, Japan. The Kampo herbal combination Shosaikoto (SST) has been used extensively in China and Japan to treat chronic liver disease and other inflammatory diseases. Over 200 research papers have demonstrated SST's therapeutic roles of anti-inflammatory, anti-fibrotic, and chemopreventive properties that both preclinical and clinical research suggest are effective for various forms of liver diseases, including chronic hepatitis.

10.4 The Korean Traditional Medicine

We cure our people with our own medicines, using our medical materials that are abundant in North Korea. (Dr Hyun Chul, Koryo Medical Hospital, N. Korea.)

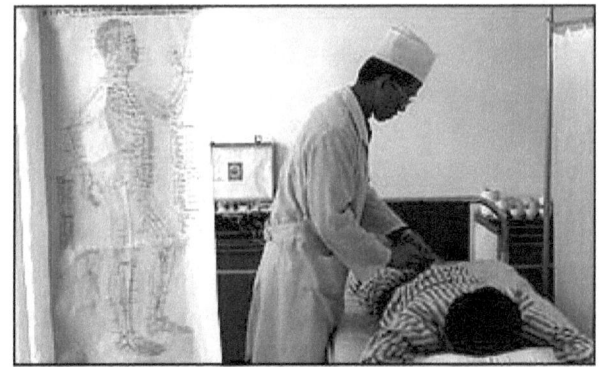

The Koryo Medicine hospital is seen as a showcase.

While countries around the world are increasingly turning to traditional and complementary medicine, Communist North Korea has had to do so more out of necessity than choice in recent years.

With many of the impoverished North's hospitals lacking essential drugs, the country's population has often had to rely on traditional medicines.

At the 500-bed General Hospital of Koryo, or traditional Korean, medicine, in Pyongyang, deputy technical director Hyun Chul shows me around.

He points out that the centre is not only a hospital, but a centre for treatment, scientific research, and training.

He says that about 1,000 people a day receive treatment and that more are turning to traditional medicine because of its benefits.

'There is no denying that there was a shortage of medicines in our country because of blockades and embargoes by foreign powers,' he says.

'But under the guidance of our leader, Kim Jong-il, we've been developing our traditional medicines and treatment.

'We cure people with our own medicines, using materials that are abundant in North Korea, with our own technology and our own doctors.'

Closed Doors

In one room of the spotlessly clean hospital, a young woman, Paek Yong-sun, tells a doctor about her health problems. She has come here to seek treatment as an outpatient. 'I was treated in the past for acute hepatitis,' she says. 'But I've come to this hospital now, as I've heard it is very good.'

The hospital is enormous, but I get no sense of bustle and activity. Most of the doors inside the huge building are closed to me. In one room, a patient is kitted out in an inflatable suit-the air pressure is increased to treat blood disorders.

In a neighbouring bed, a man is treated with a mix of injections, massage and cupping. Some of the treatments are not only plant based but include ingredients such as bear bile, says my guide. The state-run hospital now receives technical and administrative support from the World Health Organisation. WHO resident representative, Eigel Sorensen, says traditional medicine can play an important role-but points out that many of the claims are impossible to verify unless scientific research is published internationally.

I am told traditional medicine facilities exist across the country-but this hospital is clearly a showcase institution. And while many of North Korea's public hospitals are not equipped with what many would consider the basics-including clean water, medical equipment and essential drugs-much of the population is having to rely on traditional medicine in the absence of anything else.

10.5 The African Roots of Traditional Chinese Medicine

Tariq Sawandi, M. H.

Before discussing the principles of traditional Chinese medicine, I think it would be interesting to the readers and students of African holistic medicine to know of the African influence of ancient Chinese healing theory. The African role in early Asian civilisation has been submerged and distorted for centuries. Asia's African roots are well summarised in *African Presence in Early Asia* by Ivan Van Sertima/Runoko Rashidi and *African Presence in Early China* by James Brunson. The original Oriental people were blacks, and many of them still are blacks in southern China and Asia. The earliest occupants of Asia were 'small black (pygmies)' who came to the region as early as 50,000 years ago.

In *The Children of the Sun*, George Parker writes '. . . it appears that the entire continent of Asia was originally the home of many black races and that theses races were the pioneers in establishing the wonderful civilisations that have flourished throughout this vast continent.' Reports of major kingdoms ruled by blacks are frequent in Chinese documents. Chinese historians described the Fou Nanese people of China as 'small and black'. The Ainus, Japan's oldest known inhabitants, have traditions which tell of a race of dark dwarfs which inhabited Japan before they did. Historians Cheikh Anta Diop and Albert Churchward saw the Ainus as originating in Egypt! There is archaeological support for this. In addition, ancient Egypt and Mesopotamia records the 'Anu' (Ainu). The Anus are the same people who occupied Egypt for thousands of years. These same people are recorded to have made large migrations to the Asian continent taking with them thousands of years of African-Egyptian knowledge and influence.

This explains the existence of man-made pyramids in China and Japan! China's pyramids are located near Siang Fu city in the Shensi province. The Chinese do not know how they got there, but it is believed that Africans of the Nile Valley were the builders (J. Perry, *The Growth of Civilization*, p. 106, 107).

African Development of Ancient Chinese Medicine

Ancient Chinese medicine dates back to the Shang Dynasty founded by the African-Mongolian King T'ang or Ta (1500-1000 BC). The Shang (or Chiang) and Chou dynasties were credited with bringing together the elements of Chinese medical theory. The Shang were given the name of Nakhi (Na-Black, Khi-man). Under this black dynasty, the Chinese established the basic forms of a graceful calligraphy that has lasted to the present day. The first Chinese emperor, the legendary Fu-Hsi (2953-2838 BC) was a woolly haired black man. He is said to have originated the *I Ching*, or *The Book of Change*, which is the oldest most revered system of prophecy. It is known to have influenced the most distinguished philosophers of Chinese medicine and thought.

Many of the great concepts of Chinese medical science which was compiled during the Shang period were later developed during the Han Dynasty (168 BC to AD 8). During this period, medicine reflected the philosophical ideas associated in the earlier Chou and Shang period. The Han began to fuse Shang medical concepts with outlooks from the philosophical ideas of Confucius (551-479 BC). Towards that end, they generated a scheme which explained all phenomena in relation to the whole. Under this system, all natural phenomena including the human body and the organs were organised within the system of 'yin' and 'yang' and the 'five elements' or what is also called the 'five phases' theory.

Han Dynasty physicians created great classic works, such as the *Pen-ts'ao and the Nei Ching, or Yellow Emperor's Classic of Internal Medicine* (third century BC), drawing its inspiration from more ancient sources rooted in Afro-centric thought. (See diagram 1.)

Diagram 1. *The Nei Ching, The Yellow Emperor's Classic of Internal Medicine*, a medical book reportedly written in the second century BC before the birth of Hippocrates, the so-called father of Western medicine. According to Chinese legend, *The Nei Ching* was created through a dialogue between the legendary ruler Huang-Ti and his court physician, Chi Po. From *The Nei Ching*, thousands of books have been written about Chinese medicine.

Given these considerations, Chinese medicine echoes the logic of the ancient Egyptians, which viewed the universe as process-oriented in which there are no boundaries between rest and motion, time and space, mind and matter, sickness and health. The Chinese looked at reality as a unified field, an interwoven pattern of inseparable links in a circular chain called the Tao. From the Tao flowed all things and events in nature: seasons, colours, sounds, organs, tissues, emotions, climates, matters, and energies. (See diagram 2.) According to the Tao Te Ching, out of the one came the duality of Yin and Yang and the immaterial breath (chi), from which all physical matter and energy were created. This idea by Chinese philosopher Lao Tzu was borrowed from the earlier ancient Egyptian concept of 'Nu' (formless water)', the duality of Shu and Tefnut, and the Nahab Kau (tree of life).

Yin/Yang Theory and the Concept of Chi

Chinese medicine places primary emphasis on the balance of 'Chi' (Qi or Ki) or life energy constantly flowing throughout the body. There are twelve major meridians, or pathways for chi, and each is associated with a major vital organ or vital function. These meridians form an invisible network that carries chi to every tissue in the body. In health, it is properly balanced, but if it becomes unbalanced, the result is disease. It is the job of the Chinese doctor to restore the balance using diet, acupuncture, and herbal formulas.

The life energy comes in two but complementary parts: yin and yang. The yin nature includes the earth, moon, night, fall and winter, cold, wetness, the feet, the female sex, tissue growth, and a passive temperament. The yang counterparts are the heavens, the sun, day, spring and summer, heat, dryness, light, the head, the male sex, tissue breakdown, and an aggressive temperament. All individuals have both male and female polarities which consist of the combinations of yin and yang, requiring the Chinese doctor to tailor treatments to the individual's needs (See diagram 3.)

Diagram 3.

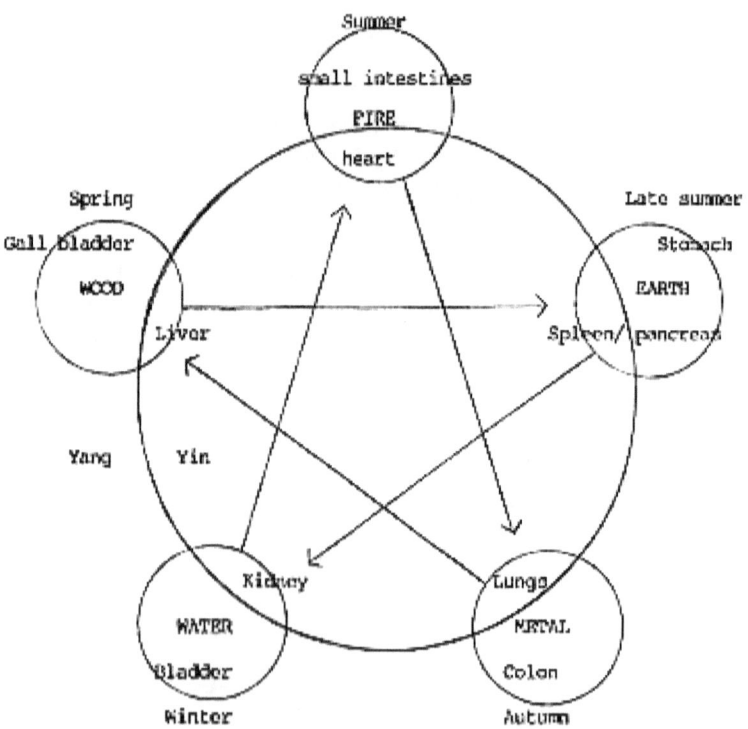

The Chinese 5-element System

The Chinese five-element system was heavily influenced by the ancient Egyptian's four-element conception. Each element relates to one season, one colour, and two organ systems, and they interact in subtle and complicated ways through the energy of chi.

An important part of the Chinese doctor's evaluation is the overall relationship between the yin and yang balance in the patient's body.

This is 'Chi'. Furthermore, we must bear in mind that yin and yang are complementary and not contradictory. There is no such thing as 'good' and the other 'bad'. Rather, one seeks to find a harmony between the two energies. The ancient Egyptians first put forward this idea, explained in terms of 'Shu' and 'Tefnut', the dual complementary energy that flows in the universe. It was later adopted by the founders of Chinese medicine to distinguish between the yin and yang qualities of a person's character or the constitution of one's illness.

The application of yin and yang is an important step in the process of making a traditional diagnosis and treatment.

Treating Conditions Through Chinese Medicine

Based on the assessment of the yin and yang energy imbalance, the Chinese herbalist looks for patterns of distress in the patient's pulse, as well as the tongue, face, and physical characteristics. The pulse system is highly developed in Chinese medicine and consists of six positions on each wrist, and various pulse beats can be determined by the trained practitioner. According to traditional Chinese medical text, the pulse corresponds to different organ networks, areas of the body, meridians or energy channels, and physiological processes like breathing, digestion, and elimination. These are thought to function in phase with yin and yang principles and also the energies represented by the five elements: earth, metal, water, wood, and fire. Some general diagnostic correspondence are:

In general, the basic treatment principles are to tonify or stimulate in a case of deficient yin or yang energy and to sedate or disperse when the energy pattern is one of excess. Herbal formulas are then tailored to fit the individual's need or designed to fit the overall condition of the patient.

Special herbal formulae have been traditionally used for thousands of years by Chinese herbalists for such ailments as fever, colds and flu, headaches, infections, menstrual problems, ulcers, high blood pressure, cancer, infertility, and diabetes to name but a few.

For example, 'Gan Mao Ling', a two-thousand-year-old formula, has been traditionally used for symptoms such as runny nose and scratchy throat. By taking six tablets of this formula every three hours, one can stop a cold in its tracks before it can take root. Chinese remedies are very effective and versatile. You can purchase Chinese herb formulas in many forms such as pills, tablets, extracts, or bulk to overcome numerous conditions and diseases. Today more than ever, Western doctors are bearing witness to the effectiveness of traditional Chinese medicine and are just beginning to realise that the Chinese masters understood profound aspects of the human mind and body without the aid of technology or sophisticated medical devices. China is heir to the secret healing arts which has been passed down by ancient Kamite (Africa). I feel that it is time that the Afrocentric roots of Chinese medicine be made public which has been ignored for too long. This and future articles seek to correct this oversight.

References

1. *The Destruction of Black Civilizations*, Chancellor Williams.
2. *The Missing Pages of History*, Indus Khamit Kush (Africa).
3. *The Five Lost Books of Africa*, Dr Khallid Al-Mansour.
4. *The Children of the Sun*, George Parker.
5. *African Presence in Early Asia*, Ivan Van Sertima/Runoko Rashidi.
6. *The Way of Herbs*, Michael Tierra.
7. *Chinese Herbal Medicine: Formulas and Strategies*, Dan Bensky and Randall Barolet.
8. *African Medicine: A guide to Yoruba divination and Herbal Medicine*, Tariq M. Sawand.

The people who live in The Bahamas are predominantly of West African descent, who were captured and forced into slavery on the cotton plantations in the Americas. Most white residents of the Bahamas are descendants of the first English settlers (English Puritans), who emigrated to Bermuda in 1647 to gain religious freedom and settled on the island of Eleuthera.

The culture is a melting pot of many native customs ranging from the indigenous 'Indian' people who populated the Bahamas, including West African, English, and other cultures who over the past three or four centuries arrived in the Bahamas. Cat's Claw, also called Uña de Gato, is a thorny liana vine reputed to be a remarkably powerful immune system booster and effective in treating a wide array of maladies. It has been proven to have anti-tumour, anti-inflammatory, and anti-oxidant properties. It has proven useful in treating arthritis, bursitis, allergies, and numerous bowel and intestinal disorders. There is some evidence that indicates effectiveness in relieving side effects of chemotherapy.

Cerasee

A tea made of the vine is used for diabetes, hypertension, worms, dysentery, and malaria and as a general tonic and blood purifier. It is also very effective to relieve constipation, colds, and fevers in children. Women in Latin American use the leaf for menstrual problems to promote discharge after childbirth. The tea is taken for nine days after giving birth to clean out and tone up all the organs involved in the delivery. Cerasee is also used as a natural method of birth control, by taking two cups each day after intercourse, for three days. It is said that women who drink Cerasee daily will not conceive during that time. As a wash, the tea is used externally for sores, rashes, skin ulcers, and all skin problems. A Cerasee bath is good for arthritis, rheumatism, gout, and other similar ailments.

Cockspur (Acacia cornigera)

Sometimes called the Bullhorn or Cow Thorn, this plant has a symbiotic relationship with an aggressive and painful species of ant (Pseudomyrmex ferruginea). The ants live in its thorns and protect the tree from encroaching plants, trying to grow near its trunk or leaves high in the canopy. The ants also emerge from the thorns to attack other insects, humans, and animals that come in contact with the tree. The Pseudomyrmex ferruginea ants have been used as a bush medicine for relief of mucous congestion in infants which are given water containing the ants (once they've been squeezed and strained). Snake doctors use the Cockspur bark and root to slow down snake venom from entering the bloodstream. Acne and other skin conditions can be treated by bathing in water in which the thorns have been boiled.

Copal (Protium copal)

This was a sacred tree of the ancient Maya who used the resin as ceremonial incense as well as to ward off evil spirits and the evil eye (it is believed that people can harm others by their envious glances). The resin was once widely used to treat tooth cavities. They would stuff it into the cavity, and several days later, the tooth broke and was removed. Bush doctors will make a powder from the bark to be applied to wounds, sores, and infections. The bark is also used in a tea (taken before each meal) to treat intestinal parasites. There are a lot of different varieties of ginger. For a more detailed description of the various plants, visit Nature Products Network's great web site.

Goat Pepper (Capsicum)

Used internally as a powerful stimulant, it is considered beneficial in exciting the appetite and also used externally as a counter-irritant. A leaf is slightly crushed and boiled to 'draw' it to a head.

Gumbo Limbo

While exploring the Belize, you may see a large tree with red shaggy bark that peels off in paper-thin strips. That's the Gumbo limbo tree, and its bark is a common topical remedy. Strips of bark are boiled in water and then used topically for skin sores, measles, sunburns, insect bites, and rashes or drunk as tea to treat backaches, urinary tract infections, colds, flu, and fevers. Young leaves rubbed on skin exposed to poison wood can prevent reaction and will soothe itching and speed recovery. The tree is a member of the same botanical species as frankincense and myrrh, both representatives of the world's oldest medicines. It is also the source of that very, very soft and light wood used for making toy airplanes and boats. In that form it is called balsa wood. Note: This tree is also known as the Gamalamee or Kamalamee tree. It is also called the sunburned tourists' tree. Tourists get burnt and peel, much like the red peeling bark on this tree. And this tree provides a cure!

Hurricane Weed (*Phyllanthus amarus*)

Called both Gale of Wind Weed and Hurricane Weed, the botanical name for this small annual herb is *Phyllanthus amarus*. It is also called the 'stone breaker plant' because it has been used for generations to eliminate gallstones or kidney stones. This plant is used for poor appetite, constipation, typhoid fever, flu, and colds. It's a popular herbal treatment because it has no side effects or toxicity. *Phyllanthus amarus* has been the focus of a great deal of research in recent years because its antiviral qualities may even be useful in treating hepatitis and the HIV virus.

Jackass Bitters (Neurolaena lobata)

Jackass Bitters is a well-respected plant that has been used widely in traditional Central American medicine. It has yellow flowers and bitter-tasting leaves which contain a potent anti-parasitic agent (sesquiterpene dialdehyde) that is active against amoebas, candida, giardia, and intestinal parasites. Traditionally, the herb is taken internally as a tea or a wine or used topically to bathe wounds and infections or as a hair wash to get rid of lice.

Jumbie Plant (wild tamarind)

The Jumbie Plant is used mostly to nourish cattle, but it is good for human ailments, too. As with most bush medicines, you boil the leaves from the plant and brew into a tea. If you've had a stressful day, a cup or two of the brew will calm you down. If, on the other hand, you're suffering from flatulence, the tea is said to have a calming effect on your stomach. Some folks drink the tea to strengthen their hearts.

Lignum Vitae (guiacum officinale)

One of the most versatile native trees is the Lignum Vitae, tree of life, or as many old folk call it 'Nigly Whitey'. Its glossy leaves are a rich green, and its abundant flowers range in colour from purple to blue. Virtually all parts of the tree are valuable, particularly its heavy, dense wood that was once used commercially in construction, until the tree became scarce. Its resin, called guaiacum, is obtained from the wood by distillation and is used to treat weakness and strengthen your back.

Limon Grass

A native from Sri Lanka and South India, lemon grass is now widely cultivated in the tropical areas of America and Asia. Its oil is used as a culinary flavouring, a scent, and a medicine. Lemon grass is principally taken as a tea to remedy digestive problems such as diarrhoea and stomachache. It relaxes the muscles of the stomach and gut and is plastered to the head to soothe a headache.

Provision Tree (Pachira aquatica)

Also known as Malabar Chestnut, Guiana Chestnut, and Saba Nut, this tree is sold commercially in the USA under the name Money Tree. It produces large, colourful flowers and fruits. The fruit can weigh up to six lbs and be a foot in diameter. The seeds can be roasted and eaten. Provision Tree bark is highly regarded as a blood tonic. A tea made by boiling its bark is used to help anaemia, low blood pressure, fatigue, and to generally build strength.

Pound-Cake Bush (Parthenium Hysterophorus)

It is used to combat 'weakness' and is also used for coughs and as a wash for skin sores. The flowers are sometimes 'parched' and sprinkled on skin sores. It is also made into a tea for diabetes.

Sarsaparilla

Brought from the New World to Spain in 1563, sarsaparilla was heralded as a cure for syphilis. In Belize, the herb has traditionally been used to treat a variety of skin problems. Sarsaparilla is anti-inflammatory and cleansing. It can bring relief to skin problems such as eczema, psoriasis, and general itchiness and help treat rheumatism, rheumatoid, arthritis, and gout. Sarsaparilla also has a progesterogenic action, making it beneficial in premenstrual problems and menopausal conditions such as debility and depression. In Mexico, the root is still frequently consumed for its reputed tonic and aphrodisiac properties. Native Amazonian peoples ta the manufacturing of birth control pills.

This write-up on the Native American traditional medicine is one of the most wonderful expositions written about the oppressor mechanism of suppression of the less privileged people. My acknowledgement of this will continue.

10.6 North Thailand Traditional Medicine

North Thailand traditional medicine is a living tradition with its roots stretching back many hundreds of years. Its tradition is oral, with training passed from traditional healers to student healers with no formal institutionalised training. The current traditional medicine base is mainly rural and within the smaller villages that make up larger centres such as Greater Chiang Mai. It is different from the more formalised Thai traditional medicine, which is centred on Wat Po in Bangkok and which has, in more recent years, attracted new students and certainly has the larger share of any 'official support'. Paralleling the North Thai traditional medicine are the traditional healers from the hill tribes. They comprise different tribal groups who have migrated to Thailand over the past few hundred years. The medicine traditions of the Lisu, Lahu, Hmong, Karen, and Akha hill tribes are also oral. Whilst each hill tribe has their own traditional medicine, they all share some commonality with each other and the Lanna Thai of North Thailand.

Traditional Medicine Specialities

Mor Muang is the general term for 'local doctor' and encompasses different traditional medicine specialities including Mor Ya (herbalist), Mor Pao (bone blower), and Mor Suang (spiritual healer). A predominantly male tradition, outsiders have to be accepted by a 'master' and then pass an initiation ceremony before being accepted into that specific traditional medicine discipline. Although an individual may be multi-skilled most individual healers focus on one particular speciality. The Mor Ya (herbalist) covers the whole disease spectrum and formulates scripts based upon herbs and other natural substances as a part of their traditional medicine. The Mor Pao (bone blower) specialises in wounds or broken bones. He often manipulates the bones and applies splints or poultices to the area around the fracture or wound and applies, by blowing, incantations to the affected area. The Mor Suang (spiritual healer) performs a series of ceremonies and incantations through calling on the spiritual essence of the client and connects with his spirit guides for assistance. Sometimes the healer may include specific referral to another traditional healer specialty and/or specific actions in order to alleviate the underlying cause of the ailment.

Other traditional Lanna Thai traditional medicine practioners include Mor Nuad (massage) whilst massage is an integral part of Thai traditional medicine home remedies; most often within the family, there are masseurs who have specialist styles and treatments. Both males and females can be Mor Nuad. Mor Tam Yae (midwives) are predominantly female and specialise in childbirth. The training is passed down through the family. In areas easily within the reach of Western medicine, this traditional medicine is rapidly disappearing. Mor Cao Baan (astrologers) are part of a mainly female healer tradition. They divine the causation of a particular ailment and may apply specific 'rubbing' ceremonies to effect a cure or refer the client to another traditional medicine specialist once the cause has been divined. Although the names for the specialists may vary, the North Thai hill tribes also feature many specialists similar to the Lanna Thai, and in addition there is a central role among many of the hill tribes for the village Shaman (Mor Pi) and soul retriever (Mor Kwan). The Mor Pi (Shaman) is the village connection with the spirit world where ancestors and spirits dwell. They are predominantly chosen by the spirits themselves through some near-death experience or divination by a group of village elders. Mostly they use trance in order to connect with their guiding ancestor spirits, and the treatment is effected in the spirit world and/or specific ceremonies are recommended to the client. Whilst similar to the Mor Pi, the Mor Kwan (soul retriever) rescues the spirit of the client when it has been 'stolen away' by a vengeful spirit causing an illness. Very specific curative rights and ceremonies are performed sometimes involving the whole family or village.

Concepts of Traditional Medicine Causality

The traditional healers have no tradition of surgery and therefore their concepts of causality of disease differ strongly from those in the Western medical tradition. Wind and blood are two strong causative factors and are often closely connected. The wind (lom) surrounds us all and is easily affected. There may be too much wind or too little, and it may turn poisonous. Diseases that cause fainting, uncontrolled movement, and heart pain are indicative of too much wind and are by far the most common. Certain foods and outside odours are said to be the cause of too much wind. Too little wind affects the mobility of limbs and is characterised by paralysis. Blood (lyad) is recognised as the basic fluid of the body, but as the healers have no tradition of surgery, the circulatory system is not well understood in a Western sense. It may be normal, hot, cold, too much, or too little and can be said to be the cause of many wind diseases.

Many diseases are affected by poison (Pid). This could be the direct poisoning from a venomous bite or ingestion of bad food but also the less tangible aspect of 'poison spirits'. This poison also has an affect on the blood and wind. Treatments are concentrated on isolating the poison, restricting its spread, and on herbal treatments for expelling it from the system. This may also involve a very prescribed diet. Diet restrictions are very integral to the whole curative process. Hot and cold, the two opposites are important in the classification of illness as well as the types of cures to apply. The client's perceptions of heat and cold are an important diagnostic tool for the healers. A fever for example may turn out to be hot, cold, or neither, and the healer proceeds with treatments indicated by these symptoms. The general rule is that hot diseases are treated with cold medicines and vice versa. The opposites of left and right, male and female, are also important in diagnosis as well as the presence of 'mother'. The 'mother' is a physical entity that enters the body and must be located and 'killed' before a cure could be affected. Most important is withholding the food that supports her, and once again diet becomes very important. Causality can be summarised as trauma, ingestion of materials alien to the body, exterior contact with materials alien to the body, bad food or food inappropriate to the client's body, noxious odours or fumes, insect and animal bites, intestinal worms, diseases caused by spirits, psychological factors, black magic, climate, seasons, age of client, and karma. In North Thai traditional medicine, the knowledge of disease has grown out of experience, and the knowledge used in their diagnosis and treatment is mainly from a symptomatic base.

The Future

Traditional medicine was, in fact, outlawed as unscientific with the advent of Western medicine in Thailand a century ago. As a result, the ancient knowledge was cast aside because practitioners were afraid of being arrested as charlatans. It was only recently that the ban was lifted and what had continued underground came slowly out into the open. The tradition of knowledge is passed on by word of mouth with no centralised teaching. Herbal remedies are closely held secrets; even to the fact that when recipes are written down some of the most potent ingredients might be deliberately left out. Students learnt from one 'master', usually in a narrow degree of specialty, and then widened their studies by working with more 'masters' as time went on and circumstances allowed. Will North Thai traditional medicine survive? In some middle-class and more educated circles traditional medicine has become 'trendy' and has received some support whilst in most government circles the support is ambivalent at best. Some see traditional medicine as a way of extending medical coverage without the cost or investment whilst in some areas traditional clinics are growing up alongside the Western medical centres. From the client's point of view, more is better. More choice!

The trend points towards clients seeking treatment along the lines of, first, visiting a pharmacy, second, a Western-style medical clinic, and third, a traditional healer. Anecdotal evidence shows clients using all forms of medical help simultaneously In the words of one healer, Phra Khru Uppakara Pattanakij, abbot of Nong Yah Nang Temple: 'We want to offer ordinary people more choices in health care. And we can do this by respecting the wisdom of our ancestors and keeping it alive by practicing it.' Although struggling, North Thai traditional medicine has every chance of survival and strengthening. A great influence on its success will be the healers and whether they can change some of their traditional secretive practices in order to create a centralised healing knowledge base and training program. We, in the West, have gone through a similar process in our past and now alternative healing and traditional medicine is gaining popularity each year. There is every reason to hope for a similar response in North Thailand.

CHAPTER 11

The Research Findings at the Portland Institute of Traditional Medicine

T his chapter discusses various research presentations at the Portland Institute of Traditional Medicine carried out by Dr Ubhut Aharmanada. This chapter also explains the uses and the relevance of the various research information exposed by each of the research findings. In each of research findings, the chapter directs us to the application of the information to the preventive therapies in question. This gives a brief background of the researcher—presenter Dr Subhuti Dharmanada.

About Dr Subhuti Dharmananda

Subhuti Dharmananda received his PhD in biology from the University of California in 1980. He travelled to China several times, the first visit was in 1977 and most recently in 2001, and has collected a large library of books and journals about traditional medicine. In addition to ITM, Subhuti Dharmananda helped initiate People's Herbs Incorporated, All-The-Tea Company, and Dharma Consulting International, and has been a consultant to several

11.1 The Portland Institute of Traditional Medicine

Portland is a city located in Maine, the Northwestern United States, near the confluence of the Willamette and Columbia rivers in the state of Oregon. The Institute for Traditional Medicine and Preventive Health Care, Inc. (ITM) is a non-profit 501(c)(3) organisation established in 1979, incorporated in 1983, and moved to its current head office in 1988. ITM was founded and is directed by Dr Subhuti Dharmananda, PhD ITM is dedicated to furthuring the knowledge, research, and education of traditional health care. Traditional medicine refers to ideas, experiences, and substances that have been handed down from generation to generation since ancient times, where the origins are obscure but where the continuity of basic understanding has been assured by a formal structure. Among the primary traditional medical systems still active today are the Chinese, Tibetan, and Indian (Ayurvedic). ITM enriches the lives of people seeking traditional medicine knowledge and services by clarifying the nature of traditional medicine and demonstrating how it can be utilised in the modern setting. To accomplish its goals, the institute performs six basic functions:

1. It operates two clinical facilities, the Immune Enhancement Project (IEP) and the An Hao Natural Health Care Clinic (An Hao). IEP is a low-cost treatment centre providing acupuncture, Chinese herb therapies, and Zen shiatsu primarily for patients with serious ailments (such as cancer and HIV), which can clearly benefit from effective adjunctive therapies, though all are welcome so long as they follow programme protocol. IEP serves as a charitable outlet for ITM's clinical activities. An Hao is a mixed therapy clinic, offering naturopathic medicine, acupuncture, chiropractic, Zen shiatsu, Chinese herbs, and modern medicine. It is a demonstration clinic that illustrates a potential new model for integrative health care. In addition, ITM provides consultation to other clinics that wish to follow the presentation method or the therapies that are available at these clinics. Selected students at local acupuncture colleges, particularly of the Chinese medical department of the National College of Naturopathic Medicine, can get advanced training at these clinics.

2. It provides numerous educational materials, primarily articles written by Subhuti Dharmananda. Currently, over 2,000 pages of such articles are in the ITM archive. Dr Dharmananda provides free consulting to practitioners who are members of the START Group to aid in their understanding of herbs, issues related to traditional medicine, individual patients, and practice methods.

3. It conducts background research in traditional medicine, including medical journal searches in China (carried out by Dr Fu Kezhi in Harbin) and computer searches here in the United States.

4. It provides specially designed herbal formulations (most in tablet form) for use in the ITM clinics and by practitioners who read ITM's literature. These formulas are described in the ITM book A Bag of Pearls and belong to the overall educational and training method of ITM, which is to integrate the study of Chinese medicine into the practice of Chinese medicine. *A Bag of Pearls* describes 200 formulas, most of them based on traditional Chinese medicine principles. ITM also maintains a pharmacy of dried extracts, following the method of herb use that is dominant in Japan, Korea, and Taiwan. These dried extracts (granules) are used to make personalised formulations or formulas that are used in doses higher than that suited to tablets.

5. ITM supports traditional environments where traditional medicine can be preserved. As funds are available, ITM has aided Tibetan, Indian, Chinese, Native American, Central, and South American groups that represent potential reservoirs of traditional medicine culture and resources. Most notably, ITM has provided funds to construct a health care clinic at the Drepung Gomang Monastic refugee camp in southern India and has helped this group of about 1,700 refugees in maintaining their traditional culture. A doctor trained in Tibet works at the clinic. ITM has also supported a licorice cultivation project in a remote area of China where the capability to develop herb cultivation is strong. Herb materials have been given to practitioners travelling to Hondurus, Guatamala, East Europe, India, and other destinations to provide traditional Chinese health care in areas of desperate need. ITM funds have aided the International Trust of Traditional Medicine in India.

6. It provides information to other organisations, such as the American Botanical Council, and to magazines, news reporters, and researchers, upon request. ITM is frequently cited as a source for reliable information on herbal therapies.

7. ITM has twenty-four employees: about half are part-time health professionals (mainly acupuncturists and massage therapists) and the other half are full-time office workers. ITM has affiliate organisations in Belgium and China. ITM is not a school and does not offer courses, certifications, or diplomas. It does not conduct clinical or laboratory research; it is not a foundation

(e.g. that might provide funding to students or others working in the field of traditional medicine). To better understand the work of ITM, please read several of the articles presented in this book below.

11.2 Amino Acid Supplements [1] Glutamine Com

Subhuti Dharmananda, PhD, Director

Background

Glutamine and the closely-related compound glutamate are two amino acids that are critical to human health. In humans, animals, and plants, glutamine and glutamate are transformed into each other as part of numerous physiological processes. The roles of these amino acids in human diseases were intensively researched during the past decade and continue to be the subject of scrutiny. One area of interest is their potential health effects when they are provided in addition to the normal dietary intake that is already several grams per day. Glutamine has been recommended by nutritionists as a dietary supplement for several serious disease conditions, and there is growing research support for this action. Hospital dietitians are aware of the value of administering glutamine in parenteral nutrition (IV nutrition) for critically ill patients, and especially for patients who have had intestinal surgery, but physicians rarely recommend glutamine supplementation in other situations for which it may be indicated. Therefore, it is valuable for other health care providers to be familiar with the over-the-counter availability and uses of glutamine for supplementation purposes.

Glutamate is also included in parenteral nutrition and is the major amino acid in certain protein-rich foods, such as eggs. Glutamate is a widely used flavouring agent, best known in the form of its sodium salt, monosodium glutamate (MSG). Harmful effects of localised high concentrations of glutamate in certain neurological disease conditions, such as multiple sclerosis and ALS, have been mentioned in recent literature. This has raised concerns about the safety of administering glutamine (which can be converted to glutamate), consuming foods with added glutamate, or including glutamate in the parenteral nutrition for such patients. In addition, there has been much concern expressed about possible allergic or other reactions to glutamate used as a flavouring agent. Therefore, it is valuable to understand the nature of its actions and its relationship to glutamine used as a supplement and the current status of the relevant research.

Glutamine

Glutamine is the most abundant of the amino acids in the human body. Its main storage site is in the musculature, where about 60 per cent of all the unbound amino acids are glutamine (glutamine makes up a smaller percentage of muscle protein, the main bound form). Glutamine has been called a 'conditionally essential' nutrient [1-6], because it is non-essential in normal situations (manufactured by the body in adequate quantities, not required in the diet), but in severe illness or injury it becomes insufficient (there is then a need for supplementation from the diet or other sources).

Dietary glutamine is especially prevalent in wheat and beans and in protein isolates, such as those used for making nutrition bars and beverages: Glutamine makes up 6-9 per cent (by weight) of soy protein and milk protein (casein, whey) isolates. Glutamine is manufactured in the body from glutamate and ammonia by the enzyme glutamine synthesis; the process takes place mainly in the skeletal muscles. The connection of glutamine to the musculature is of special interest. The amount of glutamine in reserve for release as needed is directly related to the muscle mass: More muscle mass means more glutamine is available for metabolic processes. It is possible that one of the benefits of muscle-building exercise for good health is the increased availability of glutamine during times of stress. Under conditions of metabolic stress, including injuries, illness, and even severe emotional distress, the level of glutamine in the body declines markedly, which is thought to adversely influence resistance to infectious diseases. Persons who maintain a relatively large muscle mass may have a greater ability to withstand and recover from stressful events. Chronic illness and lack of exercise work together in a vicious cycle: Poor health makes it more difficult to exercise, leading to lower muscle mass and lower glutamine stores, contributing to a higher incidence of health problems and slower recovery. Aside from lack of exercise (which may be a lifestyle choice or the result of paralytic or debilitating diseases and injuries), there are several muscle-wasting diseases, including cancer, AIDS, and pulmonary obstructive diseases. In such cases, glutamine levels can be insufficient and contribute to the overall pathology. This deficiency of glutamine, related to muscle wasting, may be partially rectified by consuming extra glutamine daily to replace the muscular manufacture of this amino acid. Additionally, glutamine administration at high doses may be associated with increased production of growth hormone, which contributes to increasing muscle mass.

The reasons that the body retains such high levels of glutamine are not fully known, though the number of biochemical reactions that take place in the body involving glutamine is quite large. Amino acids are defined, in part, by the presence of a nitrogen group in a small acidic molecule. Glutamine has two nitrogen groups, one of which, a terminal NH_2, is easily separated and transferred to other molecules (leaving glutamate as the amino acid, which has an oxygen atom in place of the extra nitrogen group). Glutamine has been described as the most important circulating nitrogen shuttle, accounting for about one-third of all amino acid nitrogen transported by the blood. By contributing to the formation of many useful compounds, the circulating glutamine brings metabolic fuel to the various organs (see Figure 1). It also transports ammonia in a non-toxic form for excretion (the ammonia is linked to glutamate to form the glutamine). In the kidneys, glutamate is the end product when the ammonia is released (to yield urea) under the control of the enzyme glutaminase. One of the well-established roles of glutamine in human health is its contribution to the integrity of the intestinal mucosa. This role is partly related to the fact that glutamine is a critical nitrogen source for rapidly dividing cells, such as those that line the gastrointestinal tract. The principal location of glutamine consumption in the body (i.e. where it is broken down to glutamate at the highest rate) is in the small intestine. During times of stress, the small intestine responds by utilising more glutamine and by more efficiently transporting glutamine that has been ingested.

One of the damaging effects of cancer chemotherapy is the inhibition of these cells that line the gastrointestinal tract, leading to a variety of adverse symptoms, such as nausea, loss of appetite, and reduced absorption of nutrients. Glutamine has been used therapeutically to protect against the toxic effects of methotrexate and other chemotherapy drugs. Glutamine is a useful adjunct to patients undergoing bone-marrow transplant procedures (e.g. intensive chemotherapy to prevent rejection), for which it is reported to improve recovery, reduce infections, and minimise complications. Intestinal surgery, such as that done to remove tumours or to remove ulcerated portions of the intestines, greatly damages the normal mucosal production, leading to slow healing. Glutamine has been used as a means of aiding recovery from intestinal surgery. Small intestine disorders, such as ulcers and bleeding (as occurs with Crohn's disease), may also benefit from extra glutamine administration. Glutamine should not be considered a cure-all for gastrointestinal disorders or any of the other conditions for which it has been indicated. Rather, if there are indications of glutamine deficiency (e.g. low muscle mass, high levels of stress, persisting and/or severe intestinal disorder), then it is a reasonable therapeutic strategy to apply. Glutamine is also considered important for the maintenance of the renal tubules, contributing to the healthy function of the kidneys. Glutamine's metabolic activities in the kidneys help assure elimination of acids from the blood. Although not yet a subject of research, kidney-damaging drug therapies might be made safer by providing extra glutamine, especially in patients who have low muscle mass.

As a fuel for rapidly dividing cells, glutamine makes a contribution to the immune system, especially in the rapid production of white blood cells during an infection. The immune system impairment that occurs after severe burns and surgical interventions is thought to be partly due to a rapid decline in glutamine that is part of the stress reaction, resulting in lowered immunological responsiveness. Supplementation of glutamine has been proposed as a means of preventing this consequence of injuries. Glutamine is already a therapy for patients with multiple organ failure and for multi-trauma patients. It has been reported that patients who require IV feedings due to advanced disease conditions show improvement in mood when glutamine is included in the solution. This change may be due to the improvements in overall physiologic conditions brought about by the higher glutamine levels.

The powerful antioxidant glutathione comprises three amino acids: glutamate, cysteine, and glycine. Glutamine is described a 'glutathione-sparing' agent, helping to maintain adequate levels of glutathione by providing adequate glutamate for its production. Glutathione deficiency tends to arise with glutamine decline (e.g. with muscle wasting) and is compensated for by administering glutamine. Glutathione is thought to contribute numerous protective effects from the adverse effects of oxidative stress and has been proposed, when administered as a supplement, to help inhibit the development of cancer, gastric ulcers, and other diseases.

While glutathione taken as a supplement is very expensive and poorly absorbed, glutamine is far less expensive and easily absorbed.

Dosage, Absorption, and Metabolism

The usual dose of orally administered glutamine for the various applications mentioned above is 0.5-0.57 g/kg of body weight, which is about 25-30 g per day for an adult who has low muscle mass (e.g. body weight of only 50 kg, about 110 lb). Recommended adult doses of glutamine taken orally range from as little as 5 g per day (roughly matching the dietary levels) to about 40 g per day (higher doses become impractical to administer and may provide no further benefits). The dosing is partly determined by body weight, with doses of 0.1-0.8 g/kg being given according to various recommendations; the largest amounts are usually reserved for cases where there is little dietary glutamine and a high need for it, such as after an intestinal surgery when the patient cannot eat ordinary foods. Because glutamine is efficiently absorbed in the small intestine, blood levels reach a peak within an hour after ingestion. IV administration of glutamine is only utilised when parenteral feeding is already required. Glutamine is available as a bulk powder that is essentially tasteless. Quantities of 5-15 g at a time can be consumed easily by mixing the powder in water, juice, or a blended drink. Encapsulated glutamine is probably ineffective due to the low dosage obtained by that method of administration (encapsulation also makes the material more expensive to use).

Glutamine is metabolised to other amino acids, including glutamate, alanine (the second-most abundant amino acid in skeletal muscle), citrulline, and arginine; in leucocytes, it can ultimately be metabolised to carbon dioxide. Following administration of glutamine, the increased blood content of the various amino acids that arises from glutamine metabolism returns to baseline after a few hours (about four hours with high dose administration). It is possible that some liver or kidney diseases may lead to difficulties in metabolism of glutamine, so that administration of the substance in high doses should only be undertaken after adequate evaluation of the patient's condition and with careful monitoring of the responses to the glutamine administration. When administered at high doses over a long period of time (e.g. for several consecutive days), the body's own production of glutamine declines in compensation. As a result, the blood levels of glutamine, though higher than they were prior to supplementation, do not rise beyond a certain point because of the compensation by lower production rates.

Glutamine and Cancer

The role of glutamine in cancer has been a topic of recent interest. On the one hand, glutamine seems to be the ideal treatment for the cachexia that accompanies tumour growth and the adverse reactions to chemotherapy. On the other hand, it has been found that tumour cells are capable of efficiently transporting glutamine and that this is one of their major respiratory fuels. Therefore, the question has been raised as to whether administering glutamine might not also be beneficial to the cancer. Thus far, all indications are that glutamine is useful as part of cancer therapy [7, 8]. In animal models, glutamine administration does not enhance the cancer growth. In order to help assure this outcome in human patients, chemotherapy can be given at the same time. As the cancer develops, it can compete with the rest of the body for the glutamine supply. The body's metabolism is forced to shift into high absorption of dietary glutamine and production of glutamine by the liver and other tissues. Attempting to block tumour growth by starving it for glutamine is not practical as the body will be starved of glutamine first. Using glutamine, analogues that will be taken up by the tumours in place of glutamine but which fail to nourish the tumour have been developed, but have not been found to be viable treatments as yet. Instead, it has been suggested that cancer patients be given supplemental glutamine so that their body levels can be maintained.

Summary of Applications of Glutamine

The potential applications for orally administered glutamine include the following: all wasting syndromes; cancer patients undergoing chemotherapy; inflammatory bowel diseases, especially of the small intestine (e.g. Crohn's disease); persons with wounds that are still healing (e.g. burns, injuries, surgeries); and persons with low muscle mass and chronic immune weakness revealed by frequent infections (note: glutamine administration is not intended to replace the recommendation for muscle-building exercise).

Glutamate

Glutamate is an amino acid similar to glutamine, but having a charged oxygen atom (making the compound negatively charged) in place of one of the neutral nitrogen groups. It is also described as glutamic acid, with glutamate being the free form (usually associated with one or more metals, such as sodium or potassium, to compensate the negative charge, making it a 'salt') and glutamic acid being the term for the bound form, in complex proteins. As described above, glutamine and glutamate are transformed back and forth during normal body metabolism. In the blood, glutamate is present at a level about 25 per cent that of glutamine. It is the third-most abundant amino acid in the blood; taurine is second (taurine is found in the free form but not in proteins). Unlike glutamine, there is little storage of glutamate in the muscles. In natural foods, glutamic acid is much more common than free glutamate, so the analysis of dietary amino acids is described in terms of glutamic acid content. It is found in all protein-containing foods, especially in animal products, such as cheese (cottage cheese provides about 6 g/cup) and meat (beef round steak provides 13 g/pound), but also in protein-rich nuts (almonds provide 8 g per cup) and beans.

Monosodium Glutamate

The glutamic acid containing foods are broken down to release glutamate in the digestive tract. Glutamate can be present in relatively large quantities in certain meals in the form of a flavouring agent, monosodium glutamate (MSG), which has found widespread use for nearly a century. Glutamate is also a significant component of hydrolysed vegetable proteins (proteins broken down to release some amino acids) used as flavourings. MSG enters some diets far more than others; for example, in the diets of Southeast Asia (e.g. Thailand, Hong Kong), the daily intake level for this compound reaches about 5 g, contributing about 4 g of glutamate to the other dietary sources. The presence of sodium in MSG is not relevant to the material's contribution of the amino acid glutamate. It does increase the total sodium in the diet, and it is relevant to the flavouring action of the compound. Because glutamate is a normal component of foods and a major amino acid in the body, there is no reason to expect any toxicity from consuming glutamate as a flavouring in the form of monosodium glutamate. However, reports of possible adverse responses to MSG, which led to the description of the 'Chinese restaurant syndrome' (a variety of discomforts described by some non-Oriental people after eating at a Chinese restaurant), gave rise to considerable research into its effects. Although a few early studies seemed to confirm the existence of a reaction (later dubbed the MSG symptom complex, since the compound can be found outside of Chinese restaurants and the reaction in the restaurants might be due to something else), almost all of the well-designed modern studies have found little or no effect.

In a frequently cited evaluation of acute toxicity, huge single doses of 10 g of MSG administered to volunteers produced no evidence of toxicity. As a result of this and long-term studies involving relatively high doses that appeared safe, there have been no limits placed on the quantities that can be used in food preparations (which are usually in amounts of only a few hundred milligrams per serving).

Rare hypersensitivity to MSG has not been ruled out, but repeated double-blind studies have shown little or no reaction to MSG among persons who considered themselves MSG-sensitive based on their own interpretations of experiences with foods. In particular, it had been suggested that MSG could worsen asthma and that it caused various allergy reactions, including skin rashes. A collection of recent research reports from around the world was published in the April 2000 issue of the *Journal of Nutrition*, and several other reports appeared in the *Journal of Allergy and Clinical Immunology* during the period 1998-2000. Among the conclusions were these: MSG has been suggested to cause postprandial symptoms after the ingestion of Chinese or Oriental meals. Therefore, we examined whether such symptoms could be elicited in Indonesians ingesting levels of MSG typically found in Indonesian cuisine . . . The study used a rigorous, randomised, double-blind, crossover design. The occurrence of symptoms after MSG ingestion did not differ from that after consumption of the placebo (Yogyakarta, Indonesia; [13]). MSG challenges in subjects with and without a perceived sensitivity to MSG failed to induce signs or symptoms of asthma. Therefore, in view of the poorly conducted studies that proposed that MSG-induced asthma and the subsequent studies that failed to confirm those findings, it is important to maintain a healthy scepticism about the existence of MSG sensitivity in individuals with asthma (La Jolla, California; [15]).

The existence of MSG-induced asthma, even in history-positive patients, has not been established conclusively (La Jolla, California; [16]).

MSG-induced asthma was not demonstrated in this study. This study highlighted the importance of adequate baseline and control data and indicated that such a rigorous protocol for individual assessment is feasible (Melbourne, Australia; [17]). In patients with chronic urticaria, the incidence of reactions to any additives, including MSG, is unknown . . . The dose of MSG given was 2,500 mg . . . We conclude, with 95 per cent confidence, that MSG is an unusual (less than 3 per cent at most) exacerbant of chronic idiopathic urticaria (La Jolla, California; [14]). Because human studies failed to confirm an involvement of MSG in the 'Chinese restaurant syndrome' or other idiosyncratic intolerance, the Joint FAO/WHO Expert Committee on Food Additives (JECFA) allocated an 'acceptable daily intake (ADI) not specified' to glutamic acid and its salts. No additional risk to infants was indicated. The Scientific Committee for Food (SCF) of the European Commission reached a similar evaluation in 1991. The conclusions of a subsequent review by the Federation of American Societies for Experimental Biology (FASEB) and the Federal Food and Drug Administration (FDA) did not discount the existence of a sensitive subpopulation, but otherwise concurred with the safety evaluation of JECFA and the SCF (Rome, Italy; [10]).

Results of surveys and of clinical challenges with MSG in the general population reveal no evidence of untoward effects. We recently conducted a multicentre, double-blind, placebo-controlled challenge study in 130 subjects (the largest to date) to analyse the response of subjects who report symptoms from ingesting MSG. The results suggest that large doses of MSG given without food may elicit more symptoms than a placebo in individuals who believe they react adversely to MSG. However, the frequency of the responses was low, and the responses reported were inconsistent and not reproducible. The responses were not observed when MSG was given with food. Controlled double-blind studies have failed to establish a relationship between the Chinese restaurant syndrome and ingestion of MSG, even in individuals reportedly sensitive to Chinese meals, and MSG did not provoke bronchoconstriction in asthmatics. Thus, high usage of MSG in ethnic cuisines does not represent a situation in which intakes might achieve unsafe levels, even among individuals claiming idiosyncratic intolerance of such foods (Surrey, United Kingdom; [11]).

In one of the earlier studies indicating the presence of a reaction to MSG [12], patients were first exposed to a very large 5 g dose of the isolated compound (as mentioned above, one could eliminate the erratic and minimal signs of reactions in careful testing when MSG is given with food). It was reported that the threshold dose (minimum amount) to get reactivity to MSG on rechallenge was 2.5 g (still a huge amount for a single ingestion). The authors of the study concluded that the symptom characteristics did not support a usual allergy-based reaction (IgE-mediated mechanism). Thus, while some evidence of reaction was found in this study, it was only with huge doses given without food; the purported basis of allergy of the reaction, which might explain claimed reactions to the small amounts present in some meals, was not apparent. Proponents of the idea that there is widespread occurrence of an MSG syndrome and overt MSG toxicity question the validity of all of the research indicating its safety, suggesting that information about adverse reactions is suppressed [18]. Nonetheless, diverse international efforts repeatedly find little or no reaction, especially when MSG is combined with food (the method of ingestion that is the basis for the claimed adverse responses). A lack of adverse reaction to glutamate, at least for most people, makes biological sense when one considers the high amounts of glutamate already in the body and its ready availability from foods as they are digested. Since glutamate is present in large concentrations in the tissues of the small intestine, where MSG and other dietary glutamate are absorbed, it is not surprising that a reaction to glutamate is elusive. In hospitalised persons who require IV nutrition, glutamate is often included in the nutrition mix to assure maintenance of normal blood levels of this nutrient; adverse reactions are not reported from that method of administration either.

Glutamate in Neurological Diseases

The other concern about glutamate is related to its essential role as a neurotransmitter. The levels of glutamate in the central nervous system (brain and spinal cord) are highly regulated, since the neurons have sensitive receptors for the compound. In some neurological diseases, it is found that glutamate levels in the central nervous system become unusually high at sites of pathology. This can occur, for example, if the rate of degradation of glutamate is slowed by an impairment of the enzymes that are involved. Also, glutamate is excreted by immune cells that take part in inflammatory processes; the result is high local concentrations at the neurons in progressive neurological diseases such as MS and ALS. Glutamate levels in the central nervous system can also increase when the blood brain barrier is substantially weakened, as occurs after neurological surgery. The excess glutamate at the neuron acts as a poison; at high enough levels, the nerves exposed to glutamate can be completely and permanently damaged so that they are no longer capable of transmitting signals. Thus, while glutamate is a major component of the body and an essential part of the nervous system, high levels localised in the nerve cells can be quite toxic, and this is readily demonstrated in animal models.

Laboratory research has revealed that in the progressive, debilitating disease ALS, one of the many processes involved in disease progression appears to be damage of nerve cells by accumulation of glutamate. In relation to multiple sclerosis, changes in control of glutamate homeostasis in the central nervous system might contribute to demyelination of the white matter of the brain [19]. Based on preliminary animal studies, it has been suggested that glutamate dumped by immune cells can exacerbate the nerve damage [20]. One of the means by which a stroke (causing blockage of blood circulation to the brain) results in brain damage is through an increase in glutamate levels in the brain cells (of course, oxygen deprivation and other effects are also contributors). These findings point to local glutamate excess as an important factor in brain diseases. The role of glutamate in neurological disorders has raised the question as to whether persons with such neurological diseases might have to be careful not to get high levels of either glutamine or glutamate via their diet and/or by taking glutamine supplements. Since glutamine is the main amino acid in the body and is produced by the body in response to deficiency, it is probably not possible to significantly lower the glutamine levels from the levels that already exist at the time of diagnosis. Indeed any attempt to significantly lower glutamine levels could lead to numerous adverse consequences. However, one can avoid excessive intake of glutamate by minimising ingestion of foods containing MSG and hydrolysed vegetable protein and by limiting the dosage of any glutamine supplementation. Glutamate levels in the blood increase slightly with high doses of supplemental glutamine administration (e.g. 15 g in a single dose) but not with moderate doses (e.g. 5 g in a single dose).

It is not known whether modification of dietary intake of glutamine and glutamate will have any effect on the degenerative brain disorders, since the mechanisms by which high glutamate content occurs in the brain may not be dependent on blood glutamate levels. However, the situation remains unclear, and questions have been raised for the case that would most likely involve alterations in blood levels: weakness of the blood brain barrier after surgery, which would allow the blood glutamate to influence the central nervous system levels and potentially exacerbate the brain oedema that occurs [21]. Until more is known about glutamine supplementation in relation to these brain diseases, it is recommended that patients who have nerve-damaging, chronic neurological diseases, such as ALS and multiple sclerosis, and those who have had recent neurological surgeries (such as for brain tumours) limit their intake of supplemental glutamine. A modest glutamine supplement level of about 5-10 g/day is likely to have some benefit in relation to muscle wasting, immune responsiveness, or intestinal disorders, without promoting increased glutamate levels in the blood. Even 10 g of glutamine is a small amount compared to the total body reserves that are already present, and studies show no significant glutamate increases in the blood after consuming such amounts. The higher levels of glutamine administration, commonly in the range of 15-30 g per day, might be reserved for patients who do not suffer from these neurological diseases.

Patients with neurological diseases who wish to avoid high glutamate levels should stay away from the meals that contain added glutamate in any large amount, but, as with glutamine, any attempt at total glutamate avoidance (including the form of glutamic acid in all protein foods) is neither possible nor necessary. The glutamate levels of the blood will be maintained at a certain level by normal metabolism even without adding dietary glutamate but can be increased significantly only by consuming large amounts of the amino acid. There may be specific chemical inhibitors of glutamate synthesis or glutamate uptake in neurons that would have a dramatic impact on the neurological diseases. It has been proposed that some drugs used experimentally to prevent brain damage from strokes (that function by inhibiting glutamate in neurons) might be of value in this regard.

Summary

Glutamine is an important body component that helps deal with several stressful situations, including the consequences of chemotherapy, burns (including radiation therapy burns), and injuries (including surgical injuries). Glutamine levels will naturally be high in persons who maintain a large muscle mass and ingest plenty of protein in their diet, but can become critically low in those who have little muscle mass (especially with muscle-wasting disease conditions) and limited dietary intake of protein. Glutamine supplementation appears to be an inexpensive, convenient, and potentially helpful means of promoting healing in those who are undergoing cancer therapies, suffering from intestinal diseases and surgeries, and recovering from injuries.

Similarly, glutamate is an important body component; it acts as a neurotransmitter, is part of the key antioxidant system glutathione, and is important for the transfer of ammonia. As with glutamine, it is present in adequate quantities in those with good muscle mass and a reasonably high protein diet. Glutamate is incidentally added to some foods in the form of MSG and hydrolysed protein flavourings, and there have been concerns raised that this leads to adverse allergy-type reactions. Thus far, a great body of research has shown that such reactions either do not exist or are very rare and not allergy-type reactions. Therefore, fear of this food component is usually unjustified. Glutamate at high enough levels in the central nervous system can cause nerve damage; these high levels are mainly the result of unusual situations such as autoimmune attacks against nervous system components (as occurs with MS and ALS) or following brain surgery. Since glutamine is converted to glutamate, supplementing glutamine at very high levels in persons who have such neurological disorders may be contraindicated. Therefore, glutamine supplementation in such individuals, if called for, should be limited to about 5-10 g per day until more is known; high glutamate meals should also be avoided in this situation.

References

1. Ziegler T. R., et al., Safety and metabolic effects of l-glutamine administration in humans, *Journal of Parenteral and Enteral Nutrition*, 1990; 14(4; supplement): 137S–46S.
2. Kaproth P. L., Glutamine: Current role in nutritional support, *RD*, 1992; 12(1): 1–8.
3. Lacey J. M. and Wilmore D. W., Is glutamine a conditionally essential amino acid? *Nutrition Reviews*, 1990; 48 (8): 287-309.
4. Young L. S., et al., Patients receiving glutamine-supplemented intravenous feedings report an improvement in mood, *Journal of Parenteral and Enteral Nutrition*, 1993; 17(5): 422-6.

5. Parry-Billings M., et al., Does glutamine contribute to immuno-suppression after major burns? *Lancet*, 1990; (336): 523-5.
6. Ziegler T. R., et al., Clinical and metabolic efficacy of glutamine-supplemented parenteral nutrition after bone marrow transplantation, *Annals of Internal Medicine*, 1992; 116(10): 821-8.
7. Souba W. W., Glutamine and cancer, *Annals of Surgery*, 1993; 218(6): 715-28.
8. Klimberg V. S., et al., Glutamine-enriched diets support muscle glutamine metabolism without stimulating tumor growth, *Journal of Surgical Research*, 1990; 48: 319-23.
9. Geha R. S., et al., Review of alleged reaction to monosodium glutamate and outcome of a multicenter double-blind placebo-controlled study, *Journal of Nutrition*, 2000; 130 (4S Suppl): 1058S–62S.
10. Walker R. and Lupien J. R., The safety evaluation of mono-sodium glutamate, *Journal of Nutrition*, 2000; 130 (4S Suppl): 1049S–52S.
11. Walker R., The significance of excursions above the ADL. Case study: monosodium glutamate, *Regulatory Toxicology and Pharmacology*, 1999; 30 (2 Pt 2): S119–21.
12. Yang W. H., et al., The monosodium glutamate symptom complex: assessment in a double-blind, placebo-controlled, randomized study, *Journal of Allergy and Clinical Immunology*, 1997; 99 (6 Pt 1): 757-62.
13. Prawirohardjono W., et al., The administration to Indonesians of monosodium glutamate in Indonesian foods: an assessment of adverse reactions in a randomized double-blind, crossover, placebo-controlled study, *Journal of Nutrition*, 2000; 130 (4S Suppl): 1074S–6S.
14. Simon R. A., Additive-induced urticaria: experience with mono-sodium glutamate, *Journal of Nutrition*, 2000, 130 (4S Suppl): 1063S–6S.
15. Woessner K. M., Simon R. A. and Stevenson D. D., Monosodium glutamate sensitivity in asthma, *Journal of Allergy and Clinical Immunology*, 1999; 1042 (2 Pt 1): 305-10.
16. Stevenson D. D., Monosodium glutamate and asthma, *Journal of Nutrition*, 2000; 130 (4S Suppl): 1067S–73S.
17. Woods R. K., et al., The effects of monosodium glutamate in adults with asthma who perceive themselves to be monosodium

glutamate-intolerant, *Journal of Allergy and Clinical Immunology*, 1998; 101 (6 Pt 1): 762-71.

18. Samuels A., The toxicity/safety of processed free glutamic acid (MSG): A study in suppression of information, *Accountability in Research*, 1999; 6: 259-310.

19. Matute C., et al., On how altered glutamate homeostasis may contribute to demyelinating diseases of the CNS, *Advances in Experimental and Medical Biology*, 1999; 468: 97-107.

20. Pitt D., Werner P. and Raine C. S., Glutamate excitotoxicity in a model of multiple sclerosis, *Nature Medicine*, 2000; 6(1): 67-70.

11.3 Appendix. Amino Acids: Exercise and Eat or Be Sedentary and Take Supplements

Most proteins found in nature comprise various combinations of just twenty amino acids. Of these, humans require eight amino acids (leucine, isoleucine, lysine, methionine, phenylalanine, threonine, tryptophan, and valine) as essential ones that cannot be manufactured in the body from other amino acids or other source materials. Some amino acids are conditionally essential, manufactured in the body and present in adequate amounts in most circumstances, but insufficient in some circumstances; examples are histidine and arginine, which cannot be produced fast enough during growth spurts in children and, therefore, are needed from the diet, and glutamine during physical stress, which may be insufficient for healing.

While all essential amino acids are found in the protein portion of foods, plant foods tend to be relatively deficient in one or more of the essential amino acids. By contrast, animal foods (meats and organs, milk, eggs) contain an amino acid profile that is fairly consistent with that required by humans. Therefore, those who consume animal foods regularly (including those vegetarians who avoid meat but consume milk and eggs) more easily get the full requirement of amino acids than those who consume no animal-source materials. In order to rely on vegetable protein sources alone and get ideal amino acid nutrition, one must skillfully combine a variety of vegetable proteins and consume an adequate quantity of them. Regardless of source, proteins are broken down to individual amino acids for metabolic use. Most modern nutrition texts suggest a daily protein intake that corresponds to 0.8 g of protein per kilogram of body weight so that an average 70 kg adult is advised to consume about 56 g of protein. With twenty amino acids in the proteins, the average amino acid intake is then about 2.8 g per amino acid. One can compare this average level to the amounts of amino acids recommended to be used as supplements, which are conservatively in the range of 0.8-1.6 g per day (higher amounts may be useful). Accordingly, one will typically add about 30-60 per cent to the dietary intake. Of course, if one relies on a lower dietary intake of protein, the supplements, at their suggested level, make up a larger percentage of the daily amino acid intake. Some amino acids are present in much larger quantities in the diet (e.g. glutamine) and are supplemented in much larger quantities (for glutamine, up to 30-40 g per day for special applications).

Advocates of vegetarian diets that limit or avoid milk and egg products have suggested that the textbook recommended level of protein intake is too high, by about a factor of two (thus, for example, suggesting a daily intake of just 30 g). Indeed, adults can survive on such low protein intake, but this is usually at the expense of not being able to carry out vigorous physical activity and with the risk of not maintaining adequate stores of amino acids that can help prevent several dysfunctions and diseases. Advocates of protein–rich diets (see, for example, *Enter the Zone* by Barry Sears, 1995 Harper Collins, New York) usually suggest high levels of physical activity, which can boost protein utilisation requirements to as much as twice the usual recommended amounts (e.g. about 100 or more grams/day for those with high body weight associated with increased muscle mass). Most of the individual amino acids have been recommended by nutritionists as supplements for alleviating various disease conditions or simply for optimising performance (e.g. athletes are told to consume certain amino acids in larger quantities to build muscles and shave time off competitive events; see Table 1). Supplementation is usually necessary only in cases where the diet has inadequate protein levels (with the correct balance of amino acid components) or where the disease condition has progressed to the point where simple dietary adjustment is not a viable option (especially in persons with limited appetite or tolerance for food).

Table 1: Sample amino acid supplement for athletes. One serving is 32.5 g of powder, derived from egg protein; *proline is technically an imino acid, similar to an amino acid. The total protein content is about 25 g per serving. Unlike other protein sources, eggs contain virtually no glutamine (glutamic acid takes its place).

Amino acid	Grams/serving
Glutamic acid	3.4
Aspartic acid	2.6
Leucine	2.1
Serine	1.8
Lycine	1.7
Valine	1.6
Phenylalanine	1.5
Alanine	1.5
Isoleucine	1.4
Arginine	1.4
Threonine	1.2
Tyrosine	1.0
Proline*	1.0
Glycine	0.9
Methionine	0.9
Cystine	0.7
Histidine	0.6
Tryptophan	0.3

The claimed benefits of amino acids, which include alleviation of depression and insomnia, reduced incidence of infections, and alleviation of inflammatory disorders, can usually be attained by following the advice of those who suggest high levels of physical activity with accompanying higher requirement for intake of foods (due to higher caloric utilisation), especially protein-rich foods. The sedentary lifestyle that has become dominant during the twentieth century and threatens the twenty-first century with increasing rates of obesity and accompanying metabolic diseases destroys health in many ways.

One of the modern concerns related to getting adequate dietary protein is that most protein sources are complexed with a considerable amount of fats. This mix of protein and fat occurs with most of the nuts, beans, and other vegetarian sources, as well as the fatty meats, dairy products, and eggs. New methods of raising food animals (reducing the fat content) and shifting to animal protein sources that normally have lower fat (such as fish) have reduced the problem of excessive fats from animal foods. Increasing evidence for benefits of the naturally occurring fats, especially those from vegetables and from fish, has reduced some of the concerns about total fat intake. Increased exercise also reduces the concern, since the fat goes into metabolic energy rather than pathological excess fat storage.

In essence, the best method of avoiding deficiencies in amino acids is through adequate exercise and the accompanying protein-balanced diet.

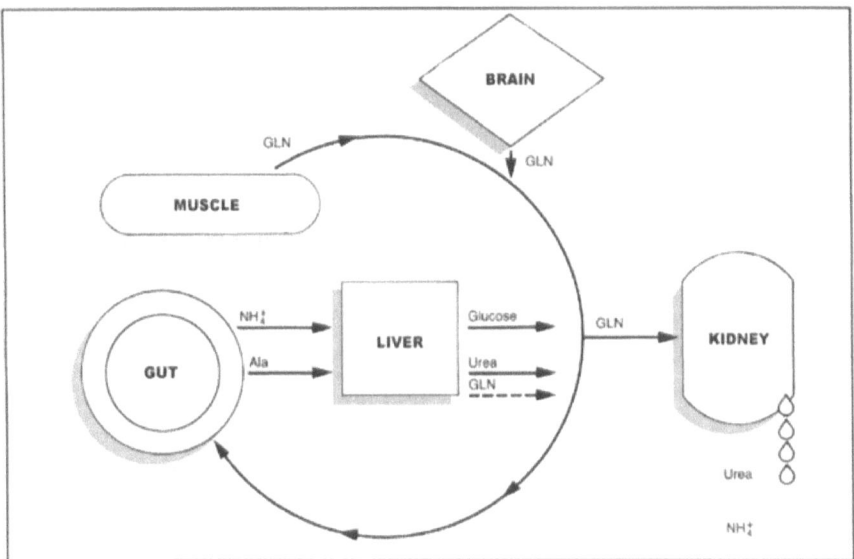

Figure 1 Some glutamine transfer pathways

11.4 Amino Acid Supplements IV: Theanine

Subhuti Dharmananda, PhD, Director

Theanine (l-theanine; see Figure 1 in the diagram below) is an amino acid found in ordinary tea leaves from *Camellia sinensis* (also known as *Thea sinensis*, hence the name theanine, pronounced like tea-anene). It is also found in other species of *Camellia* and in the edible bay boletes mushroom *Xerocomus badius* (see Figure 2 in the below diagram), but is otherwise rare in nature. L-theanine has the reputation for promoting mental and physical relaxation—decreasing stress and anxiety—without inducing drowsiness. In the beverage tea, it has an influence on taste (reducing bitterness) and is said to counteract some of the nervous agitation that can come with caffeine. Preliminary research, which needs to be carried much further before more specific claims for benefits can be properly made, suggests that l-theanine may be helpful for the following applications:

- improving learning performance, heightening mental acuity, and promoting concentration;
- acting antagonistically against high doses of caffeine;
- calming nervous agitation;
- lowering blood pressure;
- diminishing symptoms of PMS.

It has been indicated by laboratory studies that theanine produces these effects by increasing the level of GABA (gamma-amino-butyric acid), an important inhibitory neurotransmitter in the brain. GABA serves a sedative function that brings balance to excitability that can lead to restlessness, insomnia, and other disruptive conditions. Theanine also appears to increase levels of dopamine, another brain chemical with mood-enhancing effects, which can reduce blood pressure. To get adequate quantities efficiently, l-theanine is synthesised, based on the way it is synthesised in the tea plant [1-3]. The main manufacturer is Taiyo Kagaku Company of Japan, which produces 99 per cent pure amino acid. Theanine is a modification of the amino acid glutamine (see, 'Amino acid supplements I: Glutamine'), with an ethyl group added. It is simply made from glutamate as starting material:

Reaction: ATP + l-glutamate + ethylamine yields: ADP + phosphate + l-theanine. This reaction takes place in tea roots; the theanine thus produced is transported to the plant tops. The same reaction is used to synthesise l-theanine a commercial scale, using an enzymatic catalyst.

Clinical and Practical Applications of Theanine for the Nervous System

Theanine research began in the 1960s, and by 1964, the Japanese government approved use of theanine as a food additive for all foods except baby food. There are now more than fifty different food items that contain theanine sold in Japan, including soft drinks and chewing gum. It is included in these 'functional food' products to provide an anti-stress effect. The most active researcher investigating the pharmacology and applications of l-theanine is Hidehiko Yokogoshi, professor at the Food and Nutritional Sciences Department, University of Shizuoka. He has summarised the results of theanine effects this way: Of all amino acids found in green tea, l-theanine is the most prevalent. L-theanine is known as the umami component (a taste component, see next page) within green tea. When l-theanine is administered to rats, it is absorbed in the intestinal tract and delivered to each organ. It is also delivered concentration-dependently to the brain. Increase of dopamine levels and changes of serotonin levels by l-theanine have been observed. In various behavioural tests, including discrimination learning test, passive avoidance test, active avoidance test, Morris water maze test, elevated plus maze test, and locomotion tests, improvements in memory and learning performance with the administration of l-theanine have been observed. In human subjects, the activity of the parasympathetic nervous system increased. Also, alpha waves in the brain increased significantly, inducing relaxation. In addition to the relaxation, administration of l-theanine was found to alleviate the symptoms of premenstrual syndrome (PMS), especially the mental conditions associated with PMS The research on PMS was conducted at the University of Shizuoka; the comparison between l-theanine and placebo effects on the severity of symptoms has been displayed in the following graph:

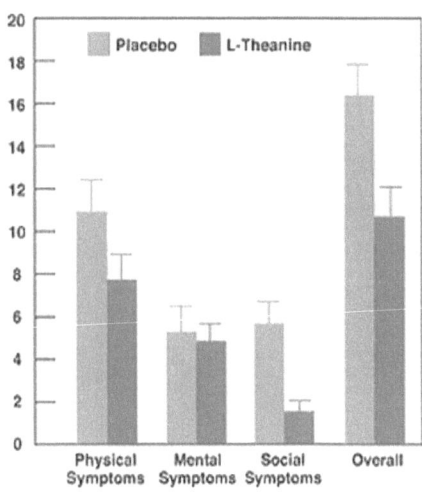

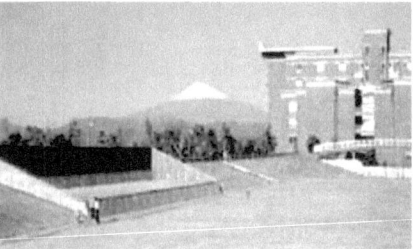

Department of Food and Nutritional Sciences at University of Shizuoka (Mt Fuji in the background)

Another important area of research is the potential of theanine to protect neurons from excesses of glutamate. Glutamate is an essential brain chemical that may be released in excess amounts with some disease conditions (e.g. ALS and cerebrovascular dementia) and with brain injuries (as occurs with strokes or physical injuries). Theanine may protect against this damage by blocking glutamine entrance to cells due to the similarity in stereochemical structures of theanine and glutamine.

In studies of isolated neuron cells and in gerbil studies, this protective effect is demonstrated. A leader in this research, and other studies of theanine neurological effects, is Dr Takami Kakuda, formerly working at the food and nutrition department with Dr Yokogoshi and now with the Central Research Institute, of Ito En, Ltd., in Shizuoka.

Umami Taste

Umami is the term for a taste that is imparted to foods by amino acids, especially the widely used food additive monosodium glutamate. The concept of this taste was first promulgated more than ninety years ago in Japan and is of such interest that there is a Society for Research on Umami Taste in Japan (founded in 1982). The taste is pictorially displayed in relation to the standard taste groups (bitter, sweet, salty, sour) as follows (the three-dimensional distribution indicates the relationships between the tastes; umami is depicted here as a receptor that fits most closely to the sweet and salty taste and is opposite to the bitter taste):

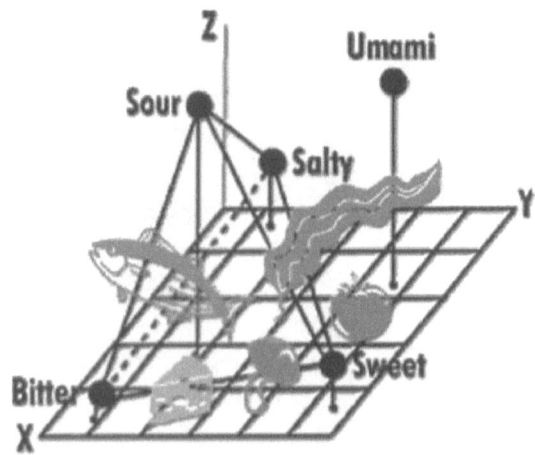

In the case of theanine in tea, it is thought that this amino acid makes a significant contribution to the flavour of the beverage, which is dominated by the bitter taste of the polyphenols and caffeine, but is mellowed and broadened by the umami taste. As tea is brewed longer, the umami taste is overcome by both the bitter taste and an astringent quality of the polyphenols, so it is important to use a proper brewing time.

In the description of Oriental herbs and foods, there are five tastes traditionally listed, including the four that are usually described in relation to taste receptors plus the taste described interchangeably as acrid, pungent, or spicy. Flavour researchers generally place this quality not as a taste but as a general impact on the tongue (and mouth), which produces a tingly, numbing, or hot sensation. Further, in the herbal system, the sour quality is sometimes broadened to include astringency as a general feature, but the astringent quality can be given a separate designation. The astringent nature of the non-sour items (like pomegranate rind) is an effect on the tongue and mouth rather than an actual taste. Meats, and other foods high in glutamine and related amino acids, are classified in the traditional system as having a sweet taste. This designation indicates that the taste is pleasant and desirable. Humans and animals are naturally attracted to foods that have pleasant tastes, which include sweet and umami tastes, as these food substances play critical nutritional roles (by contrast, bitter tastes are often avoided as they signal the potential for toxicity). The sweet and umami taste receptors have similar subunits. Only about three of four adults can distinguish the umami taste, based on glutamate, the others having weak receptor function. The umami receptors of the tongue have been isolated in rats. They respond most strongly to glutamate but also demonstrate response to each of the twenty amino acids, suggesting that they function as amino acid taste receptors that are most sensitive to glutamate (and amino acids of similar structure). Amino acid tastes range from bland to umami to sweet, depending on the particular amino acid.

Investigations of Theanine as Adjunct to Cancer Chemotherapy

There has been a developing interest, with accelerated research that is still in the laboratory stage, into the potential of theanine as an adjunct to cancer chemotherapy. The lead researcher in this field is Yasuyuki Sadzuka, working at the School of Pharmaceutical Sciences, University of Shizuoka. In an abstract of one of his recent articles, examples of the application for theanine were presented with a description of the proposed mechanism: We have confirmed that theanine, a major amino acid in green tea, enhances the antitumour activity of doxorubicin (DOX) without an increase in DOX-induced side effects. We believe that the action of theanine is due to decreases in glutamate uptake via inhibition of the glutamate transporter and reduction of glutathione and DOX export from the cell . . . To increase our knowledge of the potential clinical usefulness of theanine, we examined its effects on the antitumour activity of cisplatin and irinotecan (CPT-11), which is known to be transported out of tumour cells by the (same system). Cisplatin decreased the tumour volume in M5076 tumour-bearing mice. Furthermore, the combination of theanine with cisplatin enhanced the decrease in the tumour volume as compared with the cisplatin-alone group. Tumour volume in the CPT-11-alone group did not show a decrease, but the combination of theanine with CPT-11 significantly reduced the tumour volume.

The concentration of cisplatin in the tumour was significantly increased by combination with theanine, and thus we assume that it correlated with the enhancement on the antitumour activity by theanine. On the other hand, changes in drug concentrations with theanine were not observed in normal tissues, but rather it is indicated that theanine tends to reduce their concentrations. Therefore, theanine enhances the antitumour activity not only of DOX but also of cisplatin or CPT-11.

In essence, Sadzuka has found that theanine could block the export of doxorubicin (Adriamycin) (see Figure 6 below) from cancer cells by blocking the glutamate and glutathione transporter mechanisms; the elevated level of the drug within cancer cells strongly inhibits the tumour. At the same time, non-cancerous cells treated with the chemotherapy drug plus theanine did not accumulate the drug. There have been several studies of this nature, and if confirmed, it suggests that by either consuming green tea (several cups per day) or taking supplemental l-theanine, the anticancer effects of at least some of the chemotherapy drugs may be improved. Doxorubicin also poses some threat to the cardiac tissue, for which coenzyme Q10 is a recommended protective therapy.

Bibliography

Theanine Synthesis

1. Sasaoka K., Kito M., and Inagaki H., Studies on the biosynthesis of theanine in tea seedlings: synthesis of theanine by the homogenate of tea seedlings, *Agricultural Biology and Chemistry*, 1963; (27): 467-8.
2. K., and Kito M., Synthesis of theanine by tea seedling homogenate, *Agricultural Biology and Chemistry*, 1964; (28): 313-17.

3. Sasaoka K., Kito M., and Onishi Y., Some properties of the theanine synthesizing enzyme in tea seedlings, *Agricultural Biology and Chemistry*, 1965; (29): 984-8.

Theanine Neurological Effects

4. Yokogoshi H., et al., Reduction effect of theanine on blood pressure and brain 5-hydroxyindoles in spontaneously hypertensive rats, *Bioscience, Biotechnology, and Biochemistry*, 1995; 59: 615-18.
5. Terashima T., Takido J., and Yokogoshi H., Time-dependent changes of amino acids in the serum, liver, brain and urine of rats administered with theanine, *Bioscience, Biotechnology, and Biochemistry*, 1999; 63(4): 615-18.
6. Yokogoshi H., Mochizuki M., and Saitoh K., Theanine-induced reduction of brain serotonin concentration in rats, *Bioscience, Biotechnology, and Biochemistry*, 1998; 62(4): 816-17.
7. Yokogoshi H., et al., Effect of theanine on brain monoamines and striatal dopa-mine release in conscious rats, *Neurochemical Research*, 1998; 23(5): 667-73.
8. Yokogoshi H. and Terashima T., Effect of theanine on brain monoamines, striatal, dopamine release and some kinds of behavior in rats, *Nutrition*, 2000; 16(9): 776-7.
9. Kobayashi K., et al., Effects of l-theanine on the release of alpha-brain waves in human volunteers, *Nippon Noegikagako Kaishi*, 1998; 72 (2): 153-7.
10. Kakuda T., et al., Inhibiting effect of theanine on caffeine stimulation evaluated by EEG in the rat, *Bioscience, Biotechnology, and Biochemistry*, 2000; 64: 287-93.
11. Yokogoshi H., et al., Theanine effects on premenstrual syndrome, *Proceedings of the Nogei Kagaku Kai, Bioscience, Biotechnology, and Biochemistry*, 2001; 75: 166.
12. Yokogoshi H. and Kobayashi M., Hypotensive effect of gamma-glutamylmethylamide (theanine) in spontaneously hypertensive rats, *Life Sciences*, 1998; 62 (12): 1065-8.
13. Lekh R. J., et al., L-theanine-a unique amino acid of green tea and its relaxation effect in humans, *Trends in Food Science and Technology*, 1999; 10 (6-7): 199-204.

14. Kakuda T., et al., Protective effect of gamma-glutamylethylamide (theanine) on ischemic delayed neuronal death in gerbils, *Neuroscience Letters*, 2000; 289(3): 189-92.

Umami Taste

15. Li X., et al., Human receptors for sweet and umami taste, *Proceedings National Academy of Sciences USA*, 2002; 99(7): 4692-6.
16. Nelson G., et al., An amino acid taste receptor, *Nature*, 2002; 416 (6877): 199-202.
17. Lugaz O., Phillias A. M., and Faurion A., A new specific ageusia: some humans cannot taste l-glutamate, *Chemical Senses*, 2002; 27(2): 105-15.

Theanine and Cancer Therapy

18. Sadzuka Y., et al., The effects of theanine, as a novel biochemical modulator, on the antitumor activity of adriamycin, *Cancer Letters*, 1996; 105(2): 203-9.
19. Sadzuka Y., Sugiyama T., and Hirota S., Modulation of cancer chemotherapy by green tea, *Clinical Cancer Research*, 1998; 4(1): 153-6.
20. Sadzuka Y., et al., Efficacies of tea components on doxorubicin induced antitumor activity and reversal of multidrug resistance, *Toxicology Letters*, 2000; 114 (1-3): 155-62.
21. Sadzuka Y., et al., Improvement of idarubicin induced antitumor activity and bone marrow suppression by theanine, a component of tea, *Cancer Letters*, 2000;158(2): 119-24.
22. Sadzuka Y., et al., Enhancement of the activity of doxorubicin by inhibition of glutamate transporter, *Toxicology Letters*, 2001; 123 (2-3): 159-67.
23. Sadzuka Y., et al., Effect of dihydrokainate on the antitumor activity of doxorubicin', *Cancer Letters*, 2002; 179(2): 157-63.
24. Sugiyama T., et al., Inhibition of glutamate transporter by theanine enhances the therapeutic efficacy of doxorubicin, *Toxicology Letters*, 2001; 121(2): 89-96.

25. Sugiyama T. and Sadzuka Y., Combination of theanine with doxo-rubicin inhibits hepatic metastasis of M5076 ovarian sarcoma, *Clinical Cancer Research*, 1999; 5(2): 413-4166.
26. Sugiyama T. and Sadzuka Y., Enhancing effects of green tea components on the antitumor activity of adriamycin against M5076 ovarian sarcoma, *Cancer Letters*, 1998; 133(1): 19-26.
27. Zhang G., Miura Y., and Yagasaki K., Effects of dietary powdered green tea and theanine on tumor growth and endogenous hyper-lipidemia in hepatoma-bearing rats, *Bioscience, Biotechnology, and Biochemistry*, 2002; 66(4): 711-16.

Note: This article is part of a series of reports on amino acids used as supplements. The previous three reports in the amino acid series are as follows:

I. Glutamine (with reference to glutamate)
II. SAM-e (with reference to methionine)
III. Carnitine (with reference to taurine)

December 2002

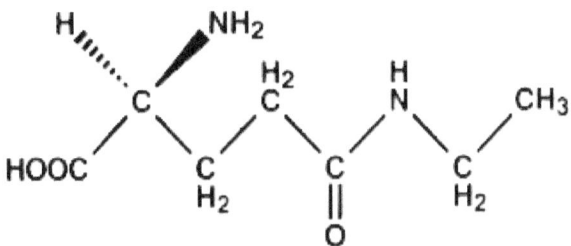

Figure 1. Theanine (5-N-ethyl gluatmine). This molecule differs from glutamine by the CH2-CH3 (ethyl) group (replacing hydrogen), drawn on the right side of this molecular structure.

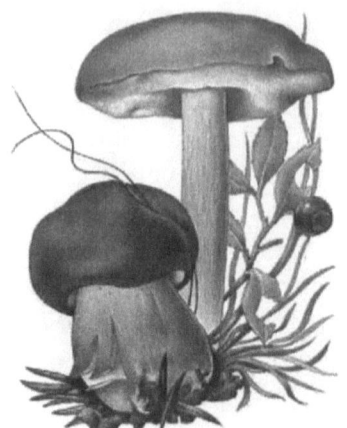

Figure 2. *Xerocomus badius.*

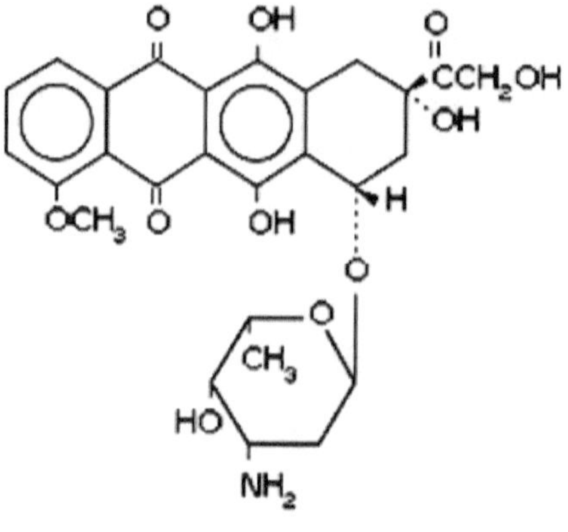

Figure 6. Doxorubicin, commonly called adriamycine.

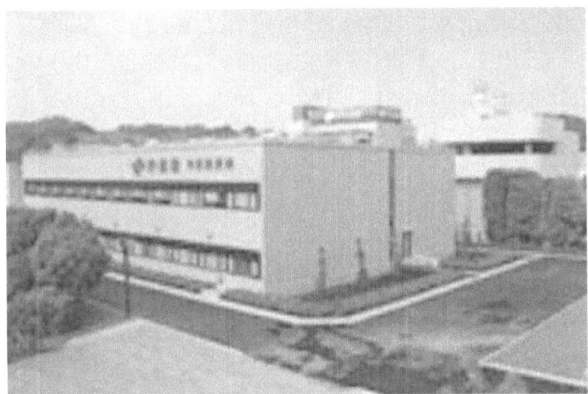

Figure 7. Central research institute of ITO EN, Ltd., in Shizuoka, Japan, where several studies of theanine and other tea leave constituents are carried out.

11.5 The Uses of Aromatic Agents for Regularising Qui: Vitalising Blood and Relieving Pains

Subhuti Dharmananda, PhD, Director, May 1997

Fragrant Herbs of Aromatherapy

Herbs with a strong fragrance often have a remarkably powerful effect on the body. The word *fragrance* (Chinese: *xiang*) conveys the sense that something is reaching out to you. Herbs that are strongly fragrant are frequently described as such by their common Chinese names: Murraya is known as *jiulixiang* (fragrance that reaches 9 *li*–about three miles); cyperus is known as *xiangfuzi* (fragrant tuber); saussurea is known as *muxiang* (fragrant wood); aquilaria is known as *chenxiang* (fragrant dense herb); and elsholtzia is known as *xiangru* (fragrant soft herb). In fact, several dozen Chinese medicinal materials, many of them imported for centuries from other lands, are designated by the term *xiang*. In addition to their uses as internal medicines, many are included in incenses used for traditional ceremonies and as fumigants to get rid of insects and to alleviate skin diseases.

When ingested, the aromatic substances contained in the fragrant herbs dissolve mucus (mucolytic; they cause the mucus to flow more freely), open up congested and contracted blood vessels (reducing atheromas and vasodilating), and regulate the flow of chi (alleviate chi stagnation and with that disperse accumulated fluids). If the essential oils or isolated constituents are applied topically, they can have an irritating effect; up to a point, this is desired: The therapeutic action is called counter-irritation (it promotes local circulation and alleviates pain) and is the basis for many Chinese liniments used for treating arthralgia and other pain syndromes. The aromatics are disruptive to the membranes of micro-organisms, placing them among the most potent of the topical antibacterial agents. Aromatics are generally said to have a spicy, pungent, or acrid taste, and this refers to a hot sensation experienced when the aromatic agents come in contact with the tongue. Peppermint, with its main component menthol, is one of the best-known aromatics; the spicy taste is familiar to almost everyone. The aromatic herbs often have a medicinal potency related to the strength of the taste and fragrance as these sensory effects are directly related to the total content of the aromatic constituents.

Early in the history of Chinese medicine, the aromatic agents were investigated and considered of importance not only in treating diseases but also for prolonging life and maintaining youthful vigour. Likewise, aromatic agents were important in Egyptian, Byzantine, and Indian medicine. A major study of the herbal constituents in China began during the Tang Dynasty and continued through the Song Dynasty (revived again towards the end of the Qing Dynasty and continued to the present). As described by Edward Schafer in the book *Food in Chinese Culture* (edited by K. C. Chang, 1977, Yale University Press, New Haven), the pharmacologists of Tang studied all potential foodstuffs hoping to ascertain their virtues and the complex effects they had on the human body, especially in conjunction with or in reaction against other edibles. They were particularly concerned with the prolongation of youth, the lengthening of life, the blackening of hair (prevention of premature greying), the restoration of waning sexual powers, and other such blessings. Pungent and spicy materials seemed especially likely to have these desirable properties in more concentrated form than did ordinary materials . . . The recommendations of learned pharmacologists must have had an immense effect on the practices of cooks, whose recipes thus modified came in time to be regarded as the authoritative designs for gourmet dishes. Venison with ginger and vinegar was first recommended for its tonic properties but was ultimately appreciated as an ambrosial delight . . . These influences are easily seen today in relation to the aromatic agents with such famous dishes as Camphor Wood and Tea Smoked Duck.

Medicinal Functions and Classifications

One can generalise the descriptions found in Chinese materia medica books to say that the aromatics are used to remove congestion and normalise the flow of chi and blood. Congestion, a stagnation of circulation accompanied by accumulation of the non-circulating substances, has become a major health problem in the modern world. This is partly a result of more sedentary lifestyle, richer diets, and confined living that arises from population growth and industrialisation. Diseases related to congestion and abnormal circulation of chi and blood are exemplified by atherosclerosis (a major source of heart attack and stroke), cancer (from the traditional Chinese perspective, an accumulation in the form of tumour growth), digestive disorders (including ulcer, constipation, and flatulence), persistent sinus and/or lung congestion, and autoimmune diseases characterised by accumulations of antibodies (such as rheumatoid arthritis). These conditions are readily recognised as among the most widespread in the modern world. Although numerous plant materials used in Chinese medicine have a strong fragrance, the ones usually considered to be 'aromatics' are mainly those that appear in five of the standard materia medica categories (based on fundamental therapeutic actions; see 'Enumerating the methods of therapy').

Fragrant herbs for dissolving wetness: examples include alpinia, cardamon, red atractylodes, kaemferia, magnolia bark, and pogostemon.

Herbs for regulating qi: examples include acronychia, aquilaria, citrus, cyperus, lindera, sandalwood, and saussurea.

Herbs for warming the interior and eliminating cold: examples include galanga, clove, cinnamon bark, evodia, fennel, and zanthoxylum.

Fragrant herbs for opening the orifices: examples include benzoin, borneol, and styrax.

Herbs for warming and releasing the surface: examples include elsholtzia, chiang-huo, perilla leaf, schizonepeta, and thyme. Some of the fragrant herbs are found in other categories, such as myrrh and frankincense among the blood-vitalising herbs and nutmeg in the category of astringents. In Ayurvedic and Tibetan medicines, the aromatics also play a primary role. Some of the Chinese herbs mentioned above were originally obtained from Tibet and India and even from the Middle East.

Active Constituents of Aromatic Herbs

Although one can successfully study Chinese herbs from a theoretical and clinical viewpoint without examining active constituents, in the case of aromatic herbs, the study of these constituents proves useful. This is because there is a class of chemical components that are common to many of the aromatic agents. Of the large number of aromatic constituents found in Chinese herbs, the volatile components in cardamon (*sharen* and *doukou*) are among the most important and widely occurring. These aromatic constituents belong to a large class of chemicals known as terpenoids, subdivided by chemists into monoterpenoids, diterpenoids, triterpenoids, and sesquiterpenoids. Terpenoids are relatively simple hydrocarbons (made up of only hydrogen and carbon), sometimes with a single oxygen molecule attached. Hydrocarbons are lipophyllic, meaning that they are not soluble in water and that in the body they tend to migrate to the fatty tissues and cell membranes. Good examples of the simple monoterpenes are limonene and pinene and of oxygenated monoterpenes are menthol and borneol. When making a herbal tea, these compounds are not solubilised in water but rather forced out of the herb by the heat. They quickly rise to the surface layer and then evaporate. For that reason, aromatic herbs are often only steeped in the tea after decoction or only decocted for a few minutes (or not decocted at all, but given in pills). Cardamon is included in numerous traditional and modern prescriptions for relief of congested qi, moisture, and blood. Cardamon (see Figure 1 for spectrographic constituent analysis of the volatile oil from *Aromatic Plants and Essential Constituents*, by South China Institute of Botany, 1993) contains the following terpenoids:

Camphor	Camphene	Terpinene	Myrcene
Bornyl acetate	Linalool	Caryophyllene	Nerolidol
Borneol	Pinene	Limonene	

There are numerous species of cardamon used in Chinese medicine. These include *baidoukou* (cluster, *Amomum cardamomum* or *Amomum kravanh*), originally produced in the countries now known as Thailand and Vietnam; *caoguo* (Tsao-kou; *Amomum tsao-ko*); and *sharen*, also known as *suosha* (cardamon; from *Amomum villosum*, *Amomum xanthioides*, and other species). Cardamon and cluster are the ones most commonly used in making Chinese herbal prescriptions, and they have similar ingredients, with borneol and bornyl acetate being the principal substance in their volatile oils. The specific amounts and range of active constituents vary among the cardamons, but the uses of the herbs in medicine are similar. For purposes of this article, I use the term 'cardamon' to refer to *Amomum villosum*, the primary source for *sharen*. Borneol and the compound that usually accompanies it in herbs, bornyl acetate, is a powerful agent for regulating chi and alleviating pain. However, more is known, historically, about the therapeutically similar camphor oil than about borneol, the latter called Borneo camphor. Borneol is a major component of camphor oil. Camphor oil is obtained from a tree (*Cinnamomum camphora*), and like cardamon, the essential oil of the tree contains a large number of terpenoids (mostly, the same ones as in cardamon, but in different proportions). Camphor was collected at least as early as the ninth century. In 1676, the trees were brought to Europe for cultivation. In the following century, it was also introduced to several other countries, including the United States.

Prior to World War II, the world use of camphor was about 5,000 tons per year; 80 per cent of this came from Taiwan (the Taiwan camphor tree yields 44 per cent camphor from its leaves, a particularly high level). During the U.S. Civil War, the demand for camphor (used primarily as a medicinal) was so high that the United States contracted for the entire Taiwan supply. It was even proposed that an effort be made to purchase Taiwan (then called Formosa) in order to monopolise the camphor trade. It is perhaps for this reason that Japan acquired Formosa in 1895. Camphor oil was a popular medicinal in the United States until about twenty years ago when several instances occurred in which children were fed camphor oil by parents who failed to distinguish it from castor oil. The pure camphor oil is toxic in the doses for which castor oil is used. Also, the U.S. Food and Drug Administration worried that topically applied camphor oil would penetrate the skin in sufficient amounts that it could cause trouble for persons with cardiac disorders who were taking various medications. As a result, it is no longer possible to purchase camphor oil for household use in the United States.

Like borneol, camphor has been used as an antiseptic, antispasmodic, carminative, cardiac stimulant, respiratory aid, and anthelmintic. It is often used in treating congestive problems such as bronchitis and emphysema. Camphor is also used in preparation of foods, being an ingredient of vanilla and peppermint flavours and incorporated into formulations of soft drinks, baked goods, and condiments. In modern Chinese medicine, camphor is most often reserved for external application, while borneol is used both internally and externally. Synthetic camphor, often made from chemically modifying pine tree resins (turpentine), is now widely used as a substitute for the natural product. The Chinese traditionally obtained their borneol (as an isolate) mainly from *Dryobalanops aromatica* and from *Blumea balsamifera*. The latter is used as the herb *ainaxiang* (fragrant herb that looks like artemisia), which is rich in borneol and also contains limonene, camphor, and other terpenoid compounds. The extracted borneol (*longnaoxiang*; fragrant dragon's brain; also known as *bingpian* (ice slice) referring to the appearance of the finished product) is considered to be suitable for abdominal and chest pains, intestinal parasites, phlegm congestion, and fevers. Blumea is in the same plant family (*Labiatae*) as capillaris, chrysanthemum, and saussurea, which also contain important terpenes.

Borneol and bornyl acetate are ingredients in the following herbal materials:

Cardamom	Magnolia
Nutmeg	Turmeric
Ginger	Liquidambar
Lindera	Camphor oil

These herbs are all used in the treatment of pain syndromes. Camphor oil is sometimes used internally for pain due to blood stasis. All have a warming quality. Many of these herbs, notably nutmeg, ginger, cardamon, turmeric, and camphor oil, are traditionally used in Ayurvedic and Tibetan medicines for the treatment of pain syndromes; these same herbs are recognised as common ingredients in the preparation of foods.

The In:

Cardamom	Frankincense	Citrus
Magnolia	Cyperus	Perilla
Myrrh	Cinnamon	Lindera
Pogostemon	Piper	Camphor oil

These herbs are all deemed warming. Citrus, cyperus, lindera, and perilla leaf are classified as qi-regulating herbs used in the treatment of digestive disorders, pain, and moisture and phlegm congestion. They are often combined together in the treatment of emotional disturbance, abdominal bloating, and asthmatic breathing. Cinnamon, lindera, and piper are used for dispelling cold that causes abdominal pain. Pogostemon (*huoxiang*) is a herb that replaced agastache; pogostemon is the source of the natural fragrance known as patchouli oil.

Camphor and the chemically related compound camphene are found in the following:

Cardamom	Ginger	Nutmeg
Saussurea	Curcuma	Cyperus
Magnolia	Cinnamon	Camphor oil

As with the previous listings, these herbs are warming and regulate circulation of chi and moisture. Myrcene is found in magnolia, capillaries, and citrus.

These three herbs are commonly used to treat gallbladder stagnation, including gallstones and aching in the area of the gallbladder.

Limonene and the chemically similar phellandrene are found in many fragrant herbs:

Limonene		Phellandrene	
Agastache	Magnolia	Frankincense	Saussurea
Camphor oil	Myrrh	Ginger	Turmeric
Cardamom	Nutmeg	Piper	Zanthoxylum
Citrus	Perilla		
Cyperus	Pine resin		
Fennel	Zanthoxylum		
Piper			

Linalool is a terpene alcohol found in the following:

Pogostemon	Lindera
Citrus	Magnolia
Ginger	Nutmeg

The chemical constituents mentioned for the above herb lists are all monoterpenes. Nerolidol, copaene, farnesene, and sesquiterpenoids are found incardamom, camphor oil, magnolia, capillaries, and citrus.

They are all useful in treating central stagnation of chi and dampness and relieving abdominal pain. Other sesquiterpenoid compounds are found in the *following herbs*:

Acorus	Myrrh
Aquilaria	Sandalwood
Cardamom	Piper
Cyperus	Pogostemon
Lindera	Saussurea
Magnolia	

These lists of herbs containing specified terpenoids (in this case, the same ingredients as found in cardamon) illustrate three points: Some herbs contain numerous terpenoids as active constituents (examples are cardamon, magnolia, citrus, cyperus, piper, camphor, ginger, frankincense, myrrh); the herbs that contain terpenoids have similar actions from the traditional viewpoint (mainly regulating circulation of qi, moisture, and blood and usually dispelling chill); the studies of active constituents, modern pharmacology, and traditional therapeutics can, at least in the case of these herbs, be joined together in providing a deeper understanding of herbal healing.

Pharmacology of Terpenoids

Pharmacologically, the terpenoid compounds have the following effects (with examples of herbs used for those effects):

- Stimulate blood circulation: frankincense, myrrh, turmeric, curcuma, and liquidambar.
- Permeate congestion: piper, citrus, saussurea, magnolia, cardamon, borneol, and camphor.
- Relieve pain: most of these herbs have this property; cardamon, aquilaria, saussurea, myrrh, and frankincense.
- Relieve inflammation: borneol, camphor, saussurea, and aquilaria.
- Improve digestion: ginger, sandalwood, clove, galanga, cyperus, magnolia, saussurea, and agastache.
- Enhance mental function: saussurea and acorus.
- Prevent and aid resolution of tumours: saussurea, clove, cardamon, myrrh, frankincense, and borneol.
- Dispel intestinal parasites and infecting organisms: saussurea, clove, zanthoxylum, capillaris, and magnolia. There are some aromatic medicinal agents that do not contain terpenoids but have some similar effects, such as styrax (liquid extract), musk, ox gallstone, and benzoin: These are classified as aromatic agents for opening the orifices.

Incorporation of Aromatics in Prescriptions

Most prescriptions for atherosclerosis, angina pectoris, stroke, injuries, intestinal parasites, children's congestive disorders, and impaired circulation contain aromatic agents. Because the aromatic components are quite strong in their pharmacologic action, and because they are easily evaporated or damaged by cooking, the majority of prescriptions are made up as pills comprising powdered crude herbs or, in the cases of myrrh, frankincense, camphor, borneol, and benzoin, as crude resins. In the formula names that include the names of one or two key herbs (OHAI common names system), the term 'formula' usually indicates a pill or a powder (swallowed whole or made into tea with minimal cooking time); the term 'combination' designates a decoction. In the case of patent medicines, the terms *wan* and *dan* mean pills.

Aromatic agents are usually quite versatile in their applications, but I have grouped the following prescriptions very roughly into categories for easier study. These formulas are derived from Chinese, Tibetan, and Ayurvedic prescriptions.

Formulas predominantly used for abdominal and chest pains are as follows:

1. Saussurea and Mastic formula [1] contains saussurea, borneol, cardamon, aquilaria, clove, sandalwood, frankincense, cinnamon, piper, musk, terminalia, licorice, platycodon, and cinnabar. It is used for angina pectoris, ulcer, and other abdominal and chest pains.

2. *Guan Xin Su Ho Wan* [2] comprises sandalwood, borneol, myrrh, styrax resin, and aristolachia root and is used for chronic heart disease, especially atherosclerosis. It is reported to have good results in treating angina and myocardial infarction in clinical studies in China. This prescription, with its very large doses of borneol (15 per cent) and styrax (8 per cent), borders on the action of a drug rather than a food supplement and so should be taken with the advice of a practitioner.

3. *Su He Xiang Wan* [2] is a patent medicine comprising borneol, styrax resin, musk, aquilaria, frankincense, piper, benzoin, saussurea, cyperus, sandalwood, clove, terminallia, aristolachia fruit, rhino horn, and cinnabar. The formula is used for atherosclerosis and apoplexy. This ancient prescription is called Styrax Formula by Dr Hsu [3]; it was recorded in the *He Ji Ju Fang* of the Song Dynasty. The formula is effective in treating angina, coma, stuttering, and limb pains. Because it contains rhino horn and cinnabar, it is not appropriate for use in the West.

4. Padma 28, comprising the aromatics cardamon, clove, camphor, saussurea, cluster, chih-shih, and sandalwood, plus other plants (most of which are non-aromatic agents), such as terminallia, melia, and licorice, is a Tibetan remedy manufactured in Switzerland that is used for the treatment of angina, atherosclerosis, and peripheral arterial occlusion. There have been more clinical studies of this herbal prescription in the West than any other

Tibetan formula. It maintains a 70 per cent efficacy rate for most disorders for which it is indicated.

5. Aquilaria 8 [4], comprising aquilaria, nutmeg, frankincense (from Sal tree), saussurea, terminallia, spondias, bamboo sap, and ironwood, is used for angina and tachicardia, myocardial insufficiency, and pulmonary arterial occlusion. It is also indicated for the treatment of pains in the breast or liver. This is a traditional Tibetan remedy made entirely of herbal ingredients (the majority of Tibetan remedies include animal substances and minerals). It is available in India but difficult to obtain in the West.

6. Cinnamon and cardamon combination [1] contains cinnamon, aurantium, cardamon, aquilaria, magnolia bark, saussurea, ginger, plus perilla fruit and licorice. Perilla fruit also contains terpenoid compounds; it is usually used in the treatment of allergy, especially in persons with weak constitution. This prescription is used for chest pain and asthma.

7. Aquilaria and hoelen combination [1] contains aquilaria, carda-mon, aurantium, evodia, coptis, licorice, and hoelen. It is used for stomach and chest pain.

8. Chih-shih and cardamon combination [3] contains cardamon, magnolia bark, ginger, citrus, saussurea, Chih-shih, cyperus, fennel, tsao-tou-kou, pinellia, hoelen, corydalis, and licorice. This ancient prescription was first recorded in *Wan Bing Hui Jun* of the Ming Dynasty. It is used for stomachache, gastric ulcer, angina pectoris, and back pain.

9. Bi-ma-mi-tra pills [4] contain nutmeg, frankincense, clove, cardamon, sandalwood, and fourteen other ingredients, including terminallia, melia, and licorice. It is indicated for heart disease, heart pain, mental disturbances, aches and pains, nervousness, and fainting. The formula is currently not available in the West.

Formulas for the treatment of arthritis, rheumatism, and injuries are as follows:

1. *Da Huo Luo Dan* [2], a patent medicine from China, comprising lindera, aquilaria, saussurea, clove, cinnamon, frankincense, oxstone, blue citrus, musk, myrrh, benzoin, cluster, cyperus, pine resin, borneol, and about two dozen other ingredients (mostly non-aromatic agents), is used as a general treatment

for pain syndromes. It is especially good for pain in the limbs. As it is produced by several different factories, the formula will vary slightly depending upon its source. The gold-leaf-coated pills are relatively expensive, but are one of the strongest of the pain-relieving formulas for arthritic problems. The product label lists rhino horn and tiger bone, but the product does not contain these ingredients. This formula, called clematis and gastrodia combination by Dr Hsu, is described in OHAI Bulletin #16 along with other therapies for arthritis, rheumatism, neuralgia, and apoplexy.

2. Musk and catechu formula [3], comprising musk, myrrh, borneol, frankincense, catechu, calamus gum, cinnabar, and carthamus, is used for severe pain, especially that caused by traumatic injury. This is a famous traditional remedy known as Qi Li San.

3. Musk-tiger bone pills [2], a patent medicine from China, is used for pains in the bones, muscles, and joints; paralysis; and muscle spasms. It contains agastache, oxstone, cyperus, cardamon, myrrh, blue citrus, pine resin, lindera, aquilaria, frankincense, benzoin, borneol, musk, and plus forty-five other ingredients. Although the formulation is overly complex, the 10 per cent aromatic components (50 per cent of the pill is honey) are quite effective. The product lists rhino horn and tiger bone, but does not contain these ingredients.

4. *Zai Zao Wan* [2], a patent medicine for treating injuries, contains musk, oxstone, cardamon, myrrh, aquilaria, frankincense, agastache, plus numerous other ingredients; many of them are aromatics. This product lists rhino horn and tiger bone on its label, but does not contain them.

Formulas for aiding digestion and relieving stomachaches:

1. *Shu Gan Wan* [2] is a patent formula from China that contains cyperus, chih-shih, citrus, aurantium, curcuma, magnolia bark, cardamon, aquilaria, sandalwood, and nine other ingredients. The product is made at several factories and the composition may vary depending on the source. It is used for abdominal pains and digestive disturbances.

2. Saussurea and cardamon formula [1] contains saussurea, cloves, sandalwood, cardamon, cluster, agastache, ginger, licorice, and salt. This prescription should not be confused with the similarly named saussurea and cardamon combination [3]. The formula treats digestive disturbance, diarrhoea, constipation, and stomachache.

3. Cyperus, cardamon, and atractylodes formula [1] contains ginger, cyperus, magnolia bark, agastache, citrus, cardamon, jujube, atractylodes, and licorice. It is used for digestive disturbances in persons with weak constitution.

4. Atractylodes and cardamon combination [3] contains citrus, magnolia bark, saussurea, cardamon, aquilaria, licorice, tang-kuei, atractylodes, morus, perilla fruit, hoelen, and ginseng. It treats weak digestion with production of excessive sputum and wheezing.

5. Pueraria flower combination [3] contains saussurea, blue citrus peel, citrus, ginger, cardamon, cluster, hoelen, alisma, pueraria flower, ginseng, polyporus, atractylodes, and shen-chu. It is indicated for nausea, vomiting, and hangover.

6. *Drachsha* contains cardamon (green and black), cinnamon, clove, fennel, ginger, nutmeg, piper (two types), turmeric, coriander, cumin, mace, oregano, and saffron. All the herbs in this formula, except for saffron, are classified as aromatics. This is an Ayurvedic remedy based on a traditional formula; it is used to improve digestion. The preparation, in the form of liquid extract, has been sold in the United States for more than a decade.

7. Minor bupleurum combination modified [1] contains citrus, saussurea, cardamon, agastache, aquilaria, ginger, fennel, licorice, kaki, mume, scute, gardenia, and pinellia. It is used for stomach distress and subcostal pains.

8. *Hingwasthaka* contains asafoetida, ginger, two types of piper, three types of cumin, and rock salt. This spicy and aromatic blend is a well-known Ayurvedic remedy for digestive disturbances, especially to be used in cases where phlegm congestion arises as the result of weak digestive activity. It is added as a powder to cooked food or taken as a pill.

Formulas used for lumps, swellings, and tumours:

1. Saussurea and lindera combination [5] contains saussurea, chih-ko, frankincense, myrrh, curcuma, citrus, cardamon, lindera, hoelen, and peony. It is used in the treatment of tumours.
2. Clove and cardamon formula [5] contains cardamon, clove, cyperus, saussurea, cluster, licorice, ginseng, malt, and atractylodes. It is used in the treatment of stomach tumours.
3. Clove and hoelen combination [3] contains citrus, clove, ginger, cinnamon, cardamon, hoelen, pinellia, and aconite. It is used for stomach cancer and gastric ulcers.
4. Scirpus combination [5] contains blue citrus peel, citrus, chih-shih, cyperus, magnolia bark, saussurea, ginger, plus 12 other herbs. It is used for treating abdominal masses.
5. Inula and haematite combination modified [5] contains citrus, evodia, cyperus, aquilaria, chih-ko, inula, coptis, haematite, pinellia, hoelen, bamboo, peony, and oyster shell. It is used for treating oesophageal cancer.

Formulas used for intestinal pains and parasites are as follows:

1. Mume and zanthoxylum combination [1] contains chih-shih, cyperus, magnolia bark, saussurea, cardamon, cinnamon, zanthoxylum, ginger, licorice, melia, areca seed, and mume. It is used for treating digestive disturbance, intestinal pains, and intestinal parasites.
2. Tang-kuei and saussurea combination [1] contains saussurea, cardamon, black cardamon, ginger, cyperus, fennel, lindera, evodia, licorice, atractylodes, juncus, tang-kuei, corydalis, and gardenia. It is used for uterine pain and intestinal pain.
3. Areca seed combination [3] contains aurantium, ginger, evodia, magnolia bark, perilla, saussurea, cinnamon, hoelen, areca seed, licorice, and rhubarb. It is indicated for constipation, abdominal fullness, swelling in the legs, chest pain, tension in the legs and arms, and emotional disorders.

Formula source texts:

1. Otsuka Keisetsu, et al., *Natural Healing with Chinese Herbs*, 1982, Oriental Healing Arts Institute, Long Beach, CA.
2. Fratkin J., *Chinese Herbal Patent Formulas*, 1986, Shya Publications, Santa Fe, NM.
3. Hsu H. Y. and Hsu C. S., *Commonly Used Chinese Herb Formulas with Illustrations*, 1980, Oriental Healing Arts Institute, Long Beach, CA.
4. Rechung Rinpoche, *Tibetan Medicine*, 1973, University of California Press, Berkeley, CA.
5. Hsu H. Y., *Treating Cancer with Chinese Herbs*, 1990, Oriental Healing Arts Institute, Long Beach, CA.

Appendix 1. Botanical Sources of Terpenoids

1. Terpenoids are found in a very wide range of plant species. They are predominantly found in seven plant families:
2. Pinaceae: pine resin, biota, and juniper are the principal herbs used as aromatics in this family.
3. Umbelliferae: fennel, anise, and coriander are aromatics from this family.
4. Lauraceae: camphor, cinnamon, lindera, and benzoin (a derivative of another species of Lindera) are the main aromatics of this family.
5. Rutaceae: citrus, blue citrus, chih-shih, and zanthoxylum are aromatic agents from this family.
6. Labiatae: agastache, perilla, pogostemon, and prunella are examples.
7. Compositae: saussurea, capillaris, and blumea are examples.
8. Zingiberaceae: galanga, cardamon, curcuma, and turmeric are examples.
9. Apart from treatment and cure, the above research findings have thrown light on some of the items that can be used for preventive therapy.

11.6 Cynomorium: Parasitic Plant Widely Used in Traditional Medicine

[4] Subhuti Dharmananda, PhD, Director

Background

Cynomorium is known in Chinese as *suoyang*, which is based on the herb's medicinal effects, 'locking the yang'. It is obtained mainly from the East Asian species, *Cynomorium songaricum*, though the similar *C. coccineum* is sometimes utilised as a substitute (and is used in other countries, from Europe to Central Asia, where it is the native species). The plant harvested for Chinese medicine grows at high altitude, mainly in Inner Mongolia, Qinghai, Gansu, and Tibet. It is used to tonify the yang (treat impotence and backache), strengthen the tendons, and nourish the blood to alleviate the blood-deficiency type of constipation (typically occurring with old age). The value of cynomorium was depicted similarly in many cultures. In sixteenth century Europe, it was known as the Maltese mushroom, though it is not a true fungus. The plant was so highly regarded that the Knights of Malta often sent samples of it to European monarchs as presents. To protect the so-called Fungus Rock, where cynomorium was abundant, the grandmaster posted guards around the area and ordered the sides of the outcropping to be rendered smooth to eliminate any footholds and prevent access from the sea. The rock, rising to a sheer height of sixty metres (200 feet) from the rough sea, became virtually inaccessible.

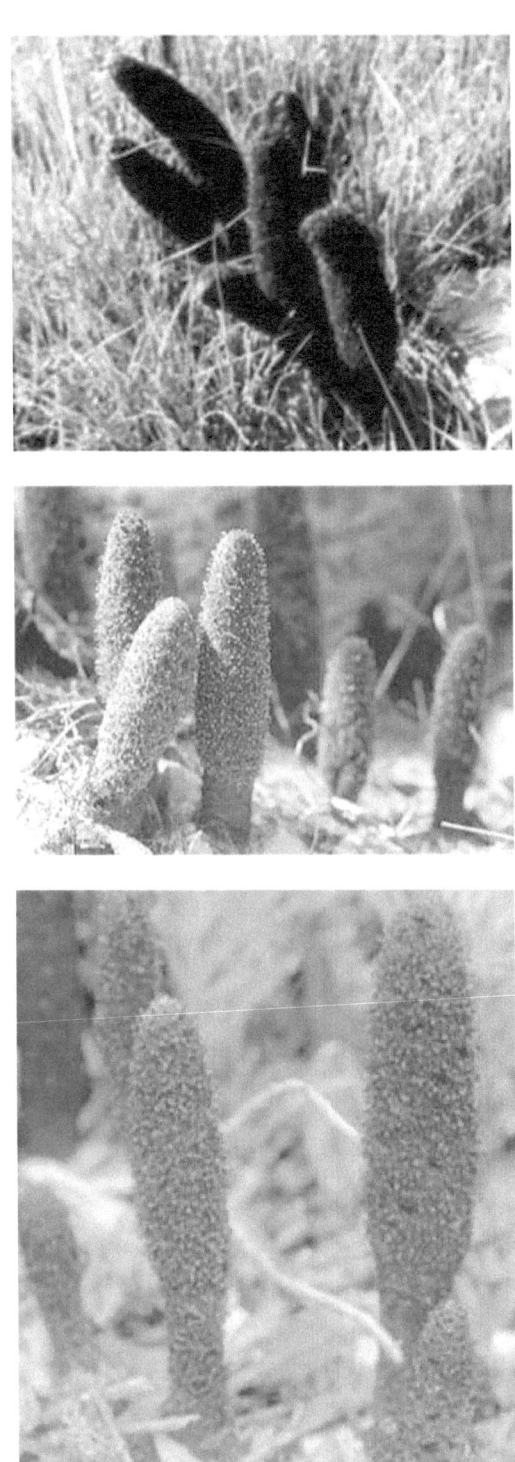

As an explanation of its uses by the doctrine of signatures, since the plant appears reddish-brown and becomes darker upon drying, herbalists thought it would be useful to treat ailments of the blood. On top of that, the phallic shape indicated the plant could also be used to treat sexual problems. The dried spikes were used by the Crusader Knights after their battles to recover strength. In Saudi Arabia, the plant is called tarthuth and is recognised to have the same properties mentioned above, as well as many others, including treatment of digestive disorders and ulcers (see Appendix for story).

Cynomorium is parasitic on the roots of salt-tolerant plants, mainly species of *Atriplex*, the 'saltbushes' (for *C. coccineum*), and on *Nitraria sibirica* (for *C. songaricum*). The plant has no chlorophyll; the fleshy red stems or spikes have tiny scarlet flowers. Its active constituents have not been fully analysed, but cynomorium is known to contain anthocyanic glycosides, triterpene saponins, and lignans. Pharmacology experiments are in the early stage with attempts to demonstrate a hormonal effect that would explain its use in impotence (its current main application in commercial products), as well as findings that the herb extracts inhibit HIV, lower blood pressure, and improve blood flow in laboratory experiments.

Cynomorium, which has a pleasant, sweet taste when raw, has long been known as a 'famine food', that is, something not frequently eaten, but nourishing enough to help people survive when the standard foods are insufficient. In fact, a city in China is named for cynomorium because of this benefit. The city is near Anxi (in today's Gansu Province), which lies at the centre of the ancient Silk Road and was long considered as the key to the West. During the Tang Dynasty, Anxi was established as a military base to gain control over Middle Asia. About forty miles away was an old Han Dynasty town called Kugucheng, also of strategic military importance. Numerous walls and gates were set up to form a line of defence. During the Tang dynasty, the famous general Xue Rengui and his army were besieged in the Anxi area while on the way to conquer the West. The soldiers had used up all their supplies and they had no hope of assistance. Yet they were able to survive by eating *suoyang*, and after that the city was renamed as Suoyang.

Cynomorium didn't enter into the Materia Medica until Zhu Danxi of the Yuan Dynasty period mentioned it in his *Bencao Yanyi Buyi* (Supplement and Expansion of Materia Medica, 1347). The Yuan Dynasty, which was the time of Mongolian rule, introduced several plants from the Mongolian area, including this one. Zhu Danxi also offered a formula with cynomorium that became quite famous, *Huqian Wan* (Hidden Tiger Pills), used for impotence and/or for weakness and atrophy of the legs. The formula is named for the tiger in the crouched position, ready to spring. In order to attain that position (which is also replicated in Gong Fu with the 'crouching tiger' technique), one must have great strength in the tendons, ligaments, and muscles of the legs. This strengthening is sometimes referred to as 'hardening' of yin (substance of the body), but that doesn't necessarily indicate lack of flexibility. The weak leg disorders were first described in the *Neijing Suwen* (*c.* AD 100), in the chapter on *wei* syndrome, which is translated as atrophy or wilting syndrome. There were five types of atrophy listed, associated with each of the five organs. The disorder was thought to derive from heat or damp heat damaging the yin.

Huqian Wan comprises anaemarrhena, phellodendron, cooked rehmannia, tortoise shell, tiger's bone (no longer used), peony, citrus, and dry ginger; sometimes cistanche (another parasitic desert plant) is added. The formula was recently described by Kong Lingqi ('Resolutely upholding the concept of hardening the kidneys method', by Kong Lingqi, *Sichuan Chinese Medicine*, 1998 (6): 8-9, translated by Bob Flaws, and edited here):

The *Suwen* chapter titled *Treatise on Wilting* says, 'The ancestral sinews rule the binding of the bones and the disinhibition of the joints.' If damp heat invades and assails the muscles and flesh and sinews and bones, the chi and blood will not move. The sinews will become slack and not pulled together and, hence, will be useless. If severe, the liver and kidneys will become debilitated and consumed, and the ancestral sinews will cease their duty. Master Ye Tianshi in his *Guide to Clinical Conditions and Case Histories* chapter titled 'Vacuity Taxation' highly praised Zhu Danxi's *Huqian Wan* for their effect of subduing yang and hardening yin. These pills use phellodendron and anemarrhena's bitterness to harden yin. This causes the source to be cleared and flow to be cleaned. Atractylodes (*cangzhu*) and coix (*yiyiren*) dispel dampness. Cistanche (*roucongrong*), cynomorium (*suoyang*), achyranthes (*niuxi*), and tiger bone (*hugu*) strengthen the sinews and bones. Peony (*baishao*) and chaenomeles (*mugua*) emolliate the sinews and relax tension. Cooked rehmannia (*shudi*) and tortoise shell (*guiban*) enrich yin and boost the marrow. Thus damp heat is discharged and transformed, yin essence is subdued and astringed, the ancestral sinews are hardened and strengthened, and the feet are able to walk. Because of these uses, the formula has been suggested by Chinese clinicians as a possible therapy for paralytic disorders, such as multiple sclerosis and ALS.

Appendix: Cynomorium Review

Following is a story about cynomorium written by Robert W. Lebling, Jr, which appeared in the March/April 2003 issue of *Saudi Aramco World*. Lebling, a graduate of Princeton, is a writer/editor and corporate communications specialist. He has lived in both Arab and Hispanic countries and has worked as a journalist. He has compiled an online handbook of Arabian medicinal herbs, which can be viewed and is currently collaborating on a book about natural remedies of Saudi Arabia. Saudi Aramco, an oil company, distributes *Saudi Aramco World* to increase cross-cultural understanding. The bimonthly magazine's goal is to broaden knowledge of the cultures, history, and geography of the Arab and Muslim worlds and their connections with the West. *Saudi Aramco World* is distributed without charge.

11.7 The Treasure of Tarthuth—Parasi

It is early spring in the Dahna, Saudi Arabia's northeastern sand desert. The winter rains have been over for several weeks, leaving a legacy of green foliage that spots the dunes and valleys—scattered arta shrubs, patches of grasses, and low saltbushes. The clumps of vegetation provide forage for the occasional flocks of sheep and goats and for small herds of camels. Where there is livestock, there is always a person to tend the animals, keep them safe, and prevent them from straying. On the slope of a dune, a Saudi youth named Ahmad settles down beside a stand of bushes and trains his eye on his father's camels, about hundred metres off, grazing on the spring bounty. He is particularly watchful of the young ones. It has been a long morning, and he now waits for the return of his brother's white pickup truck.

Suddenly a rare flash of dark red colour catches his eye. Down under the saltbushes to his left, he spies three little dark red club-like shapes poking up from the sand. *Tarthuth!* Ahmad is hungry and thirsty, and nature has furnished him with one of its tastiest snacks. Taking his pocketknife, he digs into the sand at the base of one of the stalks and cuts it off at the root. The pungent smell brings a smile to his face. Ahmad cuts away the reddish skin—tightly covered with tiny button flowers—and exposes the succulent white flesh beneath. He slices off a wet piece and pops it into his mouth. It's sweet and juicy, refreshing, like a ripe fruit. He chews contentedly. Ahmad is lucky: Tarthuth emerges from the sands only for a brief period each year, following the rains of winter. After he has finished his snack, he cuts off the remaining red clubs to take back to his family. The people of the desert have been harvesting tarthuth like this for thousands of years. It has pleased the palates of passing Bedouins and their camels, filled grocers' baskets in local markets, and served as survival food in times of dire famine. It is traditionally known for a wide range of medicinal properties as well, properties now being studied seriously by researchers in the Middle East.

Tarthuth today is barely known outside the region, though it was once harvested around the Mediterranean and was bestowed as a special gift on European royalty in the sixteenth century. In those days it was known to Arabs and Europeans alike as a wonder drug—a heritage largely forgotten in the rush of modern medicine. But things may be changing. Now, as pharmaceutical companies and medical researchers take a closer look at traditional remedies derived from plants and herbs, tarthuth may once again have an opportunity to rise to prominence. Tarthuth (pronounced tar-thooth) is the popular Arabic name for the parasitic plant *Cynomorium coccineum*. Medieval Europeans called it *fungus melitensis*—'Maltese mushroom' or 'Malta fungus,' names by which it is still known today. Sometimes it's called 'desert thumb' or 'red thumb'. The plant is found growing—usually ignored nowadays—in a wide swath that extends from southern Portugal and Spain across the Mediterranean region, including North Africa. Tarthuth even pokes above the remote sands of the Sahara. Botanists have identified it as far south as the central Hoggar range of Southern Algeria. It latches on to salt-loving bushes on Mediterranean islands like Ibiza, Sicily, and, of course, Malta. Its range passes through the Levant to the northern and eastern regions of the Arabian Peninsula and vaults across the Gulf into Iran—and perhaps beyond.

Well known in Saudi Arabia, its burgundy spikes emerged this year in late January near the colossal Ghawar oil field and at Lake Lanhardt in Dhahran; tarthuth also makes its home in Kuwait, Bahrain, Qatar, the United Arab Emirates, and Oman. In February 1999, Canadian explorer Jamie Clarke spotted the bright red flowering stems growing on a rocky shelf nearly five metres (16') up a cliff wall in Wadi Ghadun, in Oman's southern province of Dhofar. 'Traditionally the Bedu . . . ate it during long camel caravans across the Empty Quarter,' Clarke reports in his book *Everest to Arabia*. 'The entire plant is only ten inches [25 cm] high and has an awkward appeal, much like a mushroom's . . . [C]amels love to eat it and I gather this particular plant has been spared that fate by its lofty perch. In a tropical forest it would go unnoticed. Here, its vivid colour and unique character make it stand out against the starkly barren *wadi* cliff.' Tarthuth is a highly specialised parasite with some fungus-like properties. It grows underground for most of the year, feeding on the roots of saltbushes and other salt-tolerant plants. When the winter rains come, its extensive root system shoots fleshy red stems up through the sand and into the open air. The plant has no green colour because it's a parasite and thus needs no chlorophyll to feed itself. The leafless red stems or spikes, fully grown, range in height from about fifteen to thirty centimetres (6-12'). The spikes have tiny scarlet flowers so small that they can hardly be seen individually. Tightly packed and scale-like, they look somewhat like coarse fur. Pollinated by flies attracted by the plant's sweetish, somewhat cabbage-like aroma, the flowers eventually wither and the spike turns black.

When the January and February rains are good, the young fleshy stems of tarthuth can be 'sweet tasting and edible raw, with a pleasant crisp, succulent texture', reports botanist and former Aramco professional James P. Mandaville in his *Flora of Eastern Saudi Arabia*. The flesh is apple-like, with an astringent quality that freshens the mouth. Just picked, tarthuth can be very sweet; left to sit for a few days, it can be somewhat bitter on first taste, but stays tartly refreshing. The Bedouins clean the just-picked spikes, peel off the outer skin, and eat the flavourful white interior. The mature, blackened spikes are sometimes ground and made into a sweetened infusion used hot or cold to treat colic and stomach ulcers. Botanist James Duke cites tarthuth's traditional use as a medicinal tea in Qatar. Botanist Loutfi Boulos says North African medical tradition regards the entire plant as an 'aphrodisiac, spermatopoietic, tonic, [and] astringent'. In traditional medicine, it is mixed with butter and consumed to treat obstructions of the bile duct. Maltese mushroom has a close relative in the East Asia, *C. songaricum* or *suoyang*, whose brownish spikes have long been regarded as an effective medicinal agent in Chinese medicine, used to treat kidney problems, intestinal ailments, and impotence. Recent studies in China show that *Cynomorium*, like green tea, has 'very strong antioxidant effects'.

As recently as the 1920s, villagers from the Saudi coastal oasis of Qatif would head into the desert in early spring and return with their donkeys loaded with sacks of tarthuth for sale in the local *suqs* or markets, Mandaville notes. The plants are still a popular treat for Bedouins and other desert travellers, according to Saudi Aramco wellsite inspector and desert expert Geraiyan M. Al-Hajri. He says tarthuth can be found in springtime in the *suqs* of al-Hasa in the kingdom's Eastern Province. In the Maghrib, Arab North Africa, the dried and pulverised plant is used as a spice or condiment with meat dishes. The red pigment in the plants provides another benefit: It has been used as an effective fabric dye by the women of at least one Arabian tribe, the Manasir, many of whom now live in the United Arab Emirates. The dye produces a rich, colourfast crimson hue known as *dami* or 'blood-red'. Maltese mushroom's use as both foodstuff and medicine go back thousands of years. The ancient Hebrews ate the spikes in times of famine. In the Book of Job (30:4), starving Israelites consume a plant called 'juniper root', and modern botanists say this is *C. coccineum* rather than the inedible root of the juniper bush. (The use of Maltese mushroom as a famine food was most recently reported in the Canary Islands in the nineteenth century.) Arab physicians of the Middle Ages considered tarthuth 'the treasure of drugs' because it had a wealth of traditional therapeutic uses, particularly as a remedy for blood disorders, digestive ailments, and reproductive problems, including impotence and infertility. The great early philosopher of the Arabs, the polymath Al-Kindi (800–70), compiled a medical formulary, or *aqrabadhin*, that mentions tarthuth as the main ingredient of a salve used to relieve acute itching caused by foreign matter under the skin. Al-Razi (865–925), known to Europeans as Rhazes and one of the most influential of all Islamic physicians, prescribed tarthuth as a remedy for haemorrhoids as well as for nasal and uterine bleeding. The medicinal uses of tarthuth are also cited by Ibn Masawayh (777–857), a Persian Christian who directed a hospital and served as personal physician to four caliphs at Baghdad, and by Maimonides, the celebrated twelfth-century Hispanic Jewish doctor and philosopher who was court physician to Saladin in Egypt. Ninth-century Chaldean scholar Ibn Wahshiya, best known for his work *Nabataean Agriculture*, wrote a toxicological treatise called the *Book on Poisons* which includes tarthuth as a key ingredient in several antidotes.

Knowledge of the medicinal value of tarthuth was eventually passed to the Europeans, and here the plant's history takes an unusual turn. In the sixteenth century, the 'treasure of drugs' became the closely guarded treasure of the Knights Hospitaller in Malta. The Hospitallers, or Knights Hospitaller of St. John of Jerusalem, were a fighting order formed at Jerusalem during the First Crusade, some four centuries earlier. They had a dual military and medical mission and operated a 1,000-bed hospital in Jerusalem, providing care for the sick and injured. It was there, in Palestine, that Hospitaller physicians first learnt of tarthuth from their Muslim counterparts and began using the plant in their treatments. When the Muslims recaptured Palestine from the Crusaders, the Knights Hospitaller moved their headquarters to the island of Rhodes and eventually to Malta, the strategically vital island group south of Sicily, where they were pleased to find tarthuth growing on a tiny islet. Off the west coast of Gozo, the smaller of the two main Maltese islands, there is an irregular block of limestone rising from the sea, some 180 metres long and about 60 metres high (600 by 200 feet) with a flattish, sloping top and sheer cliffs on all sides. Today this islet is called Fungus Rock. It is also known to the Maltese as Gebla tal-General, General's Rock, after a Hospitaller naval squadron commander credited with discovering it. Here, on the tabletop islet, *C. coccineum*, Maltese mushroom, grew in abundance. On orders from their grand master, the knights quickly took control of Fungus Rock, placed guards on the mainland, and barred access to any but their own. They hacked all ledges from the sides of the islet to keep people from climbing the cliffs. Trespassers who tried anyway were imprisoned and made galley slaves. Thieves who managed to steal Maltese mushroom were reportedly put to death. The only way to reach the island's top was by a primitive and precarious 'cable car' rigged on ropes and pulleys and connected to poles on the mainland. A version of that cable car, a wooden box, survived into the early nineteenth century, and English traveler Claudius Shaw made the dangerous crossing in 1815:

It is not a very pleasant sensation to be suspended some hundred feet above the water, and if there is any wind, the movement of the box is anything but agreeable, and all that can be obtained are a few pieces of fungus. I was well pleased to be back again and made a determination never to risk my precious carcass in that conveyance again. Maltese mushroom was under the personal control of the Hospitaller grand master. His knights harvested the precious plant each year and stored it in a watchtower on the mainland. This structure, Dwejra Tower, was built in 1651 to guard Fungus Rock and protect the island of Gozo from pirate raids. Once harvested, the Maltese mushroom spikes were dried, pulverised, and preserved in various liquids. Hospitaller doctors used it to cure dysentery and ulcers, to stop haemorrhages, and to prevent infection. The plant was a favoured treatment for apoplexy and venereal disease and was used as a contraceptive, as a toothpaste, and as a dye to colour textiles. It was also prescribed in Malta to treat high blood pressure, vomiting, and irregular menstrual periods. Precious as it was, the grand master sent it as an appropriate special present to the kings, queens, and nobility of European countries.

In 1565, the most famous of the Hospitallers' grand masters, Jean de la Vallette—eponym of Malta's present-day capital, Valetta—was wounded by a grenade blast during a siege by Ottoman Turkish forces. Historians say his wound was dressed with Maltese mushroom and that the grand master recovered and returned to battle. The Knights Hospitaller held Malta until 1798, when they surrendered to Napoleon and lost their last territorial base in the Mediterranean. Their military role had come to an end, though they survive today as the Knights of Malta, an international non-governmental medical-service organisation recognised by the United Nations. As the order lost its military mission, so did the Maltese mushroom fade from therapeutic use in Europe. By the 1800s, the old herbal remedies of the Middle East—plant extracts known as galenicals—were largely eclipsed in the West by new, mineral-based 'drug' treatments. Today Maltese mushroom survives atop Fungus Rock, drawing its nourishment from the roots of tamarisk or sea lavender. The Maltese call it *gherq is-sinjur*, which may derive from the Arabic *irq al-sinja*, 'bayonet root'. A species of reptile found nowhere else—the Fungus Rock wall lizard, *Podarcis filfolensis generalensis*—seems to have a special affinity for the plant and can often be found climbing the succulent red spikes. But biologists say it is attracted not by the sweet juice but by the flies that help pollinate the plants. (Lizards in Saudi Arabia seem similarly drawn to tarthuth.) In recent decades, Maltese mushroom has been found growing elsewhere in Malta, but it has been declared an endangered species throughout the island group and is legally protected. Since 1992, Fungus Rock itself has been designated as a nature reserve, and the curious and adventurous are prohibited from intruding on the craggy rock, just as they were back in the sixteenth and seventeenth centuries.

Sir David Attenborough, the well-known British filmmaker and author who wrote *The Private Life of Plants*, finds Maltese mushroom a fascinating plant parasite, but he is sceptical about its medicinal value. He suggests that apothecaries may have inferred the plant's therapeutic properties from its appearance, applying the 'doctrine of the signatures', a belief going back to the ancient Greeks that a plant's external appearance indicated what its effects might be. Thus, for example, a plant with kidney-shaped leaves was good for breaking up kidney stones, and tarthuth was presumed to cure blood diseases because of its dark red, blood-like colour. But Attenborough's suggestion does not explain the range of medical uses found for the plant that had no connection with its appearance—such as its role as a treatment for ulcers and other gastrointestinal ailments—and it underestimates the Knights of Malta, who were not practitioners of magic and whose doctors employed the latest clinical and therapeutic practices, including those of Arab and Islamic medicine. The Arabs and other Muslims of the Middle Ages were the most sophisticated medical practitioners of their time and well acquainted with experimental methods. Clinical and therapeutic works written in Arabic and translated into Latin found their way into Europe's best medical schools. The massive and authoritative *Canon of Medicine* by Ibn Sina (Avicenna) was translated in the twelfth century and served as the standard textbook for medical training in European universities even well into the eighteenth century. Given their medical expertise, the Arabs may well have been correct in calling *Cynomorium coccineum* 'the treasure of drugs'. With the growing popularity of alternative and holistic medicine in recent decades—a trend now taken seriously by pharmaceutical companies and government health institutes—researchers have been exploring the claims of traditional therapies and herbal medicines, looking for new, scientifically supported treatments and applications.

'Interest in medicinal plants as a re-emerging health aid has been fuelled by the rising costs of prescription drugs in the maintenance of personal health and well-being, and the bioprospecting of new plant-derived drugs,' report Lucy Hoareau and Edgar J. DaSilva of UNESCO's Division of Life Sciences. 'Developed countries, in recent times, are turning to the use of traditional medicinal systems that involve the use of herbal drugs and remedies,' they note in the *Electronic Journal of Biotechnology* (1999). 'About 1,400 herbal preparations are used widely, according to a recent survey in Member States of the European Union.' So it is not surprising to learn that scientists have been testing the properties of tarthuth. In 1978, researchers reported in an Iranian medical journal that *Cynomorium coccineum* harvested in Iran was 'found to possess significant blood pressure lowering activity' when tested on dogs. The strong hypotensive effect occurred chiefly in tests involving the fresh juice of the plant or juice dissolved in water. Dried, powdered tarthuth was also tested but without so significant an effect. The researchers suspected the fresh samples enjoyed a 'special molecular arrangement' that caused the reduction in blood pressure. This study suggests that the traditional belief in tarthuth's value as a remedy for blood ailments warrants further investigation. Saudi researchers have also worked on some of the plant's reputed health properties. Based on their initial findings, the traditional claims that Maltese mushroom improves fertility and reproductive vigour may have a basis in truth as well. Three recent studies at King Saud University found that extracts of *Cynomorium coccineum*, administered orally, had significant positive effects on the reproductive development and fertility levels of male and female rats. The results were published in the international journals *Phytotherapy Research* (1999 and 2000) and *Ethnopharmacology* (2001). Modern scientific studies of this strange parasitic plant are clearly in their early stages. But they seem to be worth pursuing. Ethnopharmacology—the study of traditional plant and herbal remedies—is a burgeoning field with great social and commercial promise, and further research may indeed show there is much more to Maltese mushroom than a delightful desert treat.

11.8 Saffron—An Antidepressant Herb

Subhuti Dharmananda, PhD, Director

Background

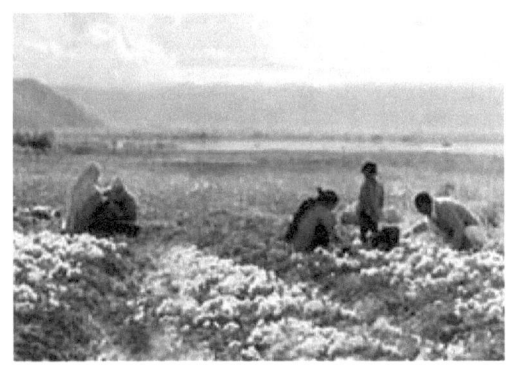

Saffron is a herb most people are unlikely to utilise, either for medicinal or culinary purposes, primarily because the material has a justified reputation for being extraordinarily expensive. Bulk quantities of relatively low-grade saffron can reach upwards of $500/pound, while retail costs for small amounts may exceed ten times that rate. But avoiding this valuable spice might be unnecessary because of the small quantity needed: In medicinal use, 1–3 g in decoction, 0.5–1.5 g ingested as powder, or 30 mg of its dried extract per day is considered adequate in standard applications (described below). For culinary use, just a few strands are sufficient to flavour food (about two to four strands per person; there are about 70,000–200,000 strands per pound).

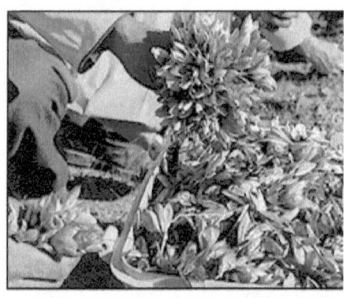

In some countries, such as Spain, Iran, and India, people know that saffron is worth its price and make good use of it. To meet the demand, world annual production is about 265 tons per year, which is grown on about 90,000 acres of land (if efficiently cultivated, each acre produces about 6 lb of saffron a year). It takes about 170–200 hours of work to collect the flowers and remove the stamens for drying in order to produce just 1 lb of saffron, which is a large part of the expense for the spice. Saffron mainly grows in arid territory with sandy soil, under hot and dry summers, often requiring irrigation.

Saffron's high cost has become an attractive factor for one potential use: as a substitute crop for opium cultivation in Afghanistan. Afghanistan is the world's second largest supplier of opium poppies used in the drug trade (the largest is the 'golden triangle' and the surrounding regions

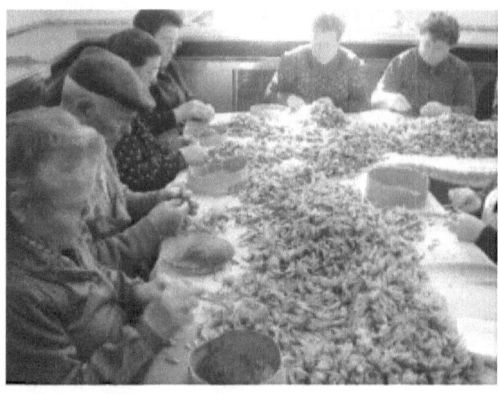

in Southeast Asia); opium is one of the major sources of income for Afghanistan. In 2002, about 3,400 tons of opium were produced there, most of it ultimately going to heroin addicts in Europe. Since Afghanistan is in the saffron-growing region, there is some potential for this crop as an economic substitute; still, saffron is estimated to bring in only about three-fourth the income of opium farming.

Iran, the world's largest producer of saffron and a neighbour to Afghanistan, has been investing in research into saffron's potential medicinal uses. Much of the work surrounds its traditional application for alleviating depression. One of the Iranian groups carrying out saffron research is headed by Shahin Akhondzadeh (pictured right), at the Roozbeh Psychiatric Hospital in the Tehran University of Medical Sciences, who has 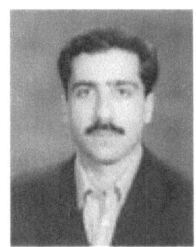 studied the use of several drugs and herbs for mental disorders, such as depression, ADHD, Alzheimer's disease, autism, opiate dependence, and epilepsy. The clinical findings suggest that saffron is a safe and effective antidepressant. For example, in a randomised, double-blind study, 30 mg of saffron extract (in capsules) given for six weeks resulted in significant alleviation of depression compared to those on placebo, and they did so without evident side effects [1]. This study was a follow-up to a preliminary trial in which the same saffron preparation performed as well as imipramine for treating depression in a double-blind trial [2]. In further preliminary work, saffron was compared to the drug fluoxetine (often known by the brand product Prozac); it was found that saffron performed as well as the drug in treatment of both depression and epilepsy [3]. Pharmacology studies done in Iran [4] and Japan [5, 6] have confirmed an anticonvulsant activity in the extract of saffron.

A potential deterrent to medicinal use of saffron comes about because erroneous information related to saffron toxicity has appeared, especially in Internet presentations, but also in books. The reports mention serious adverse effects from as little as 5 g (about three times the medicinal dose), and fatal doses of just 20 g have also been mentioned. By contrast, all recent research reports indicate that saffron is non-toxic. Why the discrepancy?

The most likely reason for this impression was writers initially confused toxic meadow saffron with non-toxic saffron; from there the reports were simply repeated. Meadow saffron, also called wild saffron or Autumn crocus (*Colchicum autumnale*), contains the toxic compound colchicine (used primarily in the treatment of gout). It appears that the literature references to saffron acting as a toxin causing severe spontaneous bleeding or even death with just a few grams are primarily the result of ingestion of meadow saffron (or other materials) but not true saffron. These reports of adverse effects are old ones; for example, this oft-repeated information is relayed in the 1987 German E Commission report, which, in turn, is based on comments in other literature now over fifty years old, which did not include an analysis of the materials ingested or other details. Meadow saffron is not a substitute for true saffron; rather, it is sometimes ingested accidentally when collected mistakenly as a source of wild garlic. However, it is often simply called saffron, and articles reporting on its toxicity may list *Crocus sativus* as the botanical name, yet refer instead to meadow saffron in the description of uses (e.g. treating arthritis and gout) and toxicity, showing how easily these two are interchanged in reporting. Today, all saffron is cultivated; the material in the market does not include adulterant herbs. The safety of saffron is important in relation to its antidepressant action because the main herb used for that purpose today, St. John's Wort, has the problem of affecting drug metabolising enzymes (thus, having a high potential for drug interactions) and for inducing photosensitivity.

The Plant and Its Cultivation

Saffron is collected from *Crocus Sativus* (*Iridaceae*), which originated in the Middle Eastern region of the Eurasian continent, from Greece to Persia (Iran). The plant does not propagate by seeds; the underground portion, corms (also called bulbs), divide to produce new plants. Flowers emerge in autumn; the outstanding feature

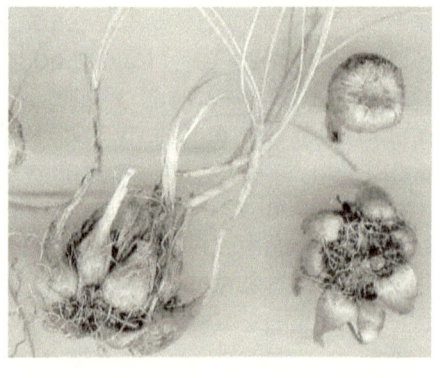

of the lilac—to mauve-coloured flower is its three stigmas 25-30 mm long, which droop over the petals: That is what is collected as saffron. There are also three yellow stamens, which lack the active compounds and are not collected. The stigma is attached to a style, which has little of the active components and is only included with the lower grades of saffron.

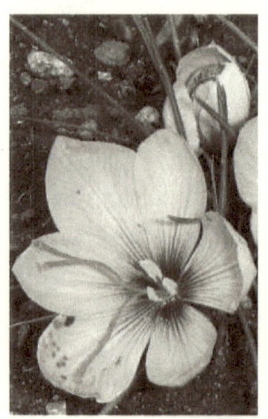

Each bulb produces from one to seven flowers. The cultivated form is thought to have originated as a naturally occurring hybrid that was selected for its extra-long stigmas and has been maintained ever since. It takes about 36,000 flowers to yield just 1 lb of the stigmas.

Saffron has been cultivated in the region from Greece to Persia for thirty-five centuries and is mentioned in early literature, such as in the fourth of the Songs of Solomon, dated to about 965 BC. Its cultivation and use spread throughout the region, moving east to Kashmir and west to Spain. The herb has been cultivated as far west as Britain and became an important medicinal product in Tibet. Saffron was described in the Chinese compendium *Bencao Gangmu* (in 1596), indicating that it was introduced from Persia and used to benefit the blood (vitalises blood, stops bleeding) and to calm fright. Th is information is very important for then preventive therapy.

Iran is the major saffron producer today, accounting for about 85 per cent of the global production. The country produced 225 tons of saffron (April 2003-March 2004) and earned $67 million from saffron exports (only 10-15 tons were used domestically; most of the export goes to Spain). This year (2011), the Iranian saffron exports may reach $100 million. Spain is the second largest producer (35-40 tons/year) but is the primary international distributor; minor producers include Portugal, France, Italy, and Turkey. Kashmir has begun large-scale production though it is not yet a major international source. Saffron has been successfully planted in several Chinese provinces, including Henan, Jiangsu, Hunan, Shanghai, and Tibet. A major problem with saffron production is that the plant grows in desert regions but needs sufficient water to thrive; irrigation in many of these areas is costly and difficult; severe draughts can cause significant crop losses.

Saffron As a Dye

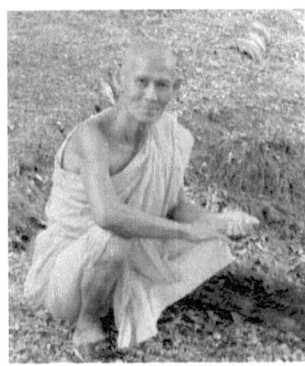

Historically, saffron was particularly important as a dye plant. Saffron dye used in small quantities will impart a yellowish-orange colour, with increasing redness as more is applied to colour the cloth.

In India, Tibet, and China, saffron has been used to produce the yellow-red colour of robes for Hindu and Buddhist monks. The main dye component, crocin, a flavonoid, has also been found in the less expensive gardenia fruit, which is now being developed as an alternative source for dye purposes in China. Inexpensive substitutes, such as the yellow colour from turmeric, do not produce a comparable colour.

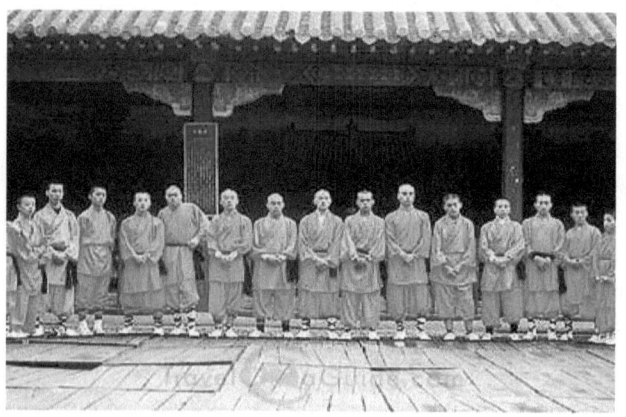

Saffron As a Medicinal Herb

The medicinal properties attributed to saffron are extensive. Topically, it is applied to improve the skin condition overall and specifically to treat acne. Internally, it is used to improve blood circulation, regulate menstruation, treat digestive disturbance, ease cough and asthmatic breathing, reduce fever and inflammation, calm nervousness, and alleviate depression. In Tibet, saffron is often an ingredient in medicinal incenses; it is considered a tonic for the heart and the nervous system. The active ingredients may be of benefit in inhibiting growth of cancer cells [7-10].

Constituents

Saffron has been analysed extensively. It contains, approximately, these common plant components:

Substance	Proportion
Simple sugars	12-15 per cent
Water	9-14 per cent
Proteins, amino acids, other nitrogen compounds	11-13 per cent
Cellulose (fibre)	4-7 per cent

Substance	Proportion
Fats	3-8 per cent
Minerals (measured as acid soluble ash)	1-1.5 per cent
Other non-nitrogen (mainly complex sugars)	About 40 per cent

These active compounds are also there:

- Essential oil (volatile oil): 0.3-1.5 per cent
- Yellow colour: crocins, derived from crocetin (about 2 per cent) and other carotenes (about 8 per cent)
- Bitter substances including picrocrocin and safranal (the main aromatic of saffron): about 4 per cent

The active constituents are degradation products of common carotenoids, mainly zeaxanthin (and, to a lesser extent, lycopene and beta-carotene), as illustrated below. Crocetin and the crocins provide far more colour than the other carotenes. Picrocrocin, derived from the terminal end of zeaxanthin, is the glycoside of safranal, which is a terpene aldehyde. Safranal is formed during the drying of the collected saffron, and it provides most of the characteristic saffron fragrance. There are other volatile components (included in the essential oil fraction) that are also derived from the carotenes and have structures similar to safranal. The following diagram shows the chemical elements present in saffron:

Zeaxanthin

Crocetin

Picrocrocin

Crocin

References

1. Akhondzadeh S., et al., Crocus sativus in the treatment of mild to moderate depression: a double-blind, randomized and placebo-controlled trial, *Phytotherapy Research*, 2005; 19(2): 148-51.
2. Akhondzadeh S., et al., Comparison of Crocus sativus and imipramine in the treatment of mild to moderate depression: a pilot double-blind randomized trial, *Biomed Central Complementary and Alternative Medicine*, 2004; 4(1): 12.
3. Noorbala A. A., Hydro-alcoholic extract of Crocus sativus versus fluoxetine in the treatment of mild to moderate depression: a double-blind, randomized pilot trial, *Journal of Ethnopharmacology*, 2005; 97(2): 281-4.
4. Hosseinzadeh H. and Khosravan V., Anticonvulsant effects aqueous and ethanolic extracts of Crocus sativus stigmas in mice, *Archives of Iranian Medicine*, 2002; 5: 44-7.
5. Abe K. and Saito H., Effects of saffron extract and its constituent crocin on learning behavior and long-term potentiation, *Phytother. Res.*, 2000; 14: 149-52.
6. Zhang Y., Shoyama Y., Sugiura M., and Saito H., Effect of Crocus sativus on the ethanol-induced impairment of passive avoidance performances in mice, *Biological and Pharmaceutical Bulletin*, 1994; 17: 217-21.
7. Escribano J., et al., Crocin, safranal and picrocrocin from saffron (Crocus sativus) inhibit the growth of human cancer cells *in vitro*, *Cancer Letters*, 1996; 100 (1-2): 23-30.
8. Tarantilis P. A., et al., Inhibition of growth and induction of differentiation of promyelocytic leukemia (HL-60) by carotenoids from Crocus sativus, *Anticancer Research*, 1994; 14(5A): 1913-18.
9. Garcia-Olmo D. C., Effects of long-term treatment of colon adenocarcinoma with crocin, a carotenoid from saffron (Crocus sativus): an experimental study in the rat, *Nutrition and Cancer*, 1999; 35(2): 120-6.
10. Abdullaev-Jafarova F. and Espinosa-Aguirre J. J., Biomedical properties of saffron and its potential use in cancer therapy and chemoprevention trials, *Cancer Detection and Prevention*, 2004; 28(6): 430-6.

11.9 Update on Soy Products: Are They Appropriate for Women Concerned About Breast Cancer?

Subhuti Dharmananda, PhD, Director

Soy products are a major nutritional food source in Japan and China. It has been uggested that high levels of consumption of these foods may contribute to certain health benefits, including reduced blood lipids, reduced oxidation of lipids, and improvements in other cardiovascular risk factors. In October 1999, the U.S. Food and Drug Administration authorised the use of food labels of health claims associated with soy protein and the reduced risk of coronary heart disease. Soy protein is one of the most complete proteins of the vegetable kingdom. Soybeans also contain substantial amounts of lecithin and vitamin E, which are understood to be very healthy components of oils. Taken together, the evidence suggests that soybeans and their *products can make a good contribution to the human diet. Complementary preventive therapist must be cautious in the use and application of these products.*

With regard to women's health, it has been suggested that high soy intake may be associated with reduction of menopausal symptoms and with reduced incidence of breast cancer. These effects, which still need to be elucidated more fully by further studies, are attributed to the soybean isoflavones. The isoflavones are found throughout the legumes (bean family), but are especially rich in soy beans. In particular, genistein, the dominant isoflavone of soy, is reported to inhibit the growth of cultured cancer cells in the laboratory, including breast cancer cells. Soy isoflavones are reported to reduce hot flashes during menopause more effectively than placebos but not as effectively as hormone replacement therapy (45 per cent, 30 per cent, and 70 per cent effectiveness, respectively). The effects of soy isoflavones on menopausal symptoms are dose–dependent, and it is possible that higher rates of effectiveness may be attained with higher isoflavone administration (currently, menopause therapies typically involve 60-80 mg/day of isoflavones).

Raw soybeans may have as much as 150 mg of total isoflavones per 100 g, and some soy flour products (such as roasted full-flat powder) may have as much as 200 mg isoflavones per 100 g. By contrast, commonly used soy food products, such as tofu, may provide only about 20-50 mg isoflavones per 100 g. During the past decade, a number of new soybean products have been designed in which the soy isoflavones are present in quantities as high or higher than in the usual soybean food products, some being comparable to the soy flour products that have the highest naturally occurring isoflavone content. These new products may have the fat and carbohydrate removed from the soybeans (removal of soy carbohydrates is often regarded as a benefit as there are polysaccharide components that are difficult for some people to digest). For example, Nutra-Soy (developed by Narula Research) provides 212 mg isoflavones per 100 g (i.e. 60 mg per one ounce serving) with half of the powder being protein. The ability to produce soy products in a desirable form with high levels of isoflavones has been made possible by commercial technologies that allow isolation of the isoflavones, which can then be added to soy products (such as soy protein powders) or simply put into capsules and tablets. One reason for this development is that most people who desire the potential benefits of these soy components are unwilling or unable to get the amounts from their diet that are said to be needed, according to research studies, to attain the desired results. Clinical studies using soy isoflavones have involved amounts that typically range from 60 to 80 mg, though higher amounts, up to 200 mg, have been tried and found to be potentially helpful. The typical doses used in such studies correspond to eating a substantial amount of soy products each day; these amounts are attainable by those who have a preference for soy foods, such as tofu, tempeh (a fermented soybean product), soy milk, and soy-based meat substitute products, but not for those who only eat soy foods occasionally or in small amounts.

A growing body of research with soy components, including soy isoflavones, lecithin, vitamin E, soy saponins, and soy protein, have pointed to significant health benefits. However, during the past couple of years, there has been a growing call for caution about consuming soy in any form, particularly in popular literature (newspaper and magazine articles) and on the Internet (non-research sites). Much of the concern that has been raised is based on misreading of the literature and on poor studies. Thus, for example, the soy isoflavones are known to be able to inhibit certain enzyme systems and thyroid hormones, a fact which is raised as a serious warning about consuming soy or its isoflavones. However, detrimental effects are not observed in adults: the problem arises when infants are fed solely soy milk formulations to replace mother's milk, cow milk, or non-soy formulations. Infants may face an adverse consequence (related to thyroid inhibition) due to their low body weight, high susceptibility, and the single substance diet. Despite the safety of use in adults, opponents of soy use have warned that this is just one of many problems that need to concern everyone interested in the health benefits of soy. A nutrition study widely reported in the news media last year suggested that people who consumed more than two servings of soy per week had a higher risk of suffering from brain shrinkage as they aged. This study has been soundly criticised with regard to this conclusion, but opponents of soy use have trotted out this inconclusive study so as to bolster a weak case against soy. In fact, other studies suggest that soy helps protect against neurodegeneration.

There is one area of concern that is very contentious and which currently remains outside of the ability of anyone to form a firm conclusion at this time. Information derived from studies of soy and soy isoflavones have yielded some conflicting implications about the possible effects of soy consumption on the risk of developing breast cancer or its suitability for women who already have breast cancer. For example, at a recent meeting on the subject of breast cancer in Portland, Oregon, two naturopathic physicians (practitioners that specialise in, among other areas, prescription of dietary and nutritional regimens to their patients) offered markedly different views. Both practitioners have a large proportion of patients dealing with breast cancer related issues and have reviewed the literature about soy so as to provide helpful advice. One doctor suggested that so long as the dosage of isoflavones is adequate, they would have a beneficial effect (a daily dosage of about 80 mg was suggested). The other doctor suggested that soy isoflavones should be avoided by adult women and that the only possible use for consuming soy regularly in relation to reducing breast cancer risk, at least as he understood the current research results, would be during the early years of life (around puberty).

While the majority of research studies support the use of soy and its isoflavones in relation to breast cancer risk (see 'Estrogen dependent tumours and herbs: how modern conditions change traditional practices'), the concern expressed by this doctor came primarily from two reports. In one case, involving a clinical evaluation of adult women, the administration of soy led to slight changes (proliferation) in the breast tissue which the researchers felt were consistent with estrogen-like changes that are believed to contribute to the risk of developing breast cancer [1]. The other case was a laboratory animal study in which soy appeared to have a protective anti-cancer effect when administered to young animals [2], whereas such effects are not as evident in studies with older animals. Put together, these two studies could be interpreted as indicating an advantage to using soy in early years that is lost, or even becomes negative, if soy is introduced in later years.

In a recent study of genistein, and the related soy isoflavone genistin, in laboratory-cultured breast cancer cells, it was shown that, although these compounds bind very weakly to the cells, they can stimulate their growth at a sufficient dosage. Generally, it is thought that these isoflavones compete for binding sites with estrogen and thereby prevent the estrogen, which is a much stronger stimulant to breast cancer cells, from having its negative impact. Thus, at the doses normally consumed (via diet or current supplementation practices), the overall risk of inducing breast cancer should be lowered. The debate about the suitability of using soy or soy isoflavones in relation to breast cancer risks is one that probably will not be resolved definitively any time soon, but continuing research appears to lend further support to a benefit of using soy, even in adults and those with breast cancer (see the listing of five abstracts at the end of this article). In fact, at this time, the only caution about using soy regularly as an adult appears to be for women who are pregnant, since a high isoflavone intake might have negative consequences for the developing fetus (suggested thus far only by laboratory animal studies). There are no evident problems in this regard from normal dietary levels of isoflavones, as are common in Japan.

One of the problems faced with making a definitive interpretation of the data is that breast cancer risk factors are very difficult to determine with specificity. Studies that appear to be conducted properly can present conflicting results with minor changes in design. In the February issue of the *Journal of the American Medical Association*, there was a review of clinical studies evaluating the risk of breast cancer in relation to consumption of fruits and vegetables [3]. The article presented information suggesting that fruit and vegetable consumption had no impact on breast cancer risk. Some early studies and reviews suggested that these foods had a notably favourable impact (more fruits and vegetables meant lower risk). The preliminary results have been one of the reasons why women who wish to avoid breast cancer are advised to eat plenty of fruits and vegetables and even to take supplements that contain what are believed to be active components of these foods (e.g. antioxidants). Similarly, there have been conflicting results regarding the contribution of fats to breast cancer. Early studies seemed to indicate that breast cancer risk was greater with a higher fat diet; more recent evaluations indicated no significant effect [5, 6]. The implication that high-fat diets contributed to breast cancer risk led to suggestions that women pursue a low-fat diet, especially by avoiding large amounts of meat and thus eating more fruits and vegetables as well as alternative protein sources, such as soy. Additionally, there have been conflicting results from studies about the increased risk of breast cancer posed by using hormone replacement therapy. Some studies find substantial increase in risk (e.g. a one-third increase in risk after using HRT for more than ten years), others find only a slight increase, and others, still, find no significant change. The hormones do not seem to increase the risk of dying of breast cancer, even if the hormone therapy is given after a diagnosis of breast cancer [6]. As pointed out in most modern literature, one of the greatest factors for breast cancer risk is delay of first childbirth or absence of child-bearing; the early differentiation of breast tissue under the hormonal effects of full-term pregnancy apparently confers lasting protection [7]. Based on current research reports, changes in breast cancer risk appear to be quite small regardless of their direction, and most reports suggest there is an improvement with soy isoflavones and soy protein. The scientific literature must still be recognised as presenting preliminary results. However, the overall conclusion that can be derived from a growing body of literature is that the impact of soy isoflavones in relation to health and longevity is a positive one.

At least, the preventive therapist can be rest assured that the above mentioned product is good for prevention oif the said potential disease.

References

1. McMichael-Phillips D. F., et al., Effects of soy-protein supplementation on epithelial proliferation in the histologically normal human breast, *American Journal of Clinical Nutrition*, 1998; 68(6 Suppl): 1431S-5S.
2. Hilakivi-Clarke L., et al., Prepubertal exposure to zearalenone or genistein reduces mamary tumorigenesis, *British Journal of Cancer*, 1999; 80(11): 1682-8.
3. Smith-Warner S. A., et al., Intake of fruits and vegetables and risk of breast cancer: a pooled analysis of cohort studies, *Journal of the American Medical Association*, 2001; 285(6): 769-76.

4. Willett W. C., et al., Dietary fat and fiber in relation to risk of breast cancer. An 8-year follow-up, *Journal of the American Medical Association,* 1992; 268(15): 2037-44.
5. Holmes M. D., et al., Dietary fat intake and endogenous sex steroid hormone levels in postmenopausal women, *Journal of Clinical Oncology,* 2000; 18(21): 3668-76.
6. Disaia P. J., et al., Breast cancer survival and hormone replacement therapy: a cohort analysis, *American Journal of Clinical Oncology,* 2000; 23(6): 541-5.
7. Chie W. C., et al., Age at any full-term pregnancy and breast cancer risk, *American Journal of Epidemiology,* 2000; 151(7):715-22.

Appendix. Sample of Recent Articles Favourable to Soy and Its Isoflavones

In the following pages five abstracts of recent articles that illustrate the direction of research on soy are given, where the indications are that soy has a favourable effect or, at the least, no unfavourable effects related to risk of breast cancer. These abstracts appear in the National Library of Medicine's worldwide web site:

Title: Genistein's 'ER-dependent and independent' actions are mediated through ER pathways in ER-positive breast carcinoma cell lines.

Authors: Shao ZM, Shen ZZ, Fontana JA, and Barsky SH.

Institution: Department of Surgery, Shanghai Medical University, P. R. China.

Source: *Anticancer Research,* 2000, July-August; 20(4): 2409-16.

Abstract: Genistein, a natural flavone found in soy has been postulated to be responsible for lowering the rate of breast cancer in Asian women. Our previous studies have shown that genistein exerts multiple suppressive effects on both estrogen receptor positive (ER+) as well as estrogen receptor negative (ER−) human breast carcinoma lines suggesting that the mechanisms of these effects may be independent of ER pathways. In the present study, however, we provide evidence that in the ER+ MCF-7, T47D and 549 lines but not in the ER-MDA-MB-231 and MDA-

MB-468 lines both presumed 'ER-dependent' and 'ER-independent' actions of genistein are mediated through ER pathways. Genistein's antiproliferative effects are estrogen-dependent in these ER+ lines, being more pronounced in estrogen-containing media and in the presence of exogenous 17-beta estradiol. Genistein also inhibits the expression of ER-downstream genes including pS2 and TGF-beta in these ER+ lines and this inhibition is also dependent on the presence of estrogen. Genistein inhibits estrogen-induced protein tyrosine kinase (PTK) activity. Genistein is only a weak transcriptional activator and actually decreases ERE-CAT levels induced by 17-beta estradiol in the ER+ lines. Genistein also decreases steady state ER mRNA only in the presence of estrogen in the ER+ lines, thereby manifesting another suppression of and through the ER pathway. Our observations resurrect the hypothesis that genistein functions as a 'good estrogen' in ER+ breast carcinomas. Since chemopreventive effects of genistein would be targeted to normal ER-positive ductal-lobular cells of the breast, this 'good estrogen' action of genistein is most relevant to our understanding of chemoprevention.

Title: Soy consumption alters endogenous estrogen metabolism in postmenopausal women.

Authors: Xu X, Duncan AM, Wangen KE, and Kurzer MS.

Institution: Department of Food Science and Nutrition, University of Minnesota, St. Paul, Minnesota.

Source: *Cancer Epidemiology Biomarkers*, 2000; 9(8):781-6.

Abstract: Isoflavones are soy phytoestrogens that have been suggested to be anticarcinogenic. Our previous study in premenopausal women suggested that the mechanisms by which isoflavones exert cancer-preventive effects may involve modulation of estrogen metabolism away from production of potentially carcinogenic metabolites [16alpha-(OH) estrone, 4-(OH) estrone, and 4-(OH) estradiol] (X. Xu, et al., *Cancer Epidemiol. Biomark. Prev.*, 7: 1101-8, 1998). To further evaluate this hypothesis, a randomised, crossover soy isoflavone feeding study was performed in eighteen healthy postmenopausal women. The study consisted of three diet periods, each separated by a washout of approximately three weeks. Each diet period lasted for ninety-three days, during which subjects consumed their habitual diets supplemented with soy protein isolate providing 0.1 (control), 1, or 2 mg isoflavones/kg body weight/day (7.1 ± 1.1, 65 ± 11, or 132 ± 22 mg/day). A 72-h urine sample was collected 3 days before the study (baseline) and days 91–93 of each diet period. Urine samples were analysed for ten phytoestrogens and fifteen endogenous estrogens and their metabolites by a capillary gas chromatography-mass spectrometry method. Compared with the soy-free baseline and very low isoflavone control diet, consumption of 65 mg isoflavones increased the urinary 2/16alpha-(OH) estrone ratio, and consumption of 65 or 132 mg isoflavones decreased excretion of 4-(OH) estrone. When compared with baseline values, consumption of all three soy diets increased the ratio of 2/4-(OH) estrogens and decreased the ratio of genotoxic: total estrogens. These data suggest that both isoflavones and other soy constituents may exert cancer-preventive effects in postmenopausal women by altering estrogen metabolism away from genotoxic metabolites towards inactive metabolites.

Title: Modest hormonal effects of soy isoflavones in postmenopausal women.

Authors: Duncan AM, Underhill KE, Xu X, Lavalleur J, Phipps WR, and Kurzer MS.

Institution: Department of Food Science and Nutrition, University of Minnesota, St. Paul, Minnesota.

Source: *Journal of Clinical Endocrinology and Metabolism*, 1999; 84(10): 3479-84.

Abstract: Soy isoflavones have been hypothesised to exert hormonal effects in postmenopausal women. To test this hypothesis, we studied the effects of three soy powders containing different levels of isoflavones in eighteen postmenopausal women. Isoflavones were consumed relative to the body weight [control: 0.11 +/– 0.01; low isoflavone (low-iso): 1.00 +/– 0.01; high isoflavone (high-iso): 2.00 +/– 0.02 mg/kg/day] for 93 days each in a randomised crossover design. Blood was collected on day 1 of the study (baseline) and days 36-38, 64-66, and 92-94 of each diet period, for analysis of estrogens, androgens, gonadotropins, sex hormone binding globulin (SHBG), prolactin, insulin, cortisol, and thyroid hormones. Vaginal cytology specimens were obtained at baseline and at the end of each diet period, and endometrial biopsies were performed at baseline and at the end of the high-iso diet period to provide additional measures of estrogen action. Overall, compared with the control diet, the effects of the low-iso and high-iso diets were modest in degree. The high-iso diet resulted in a small but significant decrease in estrone-sulphate (E1-S), a trend towards lower estradiol (E2) and estrone (E1), and a small but significant increase in SHBG. For the other hormones, the few significant changes noted were also small and probably not of physiological importance. There were no significant effects of the low-iso or high-iso diets on vaginal cytology or endometrial biopsy results. These data suggest that effects of isoflavones on plasma hormones *per se* are not significant mechanisms by which soy consumption may exert estrogen-like effects in postmenopausal women. These data also show that neither isoflavones nor soy exert clinically important estrogenic effects on vaginal epithelium or endometrium.

Title: Effect of soy protein foods on low-density lipoprotein oxidation and *ex vivo* sex hormone receptor activity—a controlled crossover trial.

Authors: Jenkins DJ, Kendall CW, Garsetti M, Rosenberg-Zand RS, Jackson CJ, Agarwal S, Rao AV, Diamandis EP, Parker T, Faulkner D, Vuksan V, and Vidgen E.

Institution: Clinical Nutrition and Risk Factor Modification Center, St. Michael's Hospital, Toronto, Ontario, Canada.

Source: *Metabolism: Clinical and Experimental*, 2000; 49(4):537-43.

Abstract: Plant-derived estrogen analogues (phytoestrogens) may confer significant health advantages including cholesterol reduction, antioxidant activity, and possibly a reduced cancer risk. However, the concern has also been raised that phytoestrogens may be endocrine disrupters and major health hazards. We therefore assessed the effects of soy foods as a rich source of isoflavonoid phytoestrogens on LDL oxidation and sex hormone receptor activity. Thirty-one hyperlipidemic subjects underwent two 1-month low-fat metabolic diets in a randomised crossover study. The major differences between the test and control diets were an increase in soy protein foods (33 g/d soy protein), providing 86 mg isoflavones/2,000 kcal/day and a doubling of the soluble fibre intake. Fasting blood samples were obtained at the start and at weeks two and four, with twenty-four-hour urine collections at the end of each phase. Soy foods increased urinary isoflavone excretion on the test diet versus the control. The test diet decreased both oxidised LDL measured as conjugated dienes in the LDL fraction (and the ratio of conjugated dienes to LDL cholesterol, even in subjects already using vitamin E supplements (400-800 mg/day). No significant difference was detected in excreted (*ex vivo*) sex hormone activity between urine samples from the test and control periods. In conclusion, consumption of high-isoflavone foods was associated with reduced levels of circulating oxidised LDL even in subjects taking vitamin E, with no evidence of increased urinary estrogenic activity. Soy consumption may reduce cardiovascular disease risk without increasing the risk for hormone-dependent cancers.

Title: Effects of genistein and synergistic action in combination with eicosapentaenoic acid on the growth of breast cancer cell lines.

Authors: Nakagawa H, Yamamoto D, Kiyozuka Y, Tsuta K, Uemura Y, Hioki K, Tsutsui Y, and Tsubura A. Institution: Department of Surgery II, Kansai Medical University, Moriguchi, Osaka, Japan.

Source: Journal of Cancer Research and Clinical Oncology 2000; 126(8):448-54.

Abstract: Genistein, a prominent isoflavone in soy products, produced dose–and time-dependent *in vitro* growth inhibition at high concentrations (at least 185 microM) with an IC50 of 7.0-274.2 microM after 72 h incubation in four breast cancer cell lines (DD-762, Sm-MT, MCF-7 and MDA-MB-231) and one breast epithelial cell line (HBL-100) of human and animal origin; it stimulated estrogen-receptor-positive MCF-7 cells at low concentrations (3.7 nM-37 microM). Genistein-exposed cells underwent apoptosis, confirmed by G2/M arrest followed by the appearance of a sub-G1 fraction in cell-cycle progression and by a characteristic cell ultrastructure. The apoptosis cascade was due to up-regulation of Bax protein, down-regulation of Bcl-XL protein, and activation of caspase-3. Genistein acted in synergism with eicosapentaenoic acid (EPA), a fish oil component, on human breast cancer MCF-7 cells (genistein > 93.2 microM and EPA > 210.9 microM) and on MDA-MB-231 cells (genistein > 176.1 microM and EPA > 609.3 microM). Dietary intake of genistein in combination with EPA may be beneficial for breast cancer control.

11.10 Tibetan Herbal Medicine: With Examples of Treating Lung Diseases Using Rhodiola and Hippophae

Subhuti Dharmananda, PhD, Director

Tibetan medicine has a rich heritage and is currently practised not only in Tibet but also in the adjacent Chinese provinces of Qinghai, Gansu, Sichuan, and Yunnan, and in the neighbouring kingdoms of Bhutan, Nepal, Ladakh, and Sikkim, where communities of Tibetan people have long been established. Many non-Tibetans also seek out treatment by this traditional system because of its good reputation. As a result of the flood of refugees from the Chinese military occupation of Tibet, Tibetan medicine extended to India and from there to many countries of the world (especially in Europe and North America) under the guidance of a small number of refugee physicians. One of the most famous of the refugee doctors is Dr Yeshe Donden, who was the personal physician of the Dalai Lama in exile from 1961 to 1969. Dr Donden has spent much time in the United States, where he has diagnosed and treated patients, given teachings to doctors and laypersons, written books and articles, and answered numerous questions about the Tibetan system of health care. Tibetan medicine has also been popularised by a lineage of the Badmajev family that originated in Russia, near Mongolia; members of the family travelled West during the twentieth century. Tibetan herbal formulas they brought with them have been available as pharmaceutical products in Europe since 1980.

Tibetan medicine originated with the local folk tradition (known as Bon) that dates back to about 300 BC and was formally recorded by Xiepu Chixi, the physician to the Tibetan King Niechi Zanpu, in 126 BC. Aspects of both the traditional Chinese and Indian (Ayurvedic) medical systems were added later; Ayurveda has had the most profound influence on

Tibetan medicine. The medicine of India was introduced to Tibet as early as AD 254 with the visit of two Indian physicians. During the following century several physicians from India reinforced the teachings. The greatest influence from India came about when Buddhism was adopted in Tibet as the state religion. This occurred as Tibet was unified under King Songzan Ganbu (AD 618-52). Buddhism had great implications for the practice of the Indian approach to medicine that evolved separately in Tibet. The Ayurvedic principles, especially the concept of tridosha, or three faults (in Buddhism, the three poisons), provided the basis for analysing physical disorders and designing treatments, while Buddhism provided a strong spiritual component. The legend of how Tibetan medicine was introduced to Tibet is relayed in the story *The Life of the Great Physician Yuthog Yonten Gonpo* (pinyin: *Yutuo Yuandan Gongbu*) which has been translated and presented in the book *Tibetan Medicine* by Rechung Rinpoche [1]. The following is the command by Tara (the Buddhist God of Compassion, who is identified in the Chinese tradition as the Goddess Guan Yin) to two famous physicians of India who are said to have become immortals (now living in the sandalwood jungles of India):

It has been prophesied by the Buddha about the country of Tibet, and all the Buddhas have discoursed on Tibet, and Avalokitesvara (also called Chenrezi, a champion of Buddhism: a boddhisatva) was made the special protector of Tibet.

Avalokitesvara is the chief protector, and I am helping him. When you go to Tibet, you will teach the people medicine, in the way the Buddha comes with his teaching. There is no doubt of success. Go quickly, and I shall look after you with my merciful eyes. And you will have the blessing of Avalokitesvara and great results. By the strength of your former prayers, the teaching of medicine will be kept up by the lineage of your families. Be of good cheer and go to Tibet!

The lineage spoken of here involved the birth in Tibet of Yuthog Yonten Gonpo (AD 708-833), who studied medicine since an early age and was exposed to Buddhism during his teen years. Yuthog made three trips to India and studied with the great masters of Buddhist and Ayurvedic medicine there, and he eventually wrote thirty classic medical works integrating the local, Indian, and Chinese medical traditions [2, 3]. The involvement of Chinese medicine came about in AD 641 when a Tang Dynasty princess, Wen Cheng, was married to the Tibetan leader Songzan Ganbu (who was also married to a Nepalese princess that introduced him to Buddhism). Wen Cheng brought with her many Chinese books, including the medical books, as well as herbal formulas and medical instruments. Seventy years later, during Yuthog's life, another Chinese princess, Jin Cheng, brought additional medical books, as well as several Chinese physicians, to Tibet. Yuthog is viewed as the father of Tibetan medicine. He became a royal court physician and established the first Tibetan medical school at Congpo Menlong; he also became a monk at the Samye Monastery. A great medical conference was held at Samye during this time, bringing together Indian, Chinese, Persian, and Greek medical experts. Yuthog received the forerunner of the Four Medical Tantras (*Sibuyidian*; in Tibetan: *rGyud-bzhi, c.* AD 770), which serve as the basis of Tibetan medical practice. The original version is thought to have been written in Sanskrit around the fourth century AD and then translated into Tibetan and given to the royal court [4]. Yuthog's work in reorganising and clarifying these books, as well as adding supplemental material (including that from other traditions described at the Samye conference), made him the true author of the Tibetan traditional text. Because of the vast contributions he made, he is considered a reincarnation of the Medicine Buddha, venerated as 'the second Medicine Buddha.'

The Four Medical Tantras were revised (AD 1573) by the 'younger Yuthog' who was a fourteenth generation descendent of the original Yuthog, now referred to as the 'elder Yuthog'. Additional revisions were made during the seventeenth century to bring forth the current version. The first two medical tantras (called the 'root tantra' and the 'explanatory tantra') have been translated and annotated by Dr Yeshi Donden [5] and translated again in expanded form by Dr Barry Clark [6]. These first two tantras make only a brief mention of herbal medicine and focus instead on behaviour, diet, diagnostics, disease categories, and other aspects of traditional medicine. The third tantra (instructions') details the cause and treatment of each major category of disease, and the fourth tantra (concluding text) is devoted to the details of diagnosis, herbs, moxibustion, and other techniques. One major obstacle to translating the section on herbs is that the identification of the original materials in this 1,200-year-old text is quite difficult. The general methods of diagnosis and therapeutics used by Tibetan doctors follow the Indian tridosha system, that is, being based on three humours (see Table 1).

Table 1: The system of three humours adopted into Tibetan medicine from India.

English	Tibetan	Pinyin	Indian	Basic Concept
Wind	rLung	*Long*	Vayu	Movement, breath, cold
Bile	mKrhispa	*Chiba*	Pitta	Metabolism, digestion, fire
Phlegm	Badkan	*Peigen*	Kapha	Restraint, lubrication, moistness

The imbalances in an individual are revealed by a combination of reported symptoms, pulse diagnosis, tongue diagnosis, and urine analysis. The overall physical appearance of the person, information about their daily habits, and consideration of seasonal influences also contribute to the analysis. The Tibetan pulse diagnosis appears to be derived from the Chinese system and is taken at the same artery of each wrist, but the method of feeling the pulse and the interpretations differ. Tongue diagnosis is simplified compared to the Chinese system (long disorders are characterised by a red and dry tongue; chiba disorders by a yellowish tongue coating; and peigen disorders by a greyish and sticky coating with a smooth and moist texture). Urine analysis is unique to the Tibetan system and may have been introduced from Persia. Physicians inspect the colour, amount of vapour, sediment, smell, and characteristics of the foam generated upon stirring, relying on the first urine excreted in the morning. Traditional Tibetan formulas are described mainly in terms of the diseases and symptoms that they treat, rather than their properties and influences on the humours. For example, in this article, several formulas that treat lung diseases are presented, and their description mainly involves characteristic symptoms (cough, colouration of sputum, fever, involvement of the throat). In order to select among various possible remedies, it is important to know if the lung disease is hot or cold in nature and to know the disturbances of the three humours that form the background to the disease in an individual patient. The humours may be either insufficient and require supplementation (invigoration) or they may be excessive and require pacification. In an attempt to correlate Tibetan and Chinese concepts, it has been suggested [3] that long corresponds roughly to concepts of chi and wind, chiba corresponds to fire or gallbladder, and peigen corresponds to moisture, the earth element, and phlegm.

The modern Materia Medica of Tibet is derived from the book *Jingzhu Bencao* (*The Pearl Herbs*), published in 1835 by Dumar Danzhenpengcuo [7]. This text has been compared to the famous Chinese herbal *Bencao Gangmu*. Its format includes two sections: one being in the style of the Buddhist sutra with praise of the medicines and the other being a detailed classification of each substance, giving the material's origin, environmental conditions where it is found, quality, parts used, and properties. The text included 2,294 materials, of which 1,006 are of plant origin, 448 of animal origin, and 840 minerals. The heavier reliance on minerals and animals than on plants—compared to other traditional medical traditions—can readily be understood for a country at such a high altitude that is very rocky and supports only small areas of plant growth over much of the terrain. About one-third of the medicinal materials used in Tibetan formulas are unique to the Tibetan region (including the Himalayan area in bordering countries), while the other two-thirds of the materials are obtained from India and China. The Tibetan population that had access to the medicines was relatively small until this century, so the total amount of pills produced were correspondingly small. Bringing herbs from India and China to Tibet has always been difficult and has limited the production of herbal formulas. Today, it is relatively easy to get Chinese herbs into Tibet, and China cultivates most of the herbs indigenous to India that might be needed.

Although Tibetan herbal medicine includes the use of decoctions and powders, for the most part, Tibetan doctors utilise pills that are usually made from a large number of herbs (typically 8-25 ingredients). Pills have the advantage of being easy to use, and they can be prepared in advance at a medical facility where all the ingredients are gathered together. Due to the vast distances, rough terrain, and limited development of Tibet, it was not possible to have the broad range of ingredients available to individual doctors who might compound formulas for decoction, as was often done in China. Instead, a relatively small variety of pills prepared at central facilities would be carried by the doctors to their patients. For many doctors, a collection of about two dozen principal formulas would have to suffice. In Lhasa, where there was a centralised population, the doctors have had access to about 200 kinds of pills.

The traditional Tibetan pills were often large, hard, and time-consuming to prepare. Dr Lobsang Dolma Khangkar [8] explained that each herb had to first be processed meticulously and then had to be mixed and preserved properly:

If we are using cardamom, we have to use only the inside, because the outside has no value and then we have to peel each one. There is no machine that can do this, it has to be done by hand. After treating each of the ingredients like this, we will mix maybe three, thirteen, or twenty-five ingredients to make one pill. The first step is to mix all of these ingredients together. If this is not done properly, then each of these ingredients will maintain their own potency without combining with the rest. So, first they have to be completely mixed and this takes a long time of grinding and mixing. After that, it has to be left at rest for a whole day. After the rest, the person who is preparing the medicines has to clean his hands and then begin again with mixing and grinding that medicine. After this, we make the pills. The pills can be made with machines . . . Then the pills are put into a very long bag made of cotton cloth. Two men hold the cloth from each side and move it back and forth so that the pills roll from one side to the other. This is done for a whole day. This last procedure is what is responsible for making Tibetan medicine pills so hard. This procedure takes out all the air that is still in the pills. If air remains in the pill, then it is prone to bacteria getting in, and for the pills to go bad.

In order to make Tibetan medicines available to more people, modern factories have worked out new methods of blending, grinding, and making the pills (see Figures 1–4) as well as producing other forms of the finished materials to make them easier to consume. There are regulations on the production of pills made in Tibet with ninety-seven different formulas formally recognised; of these twenty-five are covered under state medical insurance.

Many of the formulations that are still in use were established many centuries ago. The principles of herbal combining to yield a traditional formula are not clearly defined in the Tibetan system. There are complex methods of analysing the qualities of medicinal materials: six tastes, eight properties, and seventeen effects (see Table 2), but the precise organisational principles for compounding numerous ingredients into the formulas is lost to history.

Table 2: Classification of herbal properties in Tibetan medicine [4].

Grouping	Characteristics
Six tastes	*Sweet* (e.g. bamboo, grapes, saffron; pacifies *long* and *chiba*, increases *peigen*); *sour* (e.g. pomegranate, hippophae, crataegus; pacifies *long* and *peigen*, increases *chiba*); *salty* (e.g. salt and several minerals; pacifies long and peigen, increases *chihba*); *bitter* (e.g. gentiana, aconite, berberis; pacifies *chiba*, increases *long* and *peigen*); *acrid* (e.g. piper, ginger, garlic; pacifies *long* and *peigen*, increases chiba); and *astringent* (e.g. sandalwood, terminalia, aquilegia; pacifies *peigen*, increases *long* and *peigen*)
Eight properties	*Heavy, smooth* (these two combat *long*); *cool, soft* (these two combat *chiba*); *light, rough, acrid*, and *sharp* (these four combat *peigen*). To increase *long*, rough and cool medicines are used; to increase *chiba*, warm, sharp, and smooth medicines are used; to increase *peigen*, heavy, smooth, cool, and soft medicines are used.
Seventeen effects	*Cold, hot, warm, cool, thick, thin, moist, rough, light, heavy, steady, motive, blunt, sharp, tender, dry*, and *soft*. Disease is treated by the opposing effect; a hot disease by a cold effect, stagnant diseases by a motive effect, an accumulation by a sharp effect, a moist condition by a dry effect, etc. *Long* disorders tend to be dry, light, cool, mobile, subtle, and hard; *chiba* disorders tend to be oily, sharp, malodorous, purging, hot, flowing, and light; *peigen* disorders tend to be cold, heavy, blunt, smooth, oily, stable, and sticky.

In general, Tibetan remedies emphasise the use of spicy (acrid), aromatic, and warming herbs. The climate has a substantial influence on these choices: The high altitude of Tibet means that cold and windy conditions prevail. The warm, spicy, aromatic herbs help to compensate for this condition. Ayurvedic medicine relies heavily on spicy herbs for stimulating the digestive system functions, which is understood to be the key to health. Thus, among the commonly used Tibetan herbs are those derived mainly from the Ayurvedic system, such as peppers, cumins, cardamom, clove, ginger, and other hot spices, complemented by the local aromatics such as saussurea and musk. Also, the Tibetan system emphasises astringent herbs, possibly representing an attempt to conserve body fluids and alleviate any inflammation of the mucous membranes. The 'king' herb of Tibetan medicine is the chebulic myrobalan (*Terminalia chebula*), which is an astringent herb, but it is said to possess all the tastes (different parts of the fruit have different tastes), properties, and effects. Despite this emphasis on herbs with properties that are generally needed for the Tibetan climate, cooling and bitter herbs are often required to treat the disease manifestation as inflammatory processes finally result if the pathogenic influences are not conquered or expelled.

Tibetan medicines are today prescribed by several thousand Tibetan doctors who have been trained in recent decades in Tibet, Qinghai, Gansu, and Sichuan. Ten cities in China have set up Tibetan medical facilities (teaching and clinical units), including a large one in Lhasa and an even larger one in Beijing. There are also fifty-seven hospitals of Tibetan medicine throughout China and thirty Tibetan medicine factories. The refugee community in Dharamsala has a medical college, and there are several small manufacturers of Tibetan herb products throughout India and Nepal. Tibetan medicine, like other traditional medical systems, is highly complex and represents a comprehensive effort at dealing with health and disease. Some modern pharmacologists, herb enthusiasts, and product developers have focused on certain herbs that can be used in a general way, thus making them accessible to the world population without having to transmit the medical system itself. Two such herbs are rhodiola and hippophae.

Rhodiola

Rhodiola (see Figure 5) is mainly found on rocky slopes at 3,500-5,000 metres (11,000-16,000 feet). The Chinese name *hongjingtian* refers to the red flowers of the stonecrop—the common name given in the West (hong = red, jingtian = view of heaven or heavenly view, probably referring to its growth on high altitude stone faces). This herb is in the family Crassulaceae, which yields a small number of genera of medicinal plants, mainly rhodiola and sedum. The root of the plant is used in the current medicinal applications. The outer peel of the root has a light golden colour so that the herb is sometimes referred to as golden root; the inside of the root is pink. There are several species of rhodiola collected with the main ones being Rhodiola rosea and Rhodiola kirilowii; others are being investigated, including *R. eoccinca*, *R. crentinii*, *R. krifida*, and *R. atropurpurea*. Tibetan rhodiola has become so popular in recent years that, according to a survey by the Tibet Institute of Biology, 10,000 tons of it are collected annually, and six factories make products that have rhodiola as a key ingredient (or sole ingredient). Rather than relying on its traditional applications, rhodiola is presented as a health product of general benefit, described as an adaptogen.

The concept of an adaptogen has been attributed to the Russian pharmacologist N. V. Lazarev from his work during the period 1958-9. Basically, he defined an adaptogen as a substance that has no toxicity or side effects at normal dosages and that non-specifically increases the resistance to disease and to physical and chemical stresses. Put another way, use of an adaptogenic herb will safely assist the body in maintaining its homeostatic balance and recovering from the effects of adverse weather, emotions, and disease influences. The leading advocates of developing natural resources as adaptogens were the Russian researchers I. I. Brekhman and I. V. Dardymov. They reviewed the status of research into adaptogenic agents in the seminal article 'New substances of plant origin which increase non-specific resistance', published in 1969 [9]. The leading adaptogens identified at that time were eleutherococcus (*Eleutherococcus senticosus*), ginseng (*Panax ginseng*), rhaponticum (*Rhaponticum carthamoides*), and rhodiola (*Rhodiola rosea*). The Russians went on to develop eleutherococcus (usually simplified to eleuthero) as a major health product, used locally and exported to Western countries. The Chinese developed their own resources of this herb (which grows in abundance in northeast China), eventually becoming the world's main supplier. Ginseng had long been used in the Orient and revered as a health tonic; the Koreans developed the world market for this herb, promoting research into its pharmacology and clinical effects and cultivating huge quantities of the roots. China and the United States (providing an American species, *P. quinquefolium*) eventually became major suppliers as well. Rhaponticum is still being investigated in China and Russia; it is mainly studied in relation to antioxidant activity, but it is also reputed to improve circulation and mental acuity. Rhodiola has been researched in Russia and China and has become a common health food product which has been promoted in the West in recent years.

The development of rhodiola as an adaptogen represents one aspect of Chinese efforts to promote Tibetan medicine (as one of the Chinese indigenous medical systems).

As an adaptogen, rhodiola is considered to be like ginseng (*renshen*) and eleuthero (*ciwujia*) in terms of effects and applications; adaptogens from numerous different plant species have the same basic actions [25]. Modern promoters of rhodiola have dubbed the herb 'Tibetan ginseng.' Though some herbalists object to this off-hand use of the term *ginseng* (similarly, ashwaganda is called Indian ginseng, eleuthero is called Siberian ginseng or eleuthero ginseng), it may well represent the current intended use of the herb for consumers who are already familiar with ginseng as a general health tonic. One of the adaptogenic applications of rhodiola that has received considerable research attention recently is for aiding adaptation to high altitudes, thus, as a preventive and treatment for mountain sickness [23-25]. Information about traditional uses of rhodiola remains somewhat limited; it was used for treatment of dysentery, back pain, lung inflammation with expectoration of bloody mucus, painful and irregular menstruation, leucorrhoea, and traumatic injuries [25]. Based on the indications for use, rhodiola appears to be cooling and detoxifying and vitalises blood circulation.

By including the related genus *Sedum* in the discussion, one can get a better understanding of the herb since the two are nearly interchangeable. Some of the Chinese and Tibetan species of *Sedum* go by the name *jingtian* that is used for rhodiola: *Sedum erythrostictum* is the main species known by this name (see Figure 6). Sedum was described [10] during the Song Dynasty as 'being sweet in taste, cold and slightly toxic in nature, the plant crawls on stones of the southern side of a mountain and it is tender and lustrous . . .' *Sedum erythrostictum* was described in the *Bencao Gangmu* of the Ming Dynasty [11] as having the reputation of protecting from fire. It was grown in pots on house tops to protect the house (i.e. protecting thatched roofs), and the herb would be used to treat people burnt by fire or scalded by hot water or who suffered from the burning sensation of insect bites. It is used topically much the way we currently use *Aloe vera*, which has a similar mucilaginous quality to the leaves. Some Chinese species of *Sedum* are administered as hemostatics; this especially applies to *Sedum aizoon*, which is known as *tushanqi*, being named the same as the famous hemostatic notoginseng (*sanqi; tu* means local variety). The traditional Tibetan use of both sedum and rhodiola is for lung diseases, specifically, lung heat (generally meaning a lung infection). In fact, the two herbs are combined in a simple decoction with licorice and lacca (*zicaorong*) for treating lung heat [12].

In recent years, sedum extracts have been shown to protect the liver from damage due to chemicals, and the herb has been used in treatment of viral hepatitis. The most commonly used species for this purpose in China is *Sedum sarmentosum* (*chuipencao*). The whole plant is applied in cases of damp heat and to counteract toxic heat [13]. A tablet made from this herb, containing 8 mg of the glycoside component, was used to treat chronic hepatitis at a dosage of nine tablets per day (72 mg of glycoside). Its main effect was to lower transaminase levels within two weeks [23]. In addition to tablets, rhodiola is produced in the form of a wine, oral liquid (which includes other Chinese herbs), capsule, and tea bag.

Much of the research on rhodiola has been carried out in Lhasa. The Tibet Institute of High Altitude Biology has done research with rhodiola and confirmed that it is of benefit as an adaptogen, including use against mountain sickness. A capsule with rhodiola and hippophae (plus lycium fruit) is produced by one factory and is promoted as a treatment for altitude sickness. In Chengdu, the West China University of Medical Sciences undertook a review of the research on this herb, which was published in 1988, evaluating ninety reports on the botany, chemistry, pharmacology, toxicology, and clinical effects. They reported that *hongjingtian* was obtained from the root and rhizome of several species of *Rhodiola*, with studies conducted on the constituents of twenty of China's seventy species. The active constituents include numerous flavonoids (such as quercetin, rutin, and kaempferol), condensed flavonoids (polyphenols, mainly gallic acid and epigallocatechin), cyanoglycosides (which have histamine-inhibiting activity), and salidroside, which is deemed one of the main active constituents of interest by virtually all authorities. In concentrated extracts of rhodiola, salidroside makes up about 1–2 per cent of the content. Salidroside comprises tyrosol linked to glucose; tyrosol is one of the major flavours and aroma ingredients of the olive which confer notable antioxidant activity to olive oil. Rhodiola also contains sterols, notably daucosterol and sitosterol. According to mouse experiments conducted in China, rhodiola extract has a central stimulant action and increases the tolerance to anoxia, fatigue, microwave irradiation, poisoning by strychnine, tetanin, and other toxins; it regulates brain functions, leucocyte count, and blood glucose and promotes protein hydrolysis, and it enhances the functions of the thyroid gland, adrenals, and ovaries. According to the reports from recent clinical research efforts conducted mainly in Russia, rhodiola may prove helpful in treating depression, and its use may result in improvements in mental performance and alleviation of fatigue. All reports suggest that the toxicity of rhodiola is very low and that there are no significant side effects [24]. As can be seen, the modern research (both laboratory and clinical) is aimed at the potential of rhodiola as an adaptogen rather than its traditional function as a treatment for lung diseases.

Hippophae

Hippophae (Chinese: *shaji*, literally: sand thorn; the English common name is sea buckthorn) is a member of the Elaeagnaceae family, a family that has very few medicinal herbs, mainly *Hippophae*, *Eleaegnus*, and *Elaeocarpus*. There is one dominant species of *Hippophae* used in China and Russia: *H. rhamnoides* (see Figure 7). Hippophae is usually found at an altitude of 1,200-2,000 metres (4,000-6,500 feet) in cold climates, though it can grow at both higher and lower altitudes, in sandy soil. It has recently been planted in temperate zones worldwide to prevent soil erosion and to serve as a source of food and medicine [15]. Hippophae has been developed into a major resource for China with numerous organisations devoted to the project, including the following three that have sponsored a journal, *Hippophae*, which has been published (in Chinese) since 1988:

- China Research and Training Centre on Sea Buckthorn
- Sea Buckthorn Office of the Yellow River Water Commission
- Shaanxi Sea Buckthorn Development Office

The fruit is the main part used as food and medicine. It is one of the richest sources of vitamin C, with about 6 mg/g in the fruit and about 5 mg per ml of fruit juice [16], so the juice has been made into a health beverage on that basis. Medicinally, the flavonoids of the fruit and the oil of the seed are deemed the main active constituents. The flavonoids are present in the range 1-10 mg/g of fresh fruit. Injected into laboratory animals [17] at a dose in the range 2-5 mg/kg, they improve non-specific immunity (one of the actions of an adaptogen). In addition, the flavonoids promote bone marrow production of red blood cells and reduce allergy reactions [26]. Both the vitamin C and flavonoids are thought to help protect against carcinogenesis when ingesting food contaminated with carcinogens [18]. In a double-blind clinical trial [19], 128 patients with ischemic heart disease were given total flavonoids of hippophae at 10 mg each time, three times daily, for six weeks. The patients had a decrease in cholesterol level and improved cardiac function; also they had less angina than those receiving the control drug isosorbide dinitrate. No harmful effect of hippophae flavonoids was noted in renal functions or hepatic functions. Hippophae seed oil is rich in vitamin E and essential fatty acids, including several that inhibit inflammation. One ingredient, palmitoleic acid, is a component of skin that is considered very valuable in treating burns and healing wounds. The oil is used alone or in various preparations topically applied for a wide range of skin ailments, including burns, scalds, ulcerations, infections, and as an aid in promoting regeneration of tissues and protectant in sunblocks (hippophae oil itself has UV-blocking activity). The seed oil and the bark of the plant have been found to possess anti-tumour effects in preliminary laboratory studies [15]. For internal use, the oil is put into soft gelatin capsules, which are used for treating gastric and duodenal ulcers, liver inflammation, and skin disorders, such as atopic dermatitis. Both the seed oil and flavonoids have been used in laboratory animal studies aimed at revealing adaptogenic properties, such as protection against harmful effects of radiation, cold, fatigue from excessive activity demands, and oxygen deficits [26].

In the Indian Materia Medica, hippophae is mentioned briefly, the fruit being used for lung diseases [20]. In *Thousand Formulas and Thousand Herbs of Traditional Chinese Medicine* [21], hippophae fruit is described as sour, astringent, and warm in nature and used to eliminate phlegm, stop cough, improve digestion and remove accumulations and to move blood and remove blood stasis. Examples of uses are cough with profuse sputum; abdominal pain due to accumulation of food and indigestion; amenorrhoea due to blood stasis; and swelling and stagnation in trauma. These functions and applications are similar to those described in Tibetan medicine, where hippophae is used for lung-heat disorders and stomach-intestine disorders with bleeding. However, the emphasis of modern research and product development is on its nutritional and general health benefits rather than the traditional medical applications. Some simple formulas with more specific applications have been developed recently; for example, there is a liquid preparation of hippophae, carthamus, and licorice intended for use in treatment coronary heart disease and sequelae of heart attack and stroke, based on improving blood circulation.

11.11 Traditional Tibetan Formulas with Rhodiola and Hippophae

T. J. Tsarong outlined 175 important Tibetan formulas in his *Handbook of Traditional Tibetan Drugs* [22]. In the next two tables, formulas with rhodiola and/or hippophae are mentioned; other herbs commonly included in these formulas are sandalwood, saussurea, carthamus, bamboo, terminalia, licorice; geranium, emblica, gentiana, inula, and grapes (see also Tables 5 and 6). Of these, all are used in Chinese medicine except emblica and grapes; both are used extensively in Indian medicine. Tsarong included twelve formulas that utilise rhodiola, all of which are used for lung disorders (see Tables 3 and 4).

Table 3: Traditional Tibetan formulas with rhodiola. The number of herbs in the formula is indicated in the formula name or added in parentheses after the formula name.

Formula	Main Uses in Tibetan Tradition
Blue Garuda Bird (9)	Acute inflammation of the lungs and throat, as well as fever and dysentery
Bamboo 9	Coughing, infections, fever, and diarrhoea (this formula is usually used for paediatric cases)
Pulmonary medicine of death healing nectar (15)	Acute and chronic cough and sputum streaked with pus (formula includes hippophae)
Eliminator of lung inflammation (13)	Inflammation of the lungs, cough, chest congestion
Eliminator of all lung imbalances (11)	Chronic cough with expectoration of phlegm and fever
Blood Gentian Pill (18)	Antipyretic and expectorant for inflammation of the lungs and cough
Gentiana 15	Cough, shortness of breath, hoarseness, blood in sputum
Sandalwood 8	Inflammation of the lungs; blood and pus in the sputum

Formula	Main Uses in Tibetan Tradition
Sandalwood 9 (add cinnamon to above)	Inflammation of the lungs; pus in the sputum, fever
Yuthog's Bamboo 25	Pain and inflammation of the lungs, blood in the sputum, inflammation of the respiratory tract (formula includes hippophae)
Copper Calcine 25	All types of lung inflammation; difficulty breathing, coughing

A representative rhodiola formula is the Eliminator of Lung Inflammation. Its ingredients, in addition to rhodiola, are bamboo, carthamus, clove, white and red sandalwoods, geranium, terminalia, aconite, myrrh, musk, saussurea, and cinnabar (vermilion). Though this is considered a valuable remedy by the Tibetans, it is not a suitable preparation for use in the West as it contains raw aconite (a toxic substance, though used in small amounts), musk (obtained from the musk deer, an endangered species), saussurea (collected from wild sources; it is an endangered species), and cinnabar (contains mercury). The main characteristic of the formula is that it is very fragrant, mainly due to the clove, saussurea, sandalwood, geranium, myrrh, and musk; it has a bitter, acrid, astringent taste (sandalwood, saussurea, and terminalia are the main astringents); and the overall action is cooling. When interpreting its effects and uses, it must be understood that the classification of the herbs is often different in the Tibetan system compared to the Chinese system. As examples, both carthamus and sandalwood are deemed warming in the Chinese system but cooling in the Tibetan system; sandalwood is used to regulate chi in the Chinese system but is applied as an astringent in the Tibetan system; carthamus is used in the Chinese system to vitalise blood circulation, but it is used to stop bleeding and nourish blood in the Tibetan system. In this formulation, phlegm–fire (chiba; bile) is controlled by ingredients such as white sandalwood, carthamus, and bamboo, while phlegm–damp (peigen) is controlled by aconite and penetrated by the fragrant herbs. This formula is suited to treating lung diseases in which there is considerable difficulty breathing due to sticky phlegm. Two of the formulas in Table 3 include hippophae; there are also six formulas with hippophae that do not include rhodiola (see Table 4). Most of these are also used for lung diseases and phlegm accumulation problems, but hippophae is also included in formulas for treating blood-heat disorders (these usually manifest as bleeding disorders).

Table 4: Traditional Tibetan formulas with hippophae (see Table 3 for two additional formulas).

Formula	Main Uses in Tibetan Tradition
Blue Poppy 8	To control excess blood from the liver into the stomach lining (hematemesis)
Balancing Comforter (17)	For all types of phlegm accumulation with lack of stomach heat (symptoms of anorexia, indigestion, stomach tumours), discomfort of stomach and liver, hematamesis, lymphatic disorders, skin disorders (including itching)
Reed of Comfort (17)	For phlegm accumulation, pain along with emesis of sour and watery vomitus, inflammation of the stomach, indigestion, hematemesis, irregular menstruation, painful menstruation
White Nectar Pill (5)	To promote digestion (increases stomach fire), disintegrates stomach tumours and mucus, removes phlegm accumulations, acts like a nectar for colic and cold parasites
Amla 25	Removes bad blood, reduces blood pressure, treats dryness of throat and mouth, and redness of eyes
Hippophae 5	For chronic inflammation of the lungs, with discharge of pus and blood; it suppresses coughing and treats hidden fever

A representative formula with hippophae is Hippophae 5, which also contains licorice, grape, emblica, and saussurea. This is a formula compatible with Western requirements in terms of safety of the herbal materials, though the main Tibetan source for saussurea, *S. lappa*, is on the endangered species list (cultivated sources and a related herb used as a common substitute, *Vladimiria souliei*, can resolve this problem). Hippophae 5 has the characteristic of being sweet (mainly due to licorice and grape) and sour (mainly due to the hippophae and emblica) with only a modest fragrance (mainly contributed by saussurea) and a cooling quality (not compensated by spicy warm herbs). Sweet herbs are considered useful for controlling *chiba* (phlegm–fire), while *peigen* (phlegm) is controlled both by sour herbs and those that are coarse (hippophae). This formula is given for lung disorders with accompanying fever and with free flowing mucus. Comparing the two formulas—

Eliminator of Lung Inflammation and Hippophae 5—the former is more suited for lung disorders dominated by stuffiness and the latter is more suited for lung problems associated with fever and infection (which can lead to discharge of copious mucus including pus and blood), while both are good for the most general category of lung inflammation.

Tibetan Herbs Commonly Combined with Rhodiola and Hippophae

In traditional Tibetan formulas, rhodiola and hippophae are combined in complex formulas, as depicted above, for treatment of lung diseases. Table 5 presents these two key herbs along with several of the other herbs commonly included in the formulas. Table 6 presents information about the inclusion of these herbs in the same formulas that are listed in Tables 3 and 4. Other herbs, which are in some of these formulas but mentioned less frequently, include geranium, emblica, gentiana, inula, and grapes.

Table 5: Tibetan herbs commonly used in formulas for treating lung diseases. The Tibetan name is presented according to the transliteration system used in the *Quintessence Tantras of Tibetan Medicine* [6], and the Indian name is presented according to Indian Materia Medica [20].

Herb (common name): Botanical name	Tibetan name: Part used	Sanskrit name: Bengal name	Chinese name: Category
Bamboo resin *Bambusa sp.* or *Phyllostachys sp.*	Chu-gang Resin	Vansa Bans	*Tianzhuhuang* Resolve phlegm
Carthamus* *Carthamus tinctorius*	Gur-kum Flower	Kamalottera; kusumba Kajireh	*Honghua* Vitalise blood
Hippophae *Hippophae rhamnoides*	Star-bu Fruit	Dhurchuk (Hindi) Dhurchuk	*Shaji* Resolve phlegm
Licorice *Glycyrrhiza glabra* or *G. uralensis*	Shing-mngar Root	Madhuka, yashti-madhu Yashto-madhu	*Gancao* Tonify qi
Rhodiola *Rhodiola sp.*	Sro-lo Whole plant	Not included	*Hongjingtian* Tonify qi

Sandalwood (red) *Pterocarpus santalinus*	Tsan-dan dmar-po Heart wood	Rakta chandana Pit-sal	*Hongtanxiang* Regulate qi
Sandalwood (white) *Santalum alba*	Tsan-dan dkar-po Heart wood	Chandanam; srigandha Sada-chandan	*Tanxiang* Regulate qi
Saussurea *Saussurea lappa*	Ru-rta Root	Puskara, kushta Kashmirjagada pachak	*Guangmuxiang* Regulate qi
Terminalia *Terminalia chebula*	A-ru-ra Fruit	Haritaki, abhaya, pathya, etc. Hirda	*Hezi* Astringent

* Common substitute for saffron, the originally-specified ingredient.

Table 6: The inclusion of common Tibetan herbs in the formulas with rhodiola and/or hippophae.

Formula	Rhodiola	Hippophae	Sandalwood	Saussurea	Carthamus	Bamboo	Terminalia	Licorice
Blue Garuda Bird	•						•	
Bamboo 9	•		•		•	•		
Pulmonary Medicine of Death Healing Nectar	•	•	•	•	•	•		•
Eliminator of Lung Inflammation	•		•	•	•	•	•	
Eliminator of All Lung Imbalances	•		•				•	
Blood Gentiana Pill	•		•	•		•	•	•
Gentiana 15	•			•		•	•	•
Sandalwood 8 and 9	•		•		•	•		•
Yuthog's Bamboo 25	•	•	•	•	•	•	•	•
Copper Calcine 25	•		•		•	•		•
Blue Poppy 8		•			•	•		•
Balancing Comforter		•	•		•	•		
Reed of Comfort		•		•	•	•	•	
White Nectar Pill		•						
Amla 25		•	•	•	•		•	
Hippophae 5		•		•				•

Summary

Tibetan medicine is a derivative of the Indian and Chinese medical systems, with a dominant Buddhist influence, especially that carried over as a translation and revision of the Four Medical Tantras during the eighth century AD. Tibetan herbal medicine represents a complex system that involves a large number of medicinal substances, about a third of which are highaltitude plants (especially those that grow in dry sandy or rocky areas). The classical Tibetan Materia Medica was developed in the nineteenth century and remains the primary source of pre-scientific herb information. Rhodiola and hippophae are examples of herbs frequently included in traditional Tibetan formulas, especially for treatment of lung diseases. They have been developed into health products apart from the Tibetan tradition, with rhodiola promoted as an adaptogenic agent and hippophae as a nutritious beverage, a treatment for circulatory disorders, and as a skin protectant and healer.

Tibetan medicine has been promoted and further developed in recent years both by China and by Tibetan refugee physicians. The main Tibetan texts are being translated into other languages (mainly Chinese and English), and scholars are investigating archaeological sites and lost texts. The Tibetan medical system is experiencing a revival as the growing world population seeks solutions for difficult medical problems for which the modern system lacks adequate remedies. However, there are not enough trained physicians to support the demand. It is likely that more of the individual Tibetan herbs will be taken from this tradition and developed as health products as further research is undertaken. These general health products may stimulate interest in the preservation and further development of this unique medical tradition.

References

1. Rechung Rinpoche, *Tibetan Medicine*, 1976 University of California Press, Berkeley, California.
2. Anonymous, Survey of Tibetan medicine, *Chinese Journal of Ethnomedicine and Ethnopharmacy*, 1992; (1): 40-1.
3. Guo Jiening, et al., Tibetan medicine: historical development and theoretical system, *Chinese Journal of Ethnomedicine and Ethnopharmacy*, 1995; (14): 1-5.

4. Tsarong T. J. (translator and editor), *Fundamentals of Tibetan Medicine*, 1981; Tibetan Medical Center, Dharamsala, India.
5. Donden Y. (annotator) and Keisang J. (translator), *The Ambrosia Heart Tantra*, 1977; Library of Tibetan Works and Archives, Dharamsala, India.
6. Clark B. (translator), *The Quintessence Tantras of Tibetan Medicine*, 1995; Snow Lion Press, Ithica, New York.
7. Wang Jinhui, The characteristics of the Jingzhu Bencao, *Chinese Journal of Ethnomedicine and Ethnopharmacy*, 1995; (13): 4-5.
8. Khangkar L. D., *Lectures on Tibetan Medicine*, 1986; Library of Tibetan Works and Archives, Dharamsala.
9. Brekhman I. I. and Dardymov I. V., New substances of plant origin which increase non-specific resistance, *Annual Review of Pharmacology*, 1969; 9: 419-30.
10. Chang Minyi, *Anticancer Medicinal Herbs*, 1992; Hunan Science and Technology Publishing House, Changsha.
11. Smith F. P. and Stuart G. A., *Chinese Medicinal Herbs*, 1973; Georgetown Press, San Francisco, CA.
12. Li Yingcun, The characteristics of Tibetan medicine preparation in Sibu Yidian, *Chinese Journal of Ethnomedicine and Ethnopharmacy*, 1995; (14): 16-19.
13. Pharmacopoeia Commission of the Ministry of Public Health, *Colored Atlas of the Chinese Materia Medica*, 1995; Guangdong Science and Technology Press, Guangzhou.
14. Hson-Mou Chang and Paul Pui-Hay But (eds.), *Pharmacology and Applications of Chinese Materia Medica*, (2 vols.), 1986; World Scientific, Singapore.
15. Li TSC and Schroeder W. R., Sea buckthorn (Hippophae rhamnoides): A multipurpose plant, *Horticultural Technology*, 1996; 6(4): 370-8.
16. Ji Lanju, Free amino acids and vitamin C in the fruits of Hippophae rhamnoides, Nitraria tangutorum, and Berberis dasystachya, *Acta Botanica Sinica*, 1989; 31(6): 487-8.
17. Zhong Fei, et al., Effects of the total flavonoid of Hippophae rhamnoides on nonspecific immunity in animals, *Shanxi Medical Journal*, 1989; 18(1): 9-10.
18. Li Yong and Liu Huang, Blocking effect of the juice of Hippophae rhamnoides on synthesis of nitrosodimethylamine in rat, *Acta Nutrmenta Sinica*, 1989; 11(1): 47-53.

19. Zhang Maoshun, et al., Treatment of ischemic heart diseases with flavonoids of Hippophae rhamnoides, *Chinese Journal of Cardiology*, 1987; 15(2): 97-9.
20. Nadkarni A. K., *Indian Materia Medica*, 1908 (revised 1954); Popular Prakashan Private LTD, Bombay.
21. Huang Bingshan and Wang Yuxia, *Thousand Formulas and Thousand Herbs of Traditional Chinese Medicine*, 1993; Heilongjiang Education Press, Harbin, China.
22. Tsarong T. J., *Handbook of Traditional Tibetan Drugs*, 1986; Tibetan Medical Publications, Kalimpong.
23. Zhang Weiyun, Recent development on application of Rhodiola spp. and its preparations, *Journal of the Gansu College of Traditional Chinese Medicine*, 1997; 14(4); 41-2.
24. Wang Liang, Progress of research on the pharmacology of rhodiola, *Li Shizhen Medicine and Materia Medica Research*, 1999; 10(4): 295-6.
25. Qian Yancong, et al., Survey of research on Rhodiola kirilowii, *Acta Chinese Medicine and Pharmacology*, 1999; (5): 34-5.
26. Diao Jingli, et al., Pharmacological actions of Hippophae rhamnoides, *Li Shizhen Medicine and Materia Medica Research*, 1999; 10(12): 956-7.

May 2001

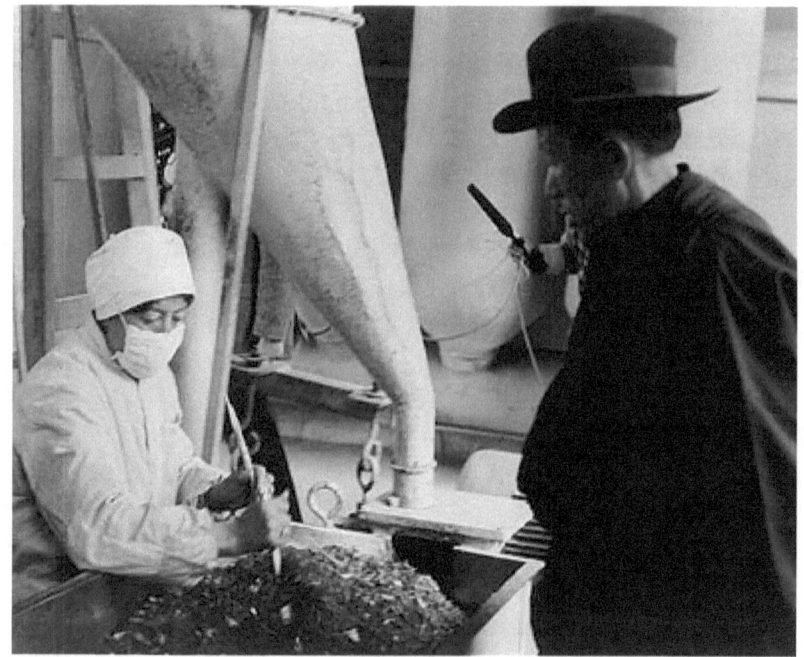

Figure 1: Blending the bulk herbs.

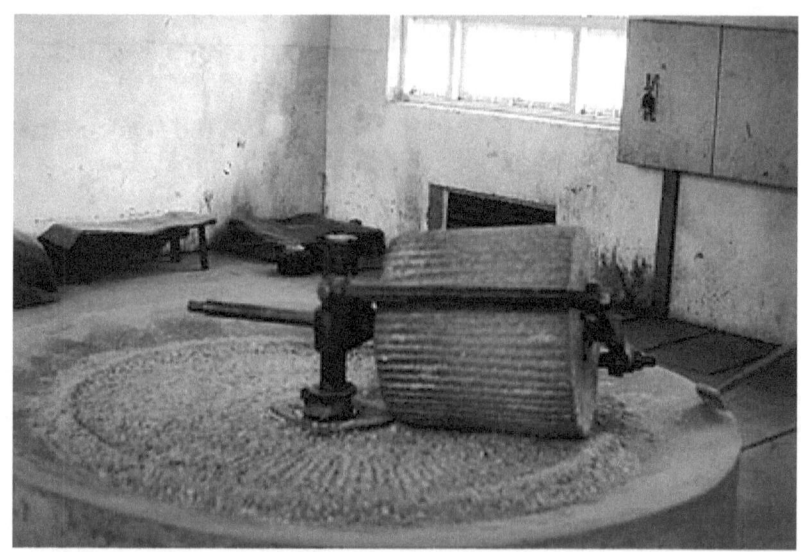

Figure 2: Grinding the herbs.

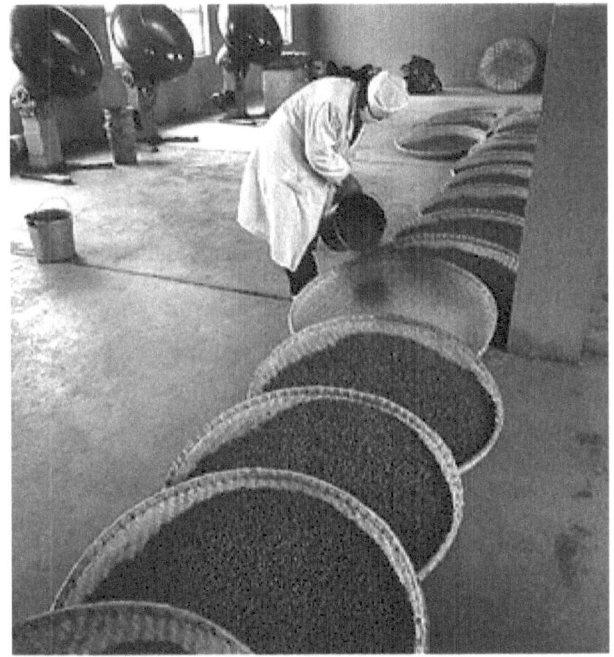

Figure 3: Setting the pills out to dry;

Note: Pill rolling machines in background.

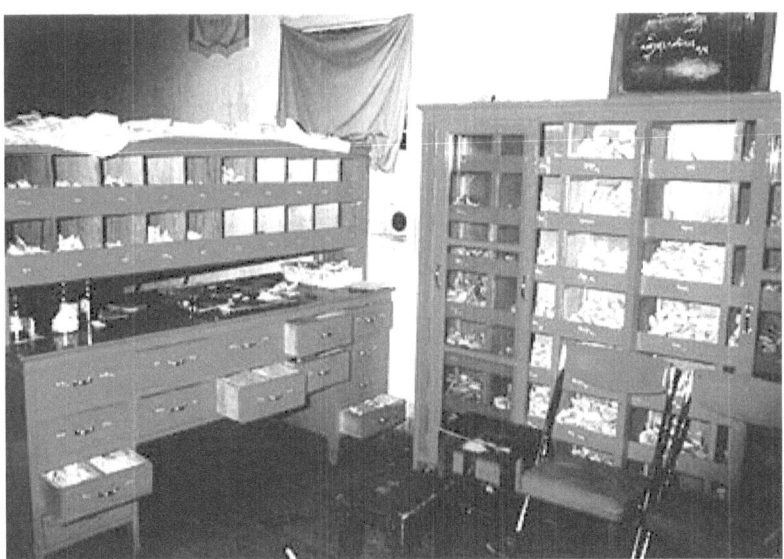

Figure 4: Tibetan dispensary; white bundles are prepackaged pills.

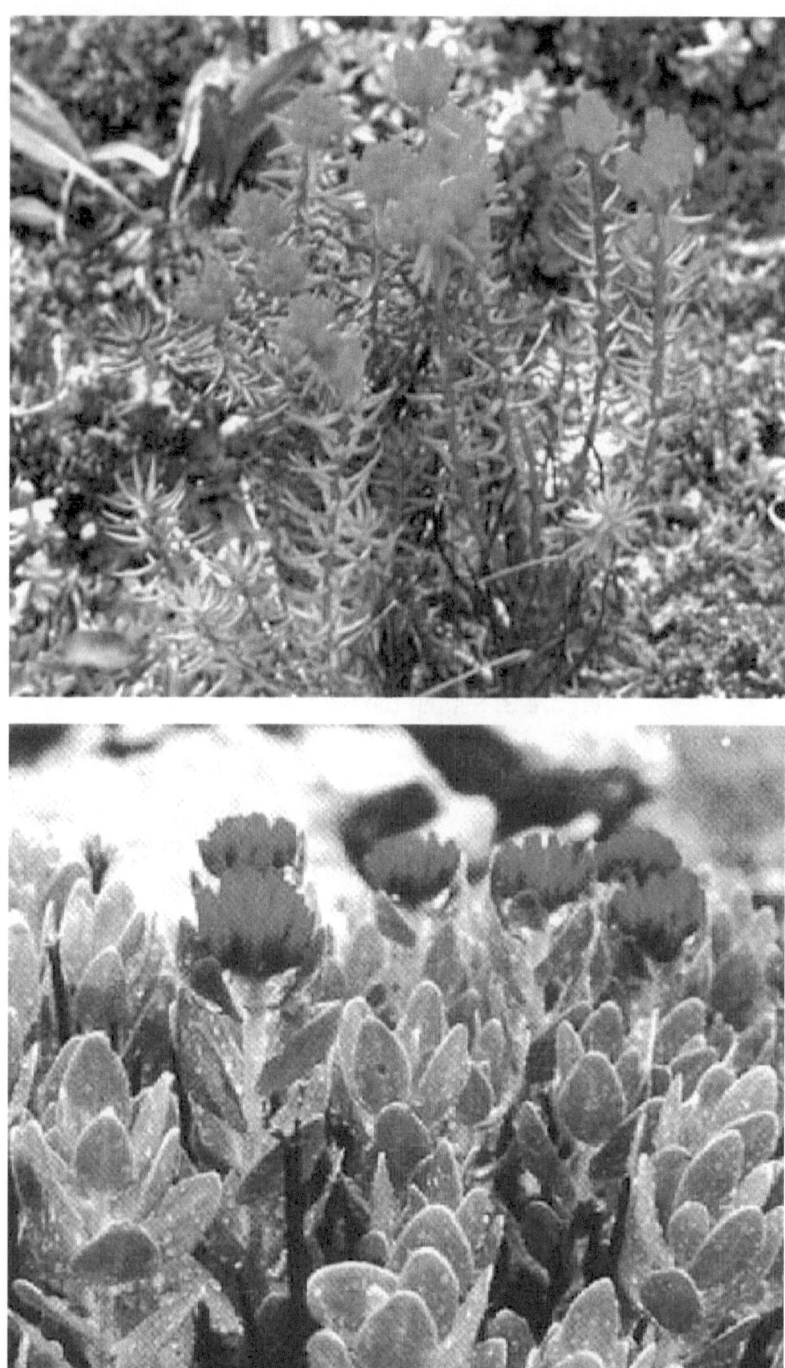

Figure 5: Two views of rhodiola (different species).

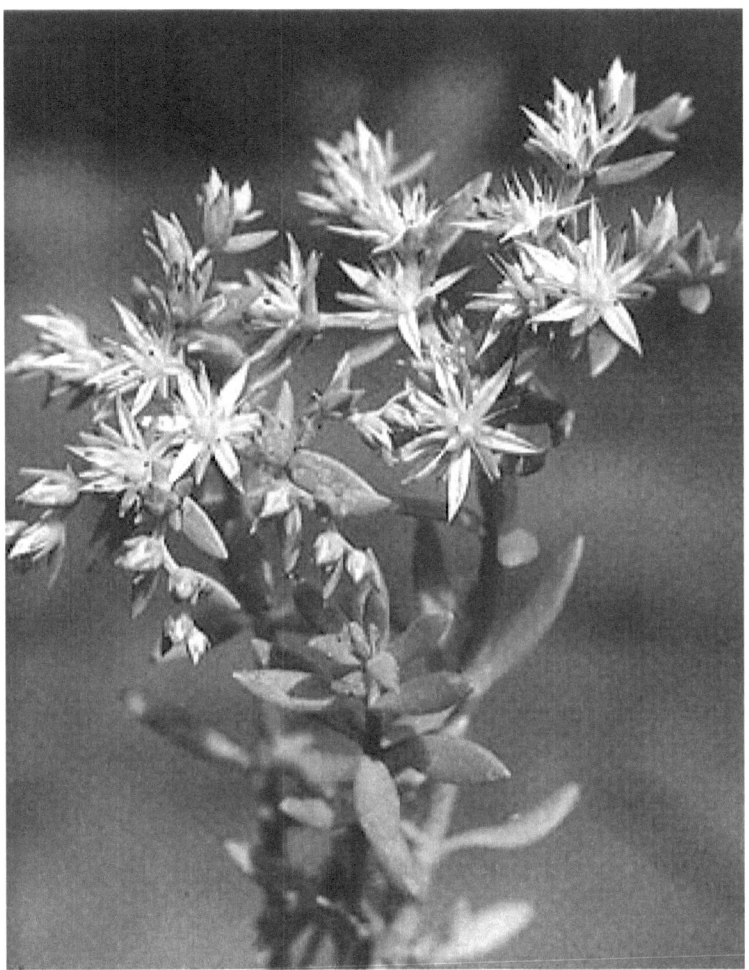

Figure 6: Sedum Sarmentosum.

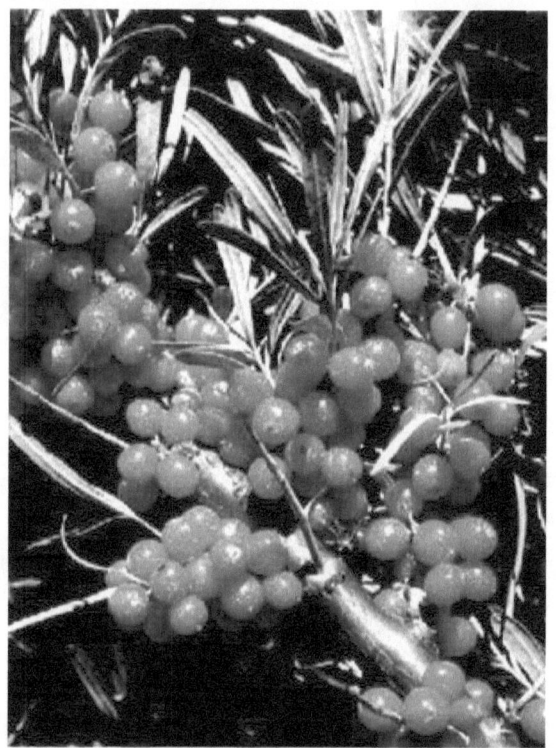

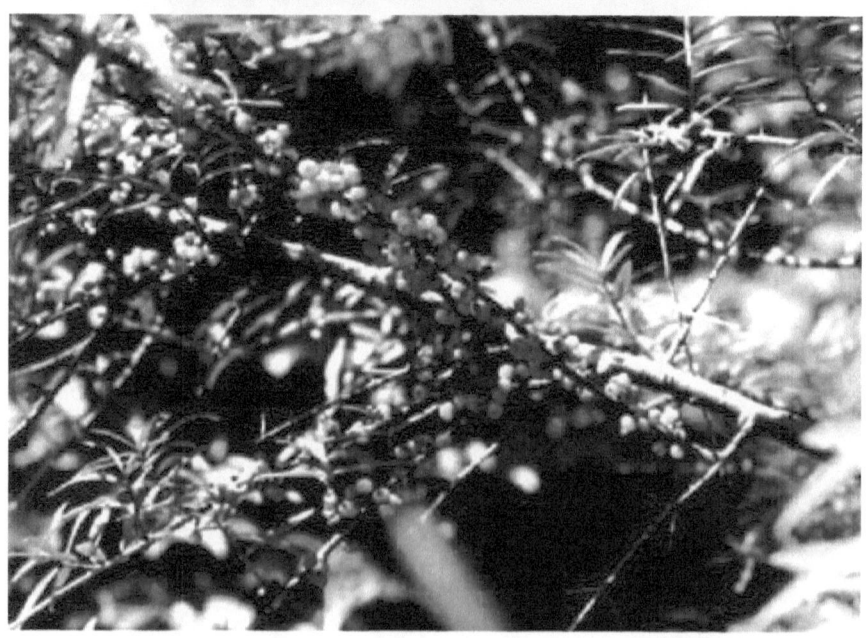

Figure 7: Two views of hippophae.

11.12 Differentiating Sulphur Compounds

Sulpha Drugs, Glucosamine Sulphate, Sulphur, and Sulphiting Agents

Subhuti Dharmananda, PhD, Director

Background

There are several misconceptions about sulphur compounds that lead to anxiety about using some natural health-care substances. A typical worry is that a person who is allergic to sulpha drugs may have problems with substances that contain sulphur. This article is aimed at clarifying the nature of the substances involved. This discussion will be of much benefit to the preventive therapist, for whom this book is meant.

First, sulphur is an element of the earth. This element is essential to life and is the eighth most prevalent element in the human body. No one is allergic to sulphur itself. Sulphur is not present as an isolated element in the body, but it is found in combination with other elements and, most often, in complex molecules. The primary placement of sulphur in the human body is in the sulphur-containing amino acids: methionine, cysteine, homocysteine (and related cystine, homocystine), and taurine.

Disulphide bonds are important to the structural integrity of the connective tissues. Sulphur is a central component of proteins that chelate and remove heavy metals from the body. The benefits of sulphur compounds used in health products are often mentioned. Popular items include alpha-lipoic acid (thiotic acid), methyl-sulphonyl-methane (MSM), allicin (the sulphur compound that is the main active ingredient of garlic), glucosamine sulphate (and its natural polymer, chondroitin), SAMe (S-adenosylmethionine), and several important antioxidants, such as glutathione, N-acetylcysteine (NAC) and dimethyl-sulphoxide (DMSO).

Composition of the Human Body	
Hydrogen	63.0
Oxygen	25.5
Carbon	9.5
Nitrogen	1.4
Calcium	0.31
Phosphorus	0.22

Composition of the Human Body	
Potassium	0.06
Sulphur	0.05
Chlorine	0.03
Sodium	0.03
Magnesium	0.01
All others	0.01

Sulpha Drugs

One of the more common drug allergies is that to sulpha drugs. Sulpha drugs are more appropriately labelled sulphonamides and are derivatives of para-amino benzoic acid. The table below lists common medications that contain a sulphonamide component.

Sulphonamide drug classes/individual drugs that may cause allergic reactions				
Sulphonamide Antibiotics	**Thiazide Diuretics**	**Loop Diuretics** furosemide	**Sulphonylureas** chlorpropamide	**Carbonic Anhydrase Inhibitors**
sulphadiazine	hydrochlorothiazide		tolbutamide	acetazolamide
sulphamethoxazole	chlorthiazide		tolazamide	
sulphasalazine	metolazone		glipizide	
sulphisoxazole	chlorthalidone		glyburide	
sulphacetamide	indapamide			
sulphanilamide	methyclothiazide			
sulphathiazole				
sulphabenzamide				

The sulpha drugs are usually not allergenic by themselves, but when a sulphonamide molecule is metabolised in the body, it is capable of attaching to proteins, thus forming a larger molecule that could serve as an allergen. Thus, the allergy is not to the original drug, but to a drug—protein complex. It is estimated that a skin rash occurs in about 3.5 per cent of hospitalised patients receiving sulphonamides, but people with HIV infection seem to have a considerably higher sensitivity to them.

A sulphanomide sample structure (see below)

sulph H₂N does contain sulphur, but the sulphur atoms are embedded in a complex molecule. The sulphur atom is not the allergenic agent, and being allergic to sulpha drugs does not imply having a propensity to allergy to other sulphur compounds. Rather, it is a unique property of this kind of compound, namely that it can form proteins that are allergenic in some individuals.

Glucosamine Sulphate

Glucosamine sulphate is an amino acid polymer that combines with sodium or potassium (depending on how it is prepared) and with sulphate (SO_4). Neither glucosamine nor sulphate is an allergenic component. Glucosamine sulphate is not known to cause allergy reactions. Glucosamine sulphate is an existing component in the human body, mainly in the connective tissues. When obtained for use in dietary supplements, glucosamine sulphate is commonly derived from shellfish, such as crabs, where it is present as chitin in the shell materials. If it were poorly prepared, persons with shellfish allergy (the allergy is mainly to the muscle portion that is eaten rather than to the shell) might have to worry about taking this product. However, purification of the glucosamine sulphate in the standard processing used for dietary supplements makes it safe for virtually everyone with a shellfish allergy problem. Glucosamine sulphate appears helpful as a dietary supplement for nourishing the joints because it is involved in the production of cartilage and synovial fluid and may help replenish depleted or damaged tissues; it has been shown to have anti-inflammatory properties and may protect against development of atherosclerosis. There is no evidence or reason to believe that those who are sensitive to sulphites (see below) or sulpha drugs are at any elevated risk of sensitivity to glucosamine sulphate, so this commonly used supplement can be enjoyed without worry. The therapist must take note of this information. We must ignore any unfounded story that has no scientific evidence to support itself.

$$\left[\begin{array}{c} \text{CH}_2\text{OH} \\ \end{array} \right]_2 \quad 2\text{Na(or K)} + \text{SO}_4 = 2\text{Cl}^-$$

Sulphites

Sulphites (or sulphiting agents) refer to a group of simple chemicals that include sulphur dioxide and sulphite salts. They are produced naturally in some foods, mainly those undergoing fermentation. Sulphites are metabolised to sulphur dioxide under certain conditions that depend on concentration, heat, and pH. Sulphur dioxide has been considered to be the offending component in cases of sulphite hypersensitivity based on the established sensitivity of asthmatics to inhaled sulphur dioxide. Even so, clinical reports of this sensitivity have involved very few people, and new analytic reports have not appeared in over a decade. This hypersensitivity is often called an allergy, but it does not involve immune mechanisms as do reactions that are properly termed allergies.

Some sulphiting agents are FDA-approved preservatives that are added to food and pharmaceuticals. The more common sulphiting agents are sodium sulphite (Na_2SO_3), sodium bisulphite (pictured below, $NaHSO_3$), and sodium metabisulphite ($Na_2S_2O_3$). Examples of foods containing sulphites are listed in the next table; these foods may only contain sulphites under certain conditions. However, the FDA has banned adding sulphites to fresh fruits and vegetables offered in restaurants and other public venues due to the concerns that were raised. Juices squeezed from lemons and limes will not have sulphites, but bottled or dehydrated juice may contain sulphites.

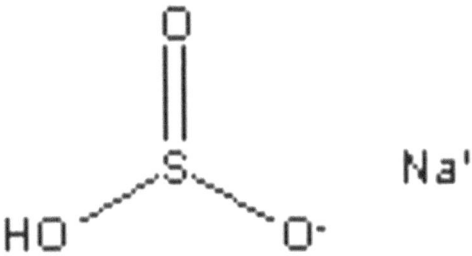

Foods that may contain sulphites		
Dried soup mixes	Dehydrated vegetables	Lemon and lime juice
Vegetable juices	Shredded coconut	Jams and jellies
Baked goods	Sauerkraut	Grape juice
Canned or dried fish	Dried noodle meals	Wine
Dried fruit	Olives	Molasses
Relishes	Pickles	Gravies
Maraschino cherries	Shrimp, lobster, scallops	Potatoes

A sulphite reaction is different from a sulphonamide allergy (a reaction to sulpha drugs) because sulphites and sulphonamides are entirely different chemicals and have unrelated mechanisms of reaction. A person sensitive to sulphites is no more likely to be allergic to sulphonamides than any other individual and vice versa. The following mechanisms of sulphite sensitivity have been proposed:

- Cholinergic reflex response
- IgE mediated delayed hypersensitivity
- Sulphite oxidase deficiency

No antibody or specific complement activity (as would be found in true allergies) has been identified in association with sulphite exposure. Sulphite sensitivity is a matter that is complicated by the fact that it is often reported by persons who display several types of hypersensitivity so that it is difficult to confirm that sulphites are actually causative factors in perceived reactions. For example, a study of asthmatics who were sensitive to wine indicated that there appeared to be a reduced sensitivity to sulphite-free wine, but that this was likely due to other differences in the wine products, since direct challenge with high-sulphite wine only rarely was associated with a reaction. Reactions to red wines, which appear to occur more often than to white wines, are apparently associated primarily with compounds in the wine other than sulphites.

The FDA estimates that about 1 per cent of the population may have some degree of sulphite sensitivity, while that figure rises to 5 per cent of asthmatics, mainly affecting those with severe, persistent asthma. Because of concerns about sulphite sensitivity, there is a requirement imposed by the FDA to label packaged foods as having sulphites if they contain as little as 10 ppm of sulphites. Generally, foods with less than 100 ppm of sulphites will not affect sensitive asthmatics, so there is a tenfold safety margin. From 1996 through mid-1999, the FDA received a total of only thirty-four reports (about ten per year) of adverse reactions allegedly due to eating foods containing undeclared sulphites. FDA specialists in the area of sulphites have not discovered the mechanism that is responsible for the apparent reactions. However, if sulphur dioxide acts in sensitive individuals to cause constriction, this could explain both the asthmatic response and the report that some people suffer headaches. Hospitals may have to consider extra precautions about sulphites used as preservatives in their drugs because people with serious illnesses may have a heightened degree of sensitivity or have more diverse reactions to sulphur dioxide, and the drugs may be introduced directly into the bloodstream or lungs.

Several years ago, a large, Western herb company began promoting the idea that Chinese herbs were problematic for those with sulphite sensitivity because many of them were treated with sulphites. Sulphur treatment is sometimes used to prevent herbs from deteriorating, usually by placing the herbs on a screen and having sulphur vapours briefly flow from below the screen, which could leave traces of sulphur dioxide (sulphur prevents the herbs from deteriorating). At the Institute for Traditional Medicine, herb formulations have been provided for nearly twenty years and administered to hundreds of thousands of people seeking Chinese medical health care. Among these people, there are many who claim to be sulphite sensitive. The institute has not received any reports of sulphite-sensitive patients having evident sulphite reactions to the herb products despite the fact that some of the herbs are 'sulphured'. It may well be that there is so little residual sulphur dioxide (and any related compounds) that it doesn't cause a reaction, or it may be that the form of sulphur residue is not one that causes the reactions, or it may be that many of the sensitivities that are described as reactions to sulphites are not actually reactions to sulphites. Nonetheless, some Chinese herb companies have described the items that they provide as 'sulphur-free' in response to the concerns that were raised. It is not known whether they routinely use different herb materials in support of those claims.

Appendix 1: Example of Using Sulphur Compounds: Allicin-DMSO Spray

A unique formulation with two sulphur ingredients is the result of collaboration between several individuals and organisations. Allicin refers to a highly concentrated extract of garlic, rich in antibiotic and mucolytic compounds (of which the sulphur compound, allicin, is the main one) that is manufactured in Shanghai, China, under strict quality-control measures and imported to the United States by Dr Qingcai Zhang. The extract comes in hermetically sealed vials that are used for intravenous applications of the garlic extract. Several clinics have used this imported allicin for respiratory therapy (in a nebuliser), for intestinal infections (by retention enema), and for systemic infections (by IV administration). DMSO is a refined component from trees that has several applications, including antioxidant therapy, though it is especially known for its highly penetrating characteristics: It is used to help carry other substances to areas of the body that are congested or difficult to penetrate. DMSO (dimethyl-sulphoxide) and its derivative compound, MSM (methyl-sulphonyl-methane), are also being used as sulphur donor molecules in treatment of several inflammatory disorders, including arthritis. Dr Stan Jacobs, at the Oregon Health Sciences University, is the leading expert in use of DMSO and MSM; he had provided the recommendations for use of DMSO for this spray. The combination has now been in use for twelve years with excellent acceptance and no adverse reports. The DMSO (pharmaceutical grade) and allicin are combined and packaged with a unique nasal sprayer by John Rawson of Flander's Pharmacy in Portland, Oregon. The allicin and DMSO are passed through microfilters to guarantee freedom from micro-organisms. The spray nozzle produces a very fine mist that penetrates the congested areas. Due to the particular characteristics of the spray unit, the glass bottles containing the allicin-DMSO mixture are not full, though they are packed with the correct amount of fluid.

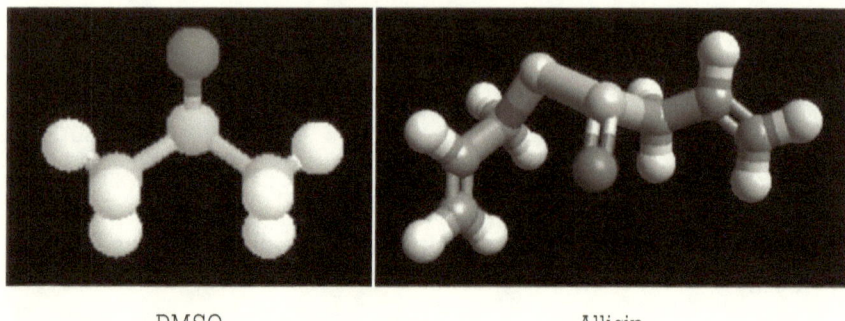

DMSO   Allicin

The primary indication for this nasal spray is for helping to alleviate persistent nasal congestion that is due to nasal infections resistant to standard antibiotics or resistant to decongestant therapies; it might also be applied in cases of persisting congestion due to allergies. The spray can be used as needed, up to six times per day, with one or two doses (sprays) delivered each time. The allicin component of the formulation may produce a temporary stinging sensation in some users. Both the allicin and DMSO have a garlic-like smell.

11.13 Updating a Valued Tradition in Natural Health Care

Father Künzle (1857-1945) was in a perfect position to observe the transitional period from an old style of life—in which most people still lived closely with nature—to a new style of life in which most people have gone to great lengths to isolate themselves from nature. This new book, written a century after he began his herbal healing practice, comes at the time when the transition that he observed proceeding slowly in the relative remoteness of Swiss villages is nearly complete throughout most of the world, and especially so in the great cities of the twenty-first century. Despite some well-deserved complaints he voiced about the rush towards the modern lifestyle, Künzle certainly did not suggest that one ought to expend one's energy resisting the entire tide of progress. The modernisation of human culture and civilisation has been going on, albeit much more slowly in past centuries, throughout history. Efforts to turn things back to the seemingly golden age of the past, a past which was never so desirable as portrayed by those who romanticise it, have always failed.

On the other hand, it is foolish to even attempt, in modern life, to leave behind the fundamental nature of human existence or the hard-won wisdom of accumulated human efforts in order to participate more fully in technological pursuits. It is for this reason that naturalists, like Father Künzle, have tried to maintain the thread of common sense and solid daily practices. Their recommendations should be given due attention, lest errors of neglect accumulate. Künzle wanted people to pay attention to their actions and to their environment and not to ignore these things as they sought the benefits of progress. There were many subjects raised by Künzle in *Herbs and Weeds* that are worth revisiting now, but in an updated manner. Künzle's focus was that one of the greatest tragedies accrued during the rush to modernisation is the impairment of human health that occurs during the earliest ages and then proceeds further, often out of sheer habit. He referred, in particular, to a trend that was already under way in his time, which accelerated in the following decades, of avoiding the proper nourishment of infants and children. He spoke of the limited duration or the absence of breastfeeding. Although he brought this subject up after outlining the properties and uses of some valuable herbs, it is here mentioned right off, because it is evident from Künzle's writing that it was a matter of great importance to him.

Medical historians agree with Künzle's depiction of the tragedy facing children during his time. 'There are regions in Switzerland,' he wrote, 'where for decades half of the newborns died in the first year of their life.' As to the cause, he writes: 'I knew a priest who searched for the reason for this mortality rate and who was soon successful. The children were deprived of the milk which God gives to mothers.' It is well confirmed now that this natural, normal, and seemingly inviolable aspect of the relationship between mother and child when discarded yields numerous problems for the child that can last throughout life. This includes intolerance and allergy to common foods, atopic dermatitis, impaired immune functions, and, perhaps, psychological irregularities that lead to an unsuccessful and unhappy life experience. While the death of infants, as occurred in Künzle's time, is largely avoided by use of antibiotics and specially designed nutrient formulas to replace the important mother's milk, the adverse effects of deleting breastfeeding are still with us. The subject may seem a strange one to lead into the topic of herbal remedies, but it is a signature act of unthinking modern people (both women and men) that one would consider this critical part of life dispensable. If this simple point isn't grasped, then the true value of herbs as a part of natural lifestyle will also not be properly understood. Whether offering natural breast milk to the newborn or a healing herbal tea to a child or adult, it is the act of living with nature, rather than against it, that captures the essence of what needs to be done to assure good health.

Künzle put it this way: 'It is God's commandment that mothers should feed their children with mother's milk as long as possible. Even the most primitive people observe this custom.' The statement is quite revealing. Today, many would think that breastfeeding is one of those things that only primitive people do, something that we can now discard in favour of the modern way of life, where the mother is too busy to be bothered by such things. Some women, because of societal messages that have become ingrained, are even repulsed by the concept of breastfeeding, while others see it as a burden to be tolerated for the shortest allowable interval. But, to Künzle, it would be the enlightened, civilised people who ought to perform this essential task, and the fact that primitive people would also do so is just a reflection of how universally important it is. At his time, mothers were not too busy, but rather, there were numerous mothers who, he said, 'neglect this holy duty or fulfil it only for a very short time of a week or two,' for regrettable reasons, like false modesty. Whatever the basis, the loss of breastfeeding is a tragedy. The replacement of breastfeeding by the use of imitation milk formulas and animal milk (or soy 'milk') from bottles, supplemented by artificial nipples (pacifiers), and then dropping off young children into the hands of strangers (childcare centres) or leaving them for hours at the television is even a step beyond what Künzle saw happening in his time, though certainly in line with it. 'They feed their infants all sorts of artificial food instead, which never replaces mother's milk, just as a servant can never replace a mother.'

The transfer of responsibility away from feeding a child appropriately is a direct correlate of another trend. This has been the move (by adults) to replace herbal remedies, exposure to nature, and healthful habits with reliance on modern drugs and turning over the care of one's health from a personal responsibility, where most of it ought to lie, to the responsibility of a medical doctor, a pharmaceutical company, and a health maintenance organisation. It must be said that maintaining one's health takes a certain amount of time, effort, and respect for the natural and traditional way of doing things, as does the care and feeding of infants. These concepts are linked. We now have generations who have grown up without the benefits of alignment to natural methods of staying healthy. Many who suffer the consequences are quick to blame other aspects of modern society—chemical pollutants, electromagnetic energy, improper medical care, the efforts of corporations to earn profits from selling unhealthy products, and the like. These things are said to be responsible for the ailments that are, for the most part, properly blamed on how individuals started out their lives under inadequate parental guidance and the fact that they were not trained to take care of themselves. This orientation to being against the trappings of society (e.g. its technology) rather than considering one's own priorities has this numbing effect: It allows one to rail against something that is outside oneself (what 'they' are doing), while passing on the same unhealthy behaviour to the next generation. It is not acceptable to simply reject drugs and seek out herbs to replace them for alleviating ailments—one must break the cycle.

With such beginnings, including, too often, failings in prenatal care, an unacceptably large portion of the population of children are diagnosed with brain defects such as attention deficit disorder, immunological disorders such as asthma, and metabolic disorders such as diabetes. Künzle saw this trend evolving even before the increase in female binge drinking, tobacco smoking, and other bad habits that had formerly been mainly to the detriment of men. He noted: 'Many children are already ill in their mother's womb. Habitual vices like confirmed drunkenness or particular sensibility . . . will be transmitted to the children.' Of course, the father, who ought to be contributing to and supporting the good habits of the mother, can't be absolved of some responsibility for the environment in which the mother lives. Today, too often, the mother is without a husband to take any daily responsibilities. For several decades, as the natural diet gave way to a processed one, a key nutrient, folic acid, became available only in reduced amounts. In its worst known cases, this leads to neural tube defects and death. Now, it is the duty of health authorities to instruct women to go back to eating fruits and vegetables, a good source of this nutrient or, at least, to take a supplement for that which may be missing in the diet. In fact, so serious is the concern, that manufacturers of certain common foods are instructed to fortify their products with folic acid, while others advertise that they uniquely do so. Modern research confirms the importance, at least in broad perspective, of dietary recommendations that Künzle had emphasised. Children are now inculcated with the idea and the experience that food does not have natural flavour and they are not aware of the basic production path of food: from the earth to the market to the kitchen stove to the plate.

Rather, food becomes a synthetically flavoured substance that appears miraculously in a packet or a box picked up at a store, or dispensed by a machine, manufactured and microwaved, or a meal served up by a stranger at a restaurant from a hidden kitchen where unknown ingredients and processes are used. The food loses its meaning and is given the role of satisfying one's palette and stomach, at least for a short time, before it causes digestive distress and worse. Food is then unrelated to the earth, just as drugs are increasingly unrelated to the earth. There is hardly a confection or a snack that has a flavour actually found in nature despite some good efforts. There is hardly a meal that doesn't include at least one item made by an industrial technique that renders the processed food tasteful to the modern palette that has now been trained to such things, but that tastes utterly bizarre to anyone used to the remarkable taste—and texture—of properly prepared natural foods. The term 'natural foods' does not refer to the strange things often sold in so-called natural food stores that are manufactured as imitations of the standard items (but having an organically grown ingredient or sea salt in place of regular salt). Rather, the term should refer to the things that are grown and raised, perhaps minimally processed (e.g. turning milk to butter), but not manufactured (e.g. chemically transforming liquid vegetable oil to solid margarine). Father Künzle, with his religious background, offered an alternative view of diet that fitted well with his spiritual side, warning against gluttony and partaking in the latest food fads: 'If you want me to express all this in a few words and to give you an unequalled absolutely sure model for a healthy and reasonable way of life at the same time, then I advise you: back to Christ, the Lord, who also wanted to have a human body like ours, who had the same natural needs as we have (with the exception of sin), who suffered from hunger, thirst, heat, and cold, who worked and got tired: Christ, the Lord, is the most perfect example for a pure and natural life, the ideal of man. *Ecco homo*, look what a man he was! The Son of God was modest and natural in his food and clothing. He partook of the meals of fisherman and day-labourers, of just what they had to offer . . . The Apostles He advised, 'Eat whatever is put before you.'

Künzle's reference to just eating what was offered had a great significance to him, and it should to us. The food that was offered at the time by fishermen and other labourers was simple, natural, and had one purpose—to provide the body what was needed in order to carry on the work at hand. What has happened in recent times is that too much of our effort is put into making the meals suit other purposes. Rather than having simple food—fish and bread was the standard fare mentioned as the foods used to serve the multitudes who had come to hear Jesus speak—many today turn to restaurants where foods that are too complicated to make at home are offered. I recall a statement from one of the oldest men to live in America; he was about 113 at the time of the interview in which he was asked about his diet, and he lucidly responded that he had lived mainly on sardines and saltines. Rather than being natural, today people usually rely on numerous foods prepared in factories from a mixture of processed foods and chemical additives. And, in place of the providing what is needed for labour, food is frequently consumed for taste and texture sensations, for comfort during times when anxious sitting replaces physical activity, and for providing a distraction while being a spectator, observing sports, movies, or television programmes. The twisted consumption patterns that have arisen during the past century have had an impact on medical practice. Young children are now routinely subjected to all kinds of drug treatments, even surgeries that might otherwise be unnecessary, and they have become used to the routine of unnatural living that is to be interrupted by medical care from time to time. Today, numerous children are obese and suffer from adult syndromes like diabetes, because their parents, often unwittingly, provide to them the wrong food, improper guidance, and are poor role models. As they become adults, this unnatural pattern is now firmly ingrained, so that people will even seek out herbal remedies that are falsely touted as substitutes for good diet and exercise, in order to control their weight with pills. They may look to herbal remedies to take the place of a growing medicine cabinet of drugs after it is almost too late to make a change. Fear of interactions between herbs and drugs now takes over as a significant concern. Worse, this pattern is passed on to the next generation. Meanwhile, the potential of research on the human genetic code is held out as an ultimate solution as if the diseases and discomforts will be wiped away once their genetic basis has been identified. The next generation is then prepared to take a step further away from nature.

The family meal, probably one of the most enduring traditions and a virtual necessity until recently, has given way to a myriad of eat-and-run experiences in many families. One not only loses the connection between cooking a meal and eating that food, but also the connection of family members to one another. As a result, there is no clear sense of tradition in consuming food, and, likewise, there is no lingering sense of tradition in taking herbs. The ability of people to succumb to peculiar diets grows as people lose connection with their larger community, starting with the family unit that was formerly united several times daily by eating together. Besides, the effect of losing this important cultural tradition can also be damaging to children beyond assuring nutritional requirements. It was reported in a recent issue (January 2002) of the *Journal of Epidemiology and Community Health*: 'Many adolescents with anxiety, depression or other mental health problems come from families that don't eat meals together or participate in similar family rituals as often as the families of adolescents without such psychological problems. Union rituals, such as sharing meals, serve to transmit belief systems and norms of behaviour. The lack of such practices can adversely affect a person's maturation, and the resolution of the crisis of adolescence may be impeded.' This being said, it is the task of the next chapter to outline a healthier way of living, in order to prepare the reader to understand and properly utilise herb.

11.14 Sea Cucumber: Food and Medicine

The pacific sea cucumber (Stichopus species and other members of the family Holothurioidea)

Subhuti Dharmananda, PhD, Director

It has been so revered by Chinese cooks since ancient times, in particular, that sea cucumber meals have been offered on special occasions, especially during the New Year celebrations. An ancient Confucian recipe, translated roughly as 'The Eight Immortals Crossing the Sea' and made with sea cucumber, shark's fin, and five kinds of fish and shellfish, is one of the classic banquet dishes. The sea cucumber is valued—along with several other delicacies, such as shark's fin, ginseng, cordyceps, and tremella—as a disease preventive and longevity tonic. It was listed as a medicinal agent in the *Bencao Congxin* (New Compilation of Materia Medica) by Wu Yiluo in 1757. The popular Chinese name for sea cucumber is haishen, which means, roughly, ginseng of the sea. It is often known in medical literature as fangcishen (fang = four-sided, ci = thorny; referring to the spiky protrusions that emanate from four sides) or, in abbreviated form, fangshen. The Asian demand for sea cucumber has been so high that these have been collected from the UnitedStates and other countries (e.g. Australia and Philippines) to get an adequate supply. The Atlantic sea cucumber, Cucumaria frondosa, has been collected primarily for food but has recently been researched as a source of medicinal components, thanks to the efforts of Coastside Bio-Resources in Maine, New England State, USA, headed by Peter Collin.

Preparation and Use of Sea Cucumber

To prepare the sea cucumber after it is collected, the internal organs are removed and dirt and sand are washed out of the cavity. It is then boiled in salty water and dried in the air to preserve it. When ready for use in making food, the hard, dried sea cucumber is softened. The process is quite lengthy, which is why this food tends to appear at special dinners and banquets more so than in day-to-day cuisine. To soften the dried sea cucumbers, the instructions are as follows: place the sea cucumbers in a pot and add cold water to cover them, soak them for at least twelve hours, and then cook over low heat for one to two hours. Add more water, as necessary, to make sure that the water always covers the cucumbers. Remove from heat, let them cool to room temperature, and then drain them. According to an analysis by principles of traditional Chinese medicine, the sea cucumber nourishes the blood and vital essence (jing), tonifies kidney chi (treats disorders of the kidney system, including reproductive organs), and moistens dryness (especially of the intestines). It has a salty quality and warming nature. Common medicinal uses of sea cucumber in China include treating the following: weakness, impotence, debility of the aged, constipation due to intestinal dryness, and frequent urination. The sea cucumber properties may be compared with certain other common Chinese tonics that are used in food therapy such as cordyceps (dongchong xiacao, which tonifies yang and is less moistening) and tremella (yiner, which nourishes yin and is moistening, but is less effective as a blood tonic). For yin and blood deficiency, especially manifesting as intestinal dryness, sea cucumber is combined with tremella to make a soup. For impotence, frequent urination, and other signs of kidney deficiency, sea cucumber is cooked with mutton. For nourishing essence and blood in persons who suffer from emaciation, it is combined in soup with pork. From the nutritional viewpoint, sea cucumber is an ideal tonic food. It is higher in protein (at 55 per cent) than most any other food except egg whites (at 99 per cent) and it has 10-16 per cent mucopolysaccharides, substances that are used to build the cartilage. Sea cucumber is lower in fat than most other foods.

Sea Cucumber as a Nutritional Supplement

From the modern medical viewpoint, sea cucumber is a valuable source of several kinds of substances that can serve as natural health products and, perhaps, be developed as drugs. Since sea cucumber is consumed as a food by a very small segment of the population outside East Asia, most people do not have access to its beneficial components. Thus, extracts of desired sea cucumber materials are put into easy-to-consume formats, such as capsules (hard and soft gelatin) and tablets. Sea cucumber, having a cartilaginous body, serves as a rich source of mucopolysaccharides, mainly chondroitin sulphate, which is well known for its ability to reduce arthritis pain, especially that of osteoarthritis As little as three grams per day of the dried sea cucumber has been helpful in significantly reducing arthralgia. Chondroitin's action is similar to that of glucosamine sulphate, the main building block of chondroitin.

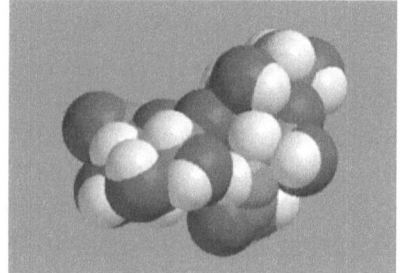

Chondroitin building blocks. On the left is the chemical layout, showing one building block that can be repeated numerous times; this is basically a glucose molecule (left portion) and glucosamine molecule (right portion), which has been sulphated (O_3S, at the top). This building block is illustrated to the right in a three-dimensional representation.

Long-chain sulphated polysaccharides, like chondroitin, also inhibit viruses; there is a Japanese patent for sea cucumber chondroitin sulphate for HIV therapy based on this action, and other sulphated polysaccharides from seaweeds have been patented as inhibitors of herpes viruses. Chondroitin is usually obtained in commercial quantities from bovine trachea or shark cartilage (including the shark fin), while glucosamine sulphate is obtained from shells of shrimp and crab. These compounds are also found in deer antler, which is not a practical source for extraction due to its rarity and cost, but it is likely that glucosamine and chondroitin are significant contributors to the medicinal action of deer antler. Russian, Japanese, and Chinese studies reveal that sea cucumbers also contain saponins (triterpene glycosides). These compounds have a structure similar to the active constituents of ginseng, ganoderma, and other famous tonic herbs. Pharmacology studies indicate anti-inflammatory and anticancer properties of the sea cucumber saponins.

One of the sea cucumber saponins, representative of the structures commonly found in these organisms.

In addition, the sea cucumber oil contains two anti-inflammatory fractions. One fraction has fatty acids characteristic of those found in fish; they can be used as a substitute for fish oil in reducing inflammatory by-products of fat metabolism and to nourish the brain and heart. The main compounds of interest in fish oil are EPA (eicosapentaenoic acid) also found in sea cucumber, and DHA (docosahaenoic acid), unique to fish:

Stereochemical representations of EPA (left) and DHA (right). The double bond locations are different, causing a different bending of the structures.

The other oil fraction is a mixture of branched–chain fatty acids, mainly 12-MTA (methyltetradecanoic acid). This compound, and the more widely studied variant, 13-MTA, are potent inhibitors of the 5-LOX (lypoxygenase) enzyme system. 5-LOX inhibitors are one of the key areas of modern drug development, with plans evolving to use the compounds in treatment of asthma, ulcerative colitis, and arthritis. In addition, cancer-inhibiting effects have been observed in preliminary studies with prostate cancer cell lines and other human cancer cells These fatty acids are thought to be produced by bacteria that live within the sea cucumbers; they are also produced by bacteria in other marine organisms, such as sponges and tunicates.

Sample branched-chain fatty acid found in sea organisms. The central chain is a simple carbohydrate.

These long chains can interact with cell membranes.

Bibliography

- Zhang Enchin (Chief Editor), *Chinese Medicated Diet*, 1988; Publishing House of Shanghai College of Traditional Chinese Medicine, Shanghai.
- Tang Weici, Chinese medicinal materials from the sea, *Abstracts of Chinese Medicine*, 1987; 1[4]: 571-600.

- Yang Peiying, et al., Inhibition of proliferation of PC3 Cells by the branched-chain fatty acid, 12–MTA, is associated with inhibition of 5–lipoxygenase, *The Prostate*, 2003; 55: 281–91.

For pictures of sea cucumbers live, dried, and prepared as food, see the tour of illustrations at cucumbe1.htm

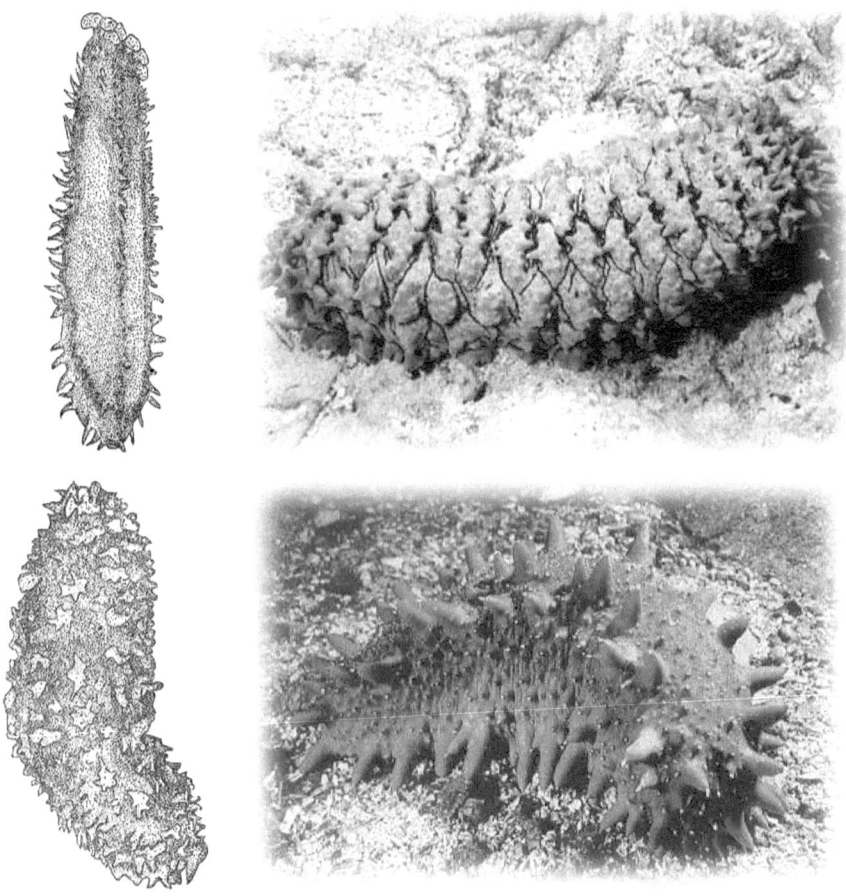

11.15 Silverweed

Subhuti Dharmananda, PhD, Director

The aim of presenting the above research information is to see where and how it can used in any therapeutic prevention in complementary therapy. Silverweed is the common name for several species of *Potentilla* (of the Rose family). Its name is based on the silvery-white colour of the leaves, particularly notable on the bottom side of the leaves of some species. This colouration is due to the presence of fine, white, downy hairs. The plant is also called cinquefoil (meaning 'five leaves'), indicating the five-part leaf groups that may be found (see photo). The genus name *Potentilla* was given to these plants in 1753 by Linnaeus, based on the powerful ('potent') healing effects attributed to the herbal medicines derived from it. The genus is a group of about five hundred hardy perennials and shrubs, and most of them found in the cooler regions of the Northern Hemisphere: North America, Europe, and Northern Asia, though they are now planted over a wider range as an attractive garden plant with bright yellow flowers. The plants vary in height from a few inches to about three feet.

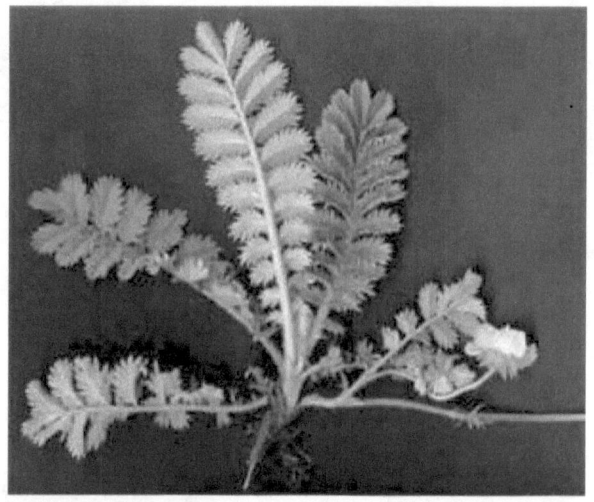

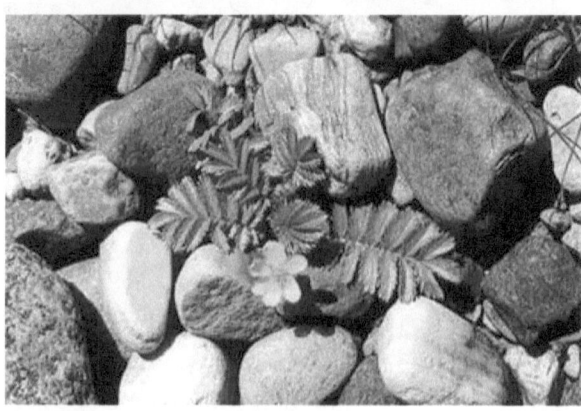

As a medicinal herb and food, the most widely used species is *Potentilla anserina*, sometimes called goosewort, goosegrass, or goose tansy because it is a favoured food of geese (anserine = goose). The leaves are also generally consumed by livestock, such as cattle, horses, and goats; sheep do not seem to like it, however. The starchy root—which is said to taste like parsnips, sweet potatoes, or chestnuts—has served as a human food, while its leaves are valued as a healthful tea. Roasted, boiled, or raw, silverweed's rootstock has been consumed as food by the Native Americans, Chinese, and Europeans for centuries. Silverweed rootstock has kept people alive when nothing else was available to eat. For the past few decades, malnutrition has been a significant problem in Tibet, especially among children, and a possible contribution to resolving the problem may be the root *Potentilla anserina*, known there as droma. It grows on grasslands throughout Tibet. In the past, Tibetans harvested droma, ground it, and fed it to their children. Bundles of the root appear in the marketplace in Tibet and Nepal (where it is also harvested from the high plateaus). A nutrient analysis of droma revealed that its amino acid profile is complementary to that of barley, a Tibetan staple. Since barley flour is mixed with tea and fed to children from a very young age, droma can easily be added to the mixture to make a complete protein food. The Tibet Child Nutrition Project, a programme of the Terma Foundation, has been introducing droma for the Tibetan diet.

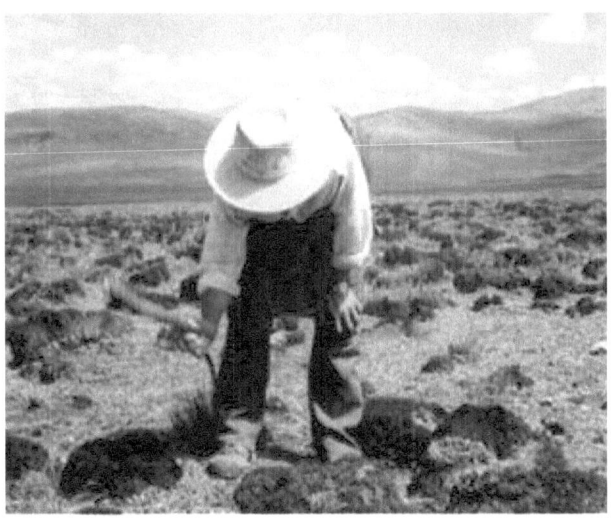

Tibetan worker using an antelope horn to dig up droma.

A project to incorporate droma into the diet to help prevent child malnutrition is run by the Terma Foundation.

In Europe, silverweed is known for its antispasmodic activity, and it has been used frequently to treat menstrual cramps. Also, its high tannin content makes it a useful treatment for sore throat, oral and skin ulcerations, bleeding, and diarrhoea. The famous Swiss herbalist Johann Künzle wrote in his 1911 booklet *Herbs and Weeds*: 'Every woman should know this herb because there hardly exists a better remedy against menstrual cramps and hemorrhages. Numerous women have found relief by drinking two cups of potentilla decoction on the ten days preceding their menstruation.' He went on to point out that 'the whole plant has therapeutic effects: it cools, fortifies, and acts as an astringent.'

The combination of astringent tannins and antispasmodic action (which is possibly due to glycosides) makes silverweed especially useful for treating diarrhoea and ulcerative colitis, since the tannins have antibacterial action and help to heal the intestines, while the antispasmodic effect reduces intestinal contractions. Künzle told of one case as follows: 'A peasant from Sion had consulted every physician all the way down to Geneva without finding relief. He weakened continuously because of the daily loss of blood in his stool. Finally, he asked a cattle dealer to drive him up to the herbalist Anna Katharine Willi [she was sometimes called 'Tormentilla' named after the herb she frequently used: Potentilla tormentilla]. She gave him half a pound of potentilla powder and she recommended he take half a tablespoonful in a glass of water three times daily. This he did, and a week later he was cured and regained his strength.'

Maude Grieve, in her 1931 *Modern Herbal*, provided a list of applications as under:

- A strong infusion of silverweed, if used as a lotion, will check the bleeding of piles, the ordinary infusion (1 oz. to a pint of boiling water) being meanwhile taken as a medicine.
- The same infusion, sweetened with honey, constitutes an excellent gargle for sore throat. A tablespoonful of the powdered herb may also be taken every three hours.
- It is also an excellent remedy for cramps in the stomach, heart, and abdomen. In addition to the infusion taken internally, it is advisable to apply it to the affected parts by compresses.
- A tablespoonful of the herb, boiled in a cup of milk, has been recommended as an effective remedy in tetanus, or lockjaw. The tea should be drunk as hot as possible.

- The dried and powdered leaves have been successfully administered in ague (an acute ailment that causes shivering or alternating chills and fever), the more astringent roots have been given in powder in doses of a scruple (about 1.3 grams) and upwards.
- As a diuretic, silverweed has been considered useful in gravel (fine urinary stones). Ettmueller extolled it as a specific in jaundice. Of the fresh plant, 3 oz. or more may be taken three or four times daily.
- The decoction has been used for ulcers in the mouth, relaxation of the uvula, spongy gums, and for fixing loose teeth, also for toothache and preserving the gums from scurvy.
- A distilled water of the herb was in earlier days much in vogue as a cosmetic for removing freckles, spots and pimples, and for restoring the complexion when sunburnt.

In Chinese medicine, *Potentilla chinensis* or *Potentilla discolor* is called *fanbaicao*; it is a commonly used remedy for diarrhoea, especially if accompanied by blood discharge; it is also given for other haemorrhages, including menstrual bleeding and blood in the urine due to infection or gravel. In India and also in Siberia, the leaves of a related plant, *Potentilla fruticosa*, are used as a substitute for tea. The combination of ordinary tea with potentilla emphasises its astringent quality.

Active Constituents

The major components of interest in potentilla species are tannins of the ellagic-acid type, with monomeric and dimeric ellagitannins, similar to those found in green tea. The herb also contains antioxidant flavonoids (quercetin and myricetin glycosides) and proanthocyanidins. Another group of components of silverweed that are being investigated is the long- and medium-chain polyprenols; they accumulate in the leaves of *Potentilla anserina* at a concentration of up to 0.3 per cent fresh weight. They appear to have antiviral activity.

Chapter 11.14

Honeybush Healthful Beverage Tea from South Africa

Subhuti Dharmananda, PhD, Director

Honeybush (*Cyclopia spp.*) is indigenous to the cape of South Africa [1, 2]. It is used to make a beverage and a medicinal tea, having a pleasant, mildly sweet taste and aroma, somewhat like honey. It has become internationally known as a substitute for ordinary tea (*Camellia sinensis*). With the dramatic growth in the use of honeybush during the past five years, export of honeybush tea products is now a major industry, following up on the success of another tea substitute from South Africa—rooibos. International interest in honeybush is traced back to the tea trade of the Dutch and the British. A settlement, which eventually became Cape Town, was established in 1652 as a supply base for the Dutch East India Company that was trading in Indian tea and Southeast Asian spices. Botanists began cataloguing the rich flora of the cape soon after; the honeybush plant was noted in botanical literature by 1705. Though there are no published reports at that time of its use as a tea by the native populations (the San and Khoi-Khoi tribes, known today as Khoisan or Bushmen), it was soon recognised by the colonists as a suitable substitute for ordinary tea, probably based on observing native practices. In 1814, the British purchased the Cape Colony from the Dutch, and English became the official language a few years later, helping to spread knowledge of South Africa to England and America. In King's American Dispensatory of 1898, under the heading of 'tea,' honeybush is already listed as a substitute with reference to a report from 1881, indicating use of honeybush as a tea in the Cape Colony of South Africa. The Khoisan of the South African Cape was also using the tea for treatment of coughs and other upper respiratory symptoms associated with infections. The plant is a shrub of the Fabaceae family (Leguminosae) that grows in the fynbos botanical zone (biome), indicated in green in the map below. It is a narrow region along the coast, bounded by mountain ranges. Fynbos is a vegetation type, characterised mainly by woody plants with small, leathery leaves (fynbos is from the Dutch, meaning fine-leaved plants).

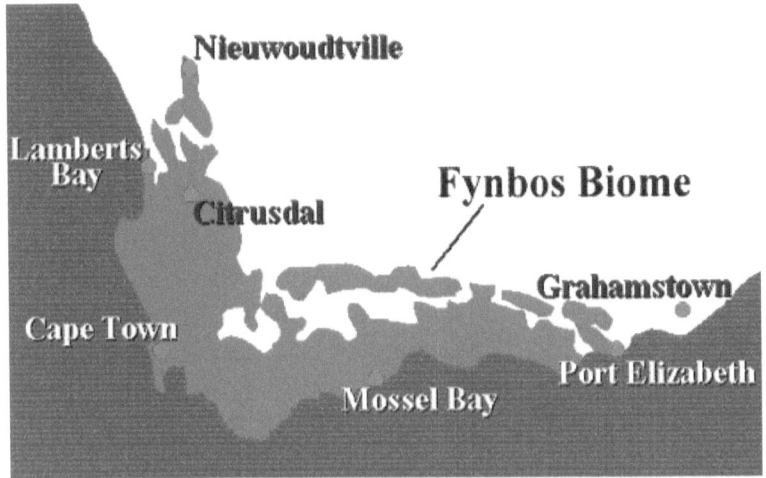

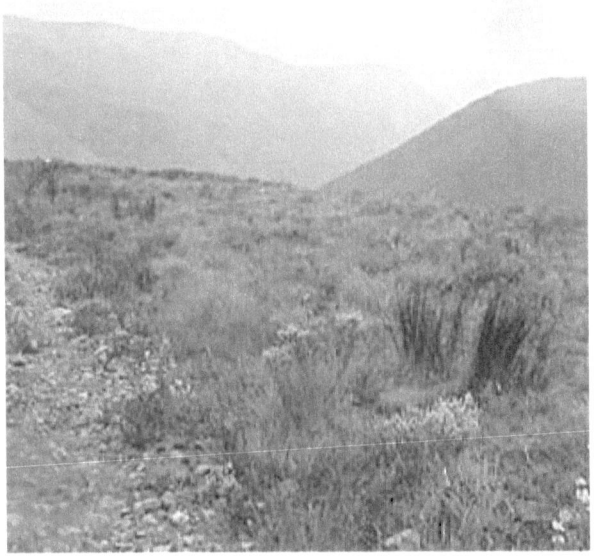

View of Typical Fynbos Terrain with
Small-leaved Vegetation.

The honeybush plant is easily recognised by its trifoliate leaves, single-flowered inflorescences, and sweetly scented, bright yellow flowers. The flowers have prominent grooves on the petals, a thrust-in (intrusive) calyx base, and two bracts fused at the base around the pedicel. The genus name *Cyclopia* alludes to the intrusive base of the calyx, which contributes to the flower's unique appearance. Honeybush plants have woody stems, a relatively low ratio of leaves to stems, and hard-shelled seeds. The most desirable components for the tea are the leaves and flowers; the relatively tasteless stems are included.

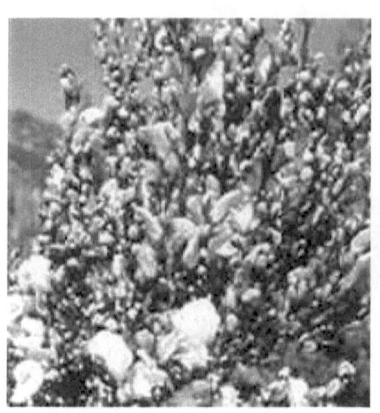

Commercial supplies of honeybush are mainly obtained from *Cyclopia intermedia* and to a lesser extent from *Cyclopia subternata*, though there are about two dozen species of *Cyclopia* identified in this narrow region of South Africa. Most of the species have very limited distribution ranges and unique habitat preferences. Some are restricted to mountain peaks, perennial streams, marshy areas, shale bands, or wet southern slopes. Some of the species, such as *Cyclopia maculata*, *Cyclopia genistoides*, and *Cyclopia sessiliflora*, have been used for home consumption. It appears that all the *Cyclopia* species are suitable for making tea, but the taste quality can vary, and some species exist in very small quantities.

Leaf shape and size differ among the species, but most are thin, needle-like to elongated leaves. All the species are easily recognised in the field as they are covered with the distinctive, deep-yellow flowers, which have a characteristic sweet honey scent. Traditionally, the tea is harvested during flowering—either in early autumn or late spring—depending on the flowering period of the species. However, with the larger demand for products, some collection is extended into the summer.

The collection of honeybush in South Africa has grown significantly in recent years. In 1997, approximately 30 tons of the plant was processed, an amount that mainly satisfied the local demand. This is enough to make about one cup of tea (2.5 g/cup) per week for the year for about 225,000 people (1/2 per cent of the South Africa population of about forty-five million). But by 2000, the amount reached about 160 tons and the amount for 2004 is likely to exceed 300 tons, the increase mainly reflecting the development of the international market for the tea, though there has also been a substantial growth in consumption domestically.

Most of the honeybush tea is still collected from wild populations, but cultivation has become necessary with the rapid growth of the industry (forcing collectors to travel further into poorly accessible areas) and with the demand for more uniform product. In 1998, a group of farmers formed the South African Honeybush Producers Association (SAHPA). In the spring of 2001, the first large-scale South African plantation dedicated to honeybush began operation in the town of Haarlem. The farm is the result of a joint partnership between South Africa and the United States (one of the potential large customers, along with Japan and Canada). The principal organisations involved are the ASNAPP (Agribusiness in Sustainable Natural African Plant Products), Rutgers University (New Jersey), and the Herb Research Foundation (Colorado). The goal is to develop a successful cooperative farm operated by local growers who will cultivate 100,000 or more honeybush plants. Based on a successful start of the Haarlem plantation, another cultivation project was started in Ericaville.

Manufacture of Tea

The manufacture of honeybush tea consists of four processing steps: harvesting, cutting, 'fermentation' (oxidation), and drying.

The gathering of material from natural field populations often takes days, since many of the plants are harvested in the mountainous regions. Cultivated fields make the harvest much easier. The bushes are often cut to the ground, as this facilitates future harvesting—the plant sprouts readily from the root base. Bushes previously harvested give better material for processing as the stems are softer and have higher leaf-to-stem ratios than older plants preserved by limited cuttings. By contrast, older bushes that are not regularly harvested give too much coarse material due to thicker stems. Ideally, the bushes are harvested every two to three years. *Cyclopia* bushes that have grown in an area subject to fire show more growth and have more flowers, thus giving good material for the making of tea. The collected shrubs are brought to the factories where they are first chopped by mechanised fodder cutters before curing. Chopping ensures the disruption of cellular integrity and facilitates fermentation, a process that turns the herb material dark brown. Leaves that are not adequately cut often retain a green to light brown colour.

There are currently two methods for honeybush tea fermentation: using a curing heap or using a baking oven. When large quantities of tea are produced, the common method of honeybush tea fermentation is the use of curing heaps. An oval-shaped heap of approximately four to five metres in diameter and two metres high is formed from 1.5 to

2.5 tons of the green honeybush material. The heap is packed firmly, covered with canvas bags, and left for three days to allow spontaneous heat generation and fermentation. Temperature build-up is quick. During the fermentation period, the material changes from green to dark brown and develops a sweet aroma. From the third day onwards, the heap is turned every twelve hours to ensure that the outer, cooler regions are mixed with the rest of the material; this also prevents oxygen deletion in the heap. The heap is inspected after three to five days of fermentation, depending on the species used. If a sweet, honey-like aroma is present and the material has a dark brown colour, the heap is spread out in a thin layer on canvas and allowed to dry in the sun. The tea normally takes one to two days to dry.

The use of a preheated oven gives a product of better and more consistent quality since more precise control over the temperature of the fermentation process is possible. Further, shorter fermentation periods (just twenty-four to thirty-six hours) are needed to obtain fully fermented tea. Baking ovens have been used for more than a hundred years. Originally, the material was preheated by scalding with hot water, and the drums used as ovens were preheated with hot coals before putting the herb material (in bags) into them. More sophisticated techniques are used today. As with the curing-heap preparation, after fermentation, the tea is dried in the sun. The final product is put through a rotating cylindrical sieve to remove all the pieces thicker than a matchstick. The finer tea material is used for making tea bags, while the coarser material is supplied in bulk for brewing as loose tea.

Health Effects

Honeybush tea is made as a simple herbal infusion. One of its early recognised benefits as a tea substitute is its lack of caffeine, which makes it especially suited for night-time consumption and for those who experience nervousness and want to avoid ordinary tea. As a result, it had a reputation as a calming beverage, though it may not have any specific sedative properties. It also has a low content of tannins, so it doesn't make a highly astringent tea, which can be a problem with some grades of black or green tea or when ordinary tea is steeped too long. The traditional use of the tea for treating cough may be explained, in part, by its content of pinitol, a modified sugar (a methyl group replaces hydrogen in one position of glucose; see diagram below) that is similar to inositol. Pinitol, named for its major source, pine trees, is also found in the leaves of several legume plants; it is an expectorant. Pinitol is also of interest for apparent blood–sugar lowering effects [3], as demonstrated in laboratory animal studies (it may increase the effects of insulin), and is being considered as a drug for diabetes. Honeybush also contains flavones, isoflavones, coumestans, luteolin, 4–hydroxycinnamic acid, polyphenols, and xanthones [4]. These ingredients serve as antioxidants and may help lower blood lipids [5]. The isoflavones and coumestans are classified as phytoestrogens, used in the treatment of menopausal symptoms [6], an application for which honeybush has recently been promoted. The flavones and isoflavones of honeybush are similar to those in soy, another leguminous plant, also used in treatment of menopausal symptoms. Luteolin is the primary yellow pigment of the flowers and has been used historically as a dye (most often obtained for this purpose from the plant called Dyer's Weld, *Reseda luteola*).

Consuming the Tea

Honeybush tea is sometimes consumed with milk and sugar as is done with black tea, but to appreciate the delicate sweet taste and flavour, no milk or sugar should be added. Adding a small amount of honey to the tea will bring out the honey–like flavour of the herb. Descriptions of the honeybush flavour include: hot apricot jam, floral, honey–like, and dried fruit mix. The overall impression is mild sweetness. The tea has the added advantage that the cold infusion can also be used as iced tea and it also blends well with fruit juices. The tea can be consumed daily, or it can be rotated with other beverage teas, such as rooibos and ordinary tea. For treatment of coughs, or as an aid in regulating blood sugar in diabetes, or helping reduce menopausal symptoms, the tea would be taken several times per day.

References

1. Smith M, et al. (compilers), Honeybush, 2001 Agribusiness in Sustainable Natural African Plant Products (ASNAPP), Dennesig, South Africa. van der Walt L. Cyclopia genistoides, 2000; National Botanical Institute, South Africa, http://www.plantzafrica.com/plantcd/cyclopiagenistoides.htm.
2. Bates S.H., Jones R.B., and Bailey C.J., Insulin-like effect of pinitol, *British Journal of Pharmacology*, 2000; 130 [8]: 1944-8.
3. Kamara BI, et al., Polyphenols from honeybush tea, *Journal Agricultural Food Chemistry*, 2003; 51[13]: 3874-9.
4. Marnewick JL, et al., Modulation of hepatic drug metabolizing enzymes and oxidative status by rooibos and honeybush, green and black (Camellia sinensis) teas in rats, *Journal Agricultural Food Chemistry* 2003; 51[27]: 8113-19.
5. Chiechi LM, Dietary phytoestrogens in the prevention of long-term postmenopausal diseases, *International Journal of Gynecology and Obstetrics*, 1999; 67[1]: 39-40.

Photo of San Tribe members gathering foods.

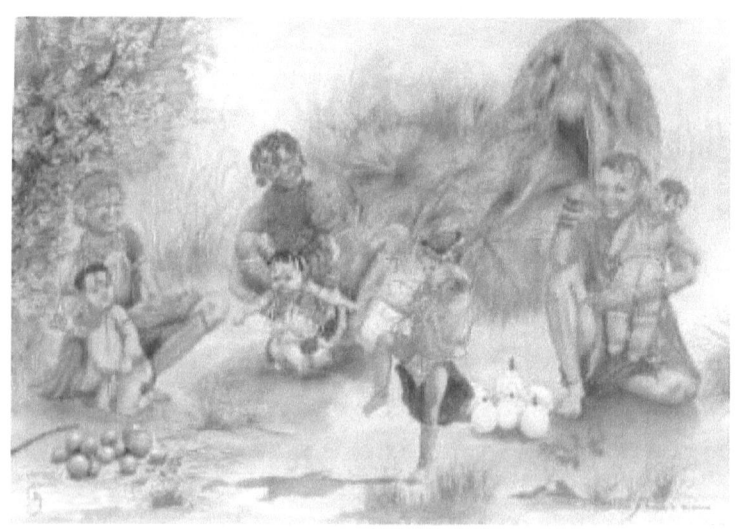

Rows of honeybush in cultivation project.

Painting of San Tribe members, with collected food, by Charlotte King.

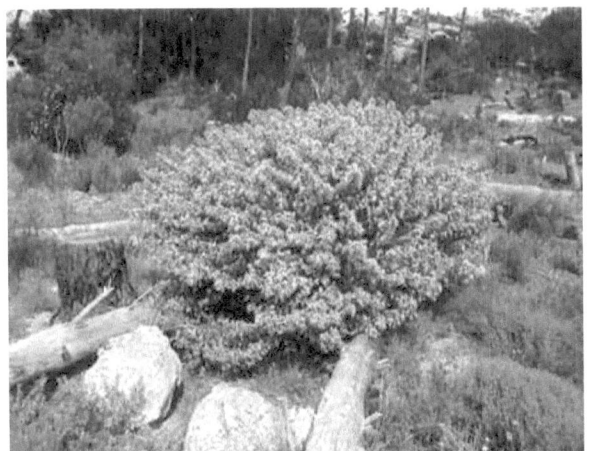

Full-grown honeybush in flower.

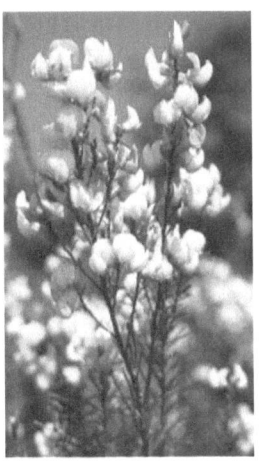

Flowers and fine
leaves of honeybush.

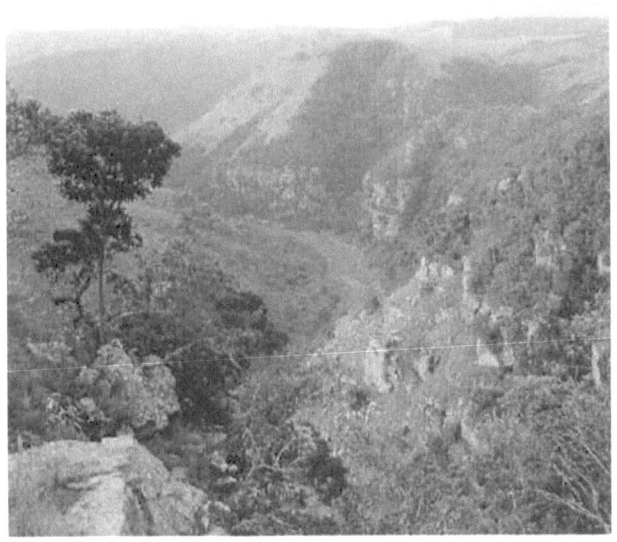

Panoramic view of Fynbos area showing difficult
mountain terrain where honeybush is collected.

11.16 The Nature of Ginseng

[11] Article Number 54, *The Journal of the American Botanical Council,* Dr Subhuti Dhanand, PhD, Director

Health Care: From Traditional to Medicine Research

The Preventive Therapy Using Ginseng Herbal Product(s) Key Chinese Medical References: chi, five viscera: hun, po, shen, spleen, and stomach Key medical terms: Diabetes, hypertension, heart failure, Hyperlipidemia, Key Chinnese herbs: ginseng, atractylodes, hoelen, liorice, codonopsis, platycodon, gynostemma, eleuthero, teen-chi, and Aerican gins Active constitutents: ginsenosides, Saponins, dammarane triteness, and oleanollic acid. Chinese formulas: Lizhong Wan, Guipi Tang, Buzhong Yigi Tang, and Shen Ling Ba.

The way in which ginseng is used depends on one's understanding of its indications, effects, and proper dosage. Unfortunately, the views expressed in today's popular literature about ginseng rarely reflect either the traditional use of the herb throughout Chinese history or the current consensus of scientific knowledge about ginseng and its active constituents. Further, research aimed at demonstrating the effectiveness of ginseng for several applications is of varying quality; the results can be misleading if study design and reporting are not critically analysed before accepting the conclusions offered by the authors. This article reviews both the traditional use and evolving modern interpretations of ginseng. In particular, the dosage of ginseng to be consumed is considered because of substantial differences between Asian and Western recommendations.

Ginseng in Traditional Chinese Literature

Ginseng was originally used as a herbal medicine in ancient China. There are written records about its properties dating back to about AD 100. Traditional Chinese medical literature is an important resource for understanding ginseng because virtually all proponents of ginseng refer to its long history of use as a reason to recommend it as a health product. Scientific investigations of ginseng are usually aimed at attempting to confirm the validity of the traditional uses. Thus, the historical basis for consuming ginseng is still relevant.

The basic framework of the traditional Chinese culture that is of such interest to the West coalesced around a group of ideas and practices that matured during the period 500 BC to about 200 BC Essential contributions included the following: development of a uniform writing system based on ideographic characters that are still recognised today; the philosophical systems derived from the trio of Confucianism, Taoism, and Buddhism; solidification of the organising principles of Yin and Yang and the Five Elements; the medical system incorporating acupuncture and herbal formulas; and institution of the Imperial government system. Then, during the Han Dynasty (203 BC to AD 220), these critical cultural developments were formalised, and the details were recorded for posterity. Any investigation of the origin of a fundamental Chinese concept, such as the meaning and value of ginseng, begins with a study of this period; the beginnings of ginseng use and the description of its effects can be traced by examining the written records.

The oldest medical document of China, buried around 170 BC, during the early Han Dynasty, was excavated from a tomb in 1973, at Mawangdui, the 'mounds of the horse emperor,' near Changsha, the capital of Hunan Province in central China. This record suggests that the traditional Chinese medical system was still forming at that time, and it had not yet reached the relatively consistent set of theories and rules that emerged soon after. For example, the system of meridians, the channels of the human body that became a central component of the acupuncture system, was different at this time. A scroll listing herb formulas found at the burial site, which has been dubbed *Wushier Bingfang* (Prescriptions for fifty-two Diseases), reveals that the early Chinese herb formulas usually employed two to three ingredients, compared to the more complex formulas used later, typically containing from six to fifteen herbs. Apparently, ginseng is not included in these early formulas. [1] The text that serves as the key source book for all of Chinese medicine, the one to which every physician refers for wise sayings of unquestionable authority, is the *Huangdi Neijing* (*Yellow Emperor's Classic of Medicine*, [2]. Based on the writing style and references to various cultural matters, this book was probably written between 100 BC and 100 AD. It describes the cause and development of diseases and specifies some acupuncture therapies for them. Herbs are barely mentioned, and only in a general way, without reference to specific herbs. Ginseng, despite its fame in years to come, is not mentioned.

The first book that serves as a compendium of herbal knowledge for the Chinese tradition is the *Shennong Bencao Jing* (*Classic Herbal of Shennong*) written around 100 AD. Shennong was a mythological figure, the divine farmer, who was said to have tasted seventy different herbs each day, determining which ones were useful for humans. Of the thousands of herbs he tasted, 360 were deemed suitable: not too poisonous, but having a nature and taste that would impart medicinal effectiveness. These were recorded in this text, a translation of which is now available [3]. This classic includes the first written record of ginseng as a medicinal agent. The use of ginseng in China, and, indeed, throughout Asia, is based largely on the description in this book, one that has been passed on from generation to generation since that time. The traditional Chinese medical system is highly conservative: rather than seeking out innovations, physicians and scholars constantly strive to stay true to the original. Thus, it is essential to know the classical understanding of ginseng to grasp its meaning in subsequent centuries.

Traditional Chinese Medicine Concepts

Each herb in the *Shennong Bencao Jing* is described by only a few sentences that, despite their brevity, convey much to the traditional physicians. In order to understand the section on ginseng, one must be familiar with the two basic descriptive categories for herbs in traditional Chinese medicine—*nature and taste*. According to classical theory, the *nature* (Chinese: *xing*) of a herb depicts not only what the herb is like inherently but also how it will interact with other herbs in a formula and the effect it will have on those who consume it. The herb's nature is classified either as cold, cool, neutral, warm, or hot. In general, warm or hot natured herbs can be used to treat disease conditions that are characterised as being cold (e.g. feeling chilled, aversion to cold environment, watery discharge, pain alleviated by warmth and pressure, and desire for warm drinks). Herbs that are cool or cold in nature can be used to treat disease conditions that are characterised as being hot (e.g. feeling feverish, aversion to hot environment, thick discharge, pain alleviated by cold and worsened by touch, and desire for cold drinks). Neutral herbs can be used for any disease condition. Because of their mild nature, both warm and cool herbs can be used with considerable flexibility and might be incorporated into treatments for either hot or cold type of diseases; by contrast, the more extreme-natured herbs, classified as hot or cold, have to be used with some caution.

The taste (*wei*) of a herb represents how the herb was formed from the basic elements of the universe, what therapeutic properties it has, and what organs it will affect. There are five basic tastes: sweet, acrid (also called pungent or spicy), bitter, sour, and salty. A herb can be described as bland (rather tasteless), which represents an added sixth category. The ancient Chinese concept of the internal anatomy involved five fundamental viscera: spleen, lung, heart, liver, and kidney—each one associated with, and particularly influenced by, one of the five tastes. The connections that were made in ancient times between the tastes and organs can be explained by simple observations; for example, the kidney yields the salty-tasting urine and is therefore associated with the salty taste. As an example of the relationship between taste and effects, sweet (pleasant tasting) herbs and foods are said to enhance the function of the 'spleen' (which refers not to the anatomical spleen but to an organ system that mainly comprises the digestive functions) and to nourish the body.

The *Shennong Bencao Jing* says this about ginseng [3]:

> Ginseng [*renshen*] is sweet and a little cold. It mainly supplements the five viscera. It quiets the essence spirit, settles the ethereal and corporeal souls, checks fright palpitations, eliminates evil qi, brightens the eyes, opens the heart, and sharpens the wits. Protracted taking may make the body light and prolong life. Its other name is *renxian*. Yet another name is *guigai*. It grows in mountains and valleys.

To appreciate fully the ancient description of ginseng, here is an elaboration of the statements made (for information about the name of the herb, see the article: 'The meaning of shen in *renshen*'):

• *Ginseng is sweet*: Anyone who tastes a ginseng root today will find it quite bitter. The freshly picked root is sweeter (has a somewhat pleasant taste compared to many other herbs), but, more importantly, the designation of the root as sweet is partly based on the idea that sweet is the underlying inherent taste within the herb that reflects its actions. Like other sweet herbs, it is believed that ginseng will supplement the spleen, calm irritation, and nourish the body. Later Chinese texts often mention the bitter taste as well.

- *A little cold*: The action of the herb is relatively mild, in contrast to a cold herb, but its nature is still like that of a cold herb—able to alleviate heat syndromes. The combination of sweet and cold together has the effect of calming nervous agitation: the sweetness alleviates irritation, and the coldness calms the internal fire that agitates the human spirit.
- *Supplements the five viscera*: Ginseng does something more than most of the sweet herbs; it benefits not only the spleen but also the other four systems of the body: liver, kidney, heart, and lung. One implication is that ginseng greatly improves the ability of the spleen to draw nutrients out of food and distribute them to the other organs. It serves as a nutritive aid but does not provide nutrients.
- *Quiets the essence spirit*: The essence spirit can be broadly interpreted as referring to the mind. Thus, ginseng quiets the mind. By taking ginseng, excessive mental chattering calms down.
- *Settles the ethereal and corporeal souls*: The ethereal soul (*hun*) and corporeal soul (*po*) refer to fundamental forces within the body. The ethereal soul is believed to reside in the liver and to be responsible for dreams; the unsettled *hun* causes one to have disturbing dreams, even nightmares. The corporeal soul is said to reside in the lungs and to be responsible for maintaining the integrity of the physical body. Persons who develop lifelong degenerative diseases are said to suffer from scattering of the corporeal soul, often the result of being frightened. It could be said that ginseng calms the distressed mind while strengthening the body.
- *Checks fright palpitations*: When a person is frightened, he or she experiences an irregular heartbeat and palpitations. Anxiety attacks and panic attacks correspond roughly to fright palpitations. Ginseng helps calm the heart (the resting place of the spirit) so that it does not overly react to external stimuli nor to internal mental worries—equanimity is restored.
- *Eliminates evil chi*: Evil chi refers to influences from the environment that cause diseases. Herbs that nourish the viscera, like

ginseng, are usually not attributed the ability to expel the evil that is causing disease; more often, such herbs are said to protect the body from evil chi (evil can't get into the strong and well-nourished body to cause disease) or to help the body recover its strength once the evil has been eliminated. Ginseng can be taken when a disease is present to help cure it by eliminating the evil chi. Some later authorities disagreed with this view, suggesting that ginseng had only tonic properties and should not be taken while evil chi was still present, for fear of enticing the evil to stay within the body.

- *Brightens the eyes, opens the heart, and sharpens the wits*: The eyes are the windows to the mind; the heart is the residence of the mind, and the wits are the expression of the mind. This section says that by taking ginseng, one's mind will not become dull. If the heart becomes closed, if the mind becomes overwhelmed with thoughts, if the spirit is clouded and the eyes, therefore, dim, then a person's fundamental nature will be prevented from attaining its ultimate expression. The person will be timid, unhappy, even depressed. When the heart opens and the mind quiets, the true nature will be expressed, and the person will display sure purpose, will, and courage, and be able to accomplish great things.

- *Protracted taking may make the body light and prolong life*: This phrase is included in reference to the intensive efforts undertaken by Taoists pursuing immortality during the Han Dynasty period. They believed that one could shed the physical body and float into the heavens as an immortal being. Most of this transformative (alchemical) process was accomplished with minerals, such as cinnabar (mercury sulphide), which slowly poisoned the Taoists' bodies due to prolonged exposure. One consequence was that they lost weight: at the time, their shrinking flesh was taken not as an indication of poisoning but as a sign that they were shedding their earthly body to leave only the heavenly body. This section does not indicate that ginseng can be used as a weight-loss herb for the obese, nor does it even suggest that one can live longer on this earth by taking the herb regularly; it refers specifically to the Taoist concept of transformation to an ethereal immortal.

Medicinal Use of Ginseng in Ancient Chinese Medicine

The first book that describes with some details the actual medical applications of herbs is the *Shanghan Lun* (*Treatise on Treatment of Diseases Induced by Cold*). *Shanghan* is the name of a disease category depicted in the *Yellow Emperor's Classic*, involving a serious illness initiated by cold evils and progressing, sometimes rapidly, from the exterior of the body (skin and muscles) to the interior (viscera). This text, written at the end of the Han Dynasty, is still studied carefully today by all who practise traditional Chinese medicine. Chinese medical scholars have cautioned physicians repeatedly to study and pay attention to the formulas mentioned in this text and to avoid straying too far from the principles described therein. There are at least three English translations currently available, of which the one by Hsu and Peacher [4] is recommended because of their attempts to stay true to the original by using an old version of the text for translation: a reprint of one first published in 1060, during the Song Dynasty (960-1279). At that time, the *Shanghan Lun* was divided into two books, the first carrying the original title, and the second given a separate title: *Jingui Yaolue*, or *Prescriptions of the Golden Cabinet*, which Hsu has also translated [5].

The *Shanghan Lun* presents 107 formulas that had been collected by the physician Zhang Zhongjing. Ginseng is an ingredient in twenty-one of the formulas, clearly being an important herb. One of the representative formulas containing ginseng is called *Lizhong Wan*, or the Pill to Rectify the Centre. Here, 'the centre' refers to the spleen system, and what is being rectified is its disturbance, marked by upper abdominal discomfort and digestive system disorders such as loss of appetite, nausea, burping, vomiting, or diarrhoea. As indicated above, the 'spleen' in traditional Chinese medicine refers, in part, to the digestive tract, *not* the specific anatomical organ called the spleen in Western medicine. In this text, the cause of the disease is thought to be excessive cold (a type of evil chi) in the environment. After entering the body, if the evil chi has not been dispelled, it penetrates to the interior and damages the function of the spleen. The formula is said to drive out this debilitating cold influence.

The formula contains equal parts of four herbs: ginseng, ginger, licorice, and atractylodes. The first three herbs are familiar to most people with even a small knowledge of Chinese herbs; atractylodes is commonly used in China for treating digestive system disorders. The herbs are prepared as a pill (*wan*). The intended effect of taking the formula is to feel warmth in the abdomen: this effect comes mainly from the ginger. If that warmth is not felt, one can increase the dosage from 1 to 2 pills to 3 to 4 pills. Alternatively, the herbs can be decocted (put in water that is then boiled). The entire batch of tea is taken in one day.

The question of how much ginseng to take in order to gain its purported beneficial effects is one that is important to the modern situation where recommendations vary widely. Estimates of ginseng dosage in its traditional applications can be derived from the ancient texts, such as the *Shanghan Lun*. The instructions for preparing *Lizhong Wan* are as follows: Grind the herbs to powder; mix them with honey, and then form pills the size of an egg yolk. Such pills are quite large, typically weighing about 9 g, of which about 6 g comes from the herbs and 3 g from honey. They cannot be swallowed whole but are either chewed up or added to hot water, dissolved, and consumed as a tea. This same type of pill is produced today by the millions at Chinese patent medicine factories, such as Beijing's Tong Ren Tang, founded in 1669 (during the Qing Dynasty), one of the largest of the hundreds of such factories in modern China. The pill, as described above, has about 1.5 g of ginseng, and the daily dose ranges from 1 to 4 pills or 1.5 to 6.0 g of ginseng. For other ginseng-containing formulas in the *Shanghan Lun* that are made in decoction rather than pill form, the ginseng dosage is about 1.3-3.9 g. Thus, the range of daily ginseng doses recommended was from as little as 1.3 g for a single dose, to as much as 6.0 g for a double dose (as might be needed in some cases).

The ginseng in use at this time (end of the Han Dynasty), and for centuries afterwards (to the end of Ming Dynasty, 1644), was all wild ginseng. Ginseng hunters would search through the forests of north-eastern China to find the plants, carefully remove them from the soil, dry them, and bring them to the herbalists who, for the most part, were working further south. Modern proponents of ginseng have argued that wild ginseng is much more potent than the cultivated type. If this is the case (and it has not been confirmed), then the dosage of cultivated ginseng to be used today, in a similar application to the ancient uses, might be even higher than that described above for the wild-harvested roots.

Unfortunately, wild ginseng plants do not flourish under pressure of collection because of limited seed germination and slow maturation. As a result, the supplies of ginseng in China gradually receded to the regions that were increasingly inaccessible in the far north-eastern mountains. The ability of herbalists to obtain ginseng declined, and the cost increased, making it available only to those who were wealthy. Despite its increasing rarity, ginseng was still mentioned in the Chinese medical literature and included in formulas to treat various ailments, especially those of the digestive system. Perhaps one of the most famous of all the ginseng-containing formulas (at least, of those in which ginseng is a primary ingredient) was recorded in an Imperial herb formula guide of the Song Dynasty (960-1279). The formula, called *Si Junzi Tang*, or the Four Gentleman Decoction (see *What's in a name? The four gentlemen decoction*), was recorded in the *Taiping Huimin Hejiju Fang* (*Formulary of the People's Benevolent Pharmacy of the Taiping Era, 1110*). This text described formulas made at the imperial pharmacy. It is the source of many of the formulas used today, especially the traditional formulas manufactured in Chinese patent medicine factories as pills. *Si Junzi Tang* is almost the same as *Lizhong Wan*. There is substitution of one herb: ginger is deleted and replaced by the fungus called *fuling* (common name: hoelen or poria). Unlike *Lizhong Wan*, which is intended to warm up the abdomen with the spicy, warming herb ginger, *Si Junzi Tang* is supposed to help assure that the water ingested, both as a beverage and as the moist part of food, is extracted and circulated (failure to do so leads to loose stool or diarrhoea). Hoelen is a bland-tasting and neutral herb that is reputed to soak up and redistribute moisture.

This formula is reported in every modern text on traditional Chinese herbal formulas; it is usually the first one listed in the section devoted to chi tonic formulas. A typical dosage pattern for *Si Junzi Tang* is [6] as below:

Ginseng	10 g
Atractylodes	9 g
Hoelen	9 g
Licorice (baked)	6 g

The dosage of ginseng in this formula, as well as the dosage of the other ingredients, is consistent with the amounts used in modern Chinese practice. In some other Chinese texts, as summarised in *Chinese Herbal Medicine Formulas and Strategies* [7], the dosage of the herbs for this particular formula is somewhat lower, with ginseng administered at 3-9 g. There are two other famous prescriptions with ginseng that deserve special mention. These were also formulated during the Song Dynasty: *Buzhong Yiqi Tang* (Decoction for Tonifying the Centre and Regulating the Qi, from a book published in 1249) and *Guipi Tang* (Decoction for Restoring the Spleen, from a book published in 1253). Both prescriptions are used to aid the digestive functions. The former is usually selected for those who have been debilitated by prolonged illness, especially when the illness has come about from poor habits: eating irregularly, working too hard without enough rest, and anxiously worrying. The latter is mainly used for those who suffer from mental agitation, anxiety, and insomnia as a syndrome secondary to deficiency of the spleen (*guipi* = restore the spleen). When prepared as a decoction, the ginseng dosage in the former is 9–12 g and, in the latter, 3–6 g [7].

In sum, ginseng was historically given mainly for syndromes that involved digestive system weakness, and the dosage of ginseng ranged from about 3–9 g in most instances, with low dose administration of about 1.3 g per time and high dose administration of up to 12 g per day. The modern Chinese materia medicas are in agreement with these amounts of ginseng, namely a recommended daily dose of 3–9 g for a one-day dose for standard applications [16, 30]. The duration of using ginseng, alone or in formulas, was not specified in the early texts. In some instances, it was understood that only one or two doses would be enough to change the course of a disease and help the patient onto the path to recovery. In other situations, it was understood that ginseng would be taken for many days to change a persistent pattern of imbalance. Due to the rarity and high cost of ginseng, it was usually used only so long as deemed necessary. The Taoists—some of whom took ginseng daily in an attempt to become an immortal—collected their own herbs to pursue their goals, spending much of their time wandering the mountains in search of ginseng and other important tonics.

Updating the Concept of Ginseng

The first known treatise devoted specifically to ginseng was written during the sixteenth century (Ming Dynasty). Excerpts of it appeared in a book that remained essential to Chinese herbalism for the next four centuries and even today: *Bencao Gangmu* (*Great Compendium of Herbs*). The author of *Bencao Gangmu*, Li Shizhen, is revered to this day for his efforts to organise herbal knowledge and sort through the morass of misinformation (see *Li Shizhen: Scholar worthy of emulation*).

The ginseng treatise had been written by his father, Li Yenwen, and the following part was published in the *Bencao Gangmu*, which was published in 1596. [24]:

> Used fresh, ginseng displays a cool nature. When it is used after preparation [steamed, red ginseng], its nature is warm. The slight sweet taste strengthens the yang; the somewhat bitter taste strengthens the yin. Nature [*xing*] controls the genesis of things: their origin is in heaven; tastes control the completion of things; their origin is in the earth. Nature and taste, genesis and completion are realizations of yin and yang. The cool nature of fresh ginseng expresses the yang influence of spring, namely, of genesis and development. This is the yang of heaven. It has the nature of rising. Sweet is a taste that has been formed through transformation of moisture and earth. These are the yang influences of earth. They have the nature of floating. The somewhat bitter taste has been formed through reciprocal interaction of fire and earth. These are the yin influences of earth. They have the nature of descending in the body.

Taste and nature are both equally weak in ginseng. Whatever has a weak nature descends in the body when fresh, and rises when prepared. Whatever has a weak taste rises in the body when fresh and descends when prepared. In case of illness in which the earth [spleen] shows a depletion and the fire [heart] shows vigor, the weak cool nature of fresh ginseng is suited to diminish the blazing of the fire and to replenishthe earth. This could be called a pure use of ginseng's nature.

In the case of illness characterised by depletion in the earth and weakness in the lung, the sweet taste and warm nature of prepared ginseng is suited to replenish the earth and to generate the metal [associated with lung]. This could be called a pure use of ginseng's taste . . .

One can take from this description that ginseng, whether 'fresh' (indicating that it is not processed i.e. dried, white ginseng that is cool in nature) or prepared (i.e. steamed ginseng, which turns red in colour and is warm in nature), has a mild quality and effect: both its nature and taste are weak. The author is illustrating that ginseng can both float and sink in the body (its taste working in one direction and its nature in the other), meaning that it can be used in treating ailments affecting both the upper and lower body. Today, some Western herbalists depict ginseng differently: as being strongly stimulating and overly heating, a view that is quite contrary to the traditional one, even for the processed (red) ginseng, described by traditional doctors as being only warm in nature. In fact, much of the red ginseng from China, such as Jilin (Kirin) ginseng, is described in China as having a nature that is neutral reflecting its mildness. Dr Shiu-ying Hu translated forty-two recipes with ginseng from Li Shizhen's compendium [60]. They are used for conditions such as having poor digestion, 'stomach trouble,' nausea, or vomiting; being thirsty all the time; feverish diseases with excessive sweating, cough, or laryngitis; bleeding disorders, including internal haemorrhage, nosebleeding, blood in the urine, and post-partum bleeding; and pregnancy disorders. Most of these disorders can be categorised as stomach and spleen problems and heat syndromes. Typical daily doses for these Ming Dynasty formulas are 8–15 g of ginseng in decoction or 6 g in powder form made into pills.

Ginseng Misuse and Ginseng Substitutes

Declining wild resources of ginseng eventually led to considerable distortions in concepts about the nature of ginseng and how it could be used. Ginseng sellers exaggerated the benefits of the herb to justify the increasing price. During the Qing Dynasty (1644–1911), ginseng was known as the herb that could restore the dying to health and restore the dead to life. Wealthy families would squander their life's savings on ginseng roots to save a dying family member. When ginseng failed to accomplish its claimed revival and the person died, ginseng was sometimes blamed for the death. Hence, ginseng gained a reputation as a highly dangerous herb—one that could save lives or snuff them out. All depended on using it correctly, so it was said that a misdiagnosis and inappropriate prescription for these terminally ill patients would be quickly fatal. The underlying concept, including both the versatility of ginseng and an allusion to dire consequences, was described by Xu Dachun [8] in his brief essay on ginseng (1757, during the Qing Dynasty) as follows:

> Since ginseng is a substance rich in influences [qi] and full
> of vigor, it is able to supplement depletion and stop the loss
> of proper influences, no matter whether a patient's illness is

related to wind, cold, summer-heat, dampness, phlegm, fire, or some binding of influences within the body. An application of ginseng is always appropriate when the evil influences that caused a patient's illness have left the body, but the proper influences are still weak; or when only a little of the evil influences remain, but the proper influences are exhausted; or when evil influences have penetrated deeply into the body and proper influences are themselves too weak to drive off the evil influences.

In order to support the elimination of evil influences by means of herbs, one must give the patient ginseng together with other herbs that are capable of driving off the evil influences. However, before one applies ginseng, one should examine whether the disorder to be treated is minor or serious [take into account the balance between the proper and evil influences], and only if this is taken into account will the effect of rescue from danger or of strengthening that which is already bent [damaged] appear as a matter of course. If one fails to investigate, though, whether evil influences are present or not, and whether the person suffers from depletion or repletion, and if one administers only warm or hot substances of a purely supplementing nature [as is common practice today due to current medical theories], then one will merely supplement the evil influences and help them settle down. In minor cases, the evil influences will, as a result of such mistaken therapy, never leave the body again. In serious cases, death is inevitable.

In other words, if the pathogenic influence has not been removed or at least tamed, one must combine ginseng with other herbs that have the effect of dispelling the evil, but not with other herbs that have a tonifying nature; otherwise, the disease can become permanent or even cause death. A common saying at that time was translated as: 'Nourishing the body with tonics when a pathogen is present is like inviting a robber into a comfortable home; he would gladly enter and not leave, taking time to steal all its valuables.' As a result of the new view of ginseng as a remedy to rescue those close to death with a potential for harm if misprescribed, Zhang Lu, a physician of the Qing Dynasty, commented: 'Some people look upon ginseng as poison or a sword [two-edged, able to provide help, but also to destroy], and stubbornly refuse to use it.' [9]

An example of this mixed thinking about ginseng was relayed by physician Cheng Maoxian at the beginning of the Qing Dynasty period. He described in detail the treatment of a very difficult case, a sixty-three-year-old woman suffering from a disease that came on suddenly and led to virtual inability to swallow; everyone was sure that she would soon die. Cheng explained his next therapeutic steps [45] as under:

> Her chest still was not free, so next I used *Shen Ling Bai Zhu San* [Ginseng and Atractylodes Combination]. The lady knew that I was using ginseng and feared that her chest would not ease but be stopped up from excessive supporting action. For this reason, over several days I added one and one-half *qian* [4.5 grams] of ginseng without letting her know. After these doses, her chest was opened and her stagnation downward abated. One day, the lady said to her son Shunian, 'In the last few days, my gullet has felt open; don't use ginseng any more.' Shunian murmured his assent but together with my unworthy self, he secretly added ginseng without ill effects for several days . . . Though the disorder was grave, she was restored to life. Half the merit was Shunian's, for the two reasons that he was a filial and friendly gentleman. First, he did not spare the ginseng; and second, he gave me complete charge. Had he looked for overnight success, or feared to use ginseng and *huangqi* [astragalus root (*Astragalus mongholicus* Bunge, Fabaceae), another tonic herb with action similar to ginseng], or, taking alarm, had changed doctors, the lady, his mother, could scarcely have preserved her life.

> Ginseng and atractylodes combination is an expanded version of *Si Junzi Tang* described previously.

> This story relays quite well the frustration that some doctors felt in the growing myths about the dangers of ginseng.

It was during this time period that ginseng gained a reputation for being excessively supplementing, and, by virtue of being linked with other supplementing herbs that were classified as warming, it also gained a reputation by some as a warming herb. A herbal published in 1757 [52] described ginseng as warm in nature and included the comment that 'the effects of ginseng are superior to all other drugs.'

An explanation of Cheng Maoxian's application of ginseng in the above case is provided by the description of ginseng in this herbal: 'It has a great ability to supplement the original qi in the lung. It drains internal fire and eliminates heat causing, in the chest, a feeling of uneasiness. It generates body fluids and quenches the thirst.' Here, it is attributed a cooling property—draining fire and eliminating heat. Stories about the rarity of ginseng during the nineteenth century were relayed by Western visitors, and several of their commentaries are told by Pamela Dixon in her book *Ginseng* [53]. The Dao Guan Emperor (1821–51) recognised that ginseng was on the verge of extinction and issued an imperial decree that forbade its collection. A report in the *Peking Gazette* of 1884 stated that twenty ginseng roots—a large quantity at that time—were sent to the Guan Xu Emperor (the last Chinese emperor to serve a full life in office).

The primary response to the rapidly diminishing supplies of ginseng was for herb collectors to flood the market with substitutes. The main one selected as a match for ginseng was codonopsis (*Codonopsis pilosula*), a herb botanically unrelated to ginseng, which, nonetheless, was said to be about the same in effects—only safer, cheaper, and abundant. Although the root just barely resembles the ginseng root, by this time in China's history virtually no one knew what ginseng looked like. So merchants could call it 'ginseng.' The Chinese name for the herb, *dangshen*, indicated that it was ginseng from the Shandang region (shen is the key term to describe ginseng or a ginseng-like herb); Shandang had been the principal source for the preferred quality *Panax ginseng*, a plant hunted to extinction in that area centuries ago. Codonopsis hadn't appeared in any of the herbals prior to the Qing Dynasty, but had received brief mention in the *Bencao Gangmu*. Some doctors of the Qing Dynasty regarded *dangshen* as the correct ginseng to use, being superior to *renshen* (ginseng) for most applications [22]. Codonopsis became an official substitute for ginseng, widely used as such today, but the Chinese market has had numerous other substitutes as well. Table 1 lists herbs that are used as substitutes for ginseng, according to recent texts [25, 29].

Table 1: Herbs used as substitutes for ginseng in traditional Chinese medicine

Botanical Name	Family	Comments
Vigna vexillata	Fabaceae (Leguminosae)	Steamed or boiled root of this type of cowpea is used in the same manner as red ginseng
Talinum paniculatum	Portulacaceae	*Turenshen* (local ginseng): Peeled and soaked in boiling water, it appears similar to red ginseng.
Physochlaina infundibularis	Solanaceae	*Huashanshen* (flower mountain ginseng) or *reshen* (warm ginseng): Henbane (*Hyoscyamus niger*) of the same plant family is also used as warm ginseng.
Pterocypsela indica (aka *Lactuca indica*)	Asteraceae (Compositae)	Taste of the root of this type of lettuce is somewhat like ginseng.
Phytolacca acinosa	Phytolaccaceae	*Shanglu*: American poke root is a close relative to this.
Mirabilis jalapa	Nyctaginaceae	*Zimoli*: It is also native to the American tropics.
Platycodon grandiflorum	Campanulaceae	*Jiegeng*: The active constituents of platycodon are similar to those found in ginseng (saponins). *Campanumoea javanica* is from the same family and used similarly.
Adenophora triphylla	Campanulaceae	*Nanshashen* (southern sand ginseng) and several other species of *Adenophora* are also used as ginseng substitutes.
Rumex madaio	Polygonaceae	The root appears somewhat like red ginseng; *Rumex hymenosepalus* has been sold improperly as 'American red ginseng.'

Several of the ginseng substitutes have a confirmed close relationship with ginseng in terms of flowering plant evolution [34]. They may contain similarly structured active components and/or present an appearance that is reminiscent of ginseng. A few of them are potentially toxic (e.g. the plants of the families Solanaceae and Phytolaccaceae), though their preparation in Chinese formulas has not been associated with any toxicity problems evident to Chinese herbalists. It is possible that some of the complaints about the dangers of ginseng raised during the Qing Dynasty arose from incidents where certain ginseng substitutes were improperly used. An illustration of this problem was presented in humorous light in the 1994 Jackie Chan film, *Drunken Master 2,*: A highly valuable ginseng root becomes lost and is hastily replaced by the root of a garden plant that nearly causes death of the patient who doesn't know what a real ginseng root looks like.

The broad range of substitution options for ginseng helps illustrate the fact that the actions of *Panax ginseng* were not seen as unique. Rather, the therapeutic effects could be attained, to some extent, from other plants. In a few cases, the active constituents of the substitute herbs are similar. For example, modern investigations reveal that the saponin components of platycodon have a structure very similar to that of the ginsenosides. By such analysis of active constituents, it was found that a plant that had only been used as a folk remedy in China, *jiaogulan (Gynostemma pentaphylla)*, contains some of the same saponins as those found in ginseng and recently has been adopted as an inexpensive ginseng substitute. Another modern ginseng substitute is *Eleutherococcus senticosus*, known as eleuthero ginseng or Siberian ginseng. Its original Chinese name, *ciwujia* (spiny *wujia*) has been updated to reflect its use as a ginseng substitute: *wujiashen* (ginseng-like *wujia*). Today, virtually all Chinese medical texts and journal articles—reflecting actual practice in Chinese clinics—describe herbal formulas with codonopsis where ginseng would formerly have been indicated as the appropriate herb. Codonopsis contains none of the active components of ginseng.

Western View of Ginseng

Among the first Westerners to attempt to penetrate the veil of Chinese herbal medicine were the British physicians F. Porter Smith and G.A. Stuart, working in China at the end of the nineteenth century and into the early twentieth century, as the Qing Dynasty came to an end. They wrote [10] as follows:

> Ginseng, with the Chinese, is the medicine *par excellence*, the *dernier resort* [last recourse] when all other drugs fail, reserved for the use of the Emperor and his household, and conferred by Imperial favor upon high and useful officials whenever they have a serious breakdown that does not yield to ordinary treatment, and which threatens to put a period to their lives

and usefulness . . . The ordinary ginseng of the markets has been studied and has not been found to possess any important medicinal properties. But the Chinese describe cases in which the sick have been practically in *articulo mortis*, when upon the administration of ginseng they were sufficiently restored to transact final items of business . . . It is prescribed in nearly every kind of disease of a severe character, with few exceptions, but with many reservations as to the stage of the disease in which it may be administered with the greatest benefit and safety. Much of the ginseng on the market consists of Campanulaceous roots [i.e. codonopsis, adenophora, platycodon], substituted for those of the Araliaceous *Panax*. The former roots, while in a general way resembling those of the true ginseng, are more or less hard and woody, and free from worms, while the latter is succulent and very liable to attack by insects.

The main use of ginseng, depicted here, was for those who were severely ill, not just those who suffered from digestive system disturbance. The ginseng used by the emperors and their households was the wild Manchurian ginseng; the market ginseng consisted mainly of cultivated roots (as used today) and substitute roots of codonopsis or other herbs. All the market samples were declared to be virtually worthless from a medicinal point of view, an opinion held by some researchers and physicians today with regard to ginseng itself. The statement by Smith and Stuart—about failing to find any important medicinal qualities in ginseng-refers to the initial investigations by the scientific method of this highly acclaimed herb. Ginseng seemed to hold great promise, based on the extravagant Chinese claims, yet little turned up when it was studied. Often, the effects reported by one researcher contradicted those of the next, and a variety of explanations were devised to explain the results. As described in the book *Korean Ginseng* [21]: 'Every investigator had his own opinion about the action of ginseng.' Even later, this concern lingered. In a report at the 1978 Ginseng Symposium in Korea, Prof. E. J. Staba of the University of Minnesota College of Pharmacy said, 'The pharmacological effects reported for ginseng and its extracts are varied and controversial [55].'

While some people simply dismissed the ginseng claims as the result of myths and superstitions, others decided to track down a basis for the reverence for ginseng.

11.17 Chemical Constituents in Ginseng

As a first step in separating the claims about ginseng from what it could actually do (from the modern scientific perspective) its active ingredients were sought. A history of these efforts was reviewed by Joseph Hou in an article and with an overview in his book: *Ginseng: The Myth and the Truth* [22]. Ginseng was found to contain none of the potent alkaloids characteristic of many plants that were being relied upon to generate new drugs. Instead, the root is comprised mainly of carbohydrates: starches, cellulose, and free sugars (the sucrose content in fresh ginseng is about 25 per cent, explaining the sweet taste, and the total sugar and starch content is over 60 per cent), the sort of things found in a carrot root [21]. In fact, like carrots, ginseng can be used fresh as a health food or vegetable [46]. Panaxynol, one of the acetylenic compounds found in ginseng, is identical to carotatoxin isolated from carrots. A small amount, less than 5 per cent of the tap roots, of a saponin (sugar bound to a triterpene molecule) was discovered in the ginseng roots. This component was shown to have some pharmacological activity. Saponins and their related triterpenes (e.g. oleanolic acid, a common component of plant oils) are found in numerous herbs and also in some food plants (e.g. soybeans, alfalfa sprouts, olives, and pumpkins). For several decades, efforts have been made to carefully isolate and identify each of the ginseng saponins, which are the main bitter components of ginseng. These saponins, formerly called panaxosides, are now called ginsenosides; there are several variants, labelled R_a, R_b, R_c and so on, and then subsets of each labelled 1, 2, 3. As of 1999, it was reported that thirty-four ginsenosides have been identified in *Panax ginseng* roots [47]; the dominant saponins in these roots are of the R_b series and are of the dammarane type. Most of the other saponins are present in miniscule amounts (the next largest group, the R_g series, also of the dammarane group, are present at about one-third the quantity of the R_b series in *Panax ginseng*; 64).

The ginsenosides are concentrated primarily in the root's cortical tissues (outer layers) compared to the quantities found in the interior portions. According to one Chinese report, the ginsenoside content of the root hairs (fibrous lateral roots which are mainly cortical type material) was 9.7 per cent, while that in the thicker, lateral roots was 6.4 per cent and that in the main tap root (which is the portion usually traded on the market, having little cortical material) was only 3.3 per cent [17]. An earlier European report gave the figures as 5-7 per cent, 2-4 per cent, and 0.7-1.7 per cent for these ginseng root parts, respectively [35].

European evaluations of ginsenosides in ginseng samples frequently generate lower figures for ginsenoside levels than Asian studies. According to Chinese studies, the range of values for total ginsenosides for *Panax ginseng* roots (taproots) is 2.2-5.5 per cent, with 4 per cent being a typical amount mentioned in the literature [11, 15]. European literature mentions 1.5 per cent and 2.0 per cent ginsenosides as a minimum level to be expected for the roots (Swiss and French Pharmacopoeias, respectively), with some studies revealing a range of levels from 0.7 to 3.0 per cent [59]. It is unclear whether the divergence in reported levels of ginsenosides between Asian investigators and European investigators is due to different selections of root material for testing, different handling of the roots prior to testing, or different testing methodology and interpretation. One possibility is that Asian researchers include a broader range of ginsenoside compounds, including some bound forms such as malonyl-ginsenosides, in their tallies. A discussion of this significant variability in reporting does not appear in the published reviews of ginseng. Higher levels of ginsenosides than found in *Panax ginseng* (with a differing mix of individual subtypes) are reported for American ginseng (*Panax quinquefolius*), at 6.2-7.4 per cent, and for Tienchi ginseng (*san qi*) of southern China (*Panax pseudoginseng*), at 3-8 per cent ginsenosides, with some reported levels of 12 per cent. In a study of ginsenosides in ginseng roots found on the Taiwanese market [40], it was reported that the highest content of ginsenosides was found in *Panax pseudoginseng*, followed, in order, by *P. quinquefolius*, *P. ginseng* root hair, and then red and white *P. ginseng* roots (tap roots, as commonly sold in stores).

Studies of ginseng processing, in which the roots are steamed soon after collection, indicate that red ginseng (often referred to in the literature as Radix Ginseng Rubra) usually has higher ginsenoside content than white ginseng. During the process to make red ginseng, malonyl-ginsenosides are converted to their corresponding ginsenosides by hydrolysis. According to a report on American ginseng, the steaming process used to produce red American ginseng increases the level of its ginsenoside Rb1 by as much as 100 per cent through conversion of malonyl-R_{b1} to R_{b1}. The acidic malonyl compounds are poorly absorbed in humans, but intestinal bacteria metabolise malonyl ginsenosides to neutral ginsenosides, which are better absorbed [44]. A small amount of acetyl-ginsenosides are also generated from the malonyl-ginsenosides when preparing red ginseng [49]. It has been proposed that some of the changes in ginsenosides that occur when white ginseng is steamed to produce red ginseng also arise during preparation of ginseng tea and ginseng extracts [57]. Another factor influencing the difference in ginsenoside content between white and red ginseng is the removal or retention of the outer root skin. White ginseng is frequently prepared by peeling the root. Since the ginsenoside content is particularly rich in the peel, this processing results in relatively low ginsenoside content. Red ginseng, on the other hand, is processed by steaming the unpeeled roots. Although ginsenosides have been the focus of research on ginseng active constituents, other compounds in the root have been discovered to have biological activity. These include acetylenic compounds, peptide glycans, polysaccharides, pyran derivatives, and flavones [17]. One can demonstrate pharmacological activity of these substances when they are isolated and concentrated; for example, the acetylenic panaxynol, panaxydol, and panaxytriol show cytotoxic activity *in vitro*. Such action is potentially of value in cancer treatments, but only if the cytotoxicity is highly specific for cancer cells. Similarly, the polysaccharides of ginseng, like those of the medicinal mushrooms, can enhance certain immune functions, as demonstrated in laboratory animal investigations [48]. The dose of immunologically active polysaccharides when isolated and used clinically is about 1-3 g. [33]. The amounts of these various non-saponin substances that are present in ginseng roots are very small: They are unlikely to significantly contribute to any of the purported clinical effects of ginseng when the roots or their extracts are consumed in ordinarily recommended quantities. Similarly, ginseng contains B vitamins (B1 and B2) and trace elements (mainly manganese), which have a therapeutic action in large doses, but the amounts consumed when taking ginseng are trivial compared to dietary sources.

Pharmacology Experiments

With proper design, pharmacology experiments can help elucidate the physiological mechanism by which the herb produces certain observed effects. Tests can be conducted on whole herb materials (e.g. by adding the powder to the diet), herb extracts, isolated active fractions (i.e. groups of chemicals), or individual chemicals from the herb. Several of the initial pharmacology studies of ginseng were based on a well-known story in China about the way to determine whether a ginseng root was genuine [22]. 'In order to test for the true ginseng, two persons would walk together, one with a piece of ginseng root in his mouth and the other with his mouth empty. If at the end of 3-5 *li* [3 *li* is about one mile], the one with ginseng in his mouth does not feel himself tired, while the other is out of breath, the ginseng is genuine.' In several of the early pharmacology experiments (during the 1960s) ginseng was given to test animals (mice and rats) that were then forced to keep moving until they became so fatigued that they had to stop (usually a forced swimming test or forced climbing test). The ones given ginseng were reported to be able to carry on longer [22].

The effect of ginseng on preventing fatigue due to overworking was viewed as an 'antistress' action, and other studies focused on ginseng's ability to protect animals from various other types of stress, such as heat and cold, low oxygen, exposure to ionising radiation, and infections. These efforts were the source of the concept of ginseng, and other herbs, as adaptogens: substances with a relatively high degree of safety that helped the organism adapt to various types of stress. Ginseng research was influenced also by the growing concern about cardiovascular diseases that had become the leading cause of death in developed nations. Since it was said in the ancient texts that taking ginseng regularly could prolong life, it seemed reasonable to demonstrate that ginseng could reduce the risk of death from cardiovascular disease. To give credence to this outcome would require massive clinical trials with people taking either ginseng or a placebo over a period of many years, but to start the investigative process, one could administer ginseng to animals in the laboratory and observe its effect on known risk factors. Researchers in China, Korea, and Japan carried out numerous laboratory animal experiments showing that ginseng could lower blood cholesterol and lipids as well as blood sugar—the key elements in the blood that were the primary focus to determine the risk of developing cardiovascular disease. Those studies led to a continuing investigation in several countries and to human clinical trials.

In order to determine the potential of a pharmacology study to predict a corresponding clinical outcome, one must translate the laboratory dosage to the clinical dosage. The pharmacology experiments with ginseng that helped animals' survival under stress and that reduced risk factors associated with cardiovascular disease appear to support the dosage of ginseng recommended in the Chinese literature. Most of the studies on laboratory animals conducted in China, Korea, and Japan were based on doses of ginseng in the range of 25 mg/kg of body weight to 250 mg/kg [17, 18], though higher doses, such as 400 mg/kg, have occasionally been used in tests (e.g. for immune stimulation purposes). It is quite difficult to convert dosages in laboratory animals to those that would be used in humans, but with proper study design and analysis of factors influencing pharmacokinetics, it is possible to estimate what might happen in humans. A detailed analysis of conversion factors for such laboratory studies to human clinical applications was carried out by J. Boik [33]. He indicates that the 25-250 mg/kg dosage range in mice corresponds to about 1-9 g of ginseng for human use and that laboratory studies of ginseng for inhibiting cancer growth utilise amounts corresponding to a human dosage of 3.2-47 g per day. The amounts of herb material used in the pharmacology testing for ginseng are similar to the amounts used in pharmacology tests of other Chinese herbs that, like ginseng, are administered to humans in doses of 3-9 g per day in traditional practices. [11] In addition to pharmacology studies that indicate reduction in factors associated with risk of heart disease, there have been investigations indicating that ginseng administration in animals improves immune functions, reduces stress-induced ulceration, provides antioxidant effects, inhibits tumour formation, and improves oxygen utilisation [18]. These diverse beneficial effects of ginseng were noted to be similar to those being reported at the same time for vitamin E [36]. Thus, while ginseng appears to be confirmed by pharmacology studies as valuable to health, it is not necessarily more interesting or more potent than vitamin supplements. In fact, one result of the research into ginseng effects was the production of nutritional supplements with ginseng added with the hope of improving upon the benefits of each component. Despite the extensive research efforts, ginseng was not accepted by the modern medical profession outside of Asia as a remedy for these health issues. It is not surprising, then, that the Western ginseng market shifted focus to a different area of concern.

Ginseng and Energy: A New Twist

The Chinese term *chi*, which has a rich meaning in the Chinese culture (see: *Drawing a Concept: Qi*), was translated by some Westerners simply as 'energy'. The concept of tonifying chi in the Chinese medical system was depicted, inaccurately, as stimulating energy. In other words, when a person was feeling run down, instead of, or in addition to, taking a cup of coffee, one could take ginseng, a chi-tonifying herb, in order to feel some immediate energy. In her book *Asian Health Secrets* [54], Letha Hadady described the situation this way: 'Most Westerners use Chinese ginseng like jet fuel, to drive themselves beyond their capacity.' The claim that ginseng increases energy has become the lead concept in the marketing of ginseng. Today's functional foods (e.g. beverages spiked with vitamins, amino acids, and/or herbs) include ginseng in the category of 'energy products', and ginseng is found in many of the herbal capsules, tablets, or liquid preparations aimed at improving energy. Ephedra, or ma-huang (*Ephedra sinica*), with its potent alkaloids, has been promoted in the same way for this purpose (typically at a dose of 20-25 mg ephedrine alkaloids each dose, up to three or more times per day). In an effort to get an energy boost from herbs, people have sometimes used extreme amounts or unusual combinations of herbs. One result can be adverse reactions and, as can be seen with the current calls for restrictions, negative publicity and fear.

For example, a 'ginseng abuse syndrome' was described in a highly controversial report published in 1979 [13]. Although the validity of this syndrome was later challenged [14], it remains a caution that is often raised about ginseng, regardless of the amount to be consumed. For the most part, the adverse reactions attributed to excessive use of ginseng, as conveyed in the 1979 article, may have been due to other products also used in excess at the same time (including high levels of caffeine). Some people, however, consumed unusually large amounts of ginseng to get an immediate reaction, and this may have generated adverse effects, especially with prolonged overdosing. The late Israel I. Brekhman, the Russian proponent of using herbs such as ginseng as adaptogens, described ginseng as having a stimulant action, and Russian researchers responded by focusing on this potential application [22]. By contrast, Chinese researchers insisted that ginseng functioned as a mild sedative and calming agent; the ability to overcome fatigue, for example, was described as the result of having less stress on the body rather than by causing an overt stimulation. One peculiar effort to resolve the differences in these viewpoints was made by a Japanese researcher, Hiroshi Saito, who suggested that ginseng did both: some of the ginsenosides, particularly the R_g series, were stimulating in nature while others, particularly the R_b series, were calming in nature [56]. He and co-worker Yien-mei Lee, pointed out that 'We noticed that multiple pharmacodynamic activities of ginseng originated from various ingredients and there are many pharmacologically antagonistic actions in ginseng.' How these apparently competing effects of some active components could explain away the difference of opinion about ginseng effects when ginseng was used as a whole preparation and not subdivided was never made clear by any subsequent authors who used the underlying concept in the attempt to cover up incompatible claims.

As an example of the confusion generated by those making claims for ginseng's effect on energy, it has been suggested that Asian ginseng is 'stimulating,' but that American ginseng is 'calming.' One origin of this concept may be traced to the Chinese view regarding yin and yang. In China, it has been said that Chinese ginseng has the ability to tonify chi and invigorate yang [corresponding roughly to metabolism and movement], while American ginseng has the ability to tonify qi and nourish yin [corresponding roughly to control and calming]. However, this analysis comes about from a peculiar historical situation rather than an inherent difference in the herbs. Chinese ginseng comes from the far north of China; American ginseng was always imported through Canton, in the far south. From this experience, the Chinese had viewed their own ginseng as a northern product and the American ginseng as a southern product. In fact, American ginseng is obtained mainly from the northern part of the Eastern United States and Canada, regions that are geographically similar to the part of China from which Asian ginseng is obtained. The north, being cold, would yield, by ancient dogma, a product that benefits yang; the south, being warm, would yield a version of the same herb that benefits yin. Although, to this day, American ginseng is classified among the yin nourishing herbs in some Chinese herb guides, it is not described as more calming than the Chinese species, which is already depicted as having a calming action. American ginseng is sometimes said to be more cooling, however, and useful in tea for the sweltering summer heat of southern China.

To quote from one Chinese herb guide detailing the uses and applications of American ginseng [15]: 'Traditional uses: nourishes yin, cleanses heat, increases salivation, supplements the lungs, moistens, and depresses fire. Applications: heat symptom-complex, pulmonary tuberculosis, dry cough due to deficiency heat.' Ignoring the historical origins of the different concepts about American and Asian ginseng, those who discuss the energising or calming effects suggest that the difference involves the precise mix or ratio of ginsenosides. At this time, there is no evidence to support the contention that the mix of ginsenosides, at the dosage ingested, has any significant influence on the effect of ginseng. There have been no valid measures for stimulant properties of ginseng as applied to humans and there have been no comparative studies of the clinical effects of the different species of herbs sold as ginseng. One cannot say with scientific certainty whether one species is better, worse, or different in effect from the others, though it is possible to assay the total amount of ginsenosides. There is no substantive evidence that any difference in proportions of ginsenoside subsets between Asian and American species produces any difference in clinical effect of consuming the roots.

11.18 Challenges Arising with Ginseng Products and Their Use

Disturbing reports began to surface in the late 1970s, and have been repeated several times since, that some ginseng products didn't contain ginseng or contained only weak or inactive ginseng, as had been suspected by ginseng experts for many years. Tests were developed to evaluate commercial products for ginsenoside content, which were found to vary considerably [19]. In the first such study, conducted by researchers at the Philadelphia College of Pharmacy and Science, some of the commercial products analysed contained so-called 'Siberian ginseng,' a herb that was being promoted initially by the Soviet Union and later by China. It was derived from eleuthero (*Eleutherococcus senticosus*), which contains no ginsenosides. In a Swiss study reported at a Chinese medicine conference in 1984 [58], six Asian ginseng products were evaluated and found to contain from as little as 0.3 mg ginsenosides per dosage unit (capsule) to 27 mg of ginsenoside per dosage unit (ampoule of ginseng extract), a ninetyfold range.

Finn Sandberg, a Swedish ginseng researcher, described the situation with product variability this way, in response to questions about the validity of ginseng clinical test results [31]: 'Does [the favorable clinical test result] apply to other ginseng preparations? From a strictly scientific point of view, it is valid only for that particular batch of capsules that was used; but it will certainly be valid for other batches of capsules, provided they have an identical composition. Here comes the problem!' Such concerns about the variability of ginseng used for both testing and for commercial products led to promotion of what has been called 'standardised ginseng'. Standardised ginseng has different meanings for different manufacturers. Some have used the term loosely, such as when simple steps have been taken to assure that the product meets a certain level in terms of amount of ginseng in the product or the amount of total ginsenosides in the product.

The first product referred to as a 'standardised ginseng' was called G115 [21, 22]. The manufacturer of G115 (Pharmaton, Lugano, Switzerland) has not described its processing method but has claimed to provide 100 mg of the ginseng extract in a capsule with 4 per cent total ginsenosides. As described in a review article on ginseng [27]: 'Each capsule of G115 contains 100 mg of a concentrated aqueous extract of *P. ginseng*, which is titrated, that is, diluted, at 4 per cent ginsenosides and equivalent to 500 mg *P. ginseng* root.' Recent testing of samples [61] indicated that recent batches of this product barely contained the claimed amount, sometimes falling short. The meaning of standardisation developed by this company (which also produces a capsule titrated to 7 per cent ginsenosides) appears to be twofold: that both the amount of ginseng extract in a capsule and its percentage of total ginsenosides are set at a certain level. However, no consistent definition of standards for such products has been utilised by the herb industry, although the American Herbal Products Association has recently developed definitions recommended to the industry. One effect of the standardisation is that it became a requisite of many Western studies to utilise standardised ginseng. A certain confidence in the value of the studies using standardised ginseng has evolved because the ginseng was well defined.

Such confidence is sometimes misplaced. Thus, for example, in the book *Herbal Prescriptions for Better Health* [50], the author, a naturopathic physician, states that: 'The best researched form of ginseng is extracts supplying approximately 4 to 7 per cent ginsenosides. The recommended dosage is 100 mg once or twice daily. Crude non-standardized extracts require a higher daily dose of 1 to 2 grams.' In fact, the standardised ginseng extracts mentioned here are the *most frequently researched* of the commercial extracts (here, he doesn't mention the brand but clearly means the Pharmaton product), but not necessarily the *best researched* in terms of quality of the studies. There is no evidence whatsoever that other non-standardised extracts need to be used in doses that are ten times higher. The author's implication is that by standardising the extract it becomes far more potent than other extracts, which is unproven and unlikely.

By gaining confidence in standardised material administered in trials, readers may ignore other potential weaknesses or flaws in the design and reporting of the studies. In a review of ginseng's potential for affecting sports performance [37], much of which relied on using the standardised ginseng preparations of Pharmaton, the authors comment that 'the published literature was characterized by numerous statistical and design problems. Much of this research failed to control for various behavioral artifacts . . .' They found that 'there is an absence of compelling research evidence regarding the efficacy of ginseng use for the purpose of improving physical performance in humans.' Similarly, in a review and meta-analysis British researchers [32] concluded that '. . . there is compelling evidence for none of the claimed indications.' One of the design flaws that was not mentioned in the reviews of ginseng trials was the low dosage of ginseng administered, levels that do not make sense from the perspective of modern knowledge of herbal pharmacology. If European ginseng research repeatedly underdoses the ginseng, then no other design characteristic will overcome this fundamental flaw.

Shrinking Dosage Recommendations and European Research

While in China the recommended dosage of ginseng for medicinal purposes has been consistent from ancient times up to the present (at several grams per day), the amount of ginseng suggested to be taken in the West has become relatively miniscule. Recommended doses of standardised ginseng products are typically one capsule each time. For the most frequently cited 4 per cent ginsenoside extract in capsule form, the daily dose of ginseng extract is just 200 mg, and the daily amount of ginsenosides is just 8 mg. This 8 mg of ginsenosides is said to be derived from 1 g of ginseng, which is the lowest daily ginseng dosage recommended in any Chinese texts, and corresponds to an extremely weak ginseng root (with 0.8 per cent ginsenoside content rather than more typical levels that are at least twice that high).

By contrast, clinical work in Asia is carried out with far higher amounts of ginseng and for uses that differ markedly from those described in the West. The *Pharmacopoeia of the People's Republic of China* [16] officially lists 3-9 g as the dosage for ginseng in decoction (tea) form. Thus, for example, in the attempt to prevent and treat cardiovascular diseases, ginseng is given in this dosage range to lower blood pressure. By contrast, Western literature cautions persons with hypertension to avoid ginseng, especially to avoid red ginseng, even in the much lower doses used in the West. In a recent report from Korea [20], red ginseng was administered at a dose of 4.5 g per day (Korean red ginseng powder, 1.5 g per dose, three times daily) and reported to have a slight blood pressure lowering effect (about 5 per cent average decline) after two months' daily administration. In reviewing prior studies of ginseng's effect on hypertension, the authors of that study noted that there had been negligble or minor effects on blood pressure previously mentioned for administration of 3 g red ginseng powder every day for three months and with 3-6 g of red ginseng powder every day for an average duration of ten months. As a reflection of this direction in ginseng research, in 1980, the Institute for Traditional Medicine of Portland, Oregon, conducted a clinical trial in Santa Cruz, California on the impact of Asian ginseng on the risk factors for cardiovascular disease: cholesterol, triglycerides, elevated blood sugar, and blood pressure [23]. In that study, the first clinical trial of ginseng in the United States., a hundred patients received red ginseng provided by the Korean Ginseng Research Institute at a dosage of either 3.0 or 4.5 g per day (others received a placebo). Only modest effects were observed after three weeks of daily administration of the ginseng capsules, with slight favourable improvements in the risk factor measurements.

Two recent Chinese clinical trials made use of closely related ginseng formulations—ginseng plus tienchi ginseng (*sanqi*) with amber [26], and ginseng plus tienchi ginseng and rhubarb root [27]—for treatment of angina pectoris and coronary heart disease, respectively. In the first study, the herbs were powdered and administered at the dose of 3 g, three times daily. The total amount of ginseng (*P. ginseng* plus *P. pseudoginseng*) ingested by the patients each day was 7.2 g. The treatment time was twelve weeks. The study report indicated that there were beneficial effects of the treatment and no adverse responses were noted. In the second study, the *P. ginseng* was a water-based extract, while the *P. pseudoginseng* was used as a powder (as is routine practice for this herb). The daily dose of the preparation administered was 2.4 g, with 1.9 g of it being a combination of the extract and powder of ginseng. Although the concentration of the extract was not stated, it is common to produce ginseng extracts that are about 4:1, meaning that the total dosage of ginseng crude materials used to make a daily dose in the treatment regimen would be about 5 g. Again, benefits were claimed without report of adverse events during a treatment time of three weeks. These studies employed about 5-7 g of ginseng, consistent with the Chinese Pharmacopoeia recommendation of 3-9 g. Even in the treatment of infants, high doses of ginseng are recommended in China. Gu Chifan described the use of ginseng for newborn babies [38]: The usual dosage is 3 g a day. For infants of low birthweight or neonates within—one to two days after delivery, reduce to 2 g a day, as a drink or nasal feeding of the steamed juice of red ginseng. Giving higher dosage is not necessary. Side effects such as tachycardia will appear if the dose is over 6 g a day. Some individuals manifest slight diarrhoea or rash after administration for three days, but it will disappear spontaneously after discontinuance.

An increasing number of European reports of ginseng effects based on small amounts of standardised ginseng appear in the literature, yet there are a few researchers using quantities comparable to those used in Asia. For example, a Canadian study investigating the reported blood sugar lowering effects of ginseng involved administration of 3 g of American ginseng [41]. The authors commented, 'In our study, we noticed our effect with a high dose (3 grams) relative to that given by others studying various types of ginseng in humans. A review of clinical studies shows that the quantity administered is typically 1.5 grams or less.' In the clinical reports from Asia cited above, the ginsenoside content of the ginseng root material used is not specified. Separate studies conducted in Asia reveal typical levels of ginsenosides of about 4 per cent, while Western studies indicate lower amounts, such as 1.5–2.0 per cent. However, whether one uses the figure of 1.5 per cent ginsenoside content for ginseng roots as the specified minimum in Europe, or uses the higher level reported in Asian sources, the doses of ginseng cited in these clinical reports correspond to from 45–135 mg (at 1.5 per cent) to 120–360 mg (at 4 per cent) of the saponin components. This is in marked contrast to recommendations for use of standardised ginseng products at doses of just 8–14 mg/day of ginsenosides.

There are only a few studies conducted in Asia in which isolated ginsenosides are given clinically. In a Chinese study [42], the saponins isolated from *P. ginseng* fruits were administered to 327 patients, aged between—fifty and seventy years to test the saponins' antisenility actions. The dosage administered was 150 mg/day. A similar clinical study was conducted with saponins isolated from *P. ginseng* rhizome: 358 patients aged from—fifty to eighty-five years were given 150 mg/day of the saponins (50 mg each time, three times a day) for two months [51]. Prolonged administration of the saponins for up to two years showed no adverse side effects. In a Korean study [43], ginsenosides of the trial series (e.g. ginsenosides of the G series, as in $R_g 1$ etc.) were given to 120 patients who had gone through gynaecological laparotomies, in an attempt to aid recovery. The dosage administered was 230 mg/day. These doses of isolated saponins are consistent with the amounts expected to be obtained from the ginseng powder and crude extracts in those studies cited above, but they are more than ten times higher than the saponin levels administered in Europe with the commonly used standardised ginseng capsules.

When using *Panax ginseng*, the consumer would generally prefer to take relatively few capsules or tablets. In fact, it is not difficult to ingest the higher levels of ginseng or its ginsenosides, at least if one can obtain high quality ginseng roots. Ginseng root powder at 500 mg per capsule will provide 3 g of ginseng in just six capsules (e.g. three capsules, two times per day). In addition, ginsenoside-rich extracts from *P. ginseng* are prepared in China with 20-85 per cent ginsenosides, making it easy to get a desired amount of ginsenosides into a single capsule. To get the higher ginsenoside concentrations, ginseng leaves and/or fruits are used as a source material. Ginseng fruits are especially rich in ginsenoside Re, which was shown to have antidiabetic activity, similar to that of the other ginsenosides [28]. These concentrated ginsenoside extracts have been subjected to clinical evaluations in China, particularly for elderly patients who may have trouble consuming large amounts of capsules or tablets, and deemed an effective substitute for crude powders [42].

Summary and Concluding Remarks

This article has reviewed the traditional understanding and uses of Asian ginseng (*Panax ginseng*), its usual recommended dosage, the type and levels of active constituents found in ginseng, and the complex situation surrounding modern research efforts. The information presented here suggests the following:

- The traditional uses of ginseng primarily revolve around promoting digestive system functions, improving nutrition, and calming agitation; the modern applications in Asia are particularly aimed at preventing and treating cardiovascular diseases and problems of aging, including diabetes. By contrast, ginseng is often described today in the West as an energising agent, a stimulant that is a healthy substitute for caffeine, though caffeine has not been shown to be harmful in normal use.

- The usual recommended dosage of ginseng in Asia is most often in the range of 3-9 g/day. By contrast, herb product manufacturers in the West may recommend using far less, with amounts that are of questionable potential to provide any of the desired ginseng actions.

- The primary active constituents in various species of *Panax* are saponins called ginsenosides. European researchers report lower levels in the roots than their Asian counterparts. The concentrations also vary according to the species of ginseng and its method of preparation. Based on the Chinese recommendations for dosage of the roots, and for the dosage of isolated ginsenosides that are sometimes given in clinical studies-the amount of ginsenosides to be taken in one day would typically be about 80-240 mg for long-term administration (several weeks or months). European recommendations for dosage of the ginsenosides are much lower, by about a factor of ten and don't correspond to the levels shown effective in most pharmacology studies.

- Modern research into ginseng and its effects has been hampered by poor quality in the study design and reporting. As a result, many physicians and researchers do not find the effects that have been reported to have a credible basis. On a precautionary basis, the reports of adverse effects appear more acceptable to many well-trained physicians than reports of beneficial effects. The research efforts have largely focused on anti-fatigue actions and reduction of risk factors for cardiovascular diseases, though other areas of interest have been pursued (e.g. radioprotective and chemoprotective effects).

- Ginseng has a long history of use in Asia that has generated interest in continuing the tradition into the present and studying, by modern methods, the constituents of ginseng and their pharmacological and clinical effects. A careful reading of both the traditional literature and modern Asian and Western research efforts is essential to help guide consumers and health care professionals towards knowing the correct indications and dosages for ginseng, selecting appropriate ginseng ma.

The reason for this extensive analysis of the research the report on ginseng is to enable us see the usefuflness of the product. Another reason is whether there exist any credible and effective medical property(s) in the herb. This information will help us in the use of ginseng as one of the sources of preventive therapy.

Complementary therapies should study this article and with experience to see where the product of ginseng can be used for the preventive benefit to their patients.

CHAPTER 12

12.1 The Iranian Traditional Medicine Integrated

About the Centre

It is supervised by Haleh Talaie, MD, MPH, Associate Professor of infectious diseases, specialist of the Shaheed Beheshti University of Medical Science, Chair of Integrative Medicine. The Center of Integrative Medicine began its programmes in 2007.

First members: Khadijeh Rahmani as a nutritionist and Simin Ahadi, who studied to be a master of Reiki, alternative medicine, joined this programme through a pilot study in 2008, and then the group was gradually formed. In 2009, Dr Hamid reza jabbari, an Internist and pulmonologist, who works on chronic respiratory diseases by alternative medicine methods, joined the group. Right now, D. Jabbari has scientific responsibility in integrative medicine group. Dr Abbas Haji Fethali hematologist, as the head of Taleghani Hospital, coordinated and organised integrative medicine clinic. He manages his cancer patients by integrative medicine approach.

Alireza Shamimi, who is trained in alternative medicine-energy therapy field and Shakiba Farahmand as a psychologist have their positions in the group. They prepared a proposal as a health research project titled 'Survey on integrative medicine, healing. oriented efficacy on people quality of life'.

This clinical trial project was accepted in the research centre of Shaheed Beheshti Medical University and also in the Ministry of Health and Medical Education, Islamic republic of Iran, 2009. We awarded the faculty members, clinician, researcher, and patients at a symposium.

Members:

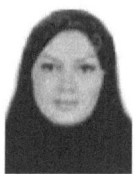

Haleh Talaie MD, MPH

- Director of Integrative Medicine Group,
- Infectious Diseases Specialist,
- Associate Professor of Shaheed Beheshti University of Medical Sciences,
- Research Fellow of Clinical Pharmacology-Toxicology, University of Toronto, and
- Vice Chancellor and Research Deputy Department of Toxicological Research Center of Loghman Hakim General Hospital.

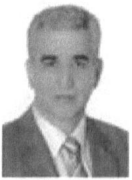

Hamidreza Jabbardarjani, MD

- Internist–Interventional Pulmonologist,
- Head of Bronchoscopes and Laser Ward of Massih Daneshvari Hospital,
- Associated Professor of Shaheed Beheshti University of Medical Sciences, and
- Member of Trachea Diseases Research Center and NRITLD.

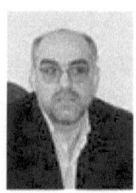

Abbas Haji Fethali MD

- Haematologist, Associate Professor of Shaheed Beheshti University of Medical Sciences, and
- Head of bone marrow transplant ward and Talaghani General Hospital.

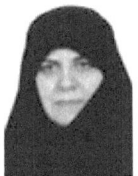

Khadijeh Rahmani

- Faculty member of community nutrition department, College of Nutrition Sciences and Food Technology, National Nutritional Science and Food Technology Research Institute, and Shaheed Beheshti University of Medical Science and health Services.

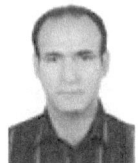

Alireza Shamimi

- A trained alternative medicine practitioner.

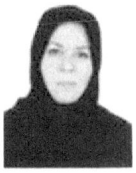

Simin Ahadi

- A trained alternative medicine practitioner.

Dependent Members

Shakiba Bashirfarahmand
    Psychologist, counselor, Director In Charge and Institutor of 7, Bavar Cultural Institute

Kiarash Saatchi M.D.
Acupuncturist and university lecturer of Complementary and Holistic Medicine

The Vision and Mission

Vision: Facilitate the opportunity for the well-being and health of the body, the mind, and the spirit of the patients and promote the quality of their life. This is achieved by using updated research and educational results of integrative medicine (conventional, alternative, and supplementary).

Mission: Create a comprehensive health care system. The aim is to achieve the well-being and the health of patients with emphasis on (contribution) participation to achieve harmony of the body, the mind, and the spirit.

About Us

We offer approaches that foster optimal wellness and healing, no matter what the health challenges. In this approach, we offer time to listen to people's stories. We review the conventional medical history as well as the use of alternative approaches. An integrative medicine plan is created that suits each individual's unique needs, offering specific recommendations for mind, body, spirit, and emotion that optimise health. Integrative therapies such as Iranian traditional medicine, holistic nutrition, relaxation techniques, acupuncture, massage, and herbs and supplements are blended with the best of medical science and technology. This is the hallmark of the Iran Difference.

One of the wonderful things about the Iranian integratesys is that it allows for the maximum use of their professional manpower in the medical field for the benefit of the public. Both the orthodox and the complementary practitioners see themselves as a united front for the ultimate common progress. Integration provides for a uniform standard in their health care delivery.

The Arabic Traditional Medicine

It is very suprising that here in the West, people do not naormally talk about the Arabic Traditional Medicine at all. It seems that the reason for this apathy can be attributable to the sense of Islamic-phobia. Whatever happens, my concern in this book is to equip the complementary medical practitioners with the knowledge and better undersanding of the technique for preventive therapy. It is improtant to understand that in a multi-ethnic society like we have in Britain, people's religious taboos should be appreciated and respected as such. Whatever information we can derive from the following will be useful to us in our daily practices and preventive therapy. In the history of medicine, *Islamic medicine* or *Arabic medicine* refers to medicine developed in the Islamic Golden Age of the Islamic civilisation and written in Arabic, the *lingua franca* of the Islamic civilisation. Some consider the label 'Arab-Islamic' as historically inaccurate, arguing that this label does not appreciate the rich diversity of Eastern scholars who have contributed to Islamic science in this era. Latin translations of Arabic medical works had a significant influence on the development of modern medicine, as did Arabic texts chronicling the medical works of earlier cultures.

Overview

Islamic medical writing was influenced by several different medical systems, including the traditional Arabian medicine of Muhammad's time, ancient Hellenistic medicine such as Unani, ancient Indian medicine such as Ayurveda, and the ancient Iranian medicine of the Academy of Gundishapur. The works of ancient Greek and Roman physicians Hippocrates, Dioscorides, Soranus, Celsus, and Galen also had a lasting impact on Islamic medicine.

Foundations

The origins of Islamic medicine can be traced back to the time of Muhammad, and a significant number of Hadiths concerning medicine are attributed to him. Several Sahaba are said to have been successfully treated of certain diseases by following the medical advice of Muhammad. [citation needed] The three methods of healing mentioned by him were honey, Hijama (wet cupping), and cauterisation, though he was generally opposed to the use of cauterisation unless it 'suits the ailment'. According to Ibn Hajar al-Asqalani, Muhammad disliked this method due to it causing 'pain and menace to a patient' since there was no anesthesia in his time. Although purported by previous physicians like Imhotep,

Hippocrates, and Galen, Muhammad appears to be the first[dubious—discuss] recorded as directly stating that there is always a cause and a cure for every disease, according to several Hadiths in the *Sahih al-Bukhari*, *Sunan Abi Dawood*, and *Al-Muwatta* attributed to Muhammad, such as: 'There is no disease that Allah has created, except that He also has created its treatment.' 'Make use of medical treatment, for Allah has not made a disease without appointing a remedy for it, with the exception of one disease, name was old age.' 'Allah has sent down both the disease and the cure, and He has appointed a cure for every disease, so treat yourselves medically.' 'The one who sent down the disease sent down the remedy.' 'For every disease, Allah has given a cure.' The belief that there is a cure for every disease encouraged early Muslims to engage in medical research and seek out cures for diseases known to them. Many early authors of Islamic medicine were primarily clerics rather than physicians and were known to have advocated the traditional medical practices of prophet Muhammad's time, such as those mentioned in the Koran and Hadith.

From the ninth century, Hunayn ibn Ishaq translated a number of Galen's works into the Arabic language, followed by translations of the *Sushruta Samhita*, *Charaka Samhita*, and Middle Persian works from Gundishapur. Muslim physicians soon began making many of their own significant advances and contributions to medicine, including the fields of allergology, anatomy, bacteriology, botany, dentistry, embryology, environmentalism, aetiology, immunology, microbiology, obstetrics, ophthalmology, pathology, pediatrics, perinatology, physiology, psychiatry, psychology, pulsology and sphygmology, surgery, therapy, urology, zoology, and the pharmaceutical sciences such as pharmacy and pharmacology. Medicine was a central part of medieval Islamic culture. Responding to circumstances of time and place, Islamic physicians and scholars developed a large and complex medical literature exploring and synthesising the theory and practice of medicine.[11] Islamic medicine was initially built on tradition, chiefly the theoretical and practical knowledge developed in Arabia, Persia, Greece, Rome, and India. Galen and Hippocrates were pre-eminent authorities, as well as the Indian physicians Sushruta and Charaka and the Hellenistic scholars in Alexandria. Islamic scholars translated their voluminous writings from Greek and Sanskrit into Arabic and then produced new medical knowledge based on those texts.[12] In order to make the Greek and Indian traditions more accessible, understandable, and teachable, Islamic scholars ordered and made more systematic the vast and sometimes inconsistent Greco-Roman and Indian medical knowledge by writing encyclopedias and summaries. It was through Arabic translations that the West learnt of Hellenic medicine, including the works of Galen and Hippocrates. Of equal, if not of greater, influence in Western Europe were systematic and comprehensive works such as Avicenna's *The Canon of Medicine*, which were translated into Latin and then disseminated in manuscript and printed form throughout Europe. During the fifteenth and sixteenth centuries alone, *The Canon of Medicine* was published more than thirty-five times.

Hospitals

Muslim physicians set up hospitals, known as Bimaristans, which were establishments where the ill were welcomed and cared for by qualified staff, and which were clearly distinguished from the ancient healing temples, sleep temples, hospices, and leper-houses that were more concerned with isolating the sick and the insane from society 'rather than to offer them any way to a true cure'. The Bimaristan hospitals later functioned as public hospitals,[14] insane asylums. In the medieval Islamic world, hospitals were built in major cities; in Cairo, for example, the Qalawun Hospital could care for eight thousand patients with a staff that included physicians, pharmacists, and nurses. One could also access a dispensary and a research facility that led to advances, which included the discovery of the contagious nature of diseases and research into optics and the mechanisms of the eye. Muslim doctors were removing cataracts with hollow needles. Hospitals were built not only for the physically sick, but for the mentally sick also. One of the first-ever psychiatric hospitals that cared for the mentally ill was built in Cairo. Hospitals later spread to Europe during the Crusades, inspired by the hospitals in the Middle East. The first hospital in Paris, Les Quinze-vingts, was founded by Louis IX after his return from the Crusade between 1254 and 1260. Hospitals in the Islamic world featured competency tests for doctors, drug purity regulations, nurses and interns, and advanced surgical procedures.[17] Hospitals were also created with separate wards for specific illnesses so that people with contagious diseases could be kept away from other patients. One of the features in medieval Muslim hospitals that distinguished them from their contemporaries and predecessors was their significantly higher standards of medical ethics. Hospitals in the Islamic world treated patients of all religions, ethnicities, and backgrounds, while the hospitals themselves often employed staff from Christian, Jewish, and other minority backgrounds. Muslim doctors and physicians were expected to have obligations towards their patients, regardless of their wealth or backgrounds. The ethical standards of Muslim physicians was first laid down in the ninth century by Ishaq bin Ali Rahawi, who wrote the *Adab al-Tabib (Conduct of a Physician)*, the first treatise dedicated to medical ethics. He regarded physicians as 'guardians of souls and bodies' and wrote twenty chapters on various topics related to medical ethics.[citation needed]Another unique feature of medieval Muslim hospitals was the role of female staff, who were rarely employed in ancient and medieval healing temples elsewhere in the world. Medieval Muslim hospitals commonly employed female nurses, including nurses from as far as Sudan, a sign of great breakthrough. Muslim hospitals were also the first to employ female physicians, the most famous being two female physicians from the Banu Zuhr family who served the Almohad ruler Abu Yusuf Ya'qub al-Mansur in the twelfth century. Later in the fifteenth century, female surgeons were illustrated for the first time in Şerafeddin Sabuncuoğlu's *Cerrahiyyetu'l-Haniyye (Imperial Surgery)*.

Encyclopedias

The first encyclopedia of medicine in Arabic was Ali ibn Sahl Rabban al-Tabari's *Firdous al-Hikmah (Paradise of Wisdom)*, written in seven parts, *c.* 860. It was the first to deal with paediatrics and child development, as well as psychology and psychotherapy. In the fields of medicine and psychotherapy, the work was primarily influenced by Islamic thought and ancient Indian physicians such as Sushruta and Charaka. Unlike earlier physicians, however, al-Tabari emphasised strong ties between psychology and medicine, and the need of psychotherapy and counseling in the therapeutic treatment of patients. Muhammad ibn Zakarīya Rāzi (Rhazes) wrote the *Comprehensive Book of Medicine* in the ninth century. The *Large Comprehensive* was the most sought-after of all his compositions, in which Rhazes recorded clinical cases of his own experience and provided very useful recordings of various diseases. The *Comprehensive Book of Medicine*, with its introduction of measles and smallpox, was very influential in Europe.

Ali ibn Abbas al-Majusi's (Haly Abbas) *Kitab Kamil as-sina'a at-tibbiya* (*Complete Book of the Medical Art*), c. 980, became better known as the *Kitab al-Maliki* (*Royal Book*, Latin: *Liber regalis*) in honour of its royal patron 'Adud al-Dawla. In twenty sections, ten of theory and ten of practice, it was more systematic and concise than Razi's *Hawi*, but more practical than Avicenna's *Canon*, by which it was superseded. With many interpolations and substitutions, it served as the basis for the *Pantegni* (*c.* 1087) of Constantinus Africanus, the founding text of the Schola Medica Salernitana in Salerno. Abu al-Qasim al-Zahrawi (Abulcasis), regarded as the father of modern surgery, contributed greatly to the discipline of medical surgery with his *Kitab al-Tasrif* (*Book of Concessions*), a thirty-volume medical encyclopedia published in 1000, which was later translated to Latin and used in European medical schools for centuries. He invented numerous surgical instruments and described them in his *al-Tasrif*. Avicenna (Ibn Sina), a Hanbali and Mu'tazili philosopher and doctor in the early eleventh century, was another influential figure. He is regarded as the father of modern medicine and one of the greatest thinkers and medical scholars in history. His medical encyclopedia, *The Canon of Medicine* (c. 1020), remained a standard textbook in Europe for centuries until the renewal of the Muslim tradition of scientific medicine. He also wrote *The Book of Healing* (actually a more general encyclopedia of science and philosophy), which became another popular textbook in Europe. Among other things, Avicenna's contributions to medicine include the discovery of the contagious nature of infectious diseases, the introduction of quarantine to limit the spread of contagious diseases, the introduction of experimental medicine, evidence-based medicine, clinical trials,[26] randomised controlled trials, efficacy tests, clinical pharmacology and the idea of a syndrome in the diagnosis of specific diseases, the first descriptions on bacteria and viral organisms, [unreliable source?] the distinction of mediastinitis from pleurisy, the contagious nature of phthisis and tuberculosis, the distribution of diseases by water and soil, and the first careful descriptions of skin troubles, sexually transmitted diseases, perversions, and nervous ailments.[16]It also included the use of ice to treat fevers, and the separation of medicine from pharmacology, which was important to the development of the pharmaceutical sciences. Abū Rayhān al-Bīrūnī's *Kitab-al-Saidana* was an extensive medical encyclopedia which synthesised Islamic medicine with Indian medicine. His medical investigations included one of the earliest descriptions on

Siamese twins. Ibn Al-Thahabi (d. 1033) was famous for writing the first known alphabetical encyclopedia of medicine.

Ibn al-Nafis (1213-88) wrote *Al-Shamil fi al-Tibb* (*The Comprehensive Book on Medicine*), a voluminous medical encyclopedia that was originally planned to comprise three hundred volumes, but he was only able to complete eighty volumes as a result of his death in 1288. However, even in its incomplete state, the book is one of the largest known medical encyclopedias in history, though only a small portion of *The Comprehensive Book on Medicine* has survived. During his lifetime, *The Comprehensive Book on Medicine* had eventually replaced Ibn Sina's *The Canon of Medicine* as a medical authority in the medieval Islamic world. Arabic biographers from the thirteenth century onwards considered Ibn al-Nafis the greatest physician in history, some referring to him as 'the second Ibn Sina', and others considering him even greater than Ibn Sina. The last major medical encyclopedia from the Islamic world was Şerafeddin Sabuncuoğlu's surgical atlas, *Cerrahiyyetu'l-Haniyye* (*Imperial Surgery*). Though his work was mostly based on Abu al-Qasim al-Zahrawi's *Al-Tasrif*, he also introduced many innovations of his own.

Legacy

George Sarton, the father of the history of science, wrote in the *Introduction to the History of Science* as under:

> Through their medical investigations they not merely widened the horizons of medicine, but enlarged humanistic concepts generally. Thus it can hardly have been accidental that those researches should have led them that were inevitably beyond the reach of Greek masters. If it is regarded as symbolic that the most spectacular achievement of the mid-twentieth century is atomic fission and the nuclear bomb, likewise it would not seem fortuitous that the early Muslim's medical endeavor should have led to a discovery that was quite as revolutionary though possibly more beneficent. A philosophy of self-centredness, under whatever disguise, would be both incomprehensible and reprehensible to the Muslim mind. That mind was incapable of viewing man, whether in health

or sickness as isolated from God, from fellow men, and from the world around him. It was probably inevitable that the Muslims should have discovered that disease need not be born within the patient himself but may reach from outside, in other words, that they should have been the first to establish clearly the existence of contagion. One of the most famous exponents of Muslim universalism and an eminent figure in Islamic learning was Ibn Sina, known in the West as Avicenna (981-1037). For a thousand years he has retained his original renown as one of the greatest thinkers and medical scholars in history. His most important medical works are the Qanun (Canon) and a treatise on cardiac drugs. The 'Qanun fi-l-Tibb' is an immense encyclopedia of medicine. It contains some of the most illuminating thoughts pertaining to distinction of mediastinitis from pleurisy; contagious nature of phthisis; distribution of diseases by water and soil; careful description of skin troubles; of sexual diseases and perversions; of nervous ailments. We have reason to believe that when, during the crusades, Europe at last began to establish hospitals, they were inspired by the Arabs of near East . . . The first hospital in Paris, Les Quinze-vingt, was founded by Louis IX after his return from the crusade 1254-1260.

Scientific Method

Like in other fields of Islamic science, Muslim physicians and doctors developed the first scientific methods for the field of medicine. This included the introduction of Mathematisation, quantification, experimentation, experimental medicine, evidence-based medicine, clinical trials,[37] dissection, animal testing, human experimentation and post-mortem autopsy by Muslim physicians, whilst hospitals in the Islamic world featured the first drug tests, drug purity regulations, and competency tests for doctors.

Mathematisation

In the ninth century, al-Kindi (Alkindus), in *De Gradibus*, demonstrated the application of mathematics and quantification to medicine, particularly in the field of pharmacology. This includes the development of a mathematical scale to quantify the strength of drugs and a system that would allow a doctor to determine in advance the most critical days of a patient's illness, based on the phases of the moon.

Experimental Method

In the tenth century, Razi (Rhazes) introduced controlled experiment and clinical observation into the field of medicine and rejected several Galenic medical theories unverified by experimentation. The earliest known medical experiment was carried out by Razi in order to find the most hygienic place to build a hospital. He hung pieces of meat in different places throughout tenth-century Baghdad and observed where the meat decomposed least quickly, and that was where he built the hospital. In his *Comprehensive Book of Medicine*, Razi recorded clinical cases of his own experience and provided very useful recordings of various diseases. He also introduced urinalysis and stool tests. Avicenna (Ibn Sina) is considered the father of modern medicine for the introduction of experimental medicine, clinical trials, risk-factor analysis, and the idea of a syndrome in the diagnosis of specific diseases in his medical encyclopedia, *The Canon of Medicine* (c. 1025), which was also the first book dealing with evidence-based medicine, randomised controlled trials, and efficacy tests. According to Toby Huff and A. C. Crombie, the *Canon* contained 'a set of rules that laid down the conditions for the experimental use and testing of drugs', which were 'a precise guide for practical experimentation' in the process of 'discovering and proving the effectiveness of medical substances'. Avicenna's emphasis on tested medicines laid the foundations for an experimental approach to pharmacology. The *Canon* laid out the following rules and principles for testing the effectiveness of new drugs and medications, which still form the basis of clinical pharmacology and modern clinical trials:

> (1) The drug must be free from any extraneous accidental quality. It must be used on a simple, not a composite, disease. (2) The drug must be tested with two contrary types of diseases, because sometimes a drug cures one disease by its essential qualities and another by its accidental ones. (3) The quality of the drug must correspond to the strength of the

disease. For example, there are some drugs whose heat is less than the coldness of certain diseases, so that they would have no effect on them. The time of action must be observed, so that essence and accident are not confused. (4) The effect of the drug must be seen to occur constantly or in many cases, for if this did not happen, it was an accidental effect. (5) The experimentation must be done with the human body, for testing a drug on a lion or a horse might not prove anything about its effect on man.

One of the earliest physicians known to have performed human dissection and post-mortem autopsy in his medical experiments was Ibn Zuhr (Avenzoar) who introduced the experimental method into surgery, for which he is considered the father of experimental surgery. There were a number of other early practitioners of human dissection and autopsy at the time, including Ibn Tufail Saladin's physicians al-Shayzariand Ibn Jumay, Abd-el-latif, and Ibn al-Nafis. The experimental method was introduced into botany, materia medica and the agricultural sciences in the thirteenth century by the Andalusian-Arab botanist Abu al-Abbas al-Nabati, the teacher of Ibn al-OBaitar. Al-Nabati introduced empirical techniques in the testing, describing, and identifing of numerous materia medica, and he separated unverified reports from those supported by actual tests and observations.[37]

Peer Review

The first documented description of a peer review process is found in the *Ethics of the Physician* written by Ishaq bin Ali al-Rahwi (854-931) of al-Raha, Syria, who describes the first medical peer review process. His work, as well as later Arabic medical manuals, states that a visiting physician must always make duplicate notes of a patient's condition on every visit. When the patient was cured or had died, the notes of the physician were examined by a local medical council of other physicians, who would review the practicing physician's notes to decide whether his/her performance have met the required standards of medical care. If their reviews were negative, the practicing physician could face a lawsuit from a maltreated patient.

Anatomy and Physiology

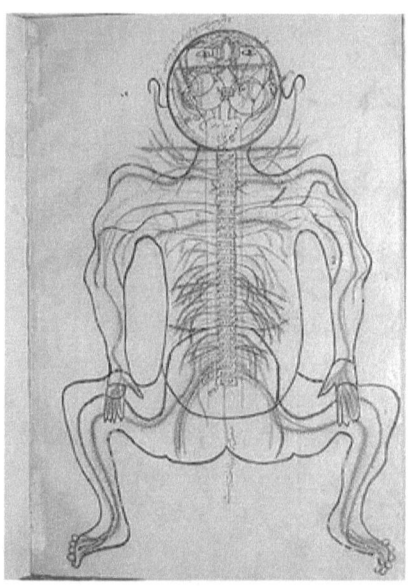

From: Mansur Ibn Ilyas: TASHRĪḤ-I BADAN-I INSĀN:
Manuscript, c. 1450, U.S. National Library of Medicine.

The above physiological picture can help to understand how such a disease as diarrhoea can act as source of blood drain on the victim. It is not sufficient just to treat the diarrhoea, the underlying causes must also be determined to prevent the future occurrence of this malady.

Experimental Anatomy and Physiology

The contributions of Ibn al-Haytham (Alhacen) to anatomy and physiology include many improvements in our understanding of the process of visual perception in his *Book of Optics*, published in 1021. Other innovations introduced by Muslim physicians to the field of physiology by this time include the use of animal testing and human dissection. The increased use of dissection in the twelfth and thirteenth centuries was influenced by the writings of the Islamic theologian, Al-Ghazali, who encouraged the study of anatomy and use of dissections as a method of gaining knowledge of God's creation.

Ibn Zuhr (Avenzoar) (1091-1161) was one of the earliest physicians known to have carried out human dissection and post-mortem autopsy. He proved that the skin disease scabies was caused by a parasite, a discovery which upset the theory of humorism supported by Hippocrates and Galen. The removal of the parasite from the patient's body did not involve purging, bleeding, or any other traditional treatments associated with the four humours. In the twelfth century, Saladin's physicians, al-Shayzariand Ibn Jumay, were also among the earliest to undertake human dissection, and they made explicit appeals to other physicians to do so as well. During a famine in Egypt in 1200, Abd-el-latif observed and examined a large number of skeletons, and he discovered that Galen was incorrect regarding the formation of the bones of the lower jaw and sacrum. The opening page of a medical work by Ibn al-Nafis, the father of the circulatory physiology. This is probably a copy made in India during the seventeenth or eighteenth century.

Circulatory Anatomy and Physiology

Ibn al-Nafis, the father of circulatory physiology, was another early proponent of human dissection. In 1242, he was the first to describe the pulmonary circulation, coronary circulation, and capillary circulation, which form the basis of the circulatory system, for which he is considered one of the greatest physiologists of the Middle Ages. The first European descriptions of the pulmonary circulation came several centuries later, by Michael Servetus in 1553 and William Harvey in 1628. Ibn al-Nafis also described the earliest concept of metabolism, and developed new Nafisian systems of anatomy, physiology, and psychology to replace the Avicennian and Galenic doctrines, while discrediting many of their erroneous theories on the four humours, pulsation, bones, muscles, intestines, sensory organs, bilious canals, esophagus, stomach, and the anatomy of almost every other part of the human body. The Arab physician Ibn al-Lubudi (1210-67), also from Damascus, wrote the *Collection of Discussions Relative to Fifty Psychological and Medical Questions*, in which he rejects the theory of four humours supported by Galen and Hippocrates, discovers that the body and its preservation depend exclusively upon blood, rejects Galen's idea that women can produce sperm, and discovers that the movement of arteries is not dependent upon the movement of the heart, that the heart is the first organ to form in a fetus' body (rather than the brain as claimed by Hippocrates), and that the bones forming the skull can grow into tumors. He also advises that in cases of extreme fever, a patient should not be released from hospital.[citation needed] In the fifteenth century, the Tashrih al-badan (*Anatomy of the Body*) written by Mansur ibn Ilyas contained comprehensive diagrams of the body's structural, nervous, and circulatory systems.

Pulsology and Sphygmology

Muslim physicians were pioneers in pulsology and sphygmology. In ancient times, Galen as well as Chinese physicians erroneously believed that there was a unique type of pulse for every organ of the body and for every disease. Galen also erroneously believed that 'every part of an artery pulsates simultaneously' and that the motion of the pulse was due to natural motions (the arteries expanding and contracting naturally) as opposed to forced motions (the heart causing the arteries to either expand or contract). The first correct explanation of pulsation was given by Muslim physicians. Avicenna was a pioneer of sphygmology after he refined Galen's theory of the pulse and discovered the following in *The Canon of Medicine*:

> Every beat of the pulse comprises two movements and two
> pauses. Thus, expansion: pause: contraction: pause. The pulse
> is a movement in the heart and arteries which takes the form
> of alternate expansion and contraction.

Avicenna also pioneered the modern approach of examining the pulse through the examination of the wrist, which is still practised in modern times. His reasons for choosing the wrist as the ideal location is due to it being easily available and the patient not needing to be distressed at the exposure of his/her body. The Latin translation of his *Canon* also laid the foundations for the later invention of the sphygmograph. Ibn al-Nafis, in his *Commentary on Anatomy* in Avicenna's *Canon*, completely rejected the Galenic theory of pulsation after his discovery of the pulmonary circulation. He developed his own Nafisian theory of pulsation after discovering that pulsation is a result of both natural and forced motions, and that the 'forced motion must be the contraction of the arteries caused by the expansion of the heart, and the natural motion must be the expansion of the arteries.' He notes that the 'arteries and the heart do not expand and contract at the same time, but rather the one contracts while the other expands' and vice versa. He also recognised that the purpose of the pulse is to help disperse the blood from the heart to the rest of the body. Ibn al-Nafis briefly summarises his new theory of pulsation as follows:

> The primary purpose of the expansion and contraction of the heart is to absorb the cool air and expel the wastes of the spirit and the warm air; however, the ventricle of the heart is wide. Moreover, when it expands it is not possible for it to absorb air until it is full, for that would then ruin the temperament of the spirit, its substance and texture, as well as the temperament of the heart. Thus, the heart is necessarily forced to complete its fill by absorbing the spirit.

Epidemiology, Aetiology, and Pathology

In aetiology and epidemiology, Muslim physicians were responsible for the discovery of infectious disease and the immune system, advances in pathology, and early hypotheses related to bacteriology and microbiology.[34] Their discovery of contagious disease in particular is considered revolutionary and is one of the most important discoveries in medicine. The earliest ideas on contagion can be traced back to several Hadiths attributed to Muhammad in the seventh century, who is said to have understood the contagious nature of leprosy, mange, and sexually transmitted disease.[60] These early ideas on contagion arose from the generally sympathetic attitude of Muslim physicians towards lepers (who were often seen in a negative light in other ancient and medieval societies), which can be traced back through Hadiths attributed to Muhammad and to the following advice given in the Koran: 'There is no fault in the blind, and there is no fault in the lame, and there is no fault in the sick.'

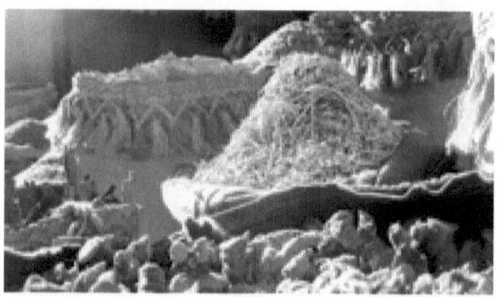

A group of Arabic spices and herbs in bowls,
usually used in medicine, and Arabic Cuisine.

This eventually led to the theory of contagious disease, which was fully understood by Avicenna in the eleventh century. By then, the pathology of contagion had been fully understood, and as a result, hospitals were created with separate wards for specific illnesses, so that people with contagious diseases could be kept away from other patients who did not have any contagious diseases. In *The Canon of Medicine* (1020), Avicenna discovered the contagious nature of infectious diseases such as phthisis and tuberculosis, the distribution of diseases by water and soil, and fully understood the contagious nature of sexually transmitted diseases. In epidemiology, he introduced the method of quarantine as a means of limiting the spread of contagious diseases[26] and introduced the method of risk-factor analysis and the idea of a syndrome in the diagnosis of specific diseases. In order to find the most hygienic place to build a hospital, Muhammad ibn Zakariya ar-Razi (Rhazes) carried out an experiment where he hung pieces of meat in places throughout tenth-century Baghdad and observed where the meat decomposed least quickly. Razi also wrote the *Comprehensive Book of Medicine* in the ninth century. The *Large Comprehensive* was the most sought-after of all his compositions, in which Razi recorded clinical cases of his own experience and provided very useful recordings of various diseases, as well as the discovery of measles and smallpox. The *Large Comprehensive* also criticised the views of Galen, after Razi had observed many clinical cases which did not follow Galen's descriptions of fevers. For example, he stated that Galen's descriptions of urinary ailments were inaccurate as he had only seen three cases, while Razi had studied hundreds of such cases in hospitals of Baghdad and Rayy. Chickenpox was also first identified by Razi, who clearly distinguished it from smallpox and measles. The *Comprehensive Book of Medicine*, especially *with its introduction of measles, smallpox, and chickenpox, was very influential in Europe.* Ibn Zuhr (Avenzoar) was the first physician to provide a real scientific aetiology for the inflammatory diseases of the ear, and the first to clearly discuss the causes of stridor. He also gave the first accurate descriptions on neurological diseases, including meningitis, intracranial thrombophlebitis, and mediastinal germ cell tumours. Averroes suggested the existence of Parkinson's disease and attributed photoreceptor properties to the retina. The Jewish Maimonides wrote about neuropsychiatric disorders.

Haematology and Heredity

In haematology, Abu al-Qasim al-Zahrawi (Abulcasis) wrote the first description on haemophilia, a hereditary genetic disorder, in his *Al-Tasrif*, in which he wrote of an Andalusian family whose males died of bleeding after minor injuries. When the Black Death bubonic plague reached al-Andalus in the fourteenth century, Ibn Khatima hypothesised that infectious diseases are caused by small 'minute bodies' that enter the human body and cause disease. Another fourteenth century Andalusian physician, Ibn al-Khatib (1313-74), wrote a treatise called *On the Plague*, in which he stated as follows:

> The existence of contagion is established by experience, investigation, the evidence of the senses and trustworthy reports. These facts constitute a sound argument. The fact of infection becomes clear to the investigator who notices how he who establishes contact with the afflicted gets the disease, whereas he who is not in contact remains safe, and how transmission is affected through garments, vessels and earrings.

Parasitology

In parasitology, Ibn Zuhr, through his dissections, was able to prove that the skin disease scabies was caused by a parasite, a discovery which upset the theory of humorism supported by Hippocrates, Galen, and Avicenna. The removal of the parasite from the patient's body did not involve purging, bleeding, or any other traditional treatments associated with the four humours.

Dentistry and Dental Surgery

Muslim dentists were pioneers in dentistry, particularly dental surgery and dental restoration. The earliest medical text to deal with dental surgery in detail was the *Al-Tasrif* by Abulcasis. He gave detailed methods for the successful replantation of dislodged teeth.

Dental Restoration

Another tenth-century Arab dentist, Abu Gaafar Amed ibn Ibrahim ibn abi Halid al-Gazzar, from North Africa, described methods of dental restoration in his *Kitab Zad al-Musafir wa qut al-Hadir* (*Provision for the traveler and nutrition for the sedentary*), which was later translated into Latin as *Viaticum* by Constantine the African in Salerno. He provided the earliest treatment for dental caries as follows:

> With caries purging must take place first, and then the teeth can be filled with gallnut, dyer's, buckthorn, terbinth resine, cedar resine, myrrh, pellitory and honey, or fumigated with colocynthis root.

Al-Gazzar also recommended arsenic compound in his prescription for holes in the teeth, as well as against dental caries, loosening, and relaxing of the nerves as a result of too many fluids. Avicenna dedicated many chapters of *The Canon of Medicine* to dentistry, particularly dental restoration. Influenced by al-Gazzar, he provided his own treatment for dental caries, stating that carious teeth should be filled with cypress, grass, mastix, myrrh, or styrox, or among others, with gallnut, yellow sulphur, pepper, camphor, and with drugs for pain relief, like arsenic or wolf's milk. He further stated that arsenic boiled in oil should be dripped into the carious defect. Both Avicenna and al-Gazzar, however, believed that dental caries were caused by 'tooth worms' like what the ancients believed. This was proven false in 1200 by another Muslim physician named Gaubari in his *Book of the Elite*, concerning the unmasking of mysteries and tearing of veils and in which a chapter was dedicated to dentistry. He was the first to reject the idea of caries being caused by tooth worms, and he stated that tooth worms, in fact, do not even exist. The theory of the tooth worm was thus no longer accepted in the Islamic medical community from the thirteenth century onwards.

Obstetrics and Perinatology

Muslim physicians made many advances in obstetrics, especially perinatology. In ancient times, Greek and Hellenistic writers such as Hippocrates, Galen, Ptolemy, and Paul of Aegina erroneously believed that uterine contractions were only an indication of the onset of childbirth and that the fetus would subsequently swim its way out of the womb and birth canal. In the tenth century, Ali ibn Abbas al-Majusi proved this theory false as he discovered that uterine contractions are in fact the cause of delivery of the fetus. Abu al-Qasim al-Zahrawi offered advice to midwives on childbirth and complex obstetrics in his *Al-Tasrif* (1000) and made a number of advances in the field. He pioneered the method of episiotomy for the delivery of obstructed labour, and he introduced the required surgical instruments for this operation. Caesarean sections were described in detail by Ferdowsi in his *Shahnameh* (1010) and by al-Biruni in his *Al-Athar al-Baliyah*.

Embryology

Further information: The relation between Islam and science: Embryology

Embryology was discussed to some extent in early Islamic literature, including the Koran and the Hadith literature (see The relation between Islam and science for more details). Ibn al-Nafis criticised previous Aristotelian, Galenic, and Avicennian explanations of embryology and proceeded to develop his own theories on embryology and generation. He believed that when a male and female semen mix, and when they create a mixed matter that has an appropriate temperament to receive an animal or human soul, God issues a soul to this matter, which then develops into an embryo that grows and generates organs. He further writes as follows:

> Galen believes that each of the two semen has in it the active faculty to fashion and the passive faculty to be fashioned, however the active faculty is stronger in the male semen while the passive in the female semen. The investigators amongst the falasifa believe that the male semen only has the active faculty, while the female only has the passive faculty. As for

our opinion on this, and God knows best, neither of the two semen has in it an active faculty to fashion.

He then shows that once the male semen and female semen are brought together in the womb, the female semen quenches the hot fire of the male semen through its own cool and wet nature. The Arab physician Ibn al-Quff (1233-1305), a student of Ibn al-Nafis, described embryology and perinatology more accurately in his *Al-Jami* as follows: sixteen days, is gradually transformed into a clot and in twenty-eight to thirty days into a small chunk of meat. In thirty-eight to forty days, the head appears separate from the shoulders and limbs. The brain and heart followed by the liver are formed before other organs. The fetus takes its food from the mother in order to grow and to replenish what it discards or loses . . . There are three membranes covering and protecting the fetus, of which the first connects arteries and veins with those in the mothers womb through the umbilical cord. The veins pass food for the nourishment of the fetus, while the arteries transmit air. By the end of seven months, all organs are complete . . . After delivery the baby's umbilical cord is cut at a distance of four fingers breadth from the body, and is tied with fine, soft woolen twine. The area of the cut is covered with a filament moistened in olive oil over which a styptic to prevent bleeding is sprinkled . . . After delivery, the baby is nursed by his mother whose milk is the best. Then the midwife puts the baby to sleep in a darkened quiet room . . . Nursing the baby is performed two to three times daily. Before nursing, the mother's breast should be squeezed out two or three times to get rid of the milk near the nipple.

Pharmaceutical Sciences

Al-Kindi was a renowned ninth-century Arab doctor who wrote many books on the subject of medicine. His most important work in the field was *De Gradibus*, in which he demonstrated the application of mathematics to medicine, particularly in the field of pharmacology. This includes the development of a mathematical scale to quantify the strength of drugs and a system that would allow a doctor to determine in advance the most critical days of a patient's illness based on the phases of the Moon. In his *Comprehensive Book of Medicine*, Razi (Rhazes) recorded clinical cases of his own experience and provided very useful recordings of various diseases. The *Comprehensive Book of Medicine*, with its introduction of measles and smallpox, was very influential in Europe. Razi also carried out an experiment in order to find the most hygienic place to build a hospital. He hung pieces of meat in places throughout tenth-century Baghdad and observed where the meat decomposed least quickly, and that was where he built his hospital. In the tenth century, Abu al-Mansur al-Muwaffak mentioned for the first time some chemical facts to distinguish certain medicines.

Clinical Pharmacology

Avicenna's contribution to pharmacology and the pharmaceutical sciences in *The Canon of Medicine* (1020s) include the following: the introduction of clinical pharmacology, experimental medicine, evidence-based medicine, clinical trials, randomised-controlled-trials-efficacy tests, the experimental use and testing of drugs, and a precise guide for practical experimentation in the process of discovering and proving the effectiveness of medical substances. It also includes the first careful descriptions of skin troubles, sexually transmitted diseases, perversions, and nervous ailments, as well the use of ice to treat fevers, and the separation of medicine from pharmacology, which was important to the development of the pharmaceutical sciences. The *Canon* laid out the following rules and principles for testing the effectiveness of new drugs and medications, which still form the basis of clinical pharmacology[1] and modern clinical trials:

> (1) The quality of the drug must correspond to the strength of the disease. For example, there are some drugs whose heat is less than the coldness of certain diseases, so that they would have no effect on them. (2) The time of action must be observed, so that essence and accident are not confused. (3) The effect of the drug must be seen to occur constantly or in many cases, for if this did not happen, it was an accidental effect. (4) The experimentation must be done with the human body, for testing a drug on a lion or a horse might not prove anything about its effect on man.

Pharmacy

The first drugstores were opened by Muslim pharmacists in Baghdad in 754 during the Abbasid Caliphate—also known as the 'Islamic Golden Age'. Due to the extraordinary advances that were made in the fields of chemistry and botany by Muslim chemists in the Middle East, it was a motive for the Muslim physicians to develop the study of pharmacology. In the beginning, medicine and chemistry were kept separate from pharmacy; the ninth century was when pharmacies were first recognised. They were not only simply stores where one could buy medicine and drugs—pharmacists had also been skilled and knowledgeable in compounding, preserving, and storing the different types of drugs. As Baghdad had been the 'central learning' region of the Middle East at the time, it was not only a place where around sixty pharmaceuticals were dispensing drugs by prescription (in Baghdad alone), but it was also the region where the first school of pharmacy was established by the Caliph al Ma'mun. The new, increasing interest in pharmacology not only benefited the process of healing those in need, but it also seemed to correlate with the increase in literary productivity—books were being written and published describing new remedies, treaties, and natural medicinal substances. Schooling, examination, and licensing were required as of AD 931 by the Caliph Al-Muqtadir in Baghdad after he had learnt that a patient had died as a result of a physician's error. Afterwards, he had ordered Sinan-ibn Thabit bin Qurrah (his chief physician) to evaluate all those who claimed to be practising the 'art of healing'. In Baghdad alone, over 860 practitioners were examined over the first year. From then on, al-Muhtasib (meaning government inspector) inspected pharmacies on regular bases, ensuring that things such as the quality of drugs sold at the pharmacies and apothecaries was good and measures and weights of the traders were well maintained.

The advances made in the Middle East by Muslim chemists in botany and chemistry led Muslim physicians to substantially develop pharmacology. Muhammad ibn Zakarīya Rāzi (Rhazes) (865-915), for instance, acted to promote the medical uses of chemical compounds. Abu al-Qasim al-Zahrawi (Abulcasis) (936-1013) pioneered the preparation of medicines by sublimation and distillation. His *Liber servitoris* is of particular interest, as it provides the reader with recipes and explains how to prepare the 'simples' from which were compounded the complex drugs then generally used. Shapur ibn Sahl (d. 869) was, however, the first physician to initiate pharmacopoeia, describing a large variety of drugs and remedies for ailments. Al-Biruni (973-1050) wrote one of the most valuable Islamic works on pharmacology, entitled *Kitab al-Saydalah* (*The Book of Drugs*), where he gave detailed knowledge of the properties of drugs and outlined the role of pharmacy and the functions and duties of the pharmacist. Avicenna, too, described no less than seven hundred preparations, their properties, mode of action, and their indications. He devoted, in fact, a whole volume to simple drugs in *The Canon of Medicine*. Of great impact were also the works by al-Maridini of Baghdad and Cairo, and Ibn al-Wafid (1008-74), both of which were printed in Latin more than fifty times, appearing as *De Medicinis universalibus et particularibus* by 'Mesue' the younger, and the *Medicamentis simplicibus* by 'Abenguefit'. Peter of Abano (1250-1316) translated and added a supplement to the work of al-Maridini under the title *De Veneris*. Al-Muwaffaq's contributions in the field are also pioneering. Living in the tenth century, he wrote *The foundations of the true properties of Remedies*, among others, describing arsenious oxide and being acquainted with silicic acid. He made clear distinction between sodium carbonate and potassium carbonate and drew attention to the poisonous nature of copper compounds, especially copper vitriol, and also lead compounds. For the story, he also mentions the distillation of sea-water for drinking.

Analgesics, Anti-Emetics, Antipyretics, Diuretics

In the medieval Islamic world, Arabic physicians discovered the diuretic, anti-emetic, antiepileptic, anti-inflammatory, analgesic (painkilling), and antipyretic properties of medical cannabis, specifically cannabis sativa, and used it extensively as medication from the eighth to eighteenth centuries.

Antiseptics

Razi (tenth century) used mercurial compounds as topical antiseptics. From the tenth century, Muslim physicians and surgeons were applying purified alcohol to wounds as an antiseptic agent. Surgeons in Islamic Spain utilised special methods for maintaining asepsis prior to and during surgery. They also originated specific protocols for maintaining hygiene during the post-operative period. Their success rate was so high that dignitaries throughout Europe came to Córdoba, Spain, to be treated at what was comparably the 'Mayo Clinic' of the Middle Ages. This is wonderful indeed.

Medical and Therapeutic Drugs

Razi, Avicenna, al-Kindi, Ibn Rushd, Abu al-Qasim, Ibn Zuhr, Ibn al-Baitar, Ibn Al-Jazzar, Ibn Juljul, Ibn al-Quff, Ibn an-Nafs, al-Biruni, Ibn Sahl, and hundreds of other Muslim physicians developed drug therapy and medicinal drugs for the treatment of specific symptoms and diseases. Their use of practical experience and careful observation was extensive. Chemotherapeutical drugs were first developed in the Muslim world. Muslim physicians used a variety of specific substances to destroy microbes. They applied (Media: sulphur) topically specifically to kill the scabies mite. Abulcasis developed a variety of medications, which he described in the cosmetics chapter of *Al-Tasrif* (*c.* 1000). For epilepsy and seizures, he invented medications called *Ghawali* and *Lafayfe*. For the relief and treatment of common colds, he invented *Muthallaathat*, which was prepared from camphor, musk and honey, similar to Vicks Vapour Rub, a modern topical cream. Abulcasis also invented nasal sprays and hand cream, and developed effective mouthwashes.[citation needed]

Medicinal Alcohol

Numerous Muslim chemists produced medicinal-grade alcohol through distillation as early as the tenth century and manufactured on a large scale the first distillation devices for use in chemistry. They used alcohol as a solvent and antiseptic.

Surgery

Abu al-Qasim al-Zahrawi (Abulcasis), regarded as the father of modern surgery, contributed greatly to the discipline of medical surgery with his *Kitab al-Tasrif* (*Book of Concessions* or *The Method of Medicine*), a thirty-volume medical encyclopedia published in 1000, which was later translated to Latin and used in European medical schools for centuries. His influential *al-Tasrif* introduced his famous collection of over two hundred surgical instruments. Many of these instruments were never used before by any previous surgeons. Hamidan, for example, listed at least twenty-six innovative surgical instruments that were not known before Abulcasis. The surgical instruments he invented include the first instruments unique to women as well as the surgical uses of catgut and forceps, the ligature, surgical needle, scalpel, curette, retractor, surgical spoon, sound, surgical hook, surgical rod, specula,[citation needed] bone saw, and plaster His work also included anatomical descriptions and sections on orthopaedic surgery and ophthalmology. The influence of the *Al–Tasrif* eventually led to the decline of the barber surgeons who were prevalent before his time, and they were, instead, replaced by physician-surgeons in the Islamic world.

Ibn al-Haytham (Alhacen) made important advances in eye surgery, as he studied and correctly explained the process of sight and visual perception for the first time in his *Book of Optics*, published in 1021. Avicenna was the first to describe the surgical procedure of intubation in order to facilitate breathing, and he also described the 'soporific sponge', an anaesthetic imbued with aromatics and narcotics, which was to be placed under a patient's nose during surgical operations. He also described the first known surgical treatment for cancer, stating that the excision should be radical and that all diseased tissue should be removed, including the use of amputation or the removal of veins running in the direction of the tumor. Ammar ibn Ali al-Mawsili is also notable for inventing the injection syringe and hypodermic needle for the extraction of cataracts in the first successful cataract surgery. Ibn al-Nafis dedicated a volume of *The Comprehensive Book on Medicine* to surgery. He described three stages of a surgical operation. The first stage is the preoperative period, which he calls the 'time of presentation' when the surgeon carries out a diagnosis on the affected area of the patient's body. The second stage is the actual operation, which he calls the 'time of operative treatment' when the surgeon repairs the affected organs of the patient. The third stage is the post-operative period, which he calls the 'time of preservation' when the patient needs to take care of himself and be taken care of by nurses and doctors until he recovers. *The Comprehensive Book on Medicine* was also the earliest book dealing with the decubitus of a patient.

Anaesthesiology

General anaesthesia and general anaesthetics were pioneered by Muslim anaesthesiologists, who were the first to utilise oral as well as inhalant anaesthetics. In Islamic Spain, Abu al-Qasim and Ibn Zuhr, among other Muslim surgeons, performed hundreds of surgeries under inhalant anaesthesia with the use of narcotic-soaked sponges that were placed over the face. Muslim physicians also introduced the anaesthetic value of opium derivatives during the Middle Ages. Laudanum was also used as an anaesthetic. Avicenna wrote about its medical uses in his works, which later influenced the works of Paracelsus. Sigrid Hunke wrote as follows:

> The science of medicine has gained a great and extremely important discovery and that is the use of general anaesthetics for surgical operations, and how unique, efficient, and merciful for those who tried it the Muslim anaesthetic was. It was quite different from the drinks the Indians, Romans and Greeks were forcing their patients to have for relief of pain. There had been some allegations to credit this discovery to an Italian or to an Alexandrian, but the truth is and history proves that, the art of using the anaesthetic sponge is a pure Muslim technique, which was not known before. The sponge used to be dipped and left in a mixture prepared from cannabis, opium, hyoscyamus and a plant called Zoan.

Cataract Surgery Ophthalmology

Experimental Surgery

Ibn Zuhr (Avenzoar) is considered the father of experimental surgery, for introducing the experimental method into surgery in his *Al-Taisir*. He was the first to employ animal testing in order to experiment with surgical procedures before applying them to human patients.[42] He also performed the first dissections and post-mortem autopsies on humans as well as animals.

Surgical Instruments, Adhesive Bandage, and Plaster

Abu al-Qasim al-Zahrawi (Abulcasis), in his *Al-Tasrif* (1000), invented the modern plaster and adhesive bandage, which are still used in hospitals throughout the world. The use of plasters for fractures became a standard practice for Arab physicians, though this practice was not widely adopted in Europe until the nineteenth century.

Cotton Dressing

Al-Zahrawi was the first surgeon to make use of cotton (which itself is derived from the Arabic word *qutn*) as a medical dressing for controlling haemorrhage.

Injection Syringe and Hypodermic Needle

The Iraqi surgeon Ammar ibn Ali al-Mawsili invented the first hollow hypodermic needle and injection syringe in *c.* 1000, using a hollow glass tube and suction to extract and remove cataracts from a patient's eye during a cataract surgery.

Aromatherapy

Steam distillation was invented by Avicenna in the early eleventh century for the purpose of producing essential oils, giving rise to aroma-therapy. As a result, he is regarded as a pioneer of aromatherapy.

Cancer Therapy

In cancer therapy, Avicenna described treatments for cancer in *The Canon of Medicine*: one was a surgical method involving amputation or removal of veins,[81] and the other was a herbal compound drug named 'Hindiba', which Ibn al-Baitar later identified as having 'anticancer' proper-ties and which could also treat other tumors and neoplastic disorders.[citation needed] After recognising its usefulness in treating neoplastic disorders, Hindiba was patented in 1997 by Nil Sari, Hanzade Dogan, and John K. Snyder.

Avicenna's *Canon* also described surgical treatment for cancer (although there was nothing new about this), stating that the excision should be radical and that all diseased tissue should be removed, including the use of amputation or the removal of veins running in the direction of the tumour.

Chromotherapy

Avicenna, who viewed colour to be of vital importance in diagnosis and treatment, made significant contributions to chromotherapy in *The Canon of Medicine*. He wrote that 'Color is an observable symptom of disease' and also developed a chart that related colour to the temperature and physical condition of the body. He further discussed the properties of colours for healing and was 'the first to establish that the wrong colour suggested for therapy would elicit no response in specific diseases.' As an example, 'He observed that a person with a nosebleed should not gaze at things of a brilliant red colour and should not be exposed to red light because this would stimulate the sanguineous humor, whereas blue would soothe it and reduce blood flow.'

Hirudotherapy

Hirudotherapy, the use of medicinal leech for medical purposes, was introduced by Avicenna in *The Canon of Medicine* (1020s). He considered the application of leech to be more useful than cupping in 'letting off the blood from deeper parts of the body.' He also introduced the use of leech as treatment for skin disease. Leech therapy became a popular method in medieval Europe due to the influence of his *Canon*. A more modern use for medicinal leech was introduced by Abd-el-latif in the twelfth century, who wrote that leech could be used for cleaning the tissues after surgical operations. He did, however, understand that there is a risk over using leech, and he advised patients that leech need to be cleaned before being used and that the dirt or dust 'clinging to a leech should be wiped off' before application. He further writes that after the leech has sucked out the blood, salt should be 'sprinkled on the affected part of the human body.'

Pharmacotherapy

Pharmaceutical sciences and Cancer therapy

Physiotherapy

Muslim physicians developed a method of therapy that began with diet and physiotherapy; if this didn't work for the patient, then prescriptions for drugs and medication were given; and if this didn't work, then they resorted to surgery. The physiotherapy prescribed by Muslim physicians usually included physical exercise and bathing. Muslim Arab physicians developed an elaborate system of dieting, in which there was an awareness of food deficiencies, and proper nutrition was an important item of treatment. Medical drugs were divided into two groups: simple and compound drugs. As they were aware of the interaction between drugs, they used simple drugs first; if these failed, then compound drugs, which are made from two or more compounds, were used; and if these conservative methods failed, then surgery was undertaken as a last resort.

Psychotherapy

Main article: Islamic Psychological Thought

Phytotherapy

In phytotherapy, Avicenna introduced the medicinal use of Taxus baccata L. in *The Canon of Medicine*. He named this herbal drug as 'Zarnab' and used it as a cardiac remedy. This was the first known use of a calcium channel blocker drug, which was not used in the Western world until the 1960s.

Urology

Muslim physicians from the Islamic world made many advances in the field of urology. Muhammad ibn Zakarīya Rāzi introduced the methods of urinalysis and stool testing, while other physicians dealt with the medical management and treatment of kidney stones, inflammations, infections, and sexual dysfunction. They pioneered advanced surgical approaches to the treatment of bladder stones as well as penile and scrotal problems, using techniques that are still used by modern physicians. They were also the first to produce tested drugs for the treatment of many urological disorders.

Lithotomy

In lithotomy, Abulcasis performed the first successful extraction of bladder and kidney stones from the urinary bladder, using a new instrument he invented—a lithotomy scalpel with two sharp cutting edges—and a new technique he invented—perineal cystolithotomy—which allowed him to crush a large stone inside the bladder before its removal, significantly decreasing the death rates previously caused by earlier attempts at this operation by the ancients.

Sexual Health

In sexual health, Muslim physicians and pharmacists identified the issues of sexual dysfunction and erectile dysfunction. They developed several methods of therapy for this issue, including the 'single-drug method' where a drug is prescribed, and a 'combination method of either a drug or food.' These drugs were also occasionally used for recreational drug use to improve male sexuality in general by those who did not suffer from sexual dysfunctions. Most of these drugs were oral medications, though a few patients were also treated through topical and transurethral means. Sexual dysfunctions were being treated with tested drugs in the Islamic world since the ninth century until the sixteenth century by a number of Muslim physicians and pharmacists, including al-Razi, Thabit bin Qurra, Ibn Al-Jazzar, Avicenna (*The Canon of Medicine*), Averroes, Ibn al-Baitar, and Ibn al-Nafis (*The Comprehensive Book on Medicine*).

Other Medieval Contributions

Other medical contributions first introduced by Muslim physicians include the discovery of the immune system, the introduction of microbiology, the use of animal testing, and the combination of medicine with other sciences (including agriculture, botany, chemistry, and pharmacology), as well as the first drugstores in Baghdad (754), the distinction between medicine and pharmacy in the twelfth century, and the discovery of at least two thousand medicinal substances. Other medical advances came in the fields of pharmacology and pharmacy, and in the following fields of the biomedical sciences:

Botany and Environmental Science

Main article: Muslim Agricultural Revolution (Further information: *Islamic geography*)

Muslims developed a scientific approach to botany and agriculture based on three major elements: sophisticated systems of crop rotation, highly developed irrigation techniques, and the introduction of a large variety of crops, which were studied and catalogued according to the season, type of land, and amount of water they required. Numerous encyclopedias on botany were produced with highly accurate precision and details. Al-Dinawari (828-96) is considered the founder of Arabic botany for his *Book of Plants*, in which he described at least 637 plants and discussed plant evolution from its birth to its death, describing the phases of plant growth and the production of flowers and fruit. In the early thirteenth century, the Andalusian-Arabian biologist Abu al-Abbas al-Nabati developed an early scientific method for botany, introducing empirical and experimental techniques in the testing, describing, and identifying of numerous materia medica, and separating unverified reports from those supported by actual tests and observations. His student Ibn al-Baitar published the *Kitab al-Jami fi al-Adwiya al-Mufrada*, which is considered one of the greatest botanical compilations in history, and was a botanical authority for centuries. It contains details on at least fourteen hundred different plants, foods, and drugs, thre hundred of which were his own original discoveries. The *Kitab al-Jami fi al-Adwiya al-Mufrada* was also influential in Europe after it was translated into Latin in 1758. The earliest known treatises dealing with environmentalism and environmental science, especially pollution, were Arabic treatises written by al-Kindi, Qusta ibn Luqa, al-Razi, Ibn Al-Jazzar, al-Tamimi, al-Masihi, Avicenna, Ali ibn Ridwan, Ibn Jumay, Isaac Israeli ben Solomon, Abd-el-latif, Ibn al-Quff, and Ibn al-Nafis. Their works covered a number of subjects related to pollution such as air pollution, water pollution, soil contamination, municipal solid waste mishandling, and environmental impact assessments of certain localities. Córdoba, al-Andalus, also had the first waste containers and waste disposal facilities for litter collection.

Child Development and Paediatrics

Ali ibn Sahl Rabban al-Tabari was a pioneer of paediatrics and the field of child development, which he discussed in his *Firdous al-Hikmah*. His student Muhammad ibn Zakariya al-Razi (Rhazes) wrote *The Diseases of Children*, the first book to deal with paediatrics as an independent field of medicine. Ibn Al-Jazzar also wrote a book on Children Medicine named *Siyaset al-Sebian*.

Endocrinology

In endocrinology, Avicenna (980-1037) provided a detailed account on diabetes mellitus in *The Canon of Medicine*, 'describing the abnormal appetite and the collapse of sexual functions' and he documented the 'sweet taste of diabetic urine.' Like Aretaeus of Cappadocia before him, Avicenna recognised a primary and secondary diabetes. He also described diabetic gangrene and treated diabetes by using a mixture of lupine, trigonella (fenugreek), and zedoary seed, which produces a considerable reduction in the excretion of sugar, a treatment which is still prescribed in modern times. Avicenna also 'described diabetes insipidus very precisely for the first time', though it was later Johann Peter Frank (1745-1821) who first differentiated between diabetes mellitus and diabetes insipidus. In the twelfth century, Zayn al-Din al-Jurjani provided the first description of Graves' disease after noting the association of goitre and exophthalmos in his *Thesaurus of the Shah of Khwarazm*, the major medical dictionary of its time. Al-Jurjani also established an association between goitre and palpitation.

Gerontology and Geriatrics

Avicenna's *The Canon of Medicine* was the first book to offer instruction for the care of the aged, foreshadowing modern gerontology and geriatrics. In a chapter entitled 'Regimen of Old Age', Avicenna wrote that 'old folk need plenty of sleep. Time spent on the couch should be liberal—more than is legitimate for adults.' He wrote that after waking up, the body should be anointed with oil 'to stimulate the sensitive faculties'. Regarding exercise, he recommended walking or horse-riding. He stated: 'The factors to consider in regard to exercise in old people are the various bodily states of different persons; the sequels likely to arise from their ailments; and their previous habits as regards exercise.'

He said that if the body is healthy, it can perform the attempted exercises, but if one part of the body is infirm, 'then that part should not be exercised until after the rest', and that exercises are to be strictly graduated 'as if the body were to be strengthened'. The *Canon* recognised four periods of life: the period of growth, prime of life, period of elderly decline (from forty to sixty), and decrepit age. He stated that during the last period, 'there is hardness of their bones, roughness of the skin, and the long time since they produced semen, blood and vaporal breath.' However, he agreed with Galen that the earth element is more prominent in the aged and the decrepit periods than in other periods. Avicenna did not agree with the concept of infirmity; however, he stated: 'There is no need to assert that there are three states of the human body—sickness, health and a state which is neither health nor disease. The first two cover everything.'

Thesis III of the *Canon* discussed the diet suitable for old people. Avicenna wrote that they should be given food in small amounts at a time and that they can have two to three meals a day, divided up according to the digestive powers and general condition of the old person in question. He also recommended fruits, such as figs and prunes. He also stated: 'Some laudable nutrition may be allowed at bedtime, [but] robust old folk may have a more liberal supper, as long as they avoid any gross aliment . . . all hot, sharp, or dessicative foods, such as dishes made with vinegar, salt, hot aromatics, seasonings and pickles. [Milk is good for the aged, being] nutritious and humectant in nature. [Yet] articles of food with a laxative action are most appropriate for the elderly.'

Ibn Al-Jazzar Al-Qayrawani (Algizar, *c.* 898-980), also wrote a special book on the medicine and health of the elderly, entitled *Kitab Tibb al-Machayikh*[110] or *Teb al-Mashaikh wa hefz sehatahom*.[111] He also wrote a book on sleep disorders and one on forgetfulness and how to strengthen memory, entitled *Kitab al-Nissian wa Toroq Taqwiati Adhakira*,[112][113][114] and a treatise on the causes of mortality, entitled *Rissala Fi Asbab al-Wafah*.[110] Another Arabic physician in the ninth century, Ishaq ibn Hunayn (died 910), the son of Hunayn Ibn Ishaq, wrote a *Treatise on Drugs for Forgetfulness* (*Risalah al-Shafiyah fi adwiyat al-nisyan*).

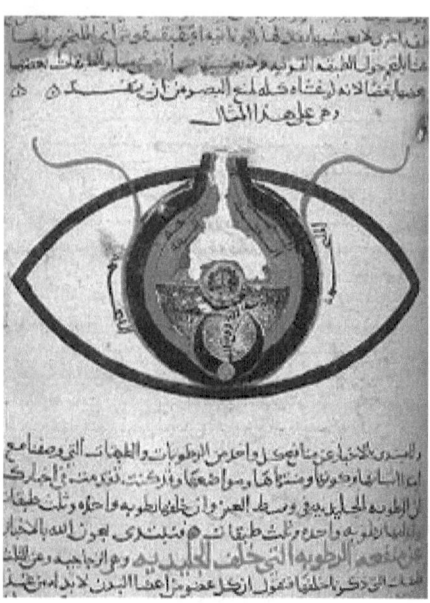

An Arabic manuscript, dated 1200 ce, titled
Anatomy of the Eye, authored by Al-Mutadibih.

12.2 Ophthalmology

Main article: Ophthalmology in medieval Islam

Of all the branches of Islamic medicine, ophthalmology was one of the foremost. The specialised instruments used in their operations ran into scores. Innovations such as the 'injection syringe', invented by the Iraqi physician Ammar ibn Ali of Mosul, which was used for the extraction by suction of soft cataracts, were quite common. In cataract surgery, Ammar ibn Ali attempted the earliest extraction of cataracts using suction. He introduced a hollow, metallic syringe hypodermic needle through the sclera and successfully extracted the cataracts through suction. Ibn al-Nafis, in *The Polished Book on Experimental Ophthalmology*, discovered that the muscle behind the eyeball does not support the ophthalmic nerve, that they do not get in contact with it, and that the optic nerves transect but do not get in touch with each other. He also discovered many new treatments for glaucoma and the weakness of vision in one eye when the other eye is affected by disease.[116]

Psychiatry and Psychology

Main Article: Psychology in Medieval Islam

The first psychiatric hospitals and insane asylums were built in the Islamic world as early as the eighth century. The first psychiatric hospitals were built by Arab Muslims in Baghdad in 705, Fes in the early eighth century, and Cairo in 800. Other famous psychiatric hospitals were built in Damascus and Aleppo in 1270. Unlike medieval Christian physicians who relied on demonological explanations for mental illness, medieval Muslim physicians relied mostly on clinical psychiatry and clinical observations on mentally ill patients. They made significant advances to psychiatry and were the first to provide psychotherapy and moral treatment for mentally ill patients, in addition to other new forms of treatment such as baths, drug medication, music therapy, and occupational therapy.

The concepts of mental health and 'mental hygiene' were introduced by the Muslim physician Ahmed ibn Sahl al-Balkhi (850-934). In his *Masalih al-Abdan wa al-Anfus* (*Sustenance for Body and Soul*), he was the first to successfully discuss diseases related to both the body and the mind, and argued that; if the *nafs* [psyche] gets sick, the body may also find no joy in life and may eventually develop a physical illness.'[118] Al-Balkhi was also a pioneer of psychotherapy, psychophysiology, and psychosomatic medicine. He recognised that the body and the soul can be healthy or sick, or 'balanced or imbalanced', and that mental illness can have both psychological and/or physiological causes. He wrote that imbalance of the body can result in fever, headaches, and other physical illnesses, while imbalance of the soul can result in anger, anxiety, sadness, and other mental symptoms. He recognised two types of depression: one caused by known reasons such as loss or failure, which can be treated psychologically; and the other caused by unknown reasons possibly caused by physiological reasons, which can be treated through physical medicine. Najab ud-din Muhammad (tenth century) described a number of mental diseases in detail. He made many careful observations of mentally ill patients and compiled them in a book that 'made up the most complete classification of mental diseases theretofore known.' The mental illnesses described by Najab include agitated depression, neurosis, priapism and sexual impotence (*Nafkhae Malikholia*), psychosis (*Kutrib*), and mania (*Dual-Kulb*). Symptoms resembling schizophrenia were also reported in later Arabic medical literature.

Muhammad ibn Zakarīya Rāzi (Rhazes) and al-Balkhi were the first known physicians to study psychotherapy. Razi in particular made significant advances in psychiatry in his landmark texts *El-Mansuri* and *Al-Hawi* in the tenth century, which presented definitions, symptoms, and treatments for problems related to mental health and mental illness. He also ran the psychiatric ward of a [Baghdad hospital]. Such institutions could not exist in Europe at the time because of fear of demonic possessions. In al-Andalus, Abu al-Qasim (Abulcasis), the father of modern surgery, developed material and technical designs that are still used in neurosurgery. Ibn Zuhr (Avenzoar) gave the first accurate descriptions on neurological disorders, including meningitis, intracranial thrombophlebitis, and mediastinal germ cell tumors, and made contributions to modern neuropharmacology. Averroes suggested the existence of Parkinson's disease and attributed photoreceptor properties to the retina. Maimonides wrote about neuropsychiatric disorders and described rabies and belladonna intoxication. Avicenna was a pioneer of psychophysiology and psychosomatic medicine. He recognised 'physiological psychology' in the treatment of illnesses involving emotions, and developed a system for associating changes in the pulse rate with inner feelings, which is seen as an anticipation of the word association test attributed to Carl Jung. Avicenna was also a pioneer of neuropsychiatry. He first described numerous neuropsychiatric conditions, including hallucination, insomnia, mania, nightmare, melancholia, dementia, epilepsy, paralysis, stroke, vertigo, and tremor.

Rheumatology

In rheumatology, Muhammad ibn Zakarīya Rāzi reported a psychotherapeutic case study from a contemporary tenth century Muslim physician who treated a woman suffering from severe cramps in her joints that made her unable to rise. The physician cured her by lifting her skirt, putting her to shame. He wrote: 'A flush of heat was produced within her, which dissolved the rheumatic humour.'

Zoology

Further Information: Early Islamic Philosophy: Evolution

The first Muslim biologist to develop a theory on evolution was al-Jahiz (781-869). He wrote about the effects of the environment on the likelihood of an animal to survive, and he first described the struggle for existence and an early form of natural selection.[121][122] Al-Jahiz was also the first to discuss food chains[123] and was also an early adherent of environmental determinism, arguing that the environment can determine the physical characteristics of the inhabitants of a certain community and that the origins of different human skin colours is the result of the environment. Ibn al-Haytham (Alhacen) wrote a book in which he argued for evolutionism (although not natural selection), and numerous other Islamic scholars and scientists, such as Ibn Miskawayh, the Brethren of Purity, al-Khazini, Abū Rayhān al-Bīrūnī, Nasir al-Din Tusi, and Ibn Khaldun discussed and developed these ideas. Translated into Latin, these works began to appear in the West after the Renaissance and appear to have had an impact on Western science.

12.3 Traditional Medicine in Ancient Rome

The basic Roman surgical instruments, found at Pompeii, include spoons, probes, spatulas, scissors, a lancet, a cautery iron, and a trocar and cannula combination. **Ancient Roman medicine** combined various techniques using different tools and rituals. Ancient Roman medicine included a number of specialisations such as intemistic, ophthalmology, and urology. The Romans favoured the prevention of diseases over the cures of them, and unlike in Greek society where health was a personal matter, Public health was encouraged by the government at the time. They built bathhouses and aqueducts to pipe water to the cities. Many of the larger cities, such as Rome, boasted an advanced sewage system, the likes of which would not be seen in the Western world again until the late seventeenth and eighteenth centuries. However, the Romans did not fully understand the involvement of germs in disease.

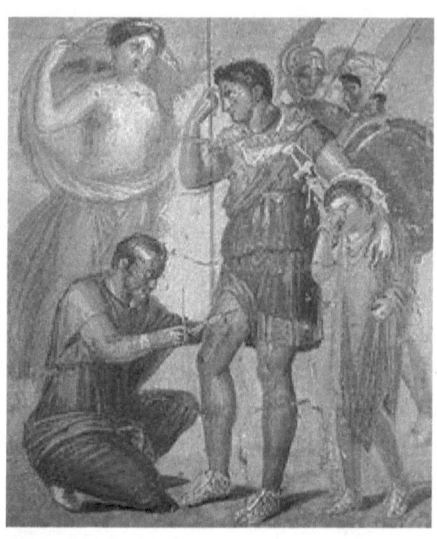

Roman painting, surgery on a soldier, from the 'Surgeon's House' in Ariminum (Rimini, Italy), mid-third century. From the above practice, it can be noticed that very primitive methods of treatment have been in use at various stages of human development. It is very clear that the pain on this Roman soldier was so severe that his daughter had nearly colapsed.

Roman surgeons carried a toolkit that contained forceps, scalpels, catheters and arrow extractors. The tools had various uses and were boiled in hot water before each use. In surgery, surgeons used pain-killers such as opium and scopolamine for treatments, and acetum (the acid in vinegar) was used to wash wounds. Romans didn't believe in the supernatural as much as the Greeks; the Greeks used temples and religious belief to try and cure someone, yet the Romans developed specific hospitals that enabled the patients to be fully rested and relaxed so that they could completely recover. By staying in the hospitals, the doctors (which now had different levels of qualification) were able to observe the illness rather than rely on the supernatural to cure him orher.

Greek Influences on Roman Medicine

Many Greek medical ideas were adopted by the Romans, and Greek medicine had a huge influence on Roman medicine. The first doctors to appear in Rome were Greek, captured as prisoners of war. Greek doctors would later move to Rome because they could make a good living there, or a better one than in the Greek cities.

The Romans also conquered the city of Alexandria, its libraries, and its universities. In ancient times Alexandria was an important centre for learning, and its Great Library held countless volumes of information, many of which would have been on medicine. Here, doctors were allowed to carry out dissections, which led to the discovery of many important medical advances such as the discovery that the brain sends messages to the body.

Greek medicine revolved heavily around the theory of the four humours and texts by Hippocrates and his followers (Hippocratic writings), who were all Greek. These ideas and writings were also used in Roman medicine.

Roman medicine also encompassed the spiritual beliefs of the Greeks (see below).

Dioscorides

Main article: Pedanius Dioscorides

Pedanius Dioscorides (*c.* 40-90) was an ancient Greek physician, pharmacologist, and botanist from Anazarbus, Cilicia, Asia Minor, who practised in ancient Rome during the time of Nero. Dioscorides is famous for writing a five-volume book *De Materia Medica* that is a precursor to all modern pharmacopeias, and is one of the most influential herbal books in history.

Soranus

Main article: Soranus of Ephesus

Soranus was a Greek physician, born at Ephesus, and who lived during the reigns of Trajan and Hadrian (AD 98-138). According to the Suda, he practised in Alexandria and subsequently in Rome. He was the chief representative of the school of physicians known as 'Methodists.' His treatise Gynaecology is extant (first published in 1838 and later by V. Rose in 1882, with a sixth-century Latin translation by Muscio, a physician of the same school).

Galen

Main article: Galen

Galen (AD 129[1]–c. 200 or 216) of Pergamon was a prominent ancient Greek[2] physician, whose theories dominated Western medical science for well over a millennium. By the age of twenty, he had served for four years in the local temple as a therapeutes ('attendant' or 'associate') of the god Asclepius. Although Galen studied the human body, dissection of human corpses was against Roman law, so instead, he used pigs, apes, and other animals. Galen moved to Rome in 162. There he lectured, wrote extensively, and performed public demonstrations of his anatomical knowledge. He soon gained a reputation as an experienced physician, attracting to his practice a large number of clients. Among them was the consul Flavius Boethius, who introduced him to the imperial court, where he became a physician to Emperor Marcus Aurelius. Despite being a member of the court, Galen reputedly shunned Latin, preferring to speak and write in his native Greek, a tongue that was actually quite popular in Rome. He would go on to treat Roman luminaries such as Lucius Verus, Commodus, and Septimius Severus. However, in 166, Galen returned to Pergamon again, where he lived until he went back to Rome for good in 169.

12.4 Ancient Roman Medicine

The ancient Romans, Like the Greeks and Egyptians, had a huge impact on health and medicine Even then, the Romans knew that poor hygiene was a constant source of disease, so public bathhouses and other public hygienic facilities were built. The Romans learnt a great deal from the ancient Greeks, whom they first came into contact with around 500 BC. By the year 27 BC, Greece and many of its surrounding islands had become Roman territory; therefore, many of the Greek medicinal methods and ways of treatment became a part of everyday Roman life. As the Romans expanded into Greece, Greek doctors came to Rome and other parts of Italy. Many of these doctors were prisoners of war and could be purchased by wealthy Romans who wanted a doctor in their household. Many of these prisoners, however, bought their freedom from their owners and started their own practices in Rome. The Greek physicians often had the support of the emperors, and they were very popular among the Roman public. Prior to this influx of medical knowledge, there was no separate medical profession in the Roman Empire. It was believed that the head of every household knew enough about herbs and medicine to treat illnesses within his family. The Romans also believed that a healthy mind meant a healthy body—If you kept fit, you would keep healthy.

Surgical tools used in ancient Rome.

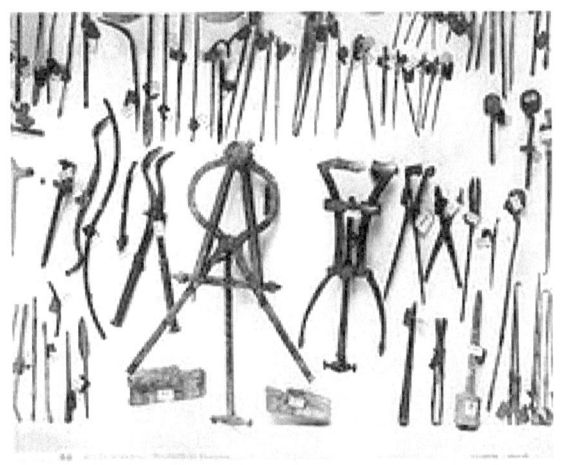

Roman surgical instruments found at Pompeii.

Scalpels could be made of either steel or bronze. Ancient scalpels had almost the same form and function as those of today. The most ordinary type of scalpels in antiquity were the longer, steel scalpels. These long scalpels could be used to make a variety of incisions, but they seem to be particularly suited for deep or long cuts. Smaller, bronze scalpels, referred to as bellied scalpels, were also used frequently by surgeons in antiquity since the shape allowed for delicate and precise cuts to be made.

Hooks were common instruments used regularly by Roman and Greek doctors. The ancient doctors used two basic types of hooks: sharp hooks and blunt hooks. Blunt hooks were used primarily as probes for dissection and for raising blood vessels. Sharp hooks, on the other hand, were used to hold and lift small pieces of tissue so that they could be extracted and to retract the edges of wounds.

Bone Drills were driven in their rotary motion by means of a thong in various configurations. Roman and Greek physicians used bone drills in order to remove diseased bone tissue from the skull and to remove foreign objects (such as a weapon) from a bone.

Forcepss were often used in conjunction with bone drills. They were used by ancient doctors to extract small fragments of bone which could not be grasped by the fingers.

Catheters were used in order to open up a blocked urinary tract which allowed urine to pass freely from the body. Early catheters were hollow tubes made of steel or bronze and had two basic designs. There were catheters with a slight S curve for male patients and a straighter one for females. There were similar-shaped devices called bladder sounds that were used to probe the bladder in search of calcifications.

Uvula crushing forceps were fine-toothed jawed forceps that were designed to facilitate the amputation of the uvula. The procedure called for the physician to crush the uvula with forceps before cutting it off in order to prevent haemorrhaging.

Vaginal Specula were among the most complex instruments used by Roman and Greek physicians. Most of the vaginal specula that have survived and been discovered consist of a screw device that, when turned, forces a crossbar to push the blades outwards.

Spatula was used to mix and apply various ointments to patients.

Surgical saw was used to cut through bones in amputations and surgeries.

Medicines

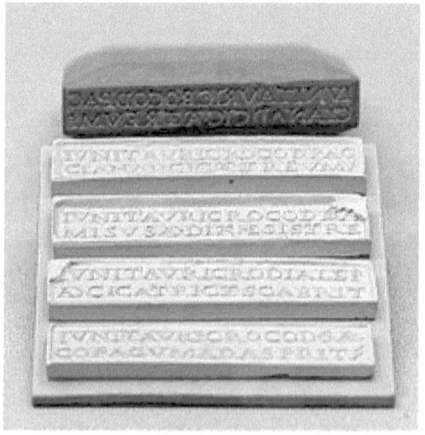

Stamp for marking semi-solid sticks of eye ointments (collyria) before they harden.

Medicinal Herbs

Some ancient Roman herbs used in medicine were as follows:

Fennel: It was thought to have calming properties.

Elecampane: It was used to help with digestion.

Sage: Although it had little medicinal value, it had great religious value.

Garlic: It was thought to be beneficial for health, particularly of the heart.

Fenugreek: It was used in the treatment of pneumonia.

Silphium: It was used for a wide variety of ailments and conditions—especially for birth control.

Willow: It was used as an antiseptic.

Asclepieions in Roman Medicine

When the Roman Army conquered Greece they adopted many of their medicinal beliefs and ideas. The cult of Asclepios had spread across much of Greece and numerous temples (asclepieions) had been built in his name. These Asclepieions (or Asklepieions) were places of healing. They contained baths, gardens, and other facilities designed to improve people's health. People who were being treated in the Asclepieions would sleep in front of a statue of the Greek god in the hope that he would heal them in their sleep. Though several accounts have been recovered, detailing the progress in health made by people admitted to the Asclepieions, it is unlikely that they were based on fact; they may simply have been used as propaganda.

Evidence of a Travelling Surgeon

At the site of the Roman Plemmirio shipwreck (c. AD 200) near Siracusa, Italy, a comprehensive instrumentarium[5] was found. Numerous other items, which could range from bone mallets to urinary catheters, remain at the site. Although it is not certain, it is highly likely that these were the tools of an oculist—an eye surgeon—and not equipment from the ship's first aid box. In support of this theory, over fifteen hundred ships have been discovered in the Mediterranean, and there is a consequent lack of evidence for surgeons in ship crews. The ship was destined for Rome, after sailing down to North Africa, where it transported amphorae, so it is a safe assumption that this surgeon was also destined for Rome. Although surgeons' kits have been found in graves, this is the first finding of a kit that was in use, before the ship was destroyed when it smashed into a cliff on its return to Rome.

Main article: Tiber Island

Tiber Island in Rome was once the location of an ancient temple to Aesculapius, the Greek god of medicine and heal accounts say that in 293 BC, there was a great plague in Rome. Upon consulting the Sibyl, the Roman Senate decided to build a temple to Aesculapius, the Greek god of healing, and sent a delegation to Epidauros to obtain a statue of the deity. They obtained a snake from a temple and put in on board their ship. It immediately curled itself around the ship's mast and this was deemed as a good sign by them. Upon their return up the Tiber River, the snake slithered off the ship and swam onto the island. They believed that this was a sign from Aesculapius, a sign which meant that he wanted his temple to be built on that island.

12.5 Traditional and Medicinal Value of Seaweeds Used in Chinese Medicine

Subhuti Dharmananda, PhD, Director

These days, Chinese Traditional medicines are approved in many parts of the world. Complementary medical practitioners are therefore free to choose the sources of remedies from anyone according to their efficacy/effectiveness.

The following research findings will prove to be very resourceful in applied preventive therapy which is theme of this book. The principal argument presented in this book is that we should not depend wholly on the uses of medicine for therapeutic treatment of health imbalance in our patients. Although the slogan used in many complementary medical books is that 'our foods are our medicine, while our medicines are also our medicine', should not be taken literally so. This claim must be applied carefully, relative to a particular individual patient or group of patients in a given health-problem situation. For example, some group of foods may prove as a remedy for a particular patient and may not be so in another person. An experienced practitioner will use his or her professional observation and skill in each case. A claim normally made by a few practitioners is that they produce their own remedies, and this can be sometimes misleading. Yes, if you are a qualified and licensed complementary pharmacist engaged in the production of herbal or homeopathic remedies, this claim can be regarded as authentic.

Four Seaweeds Commonly Used in Chinese Medicine

- Laminaria (kelp), a brown algae and Ecklonia (the more commonly used).
- Green algae as a source of *kunbu* (Laminaria is sometimes called *haidai*, to distinguish it from *Ecklonia* or other sources).
- Sargassum, a brown algae, as the source of *haizao.*
- Pyrphora, a red algae, as the source of *zicai.*

These seaweeds will form the basis of the following discussion:

12.6 Seaweed's Nutritional Value [1]

Seaweed draws an extraordinary wealth of mineral elements from the sea that can account for up to 36 per cent of its dry mass. The mineral macronutrients include sodium, calcium, magnesium, potassium, chlorine, sulphur, and phosphorus; the micronutrients include iodine, iron, zinc, copper, selenium, molybdenum, fluoride, manganese, boron, nickel, and cobalt. Seaweed has such a large proportion of iodine compared to dietary minimum requirements that it is primarily known as a source of this nutrient. The highest iodine content is found in brown algae, with dry kelp ranging from 1,500 to 8,000 ppm (parts per million) and dry rockweed (*Fucus*) from 500 to 1,000 ppm. In most instances, red and green algae have lower contents, about 100-300 ppm in dried seaweeds, but remain high in comparison to any land plants. Daily adult requirements, currently recommended at 150 µg/day, could be covered by very small quantities of seaweed. Just one gram of dried brown algae provides 500–8,000 µg of iodine and even the green and red algae (such as the purple nori that is used in Japanese cuisine) provides 100–300 µg in a single gram. The amounts of seaweed ingested as food in Japan, or in supplements, is often considerably more than 1 gram a day. Studies show that the human body adapts readily to higher iodine intake, where the thyroid gland is the main tissue involved in use of iodine (it is a component of thyroid hormones). Huge portions of the world population get insufficient iodine because the land, plants, and animals that serve as common dietary sources are very low in iodine. In many countries, iodine is added to table salt to assure that adequate levels are attained. However, some developing countries are still catching up and suffering from the effects of low iodine intake. China has the largest population with a history of low iodine intake, followed by India.

Aside from iodine, seaweed is one of the richest plant sources of calcium, but its calcium content relative to dietary requirements pales in comparison to the iodine content. The calcium content of seaweeds is typically about 4–7 per cent of dry matter. At 7 per cent calcium, one gram of dried seaweed provides 70 mg of calcium, compared to a daily dietary requirement of about 1,000 mg. Still, this is higher than a serving of most non–milk–based foods. Protein content in seaweed varies somewhat. It is low in brown algae at 5–11 per cent of dry matter, but comparable in quantitative terms to legumes at 30–40 per cent of dry matter in some species of red algae. Green algae, which are still not harvested much, also have a significant protein content, i.e. up to 20 per cent of dry matter. Spirulina, a micro–alga, is well known for its very high content, i.e. 70 per cent of dry matter.

Seaweed contains several vitamins. Red and brown algae are rich in carotenes (provitamin A) and are used, in fact, as a source of natural mixed carotenes for dietary supplements. The content ranges from 20 to 170 ppm. The vitamin C in red and brown algae is also notable, with contents ranging from 500 to 3000 ppm. Other vitamins are also present, including B_{12}, which is not found in most land plants. Seaweed has very little fat, ranging from 1 to 5 per cent of dry matter, although seaweed lipids have a higher proportion of essential fatty acids than land plants. Green algae, whose fatty acid make–up is the closest to higher plants, have a much higher oleic and alpha–linoleic acid content. Red algae have a high EPA content, a substance mostly found in animals, especially fish. Seaweed has a high fibre content, making up 32 per cent to 50 per cent of dry matter. The soluble fibre fraction accounts for 51–56 per cent of total fibers in green (ulvans) and red algae (agars, carrageenans, and xylans) and for 67–87 per cent in brown algae (laminaria, fucus, and others). Soluble fibres are generally associated with having cholesterol-lowering and hypoglycemic effects.

[1]

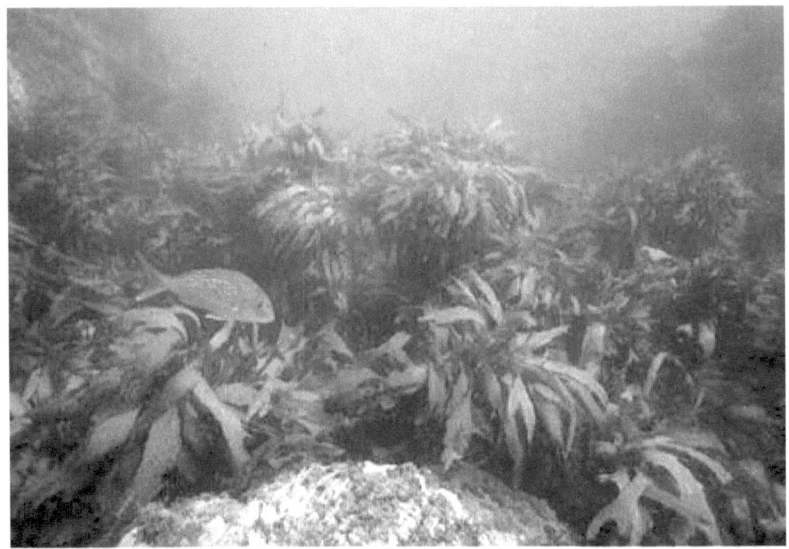

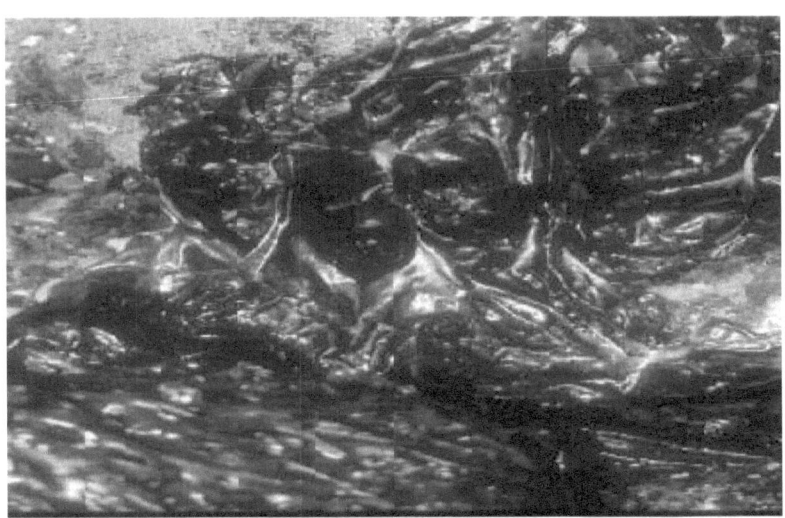

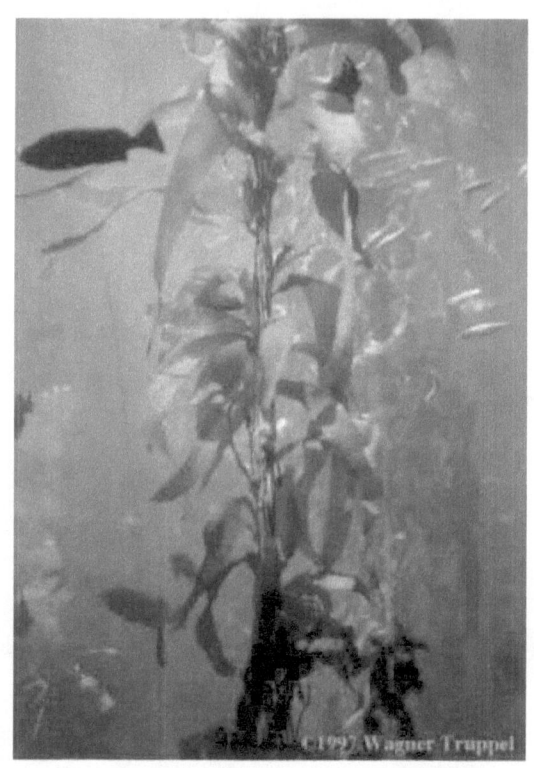

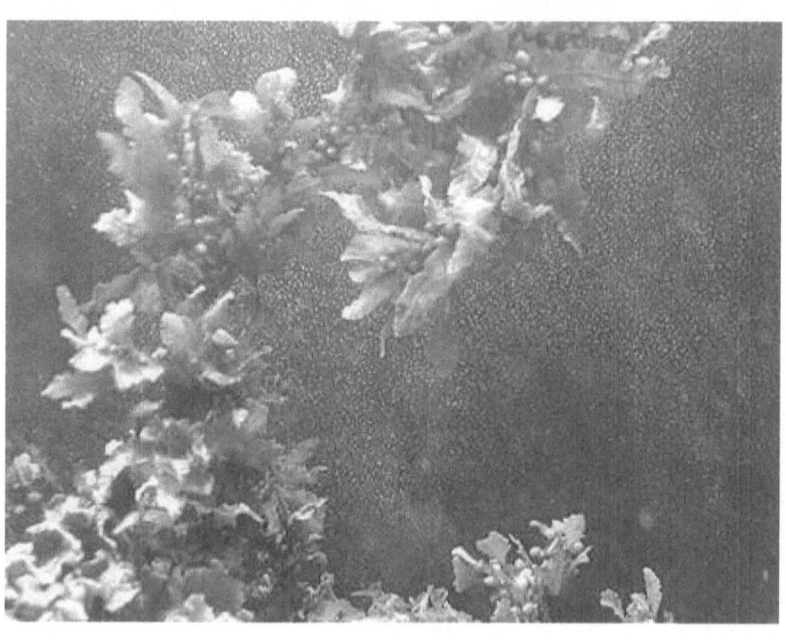

Food Uses

Probably the most widely known seaweed used for food is *Porphyra*, which literally means purple (see sample leaf below), reflecting its colour in nature. The Chinese name is *zicai*, which means purple vegetable. It is classified among the red algae, which have red to purple pigments. Upon processing to yield the food, which is know in Japan as nori, the red pigments are lost, and the final product has a dark, greenish colour. Nori is used to wrap sushi and for making numerous snacks. The other common food item is the low-cost but highly nutritious kelp (kunbu in Chinese, kombu in Japanese). Kombu is usually sold in five- to six-inch dried pieces and can be found in health food stores and Japanese groceries (see sample package below). It is also sold as kombu that cooks quickly; vinegared, shaved kombu that needs little or no cooking; boiled, soy sauce flavoured kombu; lightly pickled kombu; and powdered kombu that can be sprinkled on food or used in drinks. Dried kombu needs to be simmered for at least twenty minutes to soften it and flavour the liquid. If used only for flavouring stock, the kombu itself is removed from the liquid at the end of cooking and discarded. A third seaweed widely used in Japan is known as wakame (from *Undaria pinnatifida*). (See the Appendix for information about seaweed utilisation in Japan.)

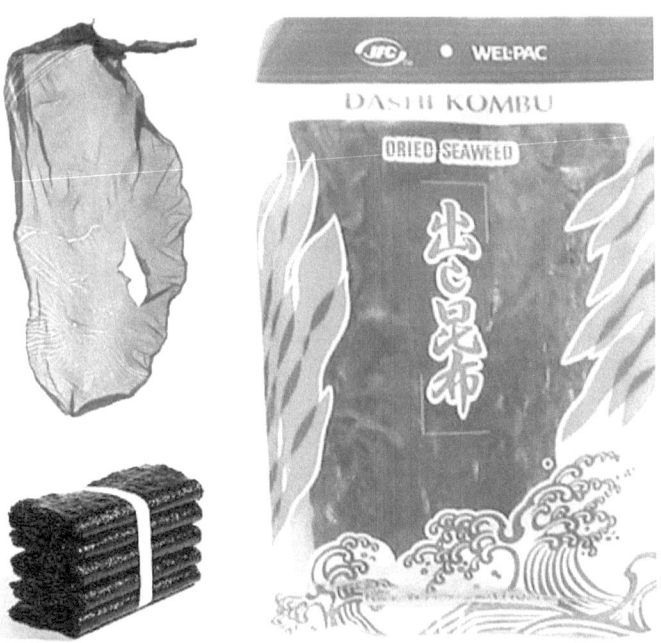

Medicinal Uses

Seaweeds have a salty taste that is an indication that the material can disperse phlegm accumulation, particularly as it forms soft masses, including goitre, the thyroid swelling that indicates severe iodine deficiency. Following are the descriptions of the seaweeds from Oriental Materia Medica [2]:

The descriptions for *kunbu* and *haizao* are quite similar. Yang Yifan (3) wrote about the differences between these commonly used seaweeds:

Haizao and *Kunbu* are salty and cold, and enter the liver, lung, and kidney meridians. Both can clear heat, transform phlegm, soften hardness, and dissipate nodules. They can also promote urination and reduce oedema. In clinical practice, they are often used together to treat nodules such as goitre and scrofula. Here are some differences between the two herbs: *Haizao* is stronger in transforming phlegm and dissipating nodules, and it is more suitable for treating goiter and scrofula. *Kunbu* is stronger in softening hardness and reducing congealed blood; it is more suitable for treating liver–spleen enlargement, liver cirrhosis, and tumours. One of the best-known formulas with the seaweeds is *Haizao Yuhu Tang*, or the Sargassum Decoction for the Jade Flask [4]. This formula of twelve ingredients includes Sargassum, Ecklonia, and Laminaria. It was used to treat a condition of goitre, which was so severe it made the throat look like a large flask. However, these seaweeds have been adopted into formulas for treating other soft swellings, including ovarian cysts, breast lumps, lymph node swellings, lipomas, and fat accumulation from simple obesity.

Appendix: Japan and Seaweed

Following is an outline report on Japanese utilisation of seaweed and seaweed products, with data from 1998, except as noted, thanks to the Fisheries Information Newsletter [1].

- Japan is the world's largest seafood producer, importer, and consumer. Annual seafood expenditures totaled 36,425 yen (~US$300) per capita.
- Total fresh seaweed production was 623,286 tons for all types of seaweed. But, this is far less than what Japan uses for certain

seaweeds, particularly those used for industrial processing of specialty seaweed products.

- Today, Japan is the leading importer of seaweed, while Korea is the premier exporter—with Japan as its main customer.
- Japanese imports stood at a total of 71,800 tons of fresh seaweed produce valued at over $150 million dollars. It consisted of 40,900 tons of *Undaria* (a seaweed that grows in the Pacific, from Korea to Japan to Australia) imported from China and Korea worth $65.3 million dollars, plus other varieties worth $38 million .
- Exports of seaweed from Japan were 1214 tons of miscellaneous seaweed, i.e. processable raw seaweed, dried kombu, and nori worth $12 million, plus 59 million dried *Porphyra* sheets (as used for making sushi) worth $4.6 million . The exports are mainly sold to the United States and Taiwan.
- There are at least twenty-one seaweed species used daily in food preparation in Japan. The Japanese consume an average of 4 kg per capita every year (~ 11 g per day). There is also a large industry built around the three common colloid compounds derived from seaweed: agar, alginate, and carrageenan. These are used to provide thickening and texture to foods and have other uses.
- The agar industry started in Japan over four hundred years ago in mountainous regions where, in cold winters, agar would set into a gel. Japan now imports the raw material, the seaweeds *Gracilaria* and *Gelidium*, from Chile and South Africa. The yearly output was 1,000–1,500 tons of agar in 1994.
- Alginate extraction in Japan is carried out using *Ecklonia* and *Durvillea* imported from Chile and South Africa. The alginate obtained is high-quality material and is used in specific biotech applications. The use of *Laminaria spp.* for kombu, moreover, has resulted in the import of another raw material so as to extract alginates. Overall production of alginate is about 1,000–1,500 tons per year (1994 figures).
- The carrageenan industry is mainly based on direct imports of seaweeds (1,718 tons in 1994). Carragenophytes are also imported from Southeast Asian aquafarms (yielding *Eucheuma* and *Kappaphycus*) and from wild stocks in North and South America and Europe (yielding *Chondrus* and *Gigartina*).

Seaweed Farming in Japan

Seaweed farming is highly developed in Japanese coastal areas. The main species grown there are *Porphyra* (nori), *Laminaria* (kombu), and *Undaria* (wakame). These alone have accounted for 98 per cent of overall Japanese seaweed production since 1984. The balance is made up of minor, traditional (*Monostroma*, *Enteromorpha* and *Cladosiphon*) or experimental (*Meristotheca* and *Grateloupia*) crops or wild stock harvests.

Nori

Nori is a traditional food used, for example, to make sushi, which has been a highly profitable crop over the past century. Since the reproduction cycle's summer phase was discovered by Dr Kathleen Drew-Baker, farming has become easier and more lucrative—so much so that no imports have occurred since 1976. *Porphyra* cultivation is the largest sub-industry in Japanese aquafarming, employing 16,800 workers. In 1998, output stood at 10,326 million nori sheets, that is, equivalent to 396,615 tons of fresh produce.

Kombu

Kombu is the most widely sold seaweed in Japan. It is an 'all-purpose' product; although it is most commonly used for bean-curd soup with kombu. Wild stock still accounts for a major share of output. Several species of the genus *Laminaria* are used in the Japanese food industry. *Laminaria japonica* takes the lion's share of kombu production with a raw-material tonnage of 141,875.

Wakame

Undaria pinnatifida cultivation is a relatively recent development in Japan, and wakame is served as a luxury food on Japanese and Korean tables. It is highly sought after for bean-curd soup or salads. Raw material production, standing at 73,508 tons, is unable to meet Japanese demand for wakame.

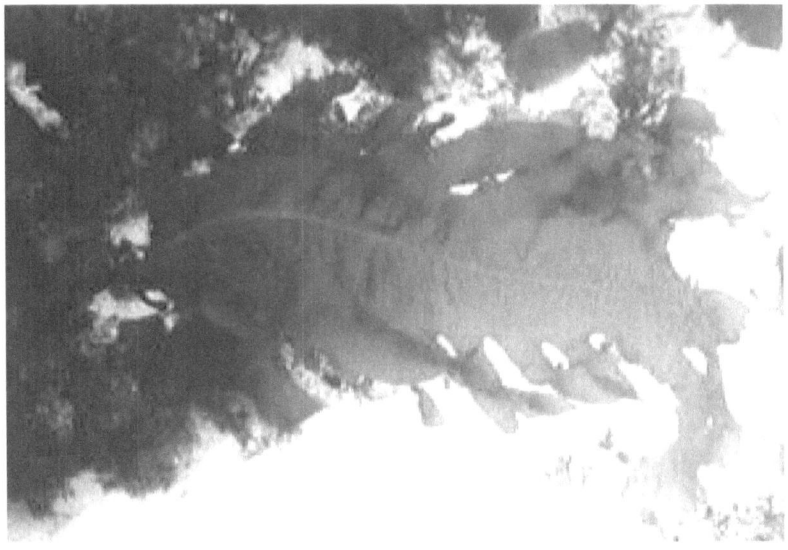

Undaria pinnatifida (wakame).

12.7 Sexual Health in the Preventive Therapy

Sexual health is another important component for anyone living a holistic lifestyle because it plays a vital role in our overall health. It should be of great interest to anyone living with a chronic illness or a health condition because of the vast amount of benefits it can brings to us both psychologically and physiologically. Sexuality is intricately tied to our mental, physical, and spiritual health. Just take a look at some of the many ways that sex is good for us.

Physical Benefits Related to Sexual Health Hormones that are released during orgasm and the physical activity of sex offer the following physical benefits:

- Alleviates joint and muscle pain, strengthens the heart, lengthens the lifespan, is a great stress reliever, and boosts our energy.
- Releases the body's natural opiates that are an extremely effective pain reliever and stimulates the immune system.
- Lowers blood pressure, improves circulation and flexibility, and the oils released are good for your skin and hair.
- Strengthens muscles and bones, lowers bad cholesterol and raises good cholesterol, and strengthens pelvic muscles.

- Improves quality of sleep, lowers the risk of prostate cancer, burns calories and aids in weight-loss, and keeps you physically fit.

Psychological and Emotional Benefits Related to Sexual Health

Now if the physical benefits alone are not enough to make you pay attention to your sexual health, the psychological benefits certainly will. The same hormones that enhance us physiologically have a powerful impact on our mental health.

They may assist with the following:

- It relieves depression, improves our mood, and we feel closer and more connected to our partner. It builds a more satisfying and fulfilling relationship. Good sexual energy between couples helps them develop a stronger relationship. It strengthens their bond on all levels and makes them less vulnerable to infidelity. It instills inner peace and harmony and enhances overall well-being
- It releases chemicals that make you feel relaxed and happy. It promotes positive feelings about yourself, your partner, and your life. It instills a sense ofcontentment and reduces stress. It enhances ability to cope and boosts self-esteem and self-concept.

12.8 Spiritual Benefits Related to Sexual Health

Last but certainly not least, our sexual health can be an amazing tool for spiritual evolution. Through sexual pleasure, connection, and energy, we can experience one of the most profound spiritual experiences available to us. It promotes feelings ofwholeness, harmony, and balance. We feel deeply connected not only to our lover, but also to ourselves and theorigin of the universe as well. Sexual energy can be used to achieve higher levels of awareness and states ofconsciousness, thus providing a gateway to finding our true self and deepening that relationship. It becomes a medium for spiritual growth, healing, and transformation. We can transcend everyday reality and have a brief rendezvous with Nirvana. Sexual pleasure, energy, and connection enhances the overall quality of our life.

Sexual Health and Being Single

What if you're single? If you're single without a partner, that doesn't mean you can't reap many of these benefits as well. Masturbation will achieve most of the same results. However, you will be missing some of the benefits that are derived fromintimacy with another human being and the benefits that require the real physical act, such as weight loss. However, if you're really creative, you can still come up with some masturbation activities that can give you a physical workout. Develop a strong and intimate relationship with nature and yourself, and you can have some very satisfying and rewarding masturbation experiences. The hormones that boost our physical and emotional health released during orgasm are released whether it is through masturbation or through sex with another person.

Sexual Health and Chronic Illness

Good sexual health is a complex combination of psycho-physiological factors and what is considered healthy sexual functioning is relative to each individual's unique situation. What works for one couple or individual may not work for another. Chronic Illness can have a profound effect on the sexual relationship. Some illnesses or conditions may inhibit energy levels, or decrease desire for sex or interfere in physical abilities to engage in intercourse. They may feel less interested in sex or may not be physically capable of enjoying it in the same manner that they are used to. Some people feel too tired, too sick, or do not have the time. There may also be fears of aggravating symptoms. In these cases, there are always many ways to work around these issues and find satisfying solutions. It can be challenging to negotiate this difficult terrain, but with communication, compromise, and the willingness to find alternatives a satisfying level of sexual health can still be achieved and maintained.

For some extreme cases, non-intercourse methods of sexual pleasure can be adopted. If you happen to be struggling with some of these issues, you may find the information on the Sex and Chronic Illness page to be helpful. On the other hand, many people with chronic conditions have no change in their sexual functioning. It can continue to be an important contributor to their quality of life and the relationship. It can be one area of life that still feels normal and comforting, when everything else is in chaos. A strong sexual bond can help the couple to weather the storms that chronic illness have on their life more effectively as a team. They will be more resistant to the possible deterioration that can occur in relationships under high stress.

They can use their sexual energy to work off their frustrations and stress and cope better with the situation.

Why so Many Sexual Health Disorders?

A very alarming issue in regard to sexual health is the rise in sexual disorders that we see in both men and women. Why is it that so many men and women are riddled with sexual health problems these days? Conditions such as erectile dysfunction, low sex drive, infertility, decreased sperm counts, endometriosis, prostatitis, genital abnormalities, prostate cancer, and hormonal imbalancescontinue to increase at terrifying rates.

Some contributing factors can be linked to work-related stress, anxiety, marital discord, past sexual trauma, concernsabout sexual performance, alcoholism, smoking, nutritional deficiencies, heart disease, lack of experience and confidence, orside effects from medications. However, many people continue to suffer with a variety of sexual disorders that have nothing to do with these factors and are, instead, directly linked to the presence of the high level of environmental toxins that we are all exposed to on a daily basis.

These toxins are called hormone disruptors or endocrine disruptors, and we are all exposed to them on a daily basis through our food, air, and water. Everything from your apples to your toothpaste contains endocrine disupters and other toxic chemicals. They are commonly found in pesticides, dioxins, phthalates, PCBs, common household cleaning products, and plastics. Endocrine disrupters interfere in normal healthy functioning of the endocrine system, which can result in severe malfunctioning of the reproductive system and deterioration of sexual health. The hormones released by the endocrine system rule our reproductive and sexual development and functioning. When environmental toxins like endocrine/hormone disrupters enter our body they wreak havoc in a variety of ways. In some cases, they may mimic our hormones like estrogen for the female and androgen for the males, which results in hormone levels that are too high. In other cases, they block hormones from producing or functioning properly.

The balance of the endocrine system is very delicate, and it takes only very low levels of these toxins to upset this balance and result in a variety of serious and detrimental health effects that may include damage to the nervous, immune, and reproductive systems. Everyone knows the powerful role of hormones in relation to sexuality. When hormone-functioning is disrupted by environmental toxins, it can lead to all kinds of sexual health issues that won't respond to the best marriage counselling in the world or the newest most powerful drug therapy for erectile dysfunction or low sex drive.

What is even more terrifying about these toxic chemicals is that the human body is not capable of breaking them down. Therefore, once they enter the body, they are very hard, if not impossible, to excrete. Instead, they get stored indefinitely in our fat cells and recirculate through our body continually, causing even more damage. One of the most important steps you can take to protect your sexual health is try and limit your exposure to hormone/endocrine disrupters. Unfortunately, these environmental toxins are found everywhere we go, so it's literally impossible to escape them completely. You can, however, reduce their presence in your life by making a variety of lifestyle changes that include eliminating the use of pesticides or herbicides, switching your household cleaning supplies and personal-care products over to natural and non-toxic products like those found with Seventh Generation, moving to a location that has cleaner air quality, and eating organic food. Living a green lifestyle is the wisest and most beneficial action we can take to safeguard not only our sexual health but also our entire life.

12.9 Multiple Chemical Sensitivity (MCS)

This health care problem is very important in preventive therapy and must be taken very seriously. Many different types of foods and medications can cause an illness to persons who are otherwise healthy.

Multiple Chemical Sensitivity, also known as MCS, is defined as 'an acquired disorder, characterised by recurrent symptoms referable to multiple organ systems, occurring in response to demonstrable exposure to many chemically unrelated compounds at doses far below those established in the general population to cause harmful effects . . . [1] or sensitivity to chemicals.' By sensitivity, we mean symptoms or signs as related to chemical exposures at levels tolerated by the population at large that is distinct from such well-recognised hypersensitivity phenomenon as IgG-mediated immediate hypersensitivity reactions, contact dermatitis, and hypersensitivity pneumonitis. Sensitivity may be expressed as symptoms and signs in one or more organ systems. Symptoms and signs wax and wane with exposure. [2] So what does this mean in lay terms? Well, basically it means that growing numbers of people, myself included, are beginning to develop serious health problems from exposures to the common, everyday chemicals we find in our environment. These chemicals can be items such as scented laundry soap or fabric softener, treated fabric, perfume, cologne, disinfectants, pesticides, herbicides, household cleansers, cigarette smoke, car exhaust, gas heat or other petroleum products, air-fresheners, bleach, shampoos, toothpaste, food supply, new carpet, remodelling materials, or cosmetics to name a few.

The symptoms of multiple chemical sensitivity are vast and numerous and usually affect many organ systems. Enzyme pathways may be inhibited, and liver detoxification pathways become overloaded. The blood-brain barrier is affected [3] and neurological, immunological, respiratory, endocrine, cardiovascular, genito-urinary, and gastrointestinal systems are likely to be affected with the central nervous system almost always being affected. [4] Symptoms may include depression, fatigue, headache, migraines, difficulty in concentrating, irritability, Short-ter memory loss, lack of coordination, shaking, trembling, visual and verbal disturbances, muscle pain, difficulty in breathing, rashes, anxiety, impaired mobility, itching, disorientation, confusion, food sensitivity, excessive drowsiness, constipation, diarrhoea, earaches, heart pounding, hypothyroidism, learning disabilities, elevated blood pressure, increased pulse and many more.

Individuals affected with multiple chemical sensitivity are forced to make profound changes in lifestyle and diet and endure multiple losses in life as they knew it, including their livelihood, identity, friends, and sometimes even family members. Most of those afflicted are no longer able to be in environments that contain the above-listed chemicals, which are found almost everywhere. Therefore, this means that most public places are off limits to them, their social life becomes extremely limited, and there are very few places, if any, where they are capable of obtaining employment. It becomes increasingly difficult to function at all in this chemicalised world. The prevalence of multiple chemical sensitivity in the population may be as high as 15 per cent at this time, [4] and yet there is incredible backlash from the medical and chemical communities who try to deny and discredit the existence of this devastating illness, because to acknowledge it would mean that global change would have to take place.

Dr Rea, the leading medical specialist in the field of multiple chemical sensitivity, calls it an environmentally triggered disease and explains that it may be acquired either by a one-time acute exposure or from low-level, long-term exposures. As well as being chemically sensitive himself, Dr Rea treats individuals with multiple chemical sensitivity in his clinic in Dallas, Texas. He points out that in 1987, the American industry poured twenty-two billion pounds of toxic chemicals into air, food, and water. He adds further that the well-being of man is a function of his environment; living in polluted surroundings adversely affects our health, and as the number of dangerous environmental pollutants continues to increase, so do the numbers of people sensitive to these contaminants. [3]

The U.S. Department of Health and Human Services states that multiple chemical sensitivity is an acquired chronic syndrome described as a severe, toxic, allergic–like reaction to extremely low levels of chemicals in our environment. It has developed over the past four decades and is caused by overexposure to some hundred thousand new, more toxic synthetic chemicals. Research contends that a victim's body becomes unable to cleanse its tissues of chemicals to which it is exposed, either in small doses over time or in a single tremendous dose. [5]

It really should come as no surprise to us that this phenomenon is occurring, as our bodies are made of the same ingredients as our earth, and the toxicity of our environment has been evident for a long time in our declining and deformed wildlife. Rachel Carson in her ground-breaking book, *Silent Spring*, first warned us of this over thirty-five years ago [6] and although we have been somewhat successful at raising some awareness of the consequences that our chemicalised society is having on our environment and wildlife, we have been leaving out a very important piece of the puzzle.

We are not pointing out that these toxins are not only poisoning nature, but our own bodies as well. We are not immune to the destruction the environment is enduring. Wildlife is smaller and more vulnerable as it is exposed to the elements continuously, and the deadly symptoms appeared in the animals first. Now we are beginning to see the same in human beings. The animals have tried to warn us, but we have not heard them. They cannot speak our language, but they have been warning us very loudly in their own language.

Another profound cutting-edge book *Our Stolen Future*, which has not received the attention it deserves, written by two leading environmental scientists and an award-winning environmental journalist, gives a staggering account of the messages our wildlife has been giving us and provides an overwhelming evidence that synthetic chemicals are endocrine disrupters, and they are not only upsetting normal reproductive and developmental processes, decreasing sperm count, increasing hormone-related cancers, endometriosis and causing birth defects and sexual abnormalities, but are also threatening actual survival.[7] Their conclusions are startling and terrifying and should serve as a wake-up call to all individuals.

Cindy Duehring, a sufferer of multiple chemical sensitivity who died at the age of thirty-six after a long struggle with complications of multiple chemical sensitivity, was a leading researcher and writer at Environmental Access Research and took this quote from *Environmental Neurotoxicity* in an article titled, 'Screening for Nervous System Damage from Chemical Exposure'—'it was a most dangerous illusion that our society has brought forth, in the false belief, that the chemical ingredients in our everyday home and office consumer products, from cosmetics and perfumes to cleaners and carpets, have been tested for health effects to protect the public. Most of the chemicals have never tested and are not under any regulation. There are three new chemical compounds introduced in the United States every day. Pre-marketing testing of compounds as potential neurotoxicants have serious deficiencies. Many of these neurotoxic compounds came into use before the passage of the Toxic Substance Control Act in 1976 and remain untested and are still not required to be tested.' [8]

As the very wise Chief Seattle said to his people in a tribal assembly in the Pacific Northwest in 1854,

> 'We are part of the Earth and it is part of us. We know the white people do not understand our ways. Our portion of land is the same to them as the next, for they are strangers who come in the night and take from the land whatever they need. This we know. The Earth does not belong to humans; humans belong to the Earth. All things are connected like the blood which unites one family. Whatever befalls the Earth befalls

the children of the Earth. Humans do not weave the web of life; they are merely a strand in it. Whatever they do to the web, they do to themselves.'

In conclusion, he added, 'When the thicket and the eagle, the swift pony and the hunt are gone from the land, it will mark the end of living and the beginning of survival.' [4]

This could not be more true and is evidenced very profoundly in multiple chemical sensitivity. As a whole, we are not hearing the warnings that the wildlife is giving us. Hopefully, we don't all have to become poisoned before we listen and learn. Multiple Chemical Sensitivity is only the tip of the iceberg, and if society does not begin to hear the messages of the earth, then someday, we will see human beings on the endangered species list.

Multiple Chemical Sensitivity Treatment

Many people have multiple chemical sensitivities but are not aware of it, because the average medical doctor is not trained in this area. They will typically tell you that your symptoms are the result of stress or depression or may even call you a hypochondriac. To find a doctor who can make a diagnosis of chemical sensitivity, you need to see a doctor of environmental medicine that can be found at the American Academy of Environmental Medicine. He or she can also be found various places by making request at the department of health. The ALCAT test is a simple test kit that can be sent to your home and test you for ten of the most common chemicals in the environment, as well as sensitivity to mould, foods, and food additives, which typically accompany MCS.

Once the body begins to break down from environmental toxins and chemical sensitivities develop, it is very difficult to make a complete recovery. The main method of treatment consists of avoiding chemicals, which means that the life of the individual is profoundly altered, permanently. So prevention is the best medicine. It is believed that malfunctioning adrenal glands, mitochondiral dysfunction, and heavy metal toxicity plays a crucial role in MCS, and some people find improvements in their condition by supporting their adrenals and supplementing the diet with glutathione and a variety of detoxification methods, like clay baths and chelation. Most people with MCS have candida overgrowth and the toxins that candida emits and overloads the liver and adds to or causes sensitivity to chemicals. Significant improvements in sensitivity levels can often be found by addressing candida with the candida diet, antifungals, etc.

The best step you can take to protect your patients from developing multiple chemical sensitivities is to adopt a green lifestyle. Environmental toxins are the cause of MCS, therefore, they must be eliminated. This means that at a minimum you should be using environmentally friendly and natural personal and health care products, cleaning supplies, and yard care products—no pesticides, herbicides, air-fresheners, perfume, or cologne—and eat an organic diet as much as possible. The construction of your home should be made as non-toxic and green as possible.

CHAPTER 13

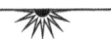

13.1 Therapeutic Sexual Health Therapy

The word *sex* can be expressed as the genric term that permeants all aspects of romantic life between men and women. In this chapter the discussion is going to fucus only on the hetrosexual aspect of life as it relates to the health care therapeutics. Once health therapists understand the crucial importance of sexuality and the role it plays in human health, this knowledge can be applied in the prevetive therapy. We thank God that in an open society like ours in Britain, people can discuss and talk about sex freely without any inhibition or the fear of being persecuted. Apart from food and beverages, sex is the next major need in human life. Sexual health and sexual therapy are the basic premise of therapeutic approach. Sexual health is dedicated to providing easy access to sexuality information, education, support, products, and other resources. Sexual health is another important component part of complementary holistic lifestyle because it plays a vital role in human overall health. It should be of great interest to anyone living with chronic illness or health condition because of the vast amount of benefits it can bring to people, both psychologically and physiologically. Sexuality is intricately tied to human mental, physical, and spiritual health. The following are some of the many ways that sex can be good for human being:

> Physical benefits related to sexual health hormones that are released during orgasm and the physical activity of sex offer the following physical benefits: It alleviates joint and muscle pain, strengthens the heart, lengthens the lifespan, is a great stress reliever, boosts the energy, and releases the body's natural opiates that are extremely effective pain relievers. It stimulates the immune system, lowers blood pressure, and improves circulation and flexibility. The oils released are good

for our skin and hair and strengthens the muscles and the bones. It lowers bad cholesterol and raises good cholesterol. It strengthens pelvic muscles, improves quality of sleep lowers the risk of prostate cancer, burns calories, and aids in losing weight, keeping you physically fit.

PSYCHOLOGICAL AND EMOTIONAL BENEFITS RELATED TO SEXUAL HEALTH

Now if the physical benefits alone are not enough to make you pay attention to your sexual health, the psychological certainly will. The same hormones that enhance us physiologically have a powerful impact on our mental health. They may assist in the following ways: It relieves depression and improves our mood so that we feel closer and more connected to our partners. A more satisfying and fulfilling relationship and good sexual energy between couples helps them to develop a stronger relationship. It strengthens their bond on all levels and makes them less vulnerable to infidelity. It also instills inner peace and harmony and enhances overall well-being. It releases chemicals that make you feel relaxed and happy, promotes positive feelings about yourself, your partner and your life, and instills a sense of contentment. It reduces stress, enhances ability to cope, and boosts self-esteem and self-concept.

SPIRITUAL BENEFITS RELATED TO SEXUAL HEALTH

Last but certainly not least, our sexual health can be an amazing tool for spiritual evolution. Through sexual pleasure, connection and energy we can experience one of the most profound spiritual experiences available to us. It promotes feelings of wholeness, harmony, and balance. We feel deeply connected to not only our lover but also to our own selves and the origin of the universe as well. Sexual energy can be used to achieve higher levels of awareness and states of consciousness, thus providing a gateway to finding our true self and deepening that relationship. It becomes a medium for spiritual growth, healing, and transformation. We can transcend everyday reality and have a brief rendezvous with Nirvana: elusive-paradise, the feeling of heaven on earth, and fantasy. Sexual pleasure, energy, and connection enhances the overall quality of our life.

SEXUAL HEALTH AND BEING SINGLE

What if you're single? If you're single without a partner that doesn't mean you can't reap many of these benefits as well. Masturbation will achieve most of the same results. However, you will be missing some of the benefits that are derived from intimacy with another human being and the benefits that require the real physical act such as weight loss. However, if you're really creative, you can still come up with some masturbation activities that can give you a physical workout. Develop a strong and intimate relationship with nature and yourself and you can have some very satisfying and rewarding masturbation experiences. The hormones released during orgasm that boost our physical and emotional health are released whether it is through masturbation or through sex with another person. But nothing surpasses the human contact—the smooth, transcelucency of a female hand and body—Just imagine how cool and soft the female breast feels to the hand!

Sexual Health and Chronic Illness

Good sexual health is a complex combination of psycho-physiological factors and what is considered healthy sexual functioning is relative to each individual's unique situation. What works for one couple or individual may not work for another. Chronic Illness can have a profound effect on the sexual relationship. Some illnesses or conditions may inhibit energy levels or decrease desire for sex or interfere in physical abilities to engage in intercourse. They may feel less interested in sex or may not be physically capable of enjoying it in the same manner that they are used to. Some people feel too tired, too sick, or have no time. There may also be fears of aggravating symptoms. In these cases, there are always many ways to work around these issues and find satisfying solutions. It can be challenging to negotiate this difficult terrain, but with communication, compromise, and the willingness to find alternatives, a satisfying level of sexual health can still be achieved and maintained.

For some extreme cases, non-intercourse methods of sexual pleasure can be adopted. If you happen to be struggling with some of these issues, you may find the information on the Sex and Chronic Illness page to be helpful. On the other hand, many people with chronic conditions have no change in their sexual functioning. It can continue to be an important contributor to their quality of life and the relationship. It can be one area of life that still feels normal and comforting, when everything else is in chaos. A strong sexual bond can help the couple to weather the storms that chronic illness has on their life more effectively as a team. They will be more resistant to the possible deterioration that can occur in relationships under high stress. They can use their sexual energy to work off their frustrations, and stress and cope better with the situation.

Sexual Health Disorders

A very alarming issue in regard to sexual health is the rise in sexual disorders that we see in both men and women. Why is it that so many men and women are riddled with sexual health problems these days? Conditions such as erectile dysfunction, low sex drive, infertility, decreased sperm counts, endometriosis, prostatitis, genital abnormalities, prostate cancer, and hormonal imbalances continue to increase at terrifying rates. Some contributing factors can be linked to work-related stress, anxiety, marital discord, past sexual trauma, concerns about sexual performance, alcoholism, smoking, nutritional deficiencies, heart disease, lack of experience and confidence, or side effects from medications. However, many people continue to suffer with a variety of sexual disorders that have nothing to do with these factors. Instead, they are directly linked to the presence of a high level of environmental toxins that we are all exposed to on a daily basis. These toxins are called hormone disruptors or endocrine disruptors, and we are all exposed to them on a daily basis through our food, air, and water. Everything from your apples to your toothpaste contains endocrine disruptors and other toxic chemicals. They are commonly found in pesticides, dioxins, phthalates, PCBs, common household cleaning products and plastics. Endocrine disruptors interfere in normal healthy functioning of the endocrine system, which can result in severe malfunctioning of the reproductive system and deterioration of sexual health.

The hormones released by the endocrine system rule our reproductive and sexual development and functioning. When environmental toxins like endocrine/hormone disrupters enter our body, they wreak havoc in a variety of ways. In some cases, they may mimic our hormones, like estrogen for the females and androgen for the males, which results in hormone levels that are too high. In other cases, it blocks hormones from producing or functioning properly. The balance of the endocrine system is very delicate, and it takes only very low levels of these toxins to upset this balance and result in a variety of serious and detrimental health effects that may include damage to the nervous, immune, and reproductive systems. Everyone knows the powerful role of hormones in relation to sexuality. When hormone functioning is disrupted by environmental toxins, it can lead to all kinds of sexual health issues that won't respond to the best marriage counselling in the world or the newest, most powerful drug therapy for erectile dysfunction or low sex drive. What is even more terrifying about these toxic chemicals is that the human body is not capable of breaking them down. Therefore, once they enter the body, they are very hard, if not impossible, to excrete. Instead, they get stored indefinitely in our fat cells and recirculate through our body continually, causing even more damage. Some of the most important steps you can take to protect your sexual health is try and limit your exposure to hormone/endocrine disrupters. Unfortunately, these environmental toxins are found everywhere we go, so it's literally impossible to escape them completely. You can, however, reduce their presence in your life by making a variety of lifestyle changes that include eliminating the use of pesticides or herbicides, switching your household cleaning supplies and personal care products over to natural and non-toxic products like those found with Seventh Generation, moving to a location that has cleaner air quality, and eating organic food. Living a green lifestyle is the wisest and most beneficial action we can take to safeguard not only our sexual health, but our entire life.

13.2 Nutrition and Healthy Functions of Water in the Body

The following information is very crucial for the pogramme of preventive therapy.

- Artificial sweeteners: Understanding these and other sugar substitutes.
- Alcohol use: If you drink, keep it moderate.
- Food pyramids: Explore these healthy diet options.
- Sodium: How to tame your salt habit now?
- Water: How much should you drink every day?
- Nutrition Facts: An interactive guide to food labels.
- Dietary fibre: Essential for a healthy diet.
- Added sugar: Don't get sabotaged by sweeteners.
- Caffeine: How much is too much?
- Dietary fats: Know which types to choose.

- Stevia: Can it help with weight control?
- MUFAs: Why should my diet include these fats?
- High-fructose corn syrup: What are the health concerns?
- Juicing: What are the health benefits?
- Low-sodium diet: Why is processed food so salty?
- Taurine in energy drinks: What is it?
- High-protein diets: Are they safe?

What are functional foods?

- Acai berry products: Do they have health benefits?
- Coffee and health: What does the research say?
- Slideshow: Guide to a high-fibre diet.
- Calorie calculator slide show: Ten great health foods for eating well.
- Energy drinks: Do they really boost energy?
- Alkaline water: Better than plain water?
- Multigrain vs whole grain: Which is healthier?
- Healthy chocolate: Dream or reality?
- Yerba mate: Is it safe to drink?
- Monosodium glutamate (MSG): Is it harmful?
- Nutrition rating system: What's behind the new food labels?
- High-fibre foods, diet soda: Is it bad for you?
- Underweight?: See how to add pounds healthfully.
- Caffeine: Is it dehydrating or not?
- Grape juice: Same heart benefits as wine?
- Water softeners: How much sodium do they add?
- Olive oil: What are the health benefits?
- Fat grams, calories, or percentages: Which are more important?
- Phenylalanine in diet soda: Is it harmful?
- Healthy diet: End guesswork with these nutrition guidelines.
- Cholesterol: Top five foods to lower your numbers.
- Nuts and your heart: Eating nuts for heart health.
- Trans fat is double trouble for your heart health.
- Salmonella: Response to latest outbreak and recall.
- Foods for healthy skin: Top picks.
- Slide show: Guide to portion control for weight loss. Can whole-grain foods lower blood pressure?
- Junk food blues: Are depression and diet related?

Nutrition in Preventive Therapy

This is one of the most important parts of preventive therapy in complementary medicine. Since we are already involved in holistic natural medicine, we would have no choice in the matter than to face our practice holistically.

Holistic nutrition uses various combinations of food and nutrients to help individuals achieve optimal mental, physical, and spiritual health. It can be used as a preventative health approach for the average person without any ailments or as a modality for healing or in symptom management for people living with chronic illness or other medical conditions. The focus is on eating foods that provide your body with the highest levels of nutritional value and supplementing the diet with vitamins, minerals, amino acids, essential fatty acids, etc., when necessary. However, it is much more than just eating a balanced diet. Diet and nutrition have a profound impact on mental and physical health. The wrong food and lack of balanced nutrients can lead to many debilitating psychological and physical symptoms and degenerative health conditions.

Holistic nutrition is Individualised. An important part of living a holistic health lifestyle and adhering to the principles of holistic nutrition is getting to know your body and what it needs. Different people need different things. It all depends on your particular body chemistry—your biochemical make-up. We want to get as many of our nutrients as we possibly can naturally in our diet; however, due to soil depletion and nutritional deficiencies, it is often necessary to supplement the diet. There is no 'one size fits all' nutritional supplement. A customised supplement designed for your unique biochemistry is the most effective method. You can learn a lot about your body by becoming very attentive to your thoughts, feelings, and reactions to specific foods and supplements. Tune into your body and learn to read the messages it provides you. Keep a journal of physical and psychological symptoms and then research their relationship to diet and nutrient levels. However, it can also be helpful to have some biochemical lab work done with something like the Priva-test that can help you pinpoint specific deficiencies or disorders and tell you how well your detoxification pathways are functioning and the ALCAT test to identify hidden food sensitivities.

Holistic nutrition is very individualised, personal, and specific to needs. It takes into account a person's overall medical and physical health, as well as the issues that he or she is trying to improve or heal. It also considers the underlying issues that are going on with the health as well as how ill a person is or how aggressive they want to be with obtaining the results that they want to achieve. Different illnesses, conditions, or diseases have different nutritional requirements, and each individual responds to diet and nutrition uniquely. This is not a 'one size fits all' diet. A diet that one person thrives on can leave another person non-functional and in a heap on the floor. You do not want to follow a diet or supplement plan that was created for someone else. A diet that was designed for someone who suffers with asthma may not be good for someone who suffers with ulcers.

A person who is deficient in magnesium or essential fatty acids will take larger doses of these nutrients than the average person, and someone who isn't deficient wouldn't want the same dosage as a person who is. One person may be allergic or sensitive to chicken, dairy, and eggs and therefore would need to eliminate these items from their diet, while another person without these allergies could thrive and benefit from the vitamins and minerals present in these particular foods. Some individuals may have a metabolic disorder such as hypoglycemia or diabetes and therefore would need to follow a diet regimen and supplementation plan that helps keep their blood sugar in balance. Another person may have many different issues going on at the same time. Perhaps they have numerous food allergies, hypoglycemia or diabetes, and several nutritional deficiencies. So they would have a very different nutritional plan from someone who has none of these issues.

The Basics of Holistic Nutrition

Although holistic nutrition is largely individualised, there are some basics that apply to all individuals who wish to follow a holistic nutritional plan. They include the following: All food should be organic as much as possible. Avoid junk food and processed food—no food with additives and preservative and no sugar or caffeine. Drink adequate amounts of pure water—filtered and free of chlorine and other contaminants. Avoid the use of microwaves. No genetically engineered food—Identify hidden food allergies and food sensitivities—address nutritional deficiencies. Eat whole foods in their natural state as much as possible. Beyond that, the key to designing a healthy diet plan lies in understanding your body and its unique biochemical needs. In my opinion, the healthiest diet for everyone is called the Paleolithic diet or a slightly modified version, because it is the diet that nature intended you to eat. Another very important part of designing a nutritious diet is to understand the difference between good carbs and bad carbs. Many people are misinformed about this aspect of diet.

Getting Started with Holistic Nutrition

If you're just getting started with holistic nutrition, it's probably best to make changes gradually so that changes won't seem so drastic and difficult to stick with. Be patient and kind with yourself, but also be self-disciplined. Change is difficult and takes time. You also want to monitor how you feel and respond to changes, so if you make too many changes all at one time, you won't be able to identify what benefits you receive from which action you've taken. When shopping at the health food store for organic and healthy foods, be sure to read the labels as not all of the foods are completely organic and pure and so you know exactly what you are putting into your body. Over time, your needs may change in response to healing or setbacks, so you may need to adjust your diet and supplements accordingly. If you have improvements in your health, then you may need lower dosages. On the other hand, if you have a setback with your health, you may need higher dosages or something entirely new. Food allergies or sensitivities may improve or get worse. They can sometimes swing like a pendulum in response to other factors in your life. So what you can eat one month is not necessarily what you can eat the next month. Whatever your situation or condition may be, you can't go wrong with holistic nutrition. It leads to a better quality of life and a higher level of functioning. You'll find more balance and harmony in your mental, physical, and spiritual well-being. In this presentation, the term 'you' has been used often; the practitioners are expected to use this information to equip themselves for consulting and guiding their clients at all times.

13.3 Mind–Body Preventive in the Therapy

Mind and body therapies not only improve overall health but also have a positive and measurable effect on specific conditions and disease. Two key principles underpin the various therapies. First, the mind can affect the body in positive or harmful ways. Second, whatever you do physically also has an impact on consciousness. A great deal of research reveals that psychological and spiritual practices, such as meditation, relaxation, guided imagery, and biofeedback can have a useful impact on physical problems, including pain.

Mind-body medicine is so widely used by the public and by the medical profession that it may be considered to belong more to conventional than to complementary medicine. According to the National Center for Complementary and Alternative Medicine (NCCAM) in the United States, 'Only a subset of mind-body interventions are considered. Many that have a well-documented theoretical basis—for example, patient education and cognitive behavioral approaches are now considered mainstream.' On the other hand, meditation therapy, dance—music and art therapy, and praying therapy, including mental healing therapy, are categorised as alternative. Generally speaking, mind-body practices, which include biofeedback, produce a beneficial, biologically regenerative, and relaxed state in which the body is more able to heal itself and function optimally. Under the direction of a skilled clinician, these therapies can be used to treat a wide array of medical and psychological conditions. However, they can also be safely used by everyone as 'self-care practices' to prevent and reverse the harmful effects of stress and to complement conventional treatments.

The extensive research into the efficacy of mind-body medicine focuses on major chronic diseases such as general pain syndromes and insomnia (see below); practice is the most effective way of achieving the maximum improvement in health and well-being.

The-Mind-Body in Preventive Therapy

Mind-body therapy is an ancient concept. Until about three hundred years ago, virtually all philosophy and medicine treated the body and mind as an integral whole. Currently, the diseases that are killing more people in the developed nations worldwide are no longer infections, but chronic degenerative conditions such as coronary artery disease, high blood pressure, cancer, and diabetes, for which there are no chemical 'magic bullets'. These diseases are inextricably related to psychological, environmental, and lifestyle factors. Increasingly, stress is recognised as a major causal factor in both the onset of acute diseases and in chronic diseases. Mind-body practices can give people the skills to manage the inevitable stress of life and, therefore, have an increasingly important role in preventing and reversing the effects of stress and disease.

The rise in the popularity of mind-body medicine has been stimulated by the introduction of Asian healing methods and systems such as yoga and traditional Chinese therapies. Also in India as Ayurvedic and in ancient Iran with famous Hakim Like Avicenna and his pulls Therapy and Diagnose, which is well known in all the world. Mind and body medicine is so widely used by the public and by the medical profession that it may be considered to belong to conventional than to complementary medicine. According to the National Center for Complementary and Alternative Medicine (NCCAM) in the US, 'Only a subset of mind-body interventions are considered CAM. Many that have a Well-documented theoretical basis-for example, patient education and cognitive behavioural approaches are now considered mainstream.' On the other hand, meditation, dance, music and art therapy, and prayer amd, mental healing are categorised as alternative. NCCAM states that 'Many CAM therapies are called holistic, which generally means they consider the whole person, including physical, mental, emotional, and spiritual aspects.'

Generally speaking, mind-body practices, which include biofeedback, produce a beneficial, biologically regenerative, relaxed state, in which the body is more able to heal itself and function optimally. Under the direction of a skilled clinician, these therapies can be used to treat a wide array of medical and psychological conditions. However, they can also be safely used by everyone as 'self-care practices' to prevent and reverse the harmful effects of stress and to complement conventional treatments.

The extensive research into the efficacy of mind-body medicine focuses on major chronic diseases, such as general pain syndromes and insomnia(see below), practice is the most effective way of achieving the maximum improvement in health and well-being.

History of Mind–Body Medicine

Imagery	Posture
We can affect the way our body behaves just by using our imagination. For example, imagine unwrapping a chocolate. Feel the paper crinkling under your fingers, smell the aroma that is released, and then imagine the taste and feel of it melting on your tongue. This imagery will no doubt have activated your salivary glands!	Studies have established that if we stand upright, keep the head erect, smile, and breathe deeply, it is impossible to 'feel' depressed.
	Immune system
	Immune molecules known as cytokines can initiate brain actions. Some cytokines help the body recuperate by sending messages to the brain that set off a series of sickness responses, such as fever. The immune molecules also can trigger feelings of sluggishness, sleepiness, and loss of appetite—behaviours that encourage people to rest while they are ill.
	Listening
	Music can enhance mood and even have a painkilling effect through encouraging endorphin release. Biological sounds, such as a mother's heartbeat, have been used to de-stress infants. Conversely, noise can increase heart rate, blood pressure, respiration rate, and blood cholesterol levels.
	Breathing
	By controlling breathing patterns, it is possible to reduce anxiety and stress responses (see pp. 408 and 414).

* Dr Kenneth R. Pelletier, *Family Guide to Complementary and Conventional Medicine*, 2008.

Self-Care for Good Health

Eighty per cent of all medical symptoms are self-diagnosed, self-treated, and self-limiting, which means they resolve without the need for formal medical care. Nevertheless, people often need help in learning how to take care of their health (self-care) in order to avoid more serious conditions. Mind-body therapies address the kind of psychosocial issues that need to change before people can successfully implement effective self-care.

Tobacco, alcohol, poor diet and inactivity patterns, stress, certain infections, drug use, and deadly drug interactions from prescription medications often cause several medical conditions.

Many of these 'causes of death' can be avoided with better self-care practices. Mind-body therapies provide the behavioural basis for individuals to make healthy changes, and so they are the foundations for helpful self-care strategies, such as exercise, good nutritional habits, and more appropriate use of conventional medicines.

Mind-Body Approaches

In addition to this, there are a number of other therapies recommended throughout the ailment section of this book. Some therapies overlap. Relaxation and stress-management techniques, in particular, are essential components of all of the therapies. Physiological benefits of relaxing include the following:

(a) Decreased levels of adrenaline, sugar, and cholesterol in the blood; (b) reduced blood pressure and less stress on the cardiovascular system; (c) slower breathing with improved lung function and metabolic rate; (d) and relaxed muscles, which contain less lactic acid, improved digestion, and cooling of skin with less activity from the sweat glands.

Now in Taleghani General Hospital outpatient's clinic as Integrative Medicine Healing oriented group, we study on our patients with mind-body approach and therapy. We organised some Stress-management, Relationship, Dream manifestation workshops. Also by psychoanalysis, meditation, art therapy and if it is necessary, by hypnosis, we work on our patients to achieve their well-being and healthy conditions. (h) Family-Guide to-ComplementaryandConventionalMedicin

13.4 Nourishment of the Human Soul

As one the major aspects of therapy, soul nourishment is a very important part of complementary medicine and more so in preventive therapy—to feed or sustain with substances necessary for life or growth; to promote growth; to maintain or support; to nurture. *Soul*—the immaterial essence, animating principle or actuating cause of an individual; the spiritual principle embodied in human beings, all rational and spiritual beings or the universe; a person's total self. The holistic health field abounds with articles and books all teaching a variety of ways to nurture our souls.

What exactly does all these mean and why are they so important? The soul, or what I call the 'core self' or 'true self', being the very essence of who and what we are is our life force, and therefore, it needs 'food' on a regular basis to sustain us and prevent us from becoming stagnant and unfulfilled with life. So what is nourishing to the soul or the core self? The things that make you feel whole, alive, and one with the universe (or God) is your soul food. This will vary from individual to individual, as our souls or core selves are very unique and complex, although many of us have some commonalities. Some common sources of soul food are nature, music, dancing, deep relationships, meditation, walking, praying, and many more.

For example, my most important source of soul food is nature and time with my beloved ones. Doing things like spending time by the seaside, taking walks along the country rides, admiring the cloud formations, feeding and watching the birds, feeding a stray cat, gazing at the stars and the moon, and spending time discussing world peace are activities most nourishing for me. Nature is my lifeline. It rejuvenates me and helps me to go on. It makes me feel alive, full of life, and connected to the universe. There is nothing more nourishing to me than spending a day on a blanket reding my favourite book and being intimate with nature, especially on a warm hammertan evening day in West Africa when the leaves are bursting with colour. Spending it with someone I love and engaging in deep conversation is even better. Writing, reading, listening to certain types of music such as the Jim Reves and the famous

Congolese African music and singing along, dancing, deep relationships, and prayer also nurture me.

You can discover your soul food by listening to the yearnings of your soul or core self, by being still and tuning into your deepest voice within. Your core self will guide you to what it needs. Don't ignore it, and don't put it off. Once you learn what you need, nourish it on a regular basis. If you neglect your soul or core self then it becomes hungry and searches for food in the wrong places, which is destructive to your life and zaps you of your life-sustaining energy. After years and years of neglect, one becomes disconnected from their soul or core self and gets lost. Our world is sadly full of people who neglect their souls (core selves) and the consequences of this are seen all around us in the level of addictions, violence, crime, depression, suicide, lack of compassion and respect for one another, divorce, and destruction of our planet exhibited in every society. Our industrialised culture has not been very good at teaching us how to avoid this, perhaps because we were unaware for a long period of time, but slowly, this is changing one by one. Don't neglect your soul-core self! Listen to it, nourish it, and feed it every day. It is as important as feeding your hungry stomach. If you have neglected your soul-core self, it is never too late to start again. It is upon this spiritual essence that our physical well-being depends. It has an amazing ability to recover, flourish, rejuvenate, regenerate, reactivate, and restore our well-being to splendour once again.

The discussion on this topic is generic—it touches every member of every society—men and women, young and the old. The topic should form an anchor point of the preventive therapy.

13.5 Deep Breathing for Preventive Therapy

This is one of the major natural means of preventive therapy we must apply and use in the processes of the counselling and consulting with our clients. The technique may sound very simple and easy, but the aspirant preventive complementary health practitioners must develop a programme of therapeutic deep breathing induction and training for their clients. Although it is a part of transcendental meditation, it can be learnt separately.

Deep breathing exercises are about the most natural and holistic self-care strategy you can find and the single most effective, beneficial technique we can use to relieve pain, stress, and anxiety and achieve overall relaxation. It's also non-toxic; costs us absolutely nothing; requires no prescriptions, equipment, visits to the doctor, or health food store; and is available to you at all times. It produces soothing, relaxing, and pleasure-inducing alpha brainwaves; calms the excitatory neurotransmitters and stress–response system; and thus relieves anxiety and stress instantly. These alpha brainwaves also stimulate the release of beta-endorphin, the body's built-in, natural pain reliever, and stimulate creativity as well. Most of us never stop and think about what an amazing thing our breath is. It is something we take for granted. It's so simple and intrinsic to living that we never give it a second thought, and most of us are unaware that we don't know how to breathe properly or that the breath can be used as a tool for improving our health. When you don't breathe properly, your body does not receive adequate amounts of oxygen. This depletes your energy, allows toxins to accumulate, weakens your immune system, clouds your head, triggers excitatory neurotransmitters, and disconnects you from your spirituality–the inner essence that propels or animates your life.

How to Breathe Properly

Learning how to breathe in a manner that promotes health is essential for those with an already existing health condition, as well as for those who are practising prevention. We are taught at an early age to sink in our stomachs and puff out our chests, and many people breathe through their mouth instead of their nose. This is in complete contradiction to healthy breathing. Deep breathing exercises that teach us to be more conscious of our breathing will help us to unlearn these bad habits. Breathing through your mouth increases the charge of energy and facilitates the discharge of emotions. You may have noticed that when you are upset, you breathe heavy sighs out through your mouth. This is not bad during those times because it helps expel the emotions, but it isn't a state you want to remain in consistently.

Breathing through your nose keeps the charge of energy in check, increasing control and slowing your metabolism.[1] To breathe properly, when you inhale, your abdomen should protrude, not your chest. When you exhale, your abdomen should flatten. When you breathe in, you should breathe in slowly through the nose, not the mouth, until the lungs are almost full. When you exhale, it should be slow and until almost all air is expelled. Each breath should be through the nose—deep, complete, long, and slow. Place your hands on your abdomen. If it rises and falls with each breath, then you are breathing correctly. In therapeutic preventive practice, teach your clients/patients how to carry out these exercises.

Basic Deep Breathing Exercise

- Open your mouth and exhale. Close your mouth and take in a long, slow breath as described above. Keep your mouth closed and breathe out in a long, slow, and controlled manner, as described above. Each time you breathe in and out, that is considered a round. So do at least seven or eight rounds. You can stop once you begin to feel the relaxation radiate through your body and mind or continue with a few more rounds for deeper relaxation.
- Close your eyes, if possible. Closing your eyes enhances the benefits of your breath, because this immediately activates alpha brainwaves and incites relaxation. However, if it isn't possible to close your eyes, the breathing alone will work as well.

Use your breath as needed throughout your day: during times of high anxiety, stress, or disharmony. Wherever you are, just stop and take a few minutes to close your eyes and take several deep breaths, using the proper breathing procedure described above. I have provided you with a very basic outline on using the breath to improve your health that you can put to use immediately. However, if you'd like to learn more about how breath-work improves your health and eight more easy techniques, Dr Andrew Weil has an excellent beginners' CD that can be found by visiting this link:*

Breathing: As The Master Key to Self-Healing

Dr Weil's CD is a fantastic educational source on why and how your breath is important. It basically gives you a little crash course on the impact that breathing has on human health and then provides eight easy and simple techniques to achieve a variety of different goals.

Benefits of Deep Breathing Exercises

When you breathe through your nose, as described above, you can use your breath to help relieve pain, boost energy, clarify and quiet the mind, relieve tension, lesson the intensity of symptoms of any health conditions you have, improve sleep, relax, calm and soothe the body and mind, quiet the deeper self and help yourself to be more spiritually connected. You will also oxygenate your body and help your body to detoxify better and boost the immune system.

Some of the conditions that benefit the most from deep breathing exercises include, insomnia, headaches, migraines, heart disease, back pain, balancing pH, high blood pressure, emphysema, improving sports performance, unspecified chronic pain, adrenal fatigue, depression, anxiety disorders, panic attacks, PTSD, MS, food sensitivities, chemical sensitivities, fibromyalgia, and arthritis. However, there probably isn't any condition that wouldn't benefit in some way, particularly if it is accompanied by pain and stress. I personally find deep breathing to be the most effective form of stress relief, next to exercising. Deep breathing turns off the sympathetic nervous system and turns on the parasympathetic nervous system, so it is one of the most beneficial techniques you can find for adrenal disorders, anxiety, PTSD, or any condition related to the sympathetic nervous system.

Sometimes you may not be able to eliminate the pain completely, but at the very least, your patients will be able to function better within the pain or other symptoms they may be experiencing. It reduces the severity of impact and improves the quality of life. Practicing deep breathing first thing in the morning and at night right before they go to sleep is really helpful for calming down and relaxing. It will get their day off to a good start and help them fall asleep. For example, I carry out deep breathing exercises as soon as I lie down every night, and it puts me right to sleep. I'm usually out before round ten. Aside from the health conditions, because of the production of alpha brainwaves, deep breathing is also highly effective for spiritual fulfillment: it promotes simple relaxation, higher states of consciousness, high levels of creativity, and heightened awareness, so even healthy people can reap the many benefits to be found with breath. Another example is that I experience very high levels of creativity when I practise my breathing exercises. Words, ideas, and insights for books, web pages, newsletters, etc. just flow like a stream and send me running for my pencil and paper constantly. When you have time, you can take your conscious breathing one step further and find deeper relaxation by using the following breathing technique.

Extended Deep Breathing Therapy

Guide your patients to lie down somewhere comfortable and close their eyes. Thye can have some relaxing, soothing music playing in the background if they prefer or complete silence. Make them completely comfortable with pillows or whatever, and let them keep their arms at their sides. Loosen any tight clothing. Tell them to take a very deep breath in (using the proper breathing exercise described above), then exhale. Make sure that they are breathing through the nose. Let them do this several times until they begin to feel that their body is relaxed a little. Ensure that they are not thinking about anything. Let them focus their minds completely on the breath—each breath flowing in and out. This is conscious breathing at its best. Now lead them to take another deep breath, and beginning with the top of their heads, guide their breath to that area. Tell them to use their minds' eyes as they exhale, directing the breath into his or her head. With the exhalation, let them envision that the breath is penetrating into that area of the body they are focusing on. Lead them to take another deep breath, and this time, using their minds' eyes, guide the breath into their face muscles, then another deep breath into their jaw and eye muscles. Your patient should begin to feel little tingles as tension and pain melt away.

If tension is persistent and doesn't loosen, then try tightening the area by clenching and then releasing and then breathing into the area again. It may take several attempts to grasp this technique if this is new for the therapist. It's easy to get distracted and let your mind drift off into unwanted territory. As you practise breathing exercises more frequently, it will become easier and quicker to attain. After you begin to relax, do several deep breaths into the whole head and face area and enjoy the sensation. Now move to your shoulders and chest. Take a deep breath and on exhalation, breathe into your shoulders and then take another deep breath and breathe into the chest. After several deep breaths guided to these areas, imagine the breath is now radiating down the arms and into the fingers as you breathe in deeply and exhale into the chest. Don't forget to make sure that you're breathing through your nose. When you're inexperienced, it's very easy to slip back into your normal pattern of breathing without realising it.

Then move to your abdomen and hips and again guide your deep breath on exhales into each of them. As they begin to relax, imagine that the breath is now radiating down the legs and into the feet and toes as it flows into the abdomen. Again, if any particular area is resisting, then tense it up by clenching and release it and breathe into it again until it releases. If you are experiencing a headache, migraine, or pain in any particular area of your body, you can use conscious breathing to guide the breath into that particular area. Now the whole body should be relaxed, and anxiety and pain will be minimised. Your mind should be calmer and you should feel peaceful. Stay in this position for a while and continue to breathe deep breaths through your nose. Guide the exhales into the centre of your body, radiating out to each and every part of your body, and enjoy the sensation of complete relaxation. At this point, you could add a meditation session and enhance the benefits even further or just bask in the feeling of being stress free. You may get up when you feel ready.

Try to make time daily for this extended deep breathing technique at least a few times a week. Additionally, music that is designed specifically for relaxation can be used to deepen your experience and benefits as well. One of my favourite pieces of music to accompany my breathing and relaxation periods is *Music to Disappear In*. It's the perfect companion to use with breathing exercises and/or meditation, and it just melts the stress away. When you combine music designed to relax with meditation and deep breathing, you triple the depth of your benefits. I have found these deep breathing exercises to work best when I can close my eyes, but it is also very helpful at other times. After you become more skilled at it, you will be able to use them while you are driving, at the computer, in a conversation, or wherever you may be, but of course, you can't close your eyes at those times. The benefits that can be found with the breathing excises of this nature are so great and the investment required is so little that it makes this a self-care technique that should be used by everyone. The cost of zero makes it accessible to even the most financially challenged people.

13.6 The Chronic Deficiency in Vitamins and Minerals Intake Found in Various Countries

Vitamins and minerals function in a wide variety of ways within the body. For instance, they often form major parts of enzymes and coenzymes. Enzymes and coenzymes are molecules that work together as catalysts to speed up chemical reactions that might otherwise take place very slowly in the body. If an enzyme is lacking the essential mineral or vitamin, it cannot function properly. By providing the necessary mineral through diet or a nutritional supplement, the enzyme can then perform its vital function. Key to nutritional medicine is supplying the necessary support or nutrients to allow various enzymes throughout the body to work at their best.

Vitamins are of very little value without minerals. Minerals are absolutely essential for our bodies to function properly. The human body cannot produce its own minerals. A deficiency of even just one trace mineral can lead to poor health, chronic diseases, and a shortened lifespan. Very few of us get the sixty-plus minerals we need every day from our food. Because of the modern methods at all stages of today's food production—from depleted soils, to refining, and further processing and packaging—many essential nutrients are lost. Attempts are often made to replace them with man-made synthetics that are not as efficiently utilised in the body as natural nutrients. In June 1992, the Earth Summit Report by the World Health Organisation reported on the decline of nutritional minerals in farm and range soils over the last hundred years:

Continent	% depleted
Australia	55%
Europe	72%
Africa	74%
Asia	76%
South America	76%
North America	85%

The Society for complementary medicine, UK

Seventy per cent of visits to the doctor's office in the United States are due to nutritional deficiency. Fortunately, there are ways to compensate for nutritional deficiencies. One of the best is by using high-quality dietary supplements. If they're formulated and manufactured properly, these supplements will help ensure that the body's enzyme systems have the vitamins and minerals they need—the point is 'if' they are formulated and manufactured properly. Unless a complementary medical practitioner has been well trained and devoted to his or her duties, the selection of an appropriate source of food supplments will not be achieved. The above information can help us in the practice of preventive therapy.

13.7 Herbal Medicine (Herbmed)

An Alternative Medicine Research Foundation Based in India

Although there are many research finding reports presented in this book, HerbMed report presented here will provide an alternative choice reference of Garlic Herbal therapeutics to the practitioners: In complementary health care, the uses of garlic are not by a guesswork. There are research evidences for its therapeutic validity.

Clinical Trials of Garlic Product

Short-term supplementation with oily garlic formulation on lipid metabolism, glucose level, and antioxidant status was tested in seventy subjects (thirty-two males, 38 females) suffering from primary arterial hypertension and it was found to have hypoglycemic and antioxidant properties, Duda in 2008.

The meta-analysis suggests that garlic preparations are superior to placebo in reducing blood pressure in individuals with hypertension, Ried in 2008.

The systemic increase of nitric oxide due to the ingestion of garlic on the plasma interferon-alpha level in normal volunteers was investigated and showed that consumption of garlic resulted in stimulated synthesis of No and, in turn, IFN-alpha, Bhattacharyya 2007 in 2007.

The frequency of garlic usage in hypertensive population was investigated and acute effect of garlic and garlic tablets on blood pressure in patients with hypertension was evaluated. 4102 of the 7703 patients (53.3 per cent) reported that they were using garlic, Capraz in 2007.

In study of eighty males (forty aged between eighteen and sixty; forty aged sixty-one years and over) and eighty females (same age ranges) A. sativum was less effective than dry extract of G. biloba in reducing blood viscosity, Galdu. In OO7.

The clinical evidence based on rigorous trials of the effectiveness of garlic relates to cancer, common cold, hypercholesterolemia, hypertension, peripheral arterial disease, and pre-eclampsia was assessed, Pittler in 2007.

Platelet function is not impaired by single and repeated oral consumption of a dietary dose of garlic in eighteen healthy volunteers. Dishes containing socially acceptable doses of raw garlic are unlikely to increase the risk of perioperative bleeding, Scharbert in 2007.

A pilot study evaluating coronary artery calcification and the effect of garlic therapy in a group of patients who were also on statin therapy suggested incremental benefits, Budoff in 2006.

A double-blind trial with 3 interventions namely treatment with amoxicillin and omeprazole, long-term administration of garlic (aged garlic ext. and steam distilled garlic oil) and supplement (vit. E and C and selenium) to study their effects in reducing precancerous gastric lesions is described, Gail in 2006.

In a randomised double-blind trial, administration of aged garlic extract to fifty patients with advanced cancer of the digestive system improved natural-killer cell activity, but caused no improvement in quality of life, Ishikawa in 2006.

The use of whole blood platelet lumi-aggregometry was studied to optimise anti-platelet therapy comprising aspirin, clopidogrel, and/or odorless garlic in twenty-seven patients with chronic myeloproliferative disorders, Manoharan in 2006.

The review of trials on the effects of garlic on prevention of pre-eclampsia and its complications found just one study of uncertain quality (n=100), which showed no differences between dried garlic tablets and placebo, Meher in 2006.

Study on the effect of oral garlic on arterial oxygen pressure in fifteen children with hepatopulmonary syndrome shows that garlic may increase oxygenation and improve dyspnoea. Najafi Sani in 2006.

A randomised, double blind pilot study of twenty female inpatients with systemic sclerosis received a seven-day add-on therapy with either 900 mg dried garlic powder or placebo shows improved rheologic properties, [Article in German] Rapp 2006.

The effect of monascus garlic fermented extract (MGFE) on fifteen hyperlipidemic subjects indicates that MGFE attenuates hyperlipidemia, suggesting that MGFE is a potent agent for preventing arteriosclerotic diseases, Sumioka 2006.

A preliminary double-blind, randomised clinical trial using high-dose aged garlic extract (age 2.4 mL/d) as an active treatment and low-dose aged (age 0.16 mL/d) as a control, suppresses progression of colorectal adenomas in thirty-seven patients, Tanaka in 2006.

A clinical trial to examine if aged garlic extract reduces macro- and micro-vascular-endothelial dysfunction during acute hyperhomo-cysteinemia induced by oral methionine in healthy subjects suggests that it prevents a decrease in bioavailable No and endothelium-derived.

13.8 The Need for a New Medical System That Cures Sickness and Cures People

The concept which puts forward that a humanistic approach to medicine must be the system of multidimentional nature. This means that we should endeavour not only to treat the disease but also the sick individual as well. For example, this is what Dr Christian Hahnneman had in mind when he introduced the system of homeopathic medicine in 1763.

Modern medical science, both in the Occident and in the Orient, looks at patients as if they were all similar objects; that is, it treats them equally, regardless of their individual differences. So in the case of an illness, it doesn't matter who is ill. The only thing that matters is the illness that the person has. So the modern medical system consists of the process of solving such questions as what is the cause of the illness, how did it arrive, and how to cure it.

Modern medical practice first finds a name for the illness through various diagnostics and then plans a cure. Oriental medical practice isn't different, except that it understands illness mainly by the included symptoms of the illness instead of by its name, and then plans a cure. Therefore, we define oriental medical science as that which distinguishes symptoms and signs. So it is said that the essence of the oriental medical system is the analysis and identifying of symptoms according to eight principal syndromes: yin, yang, outside, inside, cold, warm, weak, and strong, and by the theory of the six meridians of Zhang Zhanjiang. Up till now, the medical systems in the Orient and the Occident are the same in that they both look at the illness as being more important than the ill person in curing people. In other words, they are systems that take illnesses as objects of curing, rather than people.

We must ask, though, can the modern medical systems that uniformly treat primarily illnesses, ignoring the ill person, really save people from all kinds of illness? Even the modern medical science, strikingly evolved through the advances of cutting-edge science, still can't completely save people from the trap of illness. This is an undeniable reality. No matter how many prisons are built, crime doesn't decrease. Likewise, it is not possible to save humanity from illness through the paradigm of modern medical systems, Oriental or Occidental, which separate the person who is ill from the illness, and take only the illness as the object to be conquered.

It is time for the medical paradigm to shift, to take the ill person as primary, rather than the illness. It should not only treat illness, but also give more attention to the person suffering from the illness. A new paradigm is needed—a paradigm that doesn't treat all people the same, but recognises and accepts individual differences in each person. For that, it is necessary to study the human being.

If that's true, we can begin with these questions: Is every person the same from birth? If they're different, what is the difference? If there is an individual difference, what is its essence? In order to understand these questions, let us first look at some concrete examples easily found around us.

Even though a group of people equally expose themselves to cold winds in a frozen environment, some of them easily catch cold, but others don't. Of course, we can think that the difference is caused by the state of health and bodily strength of each individual. But even among those who caught a cold, some complain of a cough and runny nose, others of a swollen throat and tonsils. One has a stocky build, looks very strong, and has a big appetite, yet he/she catches cold more easily than others. Another is small and looks weak, but seldom catches cold but nevertheless, habitually suffers from bad digestion.

This indicates that there really is a difference between individuals, not explainable only by the bodily strength and resistance that every person has. These kinds of examples are all around us but usually are overlooked. If all people had the same bodily conditions from birth, it would be true that this kind of individual difference should not be present. If people expose themselves equally to cold winds, they should all catch colds equally. If people overeat equally, it would be true that they should suffer identical cases of indigestion. If this isn't the case, if there is a difference between individuals, that means that each person was born with a different bodily condition.

People are different according to their face, looks, character, temperament, hobbies, talent, intelligence, emotion, taste, capabilities, and other characteristics. These differences can't be denied. Besides these, people are different also by their internal organs. Some have stronger lungs, others have stronger digestion and can tolerate even overeating. Being equally over drunk, some can handle it but others cannot. There was a television comedy programme that showed an interesting experiment. A group of students each drank two litres of beer and competed to see who could hold out the longest without having to urinate. Someone went to the toilet after only half an hour, while others held out for more than four or five hours. There was quite a variety in the results. That is an example that shows a difference between individuals even in their bladder capacities.

In the same way, people are not born with the same bodily conditions: people's bodies are different from birth. This is the viewpoint of the constitutional theory and medical practice. The dictionary defines constitution as the combination of the basic bodily temperaments. Constitutional medical theory, therefore, is defined as the theory by which the differences in people's forms and functions are researched and divided into various subgroups.

CHAPTER 14

Summary of the Book

From my training, exposure, and experience, I realised that it is not only the diseases like malaria, TB, and other infections that can be prevented. It is certain that if we apply various knowledge and skills implicit in complementary medicine, many other diseases and infections can be prevented. This book is an attempt aimed at looking through the various bodies of knowledge generically referred to as complementary medicine. The principal objective of the book is to provide a projective guiding line for preventive therapy in complementary medicine. Therapies in natural medicine include naturopathy, holistic health and healing, energy work, native and traditional medicine, aromatherapy using essential oils, nutritional and cleansing therapies, homoeopathy, and vitamins supplementary therapy. Together they are referred to as Alternative/Complementary Medical System that focuses on natural remedies and the body's vital ability to heal. Holistic health is a concept in medical practice, upholding that all aspects of people's needs—psychological, physical, social, and mental aspect should be taken into account so that the individual is treated holistically. This effort has led me to the journey of many and various national cultures where traditional/complementary medicine is being practised. The result of this exposure is an additional knowledge in this field.

The term 'Preventive Therapy' must be used with great care. It is possible that it can be misunderstood as meaning the idea of stopping diseases and infections. Anybody who produces an answer for stopping sickness entirely will be facing a tremendous barrage of attacks from the individuals and organisations engaged in the manufacture and administration of medical drugs. This will be the case anywhere in the world. A typical case of similar nature is the cigarette production industry. Even though the producers of this drug are fully aware of the inherent danger, the psychology of economic self-interest, takes precedence over all other considerations. Consequently, if the producers of medical products of any type had a say in the perpetual continuation of diseases and sicknesses, would it not be for their own interest that these human maladies should continue? Another typical example in point is the manufacturing and the sales of ammunitions of any type. Apart for the national defence, what other purposes are these incendiary products serving? But you see, for the same economic self-interest, these products will continue to be in existence.

Historically, the initial aim of the founding fathers and mothers of health and therapeutic systems (Herbs-human care) was to prevent and protect mankind from the sufferings inflected upon them by diseases and sickness. The initial approaches to diagnosis and treatment can be traced back to the medicine history of African-Egyptians beginning with Imhotep. This man lived during the African Old Kingdom and was born a commoner during the Third Dynasty. He was very skilled and was dedicated to the ideals of his nation. Imhotep manufactured herbal seed products, grapefruit seed extract, and many other alternative health products. The same approach applied even to other physicians many years after Imhotep. For example, the famous Hippocrates, physician (born: c. 460 BC, birthplace: Island of Cos, Greece, died: 377 BC. He is best known as: Author of the Hippocratic Oath.) Hippocrates was committed to fostering a natural lifestyle. H introduced complemented enzyme-rich products. He also introduced 'living' foods for vegetarian cuisine. He enhanced immunity to disease through the system of positive thinking. The old masters of natural medicine followed the same pattern of approaches. Indeed, what was most important to them was the art of preventing and protecting the people from diseases.

In modern time, as we have discovered, the characteristic of conventional medical health care system and the public demand has induced us to begin tapping into the natural vital powers of non-conventional methods of health care. In our understanding, the natural powers inherent within the herbal products and the substances transcend other sources and methods of health care. The term 'Natural Medicine' is a generic one. The system (subsystem of Medical System) can be practised anywhere by anyone who is properly trained and experienced. Indeed, the field is not the exclusive domain of the non-orthodox practitioners.

In fact, some of the well-known complementary health care practitioners are also orthodox medical doctors. However, the principal point in
preventive therapy is our ability and capability to understand the components of various herbal commodities and the therapeutic properties
and their behaviour in given health care problems. One of the important
things to understand in complementary medicine is that non-herbal
products or nutritional supplements cannot substitute for good food
nutrients. In my experience, I have discovered that the best and most
effective therapy is the combination of the appropriate food intake and
the selective sources of multi-nutritional food supplements of vitamins
and minerals. The reason is because it is not possible to obtain sufficient
amount of vitamins and minerals from food alone, especially in these
days of mechanised agriculture in food production.

It is not true that natural medicines and nutritional supplements
have no side effects on health. Every type of medication has a side
effect of a kind, depending on the type of product, the purpose for the
administration, the health situation of the client, and the knowledge
and professional skills of the practitioner (s) involved. Once we start at
this premise, this will induce us to become more careful in the diagnosis
and application, knowing that as health care professionals, we will be
held fully responsible and accountable. It is unprofessional to tell the
public or our patients that the products we are giving them have no
side effects just to run down the orthodox system of medicine. The
product(s) on its own may not have any side effect, but anything can go
wrong in the process of administering the remedy. This kind of 'street
wisdom' expression of claim must be avoided by all means. The care for
human health and handling of any type of medication are very delicate
issues. The only people who might be in a position to pass such kinds
of opinions are the pharmaceutical people, who are usually involved in
the laboratory and manufacturing of the medical products in question
and not us, the practitioners.

14.1 Food as the Principal Aspect of Preventive Therapy

It is not possible for any measure in the preventive therapy to
exist without considering the numerous dangers resulting from the
consumption of foods and beverages. Let us consider first food hygiene.
This is one of the essential parts of maintaining good health by preventing
contamination. The basic rule of this factor must start with the habit

of purchasing, storage, procuring, preparing, cooking, and the transit-storing prior to serving for human consumption. When these processes are not carefully managed and controlled, the consequences in terms of food poisoning can be sudden and severe. Although this book is not a training in the subject of bacteriology and food poisoning related to the catering profession, it is important to look at some of the food items that are vulnerable to contamination and hence an infection. Fish from the river and the sea are recognised as nutritionally very beneficial. But research has discovered that their consumption can be of life-threatening due their contamination.

For example, in Japan, a fish dish as sushi and sashimi carries worms that can easily find their way into the human body. Codfish must be cooked thoroughly well to ensure that all the worms and their eggs are killed. Fish can also be contamined by cadmium and mercury in industrial discharge from smelting works. The deposits of these heavy metals in the human body can damage the nervous system. The amount of mercury in tinned tuna fish can also cause poisoning. Altough all the people involved in the processes of food and beverages catering for human consumption are expected to be trainined in the prevetion of contamination and safety for the health care of the public (customers), the complementary health care professionals must be concerned with this problem. In 1994, in England and Wales alone, eighty-seven thousand cases of food poisoning were reported and nearly sixty-five thousand of similar cases were reported in 1992 and very many were not reported. Most food items harbour bacteria, and they can be very dangerous, especially in these days of fast food and machine-displayed beef sandwich, turkey sandwich, egg sandwich, and chicken sandwich, including cheese sandwich. The two mostcommon sources of contamination are nasal and faecal transference from the food service staff (cross-contamination) These food preparation and service staff must be regularly supervised for care and safety.

14.2 The Effect of Thought on Health and the Body

The theme of this book is preventive therapy. Apart from the obvious meaning relating to complementary health care, let us reflect over the totality or the holistic meaning of the word. From the overall contents of this bok, I am sure that readers are very clear that I am not wholly stamped to the concept of applying medicine all the time, be it homeopathic, hydrotherapy, herbal therapy, or any other approach that is geared towards physical application for health care. Let us reflect over the effects of thought on the health and the body.

The body is the servant of the mind. It obeys the operations of the mind, whether they be deliberately chosen or automatically expressed. At the bidding of unlawful thoughts, the body sinks rapidly into disease and decay; at the command of glad and beautiful thoughts, it becomes clothed with youthfulness and beauty.

Disease and health, like circumstances, are rooted in thought. Sickly thoughts will express themselves through a sickly body. Thoughts of fear have been known to kill a person as speedily as a bullet, and they are continually killing thousands of people just as surely, though less rapidly. The people who live in fear of disease are the people who get it. Anxiety quickly demoralises the whole body and lays it open to the entrance of disease; while impure thoughts, even if not physically indulged, will soon shatter the nervous system. Strong, pure, and happy thoughts build up the body in vigour and grace. The body is a delicate and plastic instrument, which responds readily to the thoughts by which it is impressed, and habits of thought will produce their own effects, good or bad, upon it. We will continue to have impure and poisoned blood so long as we propagate unclean thoughts. Out of a clean heart comes a clean life and a clean body. Out of a defiled mind proceed a defiled life and a corrupt body. Thought is the fount of action, life, and manifestation; make the fountain pure, and all will be pure.

Change of diet alone will not help a person who will not change his/her thoughts. When a person makes his/her thoughts pure, he or she no longer desires impure food. Clean thoughts make clean habits. The so-called saint who does not wash his body is not a saint. He who has strengthened and purified his thoughts does not need to consider the malevolent microbe. If you would protect your body, guard your mind. If you would renew your body, beautify your mind. Thoughts of malice, envy, disappointment, and despondency, rob the body of its health and grace. A sour face does not come by chance; it is made by sour thoughts. Wrinkles that mar are drawn by folly, passion, and pride. I know a woman of ninety-six years who has the bright, innocent face of a girl. I know a man well under middle age whose face is drawn into inharmonious contours. The one is the result of a sweet and sunny disposition; the other is the outcome of passion and discontent. As you cannot have a sweet and wholesome abode unless you admit the air and sunshine freely into your rooms, so also a strong body and a bright, happy, or serene countenance can only result from the free admittance into the mind of thoughts of joy, goodwill, and serenity.

On the faces of some of the aged, there are wrinkles made by sympathy; on otherfaces, they are caused by strong and pure thought, and still on others, the wrinkles are carved by passion: who cannot distinguish them? With those who have lived righteously, age is calm, peaceful, and softly mellowed, like the setting sun. I once saw an aged elder of African descent on his deathbed. This papa was not old except in years. He died as sweetly and peacefully as he had lived. There is no physician like cheerful thought for dissipating the ills of the body; there is no comforter to compare with goodwill for dispersing the shadows of grief and sorrow. To live continually in thoughts of ill will, cynicism, suspicion, and envy, is to be confined in a self-made prison hole. But to think well of all, to be cheerful with all, to patiently learn to find the good in all—such unselfish thoughts are the very portals of heaven; and by dwelling every day in thoughts of peace towards every creature will bring abounding peace to their possessor.

All complementary health practitioners should pay more attention to preventing the possibility of their clients' becoming sick. Always consult and advise them on the matter of their inner state of mind. The reactions to various given situations of their daily lives are very important. There is an adage which says that 'it is not the load you are carrying that is very heavy but rather the way you are carrying the load.' Let me ask you the following question: What magic do you think is changing the relationship between the white people and black people in the world today? In fact, it is not the greatness of our might nor is it our physical strenghth at all. It our love for them—whether expressed or maintained inwardly. The great messiahs of the past encouraged us to love those who have treated us wrongly. Jesus said that, Mahatma Ganhdi of India told us that, Mandela of South Africa told us that, Dr King of America told us that, and Gauntama Buddha of India told us that too. This love, which we should give instead of retaliating, has power of changing the world for good! For example, watch a peson who is always positive and very happy in all his or her daily dealings with life; you will see that they will look very healthy and attractive. In fact, what is responsible for that kind of appearance is an inner self-love, inner peace, and an inner rcognition of self-worth. This 'charity must begin at home', they say.

Tracing the History of European Herbology

In all cultures, the origins of herbal medicine are lost in the mists of time. There is little doubt that humans used herbs for healing well before anything could be written about them. At some point in an advancing culture, written documents become the repository for knowledge that had been passed on from one generation to the next. Among the earliest such documents are those describing the religious beliefs of the people and those describing the medical practices. Many authorities recognise Hippocrates (460–375 BC.) as the 'father of medicine' for the European tradition. He had little interest in the use of herbs. The primary focus of the Hippocratic School of Medicine was diet and nutrition and a reliance on calm, moderate living. These are the same foundations that herbalists such as Künzle put forth as the basis for healing (see Chapter 4). A summation of the Hippocratic approach was presented by Erwin Ackerknecht in his 1968 book (revised from the 1955 edition), *A Short History of Medicine*, as relayed below. Naturopathic physicians today will recognise the opening description as the one adopted in the definition of their profession. Reference is then made to the conditions of apepsis and pepsis, referring, basically, to inability to properly digest (apepsis) or ability to properly digest (pepsis), which is likened to cooking of the food in the stomach, relying on an innate heat. To students of Asian medicine, this is a near-perfect echo of teachings from India and China about the source of disease and the resolution of disease via invigorating this digestive fire and promoting the healthy function of the digestive system.

The treatment of the Hippocratic physician reflected his fundamental approach. It was the treatment of an individual, not a disease, and the treatment of the whole body, not any part of it. Treatment was based on the fundamental assumption that nature, *physis*, had a strong healing force and tendency of its own, and that the main role of the physician was to assist nature in this healing process, rather than to direct it arbitrarily. Health was a state of harmonic mixture of the humours, and disease was a state of faulty mixture. The disordered humours were in a state of *apepsis*, and nature itself tried to re-establish balance through a process of *pepsis* or coction through the so-called innate heat. This coction, which simply means 'cooking', usually ended with a crisis on a 'critical day' when the disease matter, the end product of coction, was eliminated. Sometimes the disease petered out slowly in lysis, instead of crisis. The main ally of the physician in assisting nature in this process was diet. More violent means of elimination, such as purging, vomiting, and bloodletting, were seldom used by the Hippocratics. Only if diet failed were drugs used, and surgery was a last resort. The great philosopher Aristotle (384–322 BC) was the son of a medical man and a medical man himself, but his main influence on the development of European medicine was through his student, Theophrastus (380–287 BC), called the 'father of botany.' He was the first known author in Europe (and the rest of the world) of a classification system for plants with accompanying comments about their medicinal properties. He described about 450 different medicinal plants. However, this text has not come down through history and is only noted in later commentaries.

The first document of herbal medicine to attain the status of a medical classic in the European tradition was by Dioscorides (AD 40–90). Known as Materia Medica, a fifth century reproduction still exists, complete with botanical illustrations that were apparently added to the original text (carefully preserved in Vienna). Dioscorides was a surgeon who accompanied the armies of Nero. He travelled far, collected much information, and gained considerable medical experience as he went. His work was later adopted by Muslim physicians, leading to the development of Unani medicine (Greek medicine as retained in the Islamic tradition). Dioscorides had compiled herb knowledge for six hundred plants. His comments on the use of herbs are sometimes relayed today to provide evidence that one or more of the current uses of herbs is the same as it had been for many centuries. The book's illustrations were considered the only authoritative ones for European medicinal plants for over a thousand years. The work was translated to English in 1655, and continued to be the primary reference on European herbs, though other herbals developed from this basic work became better known because they provided current knowledge and the idiom of the times.

Greek medicine continued to develop for several decades after Dioscorides, but it eventually began to stagnate. The last notable contributor was Galen (AD 130–201), who was born in Pergamum, the site of the temple of Ascelpius (God of Healing). He was influenced by the developing Christianity, mentioning both Moses and Christ in his writings, and believed that the Creator endowed every organ with a purpose. He had determined a route by which nutrient substances were transferred to the liver, transformed there to blood, and then circulated to the rest of the body. Unlike Hippocratic physicians, he believed in more active therapies to change the course of disease, including drawing blood and inducing laxative or diuretic action. He liked complex herbal formulas, which were later referred to as Galenicals (a term still sometimes used today). The formulas were designed to balance the different qualities of the herbs so as to produce an effect that would properly restore the body humours to harmony. His talents were so great that he was made court physician to Emperor Marcus Aurelius. During the Dark Ages that followed the collapse of the formerly well-organised and powerful Greco-Roman society, knowledge of herbs and medicine was preserved in two places. In Europe, it was retained by Christian monasteries (which also stored knowledge of other fields of human inquiry), and following the development of Islam, it was retained in the Arab and Persian regions. In France, the school at the Cathedral of Chartres was an important centre for medical studies around AD 1000 Monasteries not only retained libraries of medical books, but also were involved in maintaining herbal gardens that served as a source of medicine for the monks and their visiting patients. Monastic medicine was virtually halted in 1130, however, when its practice was forbidden because it was taking up too much time, but other clergy, not confined to monasteries, continued the work. Avicenna (980-1063), in what is today Iran, was the main proponent and developer of Greek medicine, and his *Canon of Medicine* influenced European doctors for centuries afterwards. This Unani medicine, via Avicenna's book, was brought to Europe just as monastic medicine was being shut down.

After the printing of books became standard practice during the Renaissance period, each country eventually had its own herbal publications in its own language. *The Herbal*, printed in 1530 by the German Otto Brunfels, is often singled out as marking the beginning of the new era in widely published national herbals. The Italian Mattioli wrote *Commentaries on the Six Books of Dioscorides* in 1544, and included improved information about the plant identities and added descriptions of many more plants that had become used as medicines. In England, the beginning of this period was marked by publication of *New Herbal* in 1551 by William Turner. Some of the books produced around this time attained high standing, such as that of English herbalist John Gerarde (1545-1612), who published his *General History of Plants* in 1597, followed by a revised edition published posthumously in 1633. This book included two thousand eight hundred plants, serving as a vast compendium of European herbology. The revision of Gerarde's book was illustrated with the artistic work of Jacob Dietrich (1520–90), who had produced the German language book *Neuw Kreuterbuch* (*New Herbal*) in 1588. Like the work of Dioscorides, the herbals of the sixteenth century became standards that persisted in their influence, at least until another watershed change took place in the rapid medical evolution and explosion in popular publishing during the twentieth century.

14.3 Johann Künzle and His Contemporaries

Dietrich's book was the primary reference work for Künzle, who studied it in detail as an adjunct to what he had learnt from his contemporaries and immediate predecessors. Künzle then became one of the leading herbal authorities in Europe for the twentieth century, helping usher in the modern era of herbalism as an alternative to modern medicine. At age seventeen, Künzle attended a foundation school (high school) at Einsiedeln, where one of his professors was Father Ludwig. In his book, Father Künzle writes: 'For my whole life I shall be grateful to the deceased Father Ludwig because on our afternoon walks he explained to us everything about the herbs we showed him . . . When later Father Kneipp called attention to the healing powers of herbs, it was easy for me to find them.'

Thus, the herb knowledge that Künzle began to accumulate early in life was passed on to him by the Catholic professors (Father Kneipp also became famous throughout Europe and is still mentioned today, see below). No doubt, the information they had to offer, which Ludwig had acquired from early nineteenth-century sources, was largely a reflection of what both Dietrich and Gerarde had accumulated in the sixteenth century and published for succeeding generations to learn from. But, the focus of herbal interest for these niettenth-century priests was the local plants in central Europe, which they could observe and collect. In the introduction to the republished *Herbs and Weeds* in 1975, the editor notes of Künzle that 'through the profound and fervent study of the old and best books of Detrich Jacobs [sic], as well as through personal research, experiments in the laboratory, and therapeutic experiments, he became a medical chemist [pharmacist] of immense success.'

Soon after *Herbs and Weeds* was published in 1911, a herb enthusiast in England, Maude Grieve, began compiling detailed monographs on herbs. These were eventually gathered into *A Modern Herbal*, published in 1931, with the information carefully checked by the book's editor. Grieve originally had a personal interest in growing plants, but eventually dug through several English language herbal guides to produce a comprehensive presentation of accumulated herbal knowledge. Quoting directly from numerous past authorities, she especially made references to the earlier English writers, mainly Gerarde and Culpeper. Nicholas Culpeper (1616–54) was not an academic; he wrote in a popular style that was appreciated at the time. Like Künzle, he thought that proper diet, moderate exercise, and other common sense, healthful practices, along with the use of herbs, were important to avoiding serious disease. *A Modern Herbal* was republished in 1971, and became one of the key guides for the burgeoning new interest in herbs that began about that time. In 1945, the year of Künzle's death, his students produced a grand new work on herbs, *Comprehensive Guide to Herbal Healing* (*Das Grosse Karuterheilbuch*). Compared to Künzle's earlier teachings in *Herbs and Weeds*, this text revealed a more sophisticated approach, and it is largely academic in nature. The first part of the book details human anatomy and physiology. The presentation is the same as that of standard medicine, but it is simplified to focus on the aspects of interest to the new herbal practitioners, who would now be botanical specialists interested in herbs as modern pharmacy. The book then presents information about the botanical identity, chemical constituents, and other defining features of the plants. The diagnostic aspects and treatment of specific diseases are then outlined. Each of the herbs get a brief description of medical applications. Not only were the medical subjects all carefully outlined, but also, unlike Künzle's earlier work, the main subjects of interest to herbalists were all carefully alphabetised: disease names and plant names. One section of the book (The healing method of herbal priest, Künzle), not attributed to a particular author, appears to be a direct recitation of Künzle's philosophy of disease causation and treatment, perhaps taken from notes recorded by his students during numerous lectures. The table of contents gives a good overview of the subject matter; the chapters on diseases and plant descriptions in alphabetic order were said to follow Künzle's presentations. This large and detailed book, unlike the small and folksy *Herbs and Weeds*, failed to capture the imagination of the people, though it remains a well-known text of European herbal medicine still available today. It has since been largely superceded by new texts by modern authors reporting on research developments during the past thirty years.

Modern Herbal Knowledge from This European Tradition

For America, Grieve's book, being in English and including most of the herbs that were available on the international herb market, eventually became the one authoritative guide coming from Europe to answer the demands for herbal knowledge. The old British book was made available in a new two-volume set during the 1970s, when interest in herbs was accelerating thanks to the efforts of a publisher (Dover) that has pursued the republication of older books and has an extensive listing of health titles. Also during the 1970s, books by some American herbalists, such as Jethro Kloss (who wrote *Back To Eden* in the 1930s) and the contemporary popular teachers John Christopher and John Lust, presented information and ideas based on their personal experience with herbs. They passed on knowledge that they acquired locally, without much reference to the main tradition that had been preserved in historic European books. But for detailed knowledge of the herbs they discussed, many Americans simply turned to Grieve's *Modern Herbal*, which quoted extensively from the European tradition. Künzle's two books remained unknown in America (the larger volume was never translated to English). Herb knowledge is now readily obtained from numerous sources, including both professional and lay publications and on a plethora of Internet sites. Those interested in the practical application of the herbal knowledge often can obtain an orientation and context for their herb use from an inspirational figure who has captured the popular attention through untiring work culminating in a written record. In Europe, Künzle is still mentioned in this context.

Both Grieve and Künzle had an impact on the herb industry in their respective countries. Of Grieve, it was said that 'during the War (1914-18), when there was a shortage of medicinal plants because they could no longer be imported from abroad, Mrs Grieve made practical use of her knowledge and trained pupils in the work of drying and preparing herbs for the chemists' [pharmacists'] market. She did a great deal to revive the herb industry in England.'

Of Father Künzle, who virtually single-handedly stimulated the growth of a major herbal industry in Switzerland, it was said that 'he was considered one of the greatest benefactors in Switzerland.'

The revival of interest in herbal remedies eventually led to a concern about the safety and efficacy of the herbs. In Europe, where Germany was the largest source of herbal products, a concerted effort was made to evaluate the herbs. In 1976, the West German Government defined herbal remedies as belonging to the same classification as drugs. The Federal Health Agency formed a commission for evaluating the herbs, which came to be known as the Commission E. A series of three hundred herb monographs were produced and published in German during the period 1984-91. These monographs were later translated to English and published by the American Botanical Council in 1998 as *The Complete German Commission E Monographs: Therapeutic Guide to Herbal Medicines.* At the same time as these monographs were translated and compiled into a single guidebook, an effort was made to greatly expand and update the information that had been presented in the all-too-brief monographs, as well as to add some herbs that had not yet received monographs. This work was published as *Herbal Medicine: Expanded Commission E Monographs*, also by the American Botanical Council, in 2000. The information about the twenty-seven herbs outlined in this book in Chapter 8 was compiled from a search of several herb guides, but mainly from the ones described here, such as the earlier books *A Modern Herbal* and *Herbs and Weeds*, and the recent *Complete German Commission E Monographs* and *Herbal Medicine.* Historical information was obtained also from *Health Plants of the World*, and herb safety checks were made by searching the PubMed web site, which carries titles and abstracts from hundreds of medical journals worldwide.

Contributions of Herbalist Priests in Central Europe

1. Rev. Father Sebastian Kneipp (1821-97)

It is unfortunate that in most literatures of health care and medicine, whether orthordox or complementary, the immense contributions by the early missionaries are hardly mentioned. After all, the care and treatment of people began in the antiquities of the Egyptian and the European manors (houses and the surrounding lands owned by the nobilities, known as Lord of the Manors.) In the medieval Europe, the missionaries and missions were the only places of abode for the ordinary commoners. During my research, I was able to fish out some of those priests who dedicated their time and perhaps, their life too, to ensure that people within their parish received health care of a kind. The following individuals featured prominently of my findings:

Father Sebastian Kneipp (1821-97) of Bavaria is recognised as one of the leading contributors to the modern field of natural healing. He advocated exposure to nature: sunlight, baths, fresh air, and dips in cold water, eating natural foods (rather than processed foods), and having a positive mental attitude, as a means of recovering health, and this is an origin of the 'spa' movement in central Europe that remains vibrant today. He became convinced of the efficacy of this approach when, at the age of about twenty-one, he suffered from tuberculosis and cured himself by these methods—particularly 'water therapy'—which, it was said, he found described in the Vatican archives, though it may have been from another church library. After becoming a priest, he began making recommendations for the sick parishioners. Father Kneipp had a strong influence on the development of naturopathy and herbal therapeutics in America. In 1892, one of those who sought out Father Kneipp's help was Benedict Lust, a German who had immigrated to America, but then returned home after contracting tuberculosis. He was cured using Kneipp's method of water therapy (along with healthy diet and herbs) and became convinced of its general usefulness. He returned to America to promote 'Kneippism', starting schools, societies, magazines, health food stores, and sanitariums. Lust utilised the name 'naturopathy' to describe the basic approach and founded the American Naturopathic Association and the American School of Naturopathy.

2.   Father Johann Künzle (1857-1945)

Künzle had learnt from Kneipp as well as from other priest—herbalists (such as Father Ludwig, mentioned in his autobiography), and his work stimulated considerable interest in herbalism in Europe during the first half of the twentieth century. In turn, Kneipp and Künzle both influenced the Austrian herbalist Hermann-Josef Weidinger (1918-2004). He had studied European herbalism in his youth and travelled to China as a missionary, where he lived from 1938 to 1953, and learnt of their herbal system from a Buddhist monk and also while working with an army doctor. He returned from China due to illness and continued his work as a herbalist, writing numerous books on natural health care. Until recently, he and thirty-seven assistants prepared and prescribed herbal remedies in Karlstein, Austria, at the Paracelsus House Nature Cure Center. One of his favourite remedies was elderberry juice. He pointed out that 'elderberry cleanses the digestive system and promotes healthy elimination. This is most essential to good health.' Father Weidinger believed that elderberry protects the body from serious diseases and observed: 'Elderberry reduces inflammation and relieves the body of impurities. In this manner it also balances the emotions.' Weidinger employed concentrated elderberry juice as a mainstay in his herbal cleansing and healing programmes. To complete this story of the history of the European herbal tradition, it is worth noting that the first recorded medicinal use of elderberries was by Hippocrates in the fifth century BC. The Romans believed that anyone who cultivated the elderberry would die of old age instead of sickness.

A Healthier Style of Life

One of the tenets of natural healing is that anything reducing the body's ability to remove waste materials and to fend off infections is to be avoided. A factor that was of concern to Father Künzle was exposure to cold and its adverse effects on the eliminative function of the kidneys (this is explained in some detail in the appendix). Thus, for example, he raised a concern in his herb book about the practice, apparently new and increasingly common during his time, of leaving children to play on cold cement floors. He believed that this often led to the experience of sickness, such as the common cold, flu, or bronchitis. We know today that these ailments are caused, ultimately, by an infectious agent, but we also know that exposure to cold can lower the body's immune responses and allow an existing infectious agent, kept in check by a healthy immune system, to prosper and produce a disease. While modern central heating, carpeting, and other conveniences that make exposure to cold cement floors (or the equivalent) less likely, we still have children who participate in practices that overexpose them to illness, and this applies to adults as well for whom we can no longer say that they ought to know better, because they weren't taught correctly in the first place. It thus comes about that magazines, displayed by the dozen at the market check out stands, have to give the most basic advice about steps to protect health, as if it is news.

Künzle also complained about a practice of relying on too much meat in the diet. He said that as a result of eating so much meat, even two or three different kinds in one meal, and having it with every meal and even some sausage at teatime (a European practice), 'the head is dull, the stomach full, sleep is restless, and humour (mood) detestable.' We know now that the heavy reliance on meat puts far too much saturated fat into the bloodstream and that the excessive protein puts its burden on the kidneys to eliminate the waste as uric acid. Further, we know that filling a stomach with meat leaves little room for vegetables that provide fibre, flavonoids, and other substances that promote the health of the gastrointestinal system and have a beneficial effect on the circulation. But the dull-headed feeling, the sleep that is restless, and the humour that is detestable are rarely blamed on this or other poor dietary choices, even though they are likely to be among the consequences of such eating habits. When it comes to gastric distress that might be most obviously linked to poor eating habits, modern drugs are recommended to alleviate the heartburn and other symptoms so as to permit one's choice of foods to be unimpeded by normal body reactions. Modern authorities recommend limiting the total intake of meat at any meal to a measly three ounces and to use lean meat at that. Vegetarianism, or inclusion of meatless meals several times per week, has become popular. Overall, this is a good thing. Still it is a shame that people have come to counting quantities of substances in their daily consumption instead of getting a better sense of dietary balance. Such counting has given rise to entirely ridiculous decisions, such as using a synthetic chemical sweetener in place of natural sugar (to avoid a number of calories) or consuming an imitation cheese product in place of natural cheese (to avoid a quantity of fat). It is unclear if soybeans converted by some industrial process into something that loosely resembles meat is really any healthier than eating the meat itself. Instead of enabling unmitigated consumption by creating synthetic substitutes, returning to what nature has to offer is a viable alternative, if only it would be given due attention.

Children are naturally vegetarian, distaining the idea of eating the animals that they so much enjoy seeing in their live state—that is, if the parents let children have regular exposure to a variety of (live) animals. It is not necessary to isolate them from animal-based products, such as milk, cheese, butter, and eggs. These are natural foods that are rich in nutrients, particularly calcium in milk and cheese and protein in eggs and milk products, that growing children need in such large quantities as it is difficult to get adequate amounts from other sources. Nor is it necessary to ban the intake of meats. On the other hand, there is no value in pushing a meat-eating diet on children as a requirement for health, so long as careful consideration is given to getting the essential nutritional value from other natural sources. For teenagers and adults, one should select a diet that is consistent with one's lifestyle and individual physiology. There will be some, especially those who are very physically active, who will do best having some meat and other rich foods with virtually every meal, and those people should not be said to be wrong for doing so. Similarly, there will be some, especially those who have a more sedentary lifestyle, who will remain vegetarian, to varying degrees of strictness, and they should not be said more right for doing so. What is wrong in a diet is to pursue something that is unhealthful just for a wrong-headed idea. Künzle pointed to people who ate too much meat because they deemed it a sign of being successful: if you have money, you eat meat. This is eating for appearance's sake, and the appearance is not all that grand. But those who only eat certain vegetables and nothing else—simply because someone has stated that these are superior—may likewise follow a false path, thinking oneself more righteous on account of a meagre diet, one which might leave one gaseous and sickly, rather than in glowing health.

Künzle put it this way: 'If you split wood after such a meal [of rich foods, with eggs, flour, cheese, etc.], or dig up your field, or carry home a good load of hay, you may be able to digest the food, provided your stomach is not already weakened by continuous meat eating. But, if your work requires no considerable physical exertion, you will have to avoid such heavy dishes.' The food has to match the requirements of the physical activities—it is fuel for the body. In modern times, there have been significant debates about the positive or negative effects of grains (and other carbohydrates), meats (and other proteins), and fats (saturated, unsaturated, omega-3, omega-6, etc.). Unfortunately, the discussion often is based not on a natural approach to diet, but on trying to get around problems that have been generated by the modern way of producing food, processing food, and eating meals. Otherwise, it wouldn't be necessary to worry about these issues based on laboratory analysis of food constituents.

Künzle made some specific dietary recommendations, and their value has been confirmed over time. One of Künzle's main recommendations—that people should consume legumes such as peas and beans—is now known to be a very healthful way of getting the protein benefits of the plant world. These foods provide other advantages inherent in eating vegetables, such as fibre, calcium, and flavonoids. Today, most health books promote the advantages of consuming soybean products, but this is really a benefit to be found to varying extents in all the legumes. A favoured Künzle recipe, which he attributes to Father Kneipp, was to combine barley, peas, and beans, boiled together with celery, parsley, and chives to make a nourishing, savoury soup. 'Two or three platefuls at noon will satisfy the strongest man and keep him healthy. This is the soup of our forefathers and of the good old days of natural living. This soup made men of iron and women were as strong as oaks even after having given birth to as many as a dozen children.'

Unlike some of today's advocates of natural health care, he did not shun milk and wheat but thought that they served as a good substitute for eating meat, referring to them as Lenten foods (being used during Lent when eating meat was not permitted for the religious faithful). He was very concerned with the increasing problem of constipation. This condition, which had made laxatives a best-selling over-the-counter remedy during most of the twentieth century, was due to substitution of fibreless foods for those that had long been relied upon previously, as well as loss of exercise and, as a result, deterioration of the abdominal musculature. He pointed out, as an example, the reliance on chocolate, for which his country has held a worldwide reputation. He complained:

> In factories and shops, many munch these black tablets [of chocolate] like old horses the whole day long. As a sign of our sweet civilization, one finds every street littered with chocolate wrappers and pictures . . . If you want to ruin your child's health, just give them a log of it. But, if you want them to be healthy, give them all kinds of fruit, like nuts, figs, oranges, dates, apples, pears, etc.

Today, it is the agriculture department that advises people to change habits and eat more fruits (and vegetables and grains) but less fats and sweets (which chocolate provides plenty of). The taste for and hence the desire to eat these natural treats (fruits) is lost by the continued reliance on artificial flavours and artificially produced textures of snack foods.

As a Catholic priest, Künzle was well aware of the importance of religion in maintaining a solid healthful style of living. He believed that the teachings showed that Christ 'did not want man to be ill but healed the sick instead and restored the injured nature. This He did not achieve, of course, with herbs, poisons, or baths, but with divine power. But, the very fact that He worked miracles to heal men proves that He wanted men to be healthy and that it is against the will of God to make the body sick by unreasonable living.' Faith in this basic principle guided

Künzle's efforts. This was an important observation, because in earlier centuries many people ignored their health, looking forward only to the life after this one on earth. He also stated that 'God has surrounded us with remedies on all sides by giving curative properties to herbs, flowers, fruits, and roots.' In this, he expressed the sentiment that had arisen in all cultures: that we are born into a world that has what is needed. It is up to us to take proper advantage of that. Similar ideas, from any religious faith, should be able to do the same for others who are not Catholic or Christian. For example, if the body is said to be like a 'temple', that means it is to be treated with respect and kept as clean and healthy as possible in order to accomplish spiritual goals. There were some aspects of Künzle's life that he may have taken for granted and not delineated as recommendations. I'd like to elaborate a few concerns that one can sense from his presentation, but were not outlined explicitly in the book that he left as a legacy of his learning and wise counsel. I take full responsibility for any suggestions that miss the mark. They are presented as under:

1) Get up early in the morning. This is not to gain an advantage, as expressed in the saying about the early bird, nor is it to beat the rush-hour traffic. It is to give time that is needed to taking care of the spirit and the body. In the morning, with the freshness of sleep and the crispness of the air, one can undertake spiritual practices, do some simple exercises, develop an appetite, take care of hygiene, and become truly prepared for the day by laying a good, strong foundation. Greet the sun. It is the most powerful force in nature: if you ignore it, you ignore all other natural signs. Prepare a healthful breakfast. Künzle stated that 'it is most important that our first meal in the morning is nourishing and wholesome,' a recommendation still relayed by virtually all health authorities today. In his book, Künzle relayed this about his childhood:

> We always got up early, usually at five o'clock in the morn-ing, in summer at four o'clock, and during the haymaking season, at three o'clock. We came down to the living room, dipped our hands in holy water, blessed ourselves and repeated 'Jesus Christ be praised!' Before and after every meal we said Grace . . . Meat was served on Sundays only. On the other days we ate porridge, milk, barley,

groats soup, Chas-Chnopfli (wheat farina with cheese), or potatoes.'

2) Work diligently. No matter what the task at hand, do it well, pay attention, try to excel, and don't shy away from physical labour. There is nothing to be gained by doing work half-heartedly, absent mindedly, or with no intention to improve. And, don't plan on retiring early to avoid the work of using your hard-won skills. It is reported that 'in 1922, Father Künzle, as a sixty-five-year-old student, was called before the most meticulous physician's examining board for an examination which he passed brilliantly. It is said that right at the beginning of it, he embarrassed the noble gentlemen by asking innocently whether they wanted him to answer the questions in Greek or Latin.' Künzle continued his studies, healing work, and teaching into his eighties.

3) Help others. There is no greater reward than spending one's time be helpful to others: family members, neighbours, and all who you have the power to contact. Seek no rewards for your help; they flow naturally. It is reported of Künzle that 'the vein of gold that he struck by his popularity he gave away to the poor and sick, disregarding differences in religion. Though the right hand did not know what the left was doing [meaning: while he did his charitable work, it also brought a lot of fame and fortune that was not given attention], he was considered one of the greatest benefactors in Switzerland. He did his work of charity inconspicuously and secretly and, in most cases, forgot about it soon.'

4) Study There is much to learn and so little time to learn it. Knowledge can be passed on to the next generation who will benefit greatly from your efforts. Künzle wrote: 'To help people is a Christian and social deed. Would therefore all who have people's welfare at heart, as well as time and opportunity, study the old forgotten botany and give to the suffering quick [to prepare], cheap, and harmless household remedies.'

5) Get exercise and sunshine. The human body was made for movement outdoors and has been subjected to confinement indoors by modernisation. Some balance must be attained. Künzle already revealed his experience in hard farm work during his youth and hours of study taken regularly indoors to pursue his career. In

visiting people who lived in remote areas, ministering to sickness that affected their soul and their body, he walked considerable distances, much of it in the hilly terrain characteristic of Switzerland. Already in the early twentieth century, he complained that 'no one cares to go on foot any more no matter how much time he may have at his disposal or how fine the weather may be . . . It is considered improper nowadays to carry any load whatever: and why? Because it stimulates walking, carrying loads, working, and consequently digestion and therefore good health, all of which is opposed to the modern views of the twentieth century.' He did not advocate vigorous exercises that bring people to the limits of their capability, but he advocated moderate exercise done in adequate amounts, as was suggested by all medical authorities in the past, from Hippocrates on. The sun is also important to man; its rays, we know now, convert vitamin D to an active form that puts calcium into bone and strengthens the human frame. The sunlight raises the spirit. Of course, we are all cautioned about the damaging effects of sun, but this comes from the excesses of sun exposure. Unavoidable long-term exposure to the hot sun (e.g. when labouring out of doors) can be well managed with hats and proper clothing, sunblocks (creams that halt the penetration of the most harmful rays), and avoiding excessive time in the midday sun. Today, people sit behind glass, if exposed to sunlight at all, watching TV, computer monitors, and reading books and are otherwise sheltered from both fresh air and sunlight. This is hardly conducive to health, maintenance of good vision, or a happy countenance.

A person who will arise early, eat a nutritious breakfast, work diligently (including some time out of doors, both for work and for relaxation and pleasure), study, and spend time helping others, who eats and sleeps to be able to do these things well (rather than to simply enjoy some temporary pleasures), and who eschews those activities that detract from these, will be healthy, happy, and productive. Herbs will be a help in times of trouble, and one will rarely have to rely on drugs. It is somewhat scandalous that the modern naturopathy profession has virtually ignored the recommendations of European nature doctors like Kneipp, who were influential in developing naturopathic medicine in both Europe and America. In place of recommending an approach like that outlined here on the basis of Künzle's book, there is increasingly a reliance on prescribing numerous manufactured remedies so that patients spend hundreds of dollars each month to consume highly processed materials or to get such materials injected into the body. In place of suggesting nutritious food to fuel diligent work, emphasis is placed almost entirely on avoidance of a growing list of ordinary foods. Therefore, the message of Künzle's small book is quite worthy of reconsideration at this time, even by those who are pursuing so-called natural health care.

14.4 Priests and Reverend Father Herbalists

Priets and Reverend Father herbalists within the church. (The body missionaries with the compliments of the baslica in Rome)

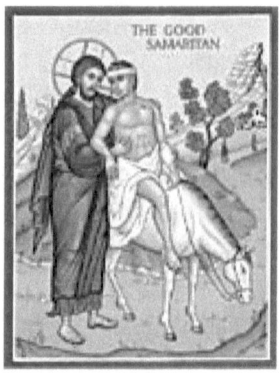

The above picture shows the good Samaritan conveying
a sick person to a priest-herbalist for treatment
as far back as eighteenth century in Europe.

For about 150 years (c. 1850-2000), several Catholic priests in central Europe (Germany, Switzerland, Austria) were involved in a 'back to nature' approach and herbal prescribing. Three of them became particularly well known and have left a legacy of natural health care methods appreciated by many today. Father Sebastian Kneipp (1821-97) of Bavaria is recognised as one of the leading contributors to the modern field of natural healing. He advocated exposure to nature: sunlight, baths, fresh air, dips in cold water, eating natural foods, and having a positive mental attitude, as a means of recovering health, and this is an origin of the 'spa' movement in central Europe that remains vibrant today. He became convinced of the efficacy of natural healing methods when, at the age of about twenty-one, he suffered from tuberculosis and cured himself, relying especially on the 'cold water method' that he had found described in a small book by a country doctor that was in King's library in Munich. After becoming a priest, he began making recommendations for sick parishioners (see the Catholic Encyclopedia for more information about Sebastian Kneipp).

Father Johann Künzle (1857-1945) of Switzerland had learnt from Kneipp as well as from other priest-herbalists (such as Father Ludwig, mentioned in his autobiography), and his work stimulated considerable interest in herbalism in Europe during the first half of the twentieth century. His work has led to production of herb formulas used in many countries. Künzle wrote a small book, *Chrut und Uchrut* (*Herbs and Weeds*) that was published in 1911 (and reprinted with additions until 1975). It captured the essence of the culture of natural living and natural healing that was still alive but struggling. Eventually, more than a million copies of the book were printed in the German language, distributed mainly in Switzerland, Germany, and Austria, and this was followed up with translations distributed to several other countries in Europe. Künzle had been first exposed to the medicinal properties of herbs during his high school years by a professor who was a Catholic priest. Künzle then attended the University of Lowen where he studied theology and philosophy and entered the seminary at St Gallen, Switzerland. He was ordained a priest in 1881. Künzle pursued herbalism in response to his experience of being a spiritual adviser to parents who were dying and about to leave behind young children. He would sometimes restore the health of his wards by administering or recommending teas, herbal baths, and other preparations. Eventually, his work as herbalist took over his daily life, and he devoted himself almost solely to this task, though never leaving behind his devotion to the Catholic faith.

Father Johann Künzle described his experiences in the following introduction:

> A spiritual adviser, I often had to visit sick fathers and mothers who according to the reports of the local physicians, were dying, leaving behind their little children. In such cases, I gathered up all my knowledge of herbs and was often able to get them back on their feet again. Among others, I was thus able to help a poor Protestant who had been lying in his bed for two years, painfully afflicted with gout and swollen

limbs. 'You must get this man out of bed again,' I told myself, and accomplished it after four weeks. Now people said, 'The parson can almost work miracles. He helps disregarding even the difference of faith!' Every evening, groups of working men and women came to me and implored me to help them and I did what I could. When someone reported me to the bishop, who at first did not want to hear anything about my doctoring activity, I sent some of the cured to him to tell the story. This satisfied the bishop, who then gave me per He recommended the use of herbs to prevent an ailment from progressing to a stage so serious that the new medical treatments were needed; to treat persons who were not able to get to a doctor due to their remote location; and to try, somet

The priest Johann Künzle set an example of unaffected and direct naturalness for the whole church and the whole Swiss people, the like of which perhaps hasn't existed since Francis of Assisi. Caring for neither popularity nor offence, throughout his whole life, he exhibited the direct frankness and honesty on which the Kingdom of Heaven could have been built and by which all stupidity and evil on this earth could have been vanquished. He always loved the people, the simplest and the most modest, and every mountain peasant meant as much to him as a cardinal. His egalitarian beliefs were carried out in actions as he was quite capable of saying what he thought in the presence of His Eminence. The Protestant was as near to him as his co-religionist. For him, faith and honesty were healing herbs for human society, and he didn't care in which meadow they were found. All this was his nature, his high moral character. And to that, I take my hat off!

The work of both Kneipp and Künzle influenced the Austrian Hermann-Josef Weidinger (1918-2004), better known as Herbal Priest Weidinger. He had studied European herbalism in his youth and travelled to China as a missionary in 1938, where he learnt also of their herbal system; he returned from China in 1953 and soon after entered the Premonstratensian Monastery of Geras. He continued his work as a herbalist and proponent of healthy lifestyle, writing some forty books on natural health care. Until recently, he and thirty-seven assistants prepared and prescribed herbal remedies in Karlstein, Austria, at the Paracelsus House Nature Cure Center. Weidinger had collaborated with the Austrian artist Adolf Blaim (1942-2004), who had contributed to the restoration of the convent of Altenburg. Blaim painted more than a thousand pictures for Weidinger as illustrations for his books as well as for use by Vereins der Freunde der Heilkräuter (Friends of Medicinal Herbs Association) that was headed by Weidinger after the death of the priest herbalist Karl Rau in 1979; the association has a membership of thirty thousand. The following are some of those paintings:

Saints Cosmas and Damien

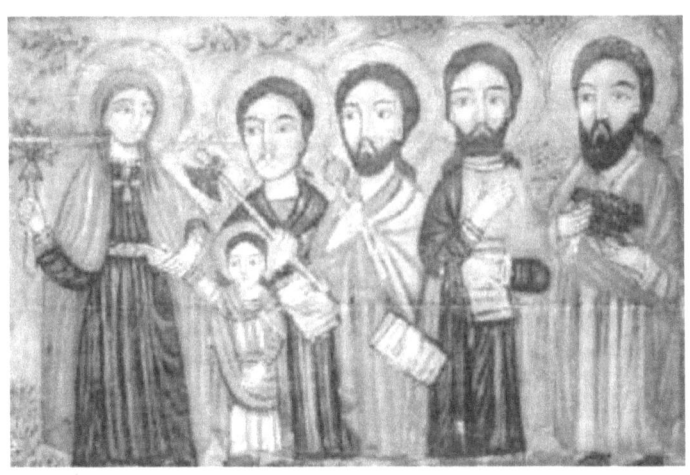

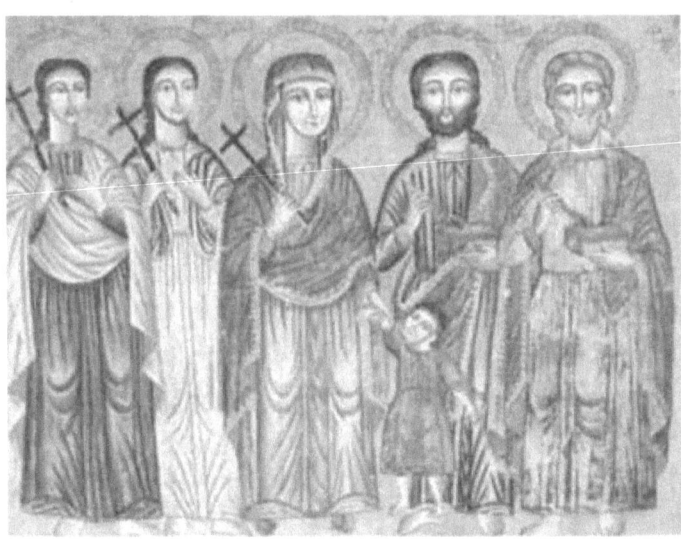

Icons of Saints Cosmas and Damien, with their brothers (Anthimus, Leontius, and Euprepius and their mother, the widow Theodota. All were martyered in the year 303.

Saints Cosmas and Damien were twin brothers born in Arabia (modern-day Syria) around AD 270. They had three younger brothers; their father died, so their mother, Theodota, was left to raise all five of them herself. Cosmas and Damien were educated in science and medicine and became physicians who were quite skilled and enthusiastic about their work. They offered their services primarily in the seaport Aegea (between Tarsus and Antioch), on the Gulf of Iskenderun in the Roman Province of Cilicia (modern-day Turkey, south-central coast). The following story of their work provides a meditation for our own lives:

> Cosmas and Damien saw in every patient a brother or sister in Christ. For this reason, they showed great charity to all and treated their patients to the best of their abilities. Yet no matter how much care a patient required, neither Cosmas nor Damien ever accepted any money for their services. For this reason, they were called *anargyroi* in Greek, which means 'the penniless ones'. Every chance they had, the two saints told their patients about Jesus Christ, the Son of God. Because the people all loved these twin doctors, they listened to them willingly. Cosmas and Damien often brought health back to both the bodies and the souls of those who came to them for help.

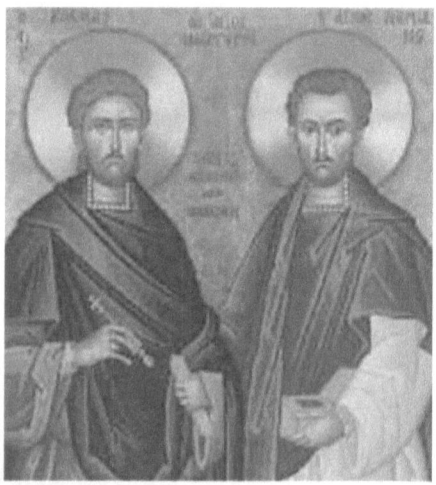

When Diocletian's persecution of Christians began in their city, the saints were arrested at once. They had never tried to hide their great love for their Christian faith. They were tortured, but nothing could make them give up their belief in Christ. They had lived for him and had brought so many people to his love. So at last, they were put to death in the year 303. Diocletian's edict in 303 demanded religious uniformity and the elimination of the Christian sacred literature. Christians who refused to cooperate could face death. It was said that Cosmas and Damien, after refusing to worship the Roman idols, had survived several devious means of torture and death and were finally beheaded. These martyrs are named in the first Eucharistic prayer of the Mass and in the Litany of the Saints.

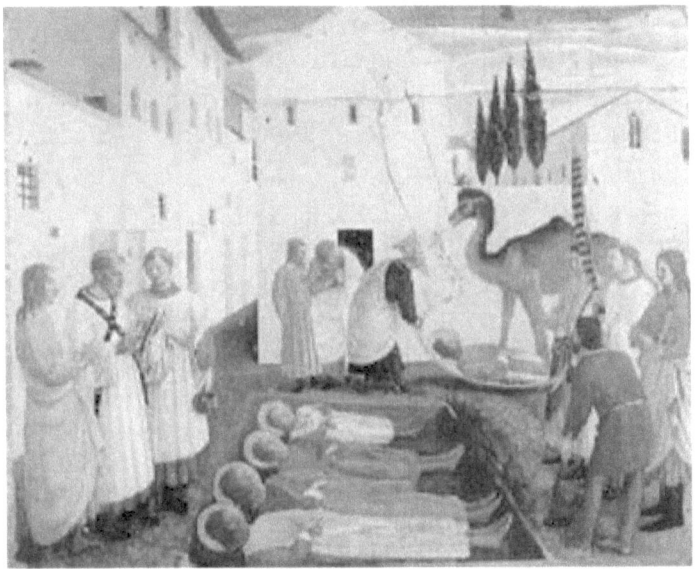

A painting depicting the burial of the martyred saints Cosmas and Damien (foreground), along with their three brothers (one in the background). They were buried in Cyrus (in Syria) and a basilica was built over their tombs. Their feast day is September 27.

Cosmas and Damien followed the instruction Jesus gave to his twelve Apostles, which was relayed in the gospels of Luke and Matthew. 'He sent them out to proclaim the kingdom of God and to heal' (Luke 9: 2), and instructed them 'Cure the sick, raise the dead, cleanse those suffering from leprosy, drive out devils. You received without charge, give without charge' (Matt. 10: 8). These two appear to have been especially revered for adhering to this latter teaching, which was rarely followed by others.

As a result, numerous churches, monasteries, and schools have been named after Cosmas and Damien. A basilica in Rome was erected in their honour two centuries after their deaths by Pope Felix IV (elected Pope 526); at the time, there were already five churches dedicated to these medical martyrs in the city. The basilica was built in an area of Rome considered the zone of medicine, replacing a structure that was part of Vespasian's Forum of Peace, and dedicated in 530. At about the same time, Emperor Justinian I restored the city of Cyrus in their honour. Although the remains of Cosmas and Damien are at Cyrus, there are also relics preserved in the crypt at the Roman basilica. Over time, the basilica went through numerous changes, with deterioration followed by restoration, with additions and reconstructions. In 1503, the basilica was consigned to the Third Order Regular of St Francis for maintenance (formally transferred in 1512), and this religious order manages the basilica to this day.

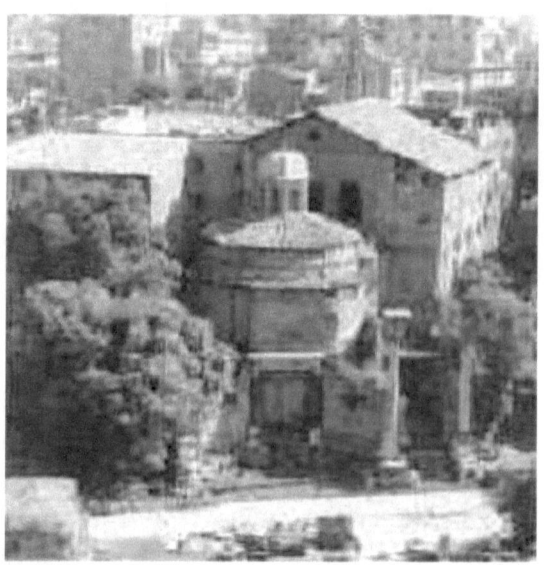

Exterior view of the basilica of Cosmas and Damien.

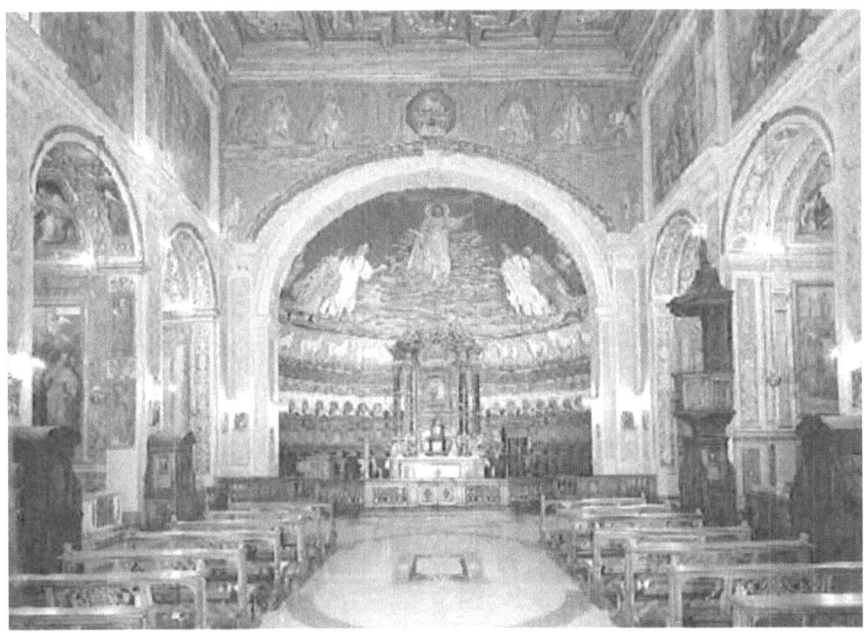

Interior view of the basilica in Rome. In the renowned mosaic from the original construction of the basilica, Christ is flanked by St Cosmas and St Damien, who stand with St Peter (next to Cosmas) and St Paul (next to Damien); the Apostles, with arms around their shoulders, are introducing them to Christ. St Theodore of Tyre (a soldier who converted to Christianity and was also martyred during the Diocletian persecution) and Pope Felix IV are also depicted, the latter with a model of the church in his hands. They stand on golden water plants, symbolising the river Jordan. Below is the Lamb of God with twelve sheep symbolising the Apostles. The Latin inscription accompanying the mosaic is translated as follows: 'God's residence radiates brilliantly in shining materials, the precious light of the faith in it glows even more. The secure hope of salvation comes to the people from the martyred doctors, and from the sanctity of this place derives honor. Felix offers this worthy gift to God, so that he might live in the heavenly abode.'

Following is an example of a prayer that is offered to saints Cosmas and Damien: O My Jesus, saints Cosmas and Damien were twins who became excellent doctors. They refused payment for their medical care because they believed that when they treated patients, they were also caring for you. By conveying great love, they won the hearts of their patients as they taught them about the faith. I ask them to pray for my special skills, that I use them for your glory. I also ask them to pray for all those in the medical field, that they grow in generosity of spirit. Bring conversion to the unsaved and teach Christians to serve you through their professional lives. Saints Cosmas and Damien, pray for us, amen.

Herbs in the Tea Formulas

The herbs in the tea formulas that were described in the previous chapter have passed numerous safety evaluations and are considered by most herbalists as effective ingredients. All of these herbs have been used for centuries; some of them were already in use during the ancient Graeco-Roman period of herbalism described in Chapter 2. In the following pages, there is a brief review of each of the herbs. The ingredients are arranged in alphabetical order.

1	Anise	15	Lemon balm
2	Birch	16	Licorice
3	Boldo	17	Meadowsweet
4	Caraway	18	Orange blossom
5	Chamomile	19	Peppermint
6	Coriander	20	Plantain
7	Echinacea	21	Rosemary
8	Elder	22	Senna leaf
9	Fennel	23	St John's wort
10	Goldenrod	24	Star anise
11	Green tea	25	Thyme
12	Hops	26	Valerian
13	Juniper	27	Yarrow
14	Lavender		

Of these, certain ingredients are included in most of the teas due to their known benefits, good taste, and common use by European herbalists: anise, fennel, hops, lemon balm, licorice, peppermint, and valerian. In particular, peppermint is in all but one of the tea blends (not in laxative tea), serving as the basic health tea. It is common practice to have a base ingredient in most blends in other herbal cultures as well: Chinese teas often use ginger, jujube, and licorice as base ingredients, while Indian blends often include myrobalans fruits (a combination of the three), and Indonesian remedies often have turmeric as their base. Here is how Künzle explains the special value of peppermint:

All varieties of mint dissolve old residues and eliminate waste matter and obstinate flatulence and are, therefore, used against almost all ailments of man and cattle. Besides, they increase and further the healing power of other herbs. To assist in understanding the therapeutic contributions of the formula ingredients, following is a table of terms used in the herbal literature to describe the actions of herbs.

Terms used to describe the action of herbs

Term	Meaning
Anodyne	Relieves pain
Anthelmintic	Inhibits intestinal worms
Anti-cattharal	Reduces excessive mucous secretions
Antidiarrhoeal	Treats diarrhoea, especially chronic condition
Anti-emetic	Reduces nausea and helps prevent vomiting
Anti-inflammatory	Reduces inflammation (e.g. in arthritis, skin diseases, infections)
Antipyretic	Reduces fever (antipyretic herbs are described as febrifuge)
Antirheumatic	Relieves joint and muscle pain due to rheumatism (as opposed to injury)
Antispasmodic	Alleviates muscle contractions
Aperient	Produces mild laxative effect
Astringent	Reduces discharge of fluids (e.g. diarrhoea, leucorrhoea, copious sputum)
Bronchodilator	Alleviates wheezing by dilating lung passages
Carminative	Alleviates gas and bloating
Cholagogue	Promotes secretion of bile
Demulcent	Provides soothing effect on mucous membranes (has slippery, coating action)
Diaphoretic	Promotes sweating, a method of therapy to treat acute infections and fevers
Digestive aid	Provides general improvement of digestive function
Diuretic	Promotes urination, usually in cases of oedema
Emenogogue	Promotes initiation of menstrual bleeding
Expectorant	Promotes release of sputum
Galactagogue	Promotes milk production in nursing mothers
Haemostatic	Reduces bleeding

Hepatoprotective	Reduces liver inflammation caused by chemicals, viruses, etc.
Hypoglycaemic	Reduces blood sugar in cases of elevated sugar levels (i.e. diabetes)
Hypolipemic	Reduces elevated blood lipids (e.g. high cholesterol, high triglycerides)
Laxative	Promotes bowel movements, usually in cases of constipation
Nervine sedative	Calms and improves nervous system functions
Refrigerant	Has a cooling effect on a non-fever condition, such as experienced on hot days
Sedative	Calming, usually has prompt effect
Stimulant	Enlivens nervous system and metabolism
Stomachic	Improves digestive function of the stomach, improves appetite
Tonic	Helps overcome weakness
Uterine sedative	Reduces uterine contractions (i.e. cramping)
Uterine stimulant	Promotes uterine contractions (i.e. during menstruation)

The Nature of Herbs Described by Rev. Father Künzle

There are a million kinds of plants, and humans have named just about every one of them. Yet, we have been able to focus attention on a small fraction that suit our needs. A few hundred are collected or cultivated in huge amounts for food, building materials, clothing, and other common applications. By far, the greatest number of plants for any use other than gardening (flowers, greenery, shade, etc.) has been to aid human health. Worldwide, about fifty thousand species of plants have been adopted as medicines. Still, only a fraction of them are relied upon in large quantity. For example, in the practice of European herbal medicine there are about 300 species that were in common use during the twentieth century, of which 175 were depicted in Künzle's *Comprehensive Guide to Herbal Healing*; about 100 of those were used frequently.

This trend towards focusing on a small number of herbs is based, in part, on the work of a few herbal practitioners and scholars who devoted considerable time to the investigation of individual species of interest. In order for a herb to enter into regular usage, it has to have been described with sufficient accuracy—and enthusiasm—so that subsequent generations can rely on what has been reported. Over time, plants with powerful effects that are too difficult to control are eliminated from routine use and described as toxic. When two herbs have similar therapeutic uses, one may be retained over the other for reasons of easier access to the medicinal material. Some herbs thought to have remarkable benefits turn out to rarely produce the effect described earlier, and they are dropped. Attention is turned to making the best of those that remain. Once a herb has been deemed reliable in beneficial effect, safe for virtually all users, and able to be found when needed, the next task is to make sure that those in future generations are able to obtain the correct materials. This has been one of the primary roles of the great herbals, especially the illustrated herbals. Still, different plants may have gross features that are similar, and herbs described in the herbals may go by numerous names, generating considerable confusion, which has limited the development of herbalism. It was easy for errors to be introduced and for remedies to go wrong.

We are fortunate that a systematic means of describing plants and naming them has emerged. In relation to the requirements for understanding medicinal plants, botanists subdivide the plants by family, then subdivide the family by genus, and genus by species (sometimes further, by variety). Plant families are marked by having similarities in their general structures; hence, the Pinaceae includes a wide variety of evergreen trees and shrubs with tight leaves, and the Asteracea has showy flowers and includes daisies, dandelions, sunflowers, and many other garden flowers and weeds. The genus links plants that form natural groupings with more similar features. Within a genus, the plants may look similar; sometimes even botanists can easily mistake two species of the same genus due to natural variability in the way the plant grows. Therefore, they must examine the detailed structure of the plant leaves, the flowers (if present), and vascular system to place a plant within one species or another. Microscopic examination may give the requisite information, revealing fibrous structural components and storage cells. This system of differentiating plants and naming them was given to us by the Swedish scientist Carl Linnaeus (1707-78), and it has been a tremendous benefit to herbalists. It was not fully utilised until the end of the nineteenth century, at which point all the European medicinal herbs were identified by these botanical names. Today, we can specify the botanical name of a plant, and it will have the same meaning everywhere in the world. The clinical experiences with using a single species or two closely related species of the same genus in entirely different cultures can now be directly compared. Some herbs have been used not only in Europe but also by the natives of America, by the Chinese, the Africans, and others. The combined knowledge of the herbs from different cultures can be a powerful tool in understanding their potential applications. Modern laboratory and clinical evaluations only make sense when the botanical species under study is clearly identified.

Most herbs have one or two main applications even though they may have dozens of minor uses. We understand that the primary uses of the herb are the direct result of particular groups of active constituents (e.g. terpenes, alkaloids, flavonoids, etc.). Each plant contains thousands of biochemicals, but most of them are either physiologically inactive (or of little activity) or are present in such small amounts as to have no significant effect (unless isolated in high concentration). Fragrant herbs frequently owe their action to the volatile oils that give them their fragrance. Bitter herbs frequently owe their action to alkaloids, saponins, or flavonoids that contribute bitterness. Yet unlike isolated chemicals used as drugs, herbal remedies often rely on numerous active ingredients from one or more plant materials that may have a general effect on the body, such as improving digestion or purifying the blood. Promoting digestive functions and relieving digestive distress is one of the central components of herbal healing across the globe because of the long-held belief in the role of diet and the importance of transforming the foods consumed into useful essences for the body. The role of blood purification is particularly important to the European tradition, where it was considered that accumulations of toxic materials in the blood could make the body susceptible to numerous diseases. Several different plants would be considered of use in treating such conditions and would be combined together. The principles of formulation are diverse and could depend on the nature of the plant materials themselves, their claimed effect in the body, or some combination thereof. As an example, Father Künzle described the following unnamed, but easily recognised, medical condition to which he also presented a unique herbal cure: 'Many persons are permanently indisposed without really being confined to bed. Lack of appetite makes them refuse even the best sausage [a treat desired by most people]. They suffer from obstinate constipation, have pressure on the chest and stomach, and their head aches and seems on fire. They rarely find sleep, and when they do, it is troubled with bad dreams or nightmares. They consult many physicians and annoy them to exasperation. They reel and totter like a victorious party leader after celebrating an election. They put forth a piteous wail of lamentation like organ pipes, often with a full orchestra into the bargain.

While this colourful explanation may not fit a particular disease recognised today, most health practitioners will sense that he was describing something akin to what is often seen today. According to Künzle, 'Such people ought to take a so-called "spring cure" for a week or a fortnight [two weeks] if they seriously wish to recover. They should send Tony and Jack out to the nearest brushwood with a basket and knife and let them cut as many sprigs as possible from all the thorny bushes that can be found: rosethorn, blackthorn, whitethorn, common barberry, shoots of blackberries, raspberries, pines, beeches, hazels, cherry trees, oaks, larches, ashes, and poplars. Shoots of currants, gooseberries, and fruit trees may be added. Put a handful of this mixture in a pan with two liters of water and let it boil. Add sugar and make your patient drink one or two liters of this tea daily. It cleans and purifies the whole body. It will restore health of persons who really are pitifully ill . . . The grave-digger can put his shovel back in the shed . . .'

I have no idea if this 'spring cure', formulated randomly from spiked sprigs and other branches and shoots as available at the locale, really works, but I must admit it sounds good to me. It is likely that these plants have little toxicity. Natural products specialists will note immediately that the list of ingredients Künzle has proposed is going to be rich in phenolic compounds, mainly flavonoids (including tannins found in the bark of branches and stems). These are understood today to be one of the most interesting groups of herbal compounds because of their low toxicity and wide-ranging therapeutic potential. Included among their actions are inhibiting viral infections, reducing allergy reactions, enhancing capillary integrity, and substantial antioxidant effects. Perhaps this would take care of some of the ailing patients. Today, similar flavonoids from pine bark, grape seeds, and other sources are claimed to have remarkable benefits for those troubled by erratic complaints.

The property attributed to these spiked sprigs by herbalists is a blood purifier. This term is sometimes rendered as alterative, implying that the use of the herbs gradually leads one towards a healthier state: altering the body from a sick condition to a healthy one. Such terms are still relayed from earlier books, but they are sufficiently vague in that they don't inform one about the herbs' activities in the modern context.

At the time Künzle was working, blood purifiers were often diuretics that purged out toxins via the urine. Today, it is common for herbalists to speak of them as stimulants to the liver's enzymatic detoxification system. If someone takes a herb or herb formula and gets better, doesn't that really mean that it served as an alterative, regardless of whether the herb has been so designated? And if illness is perceived to be a matter of impure blood, then anything that helps will serve as a blood purifier. So, the definitions may remain unclear, but a they are a reflection of the overall functions of the herbs.

Due to progress in chemistry, an investigative method first applied to herbal medicine during the nineteenth century, it is often possible to identify very precisely the components of a herb that are responsible for the effects that have long been described by herbalists. Frequently, the chemical analysis is accompanied by laboratory experiments—pharmacology studies—that confirm the connection between a herb ingredient and a specific type of effect. The active constituent, after being isolated from the rest of the plant, is tested in laboratory animals to confirm (or deny) that it produces an effect related to the claimed benefit of the whole herb. It is rare that a carefully controlled clinical trial is performed with herbs due to numerous factors that make such tests expensive, time-consuming, and subject to easy criticism. Plants are like warehouses of hundreds of chemicals, and it is of little value to list off all the types of substances present, as is sometimes done in herb guides. Surely, a herb may contain essential oils, fixed oils, tannins, flavonoids, alkaloids, sterols, glycosides, and the rest of the list (including virtually all vitamins, amino acids, and other substances common to all plants). Instead, one must identify the materials that are present in sufficient quantity to produce an effect that has been described by herbalists when the herb is given in the usual dosage. In many cases, a single, main active constituent or group of constituents of similar nature can be found. For example, anise seed contains a relatively large amount of essential oil (still only a few percentage of the whole herb material), which is believed to be responsible for most of the proclaimed benefits of using the herb. Over 90 per cent of its essential oil is one chemical constituent: anethole. Thus, whatever the laboratory researchers can find out about anethole will pretty much describe what this herb does as a crude product. A single constituent can certainly have more than one effect on the body, but it is usually the case that there will only be two or three significant actions of any biochemical. Some herbs have more than one major active constituent, and two (or more) of these constituents may contribute to each of the various therapeutic actions ascribed to the herb.

All herbs, no matter how valuable to health, have the potential for adverse effects, at least in some individuals, or in some manner of use. Some people may develop an allergy to one or more constituents of a plant, and others may simply have some hypersensitivity or intolerance to a constituent (yielding an unpredictable, idiosyncratic response). At some dosage, if one takes enough, the herb may become toxic to the body or, at the least, cause an undesired reaction (such as nausea, vomiting, diarrhoea, or headache). If a herb is taken in a moderately high dosage, not enough to cause an adverse reaction immediately, prolonged ingestion of it might still cause effects that are detrimental in rare instances. Some active constituents may accumulate over time if the amount consumed is sufficient to overwhelm the rate of elimination. It is important for herbalists to present cautions about herb use. Some cautions are based on known effects, something that may have been observed in people using the herb or something that was revealed in laboratory experiments. Others are based on lack of knowledge and a desire to avoid problems that could theoretically arise. For example, pregnant women are advised to either avoid use of herbs, use a lower dose of herbs, or use herbs only for a short time, because the potential impact of large amounts, especially if consumed regularly, is either unknown or theoretically problematic. Many people feel that herbal medicine was suppressed by those who promoted the use of drugs. This is not a true depiction of the situation. Drug therapies, when they first became widely available, were embraced enthusiastically and almost universally by both doctors and patients. The potency, reliability, and ease of use apparent in the drug therapies available during the first half of the twentieth century was sufficient to convince most people that this was certainly the direction that medicine ought to follow. The remarkable difference between the high rate of death by infection before penicillin and after its introduction could leave little doubt about its efficacy and appropriateness. Similarly, the acceptance was great for opium-derived pain relievers (morphine and its analogues), powerful anti-inflammatories (corticosteroids and non-steroidal anti-inflammatories), birth control pills, and numerous other medical achievements. It was only after almost the entire population had come to rely heavily and regularly on these drugs that the concept that this might not be the way to go became a significant concern. For those who then turned to herbs and other natural remedies, it was often an unrecognised luxury to be able to do so: these same individuals may have been saved from death, deformity, or debility by previous use of antibiotics, vaccines, and other modern medical interventions.

What had happened was not a conspiracy by doctors, pharmaceutical firms, and regulatory agencies to displace herbs and make people dependent on drugs; rather, it was an across-the-board acquiescence to the process of discarding several valuable aspects of traditional lifestyle, thus making herbs less attractive and drugs more attractive. Herbs were set aside because they were perceived as having a low efficacy, slow action, inconvenient administration, and unreliable composition. Consider Künzle's spring cure. One first has to find a 'Tony and Jack' willing to go out in the frosty early spring air and collect thorny sprigs (which are increasingly hard to find within the city). Then, one has to take the time to boil it up, and drink the bitter decoction (flavoured with sugar, but, not what modern people have come to like in a medicine). This has to be continued for a week or more. Consider how much more convenient it is to take a single analgesic drug tablet for a headache, and a couple of capsules of fibre for the constipation. Further, one expects from these pills to get results right away, not after a week or two. What people are slowly coming to realise is that a gentle action is not the same as low efficacy, a slow action does not imply an undesirable outcome, and inconvenient administration can be largely resolved, as long as one is able to tolerate things in a more natural form. Increasingly, drugs are being viewed not just as powerful remedies but as harsh remedies. The gentle action of herbs, therefore, has attained a certain degree of attractiveness. Why stop the body from producing stomach acid that is otherwise needed for good digestion, when one can eat right and take a herb that will improve the digestive function?

Few can argue with the desirability of fast action, but many more are awakening to the fact that something that works quickly often leaves the disease intact, there to be treated again and again and again, each time with increasing threat of drug side effects. The slow action of herbs is just right for an accompaniment to a gradual change in lifestyle (even a temporary change) until more solid health is attained. While it may be increasingly inconvenient to go out and collect herbs and cook them up, large herbal companies have arisen to address the demands of a huge global market. They have hired people to raise, harvest, and process the herbs into a form that is ready to use. By carefully selecting from the full range of available herbs, the manufacturer can often produce remedies that have a tolerable taste (if not actually pleasant) or they can be prepared in ready-to-ingest forms, such as tea bags for brewing a tea or powders and extracts made into convenient pills. Consider the use of orange blossom, an ingredient of some of Kunzle's herbal teas. In the addendum to *Herbs and Weeds* that was added in 1975, it is mentioned that 'orange blossoms are considered to be a pleasant and absolutely harmless sedative for the nerves', which explains why they are mainly used as an ingredient in teas to calm the nerves and to encourage sleep. They are also suitable for correcting the scent and taste in remedies.

These blossoms would be difficult to come by in many locations, so the modern effort to gather herbs from around the globe resolves that problem. The safety and mild action are desired by those who worry about the potency of drug sedatives or potential adverse effects of strong-acting herbs, and the blossoms make the herb tea more pleasant to drink. The problem of unreliability of herb resources—variability in the origin and quality of the herb materials—has been addressed by applying advanced quality control measures in making herbal products. Manufacturers are able to employ botanist consultants to confirm the identity of materials and chemical analysts to assure that key active ingredients are present (and in adequate quantity). Food safety laboratories or in-house scientists are able to check for bacteria, yeasts, heavy metals, and pesticides. Pharmacy authorities have surveyed the known literature to determine which herbs are generally recognised as safe and what cautions should be pursued (as was done for the German Commission E). Nowhere are these quality control efforts more intensively pursued than in Europe, where herbs have remained a part of the health care system throughout the twentieth century, when the stringent drug standards were developed.

How Herbs Are to Be Used

Even the most ancient documents about the use of herbs present numerous methods of applying the various plants to produce a desired effect. Some are ground to powder and swallowed down much as one uses black pepper with foods; some are boiled in water, as one would boil beans in making a soup, and others are steeped in hot water to make a tea; some are extracted in a liquor to make a tincture. Yet others are applied topically in various forms, including baths, poultices, and plasters. All of these methods of application have come down to the present time, and Künzle had mentioned them in his book.

In the twenty-first century, herbal preparations are being altered somewhat to address concerns about their lack of convenience. Preparation time, which could easily be an hour or two for cooking up tough herbs in decoction, or which could involve a week or two for soaking herbs in a wine to make a tincture, is virtually eliminated by purchasing prepared forms of herbs. Topical applications that are messy, that stain clothes or bedding, and that are smelly, greasy, or sticky are mostly rejected. They are being replaced by conveniently packaged liquids and creams that soak into the skin immediately and leave little or no residue, having been reformulated to eliminate ingredients that produce unpleasant results.

For example, Künzle was an advocate of healing baths to be given along with therapeutic teas, for which he eventually developed a simpler method. For rheumatoid arthritis, he wrote:

Suddenly, you can no longer walk. You feel a stinging and gnawing pain in your knees or thighs or you can no longer raise your arm. There is a tormenting rheumatic pain in your should blade and joints . . . If you want to get rid of this malicious visitor quickly, in just five to seven days, just proceed as follows:

> Take one or two fern roots (*Dryopteris filix*) which are still fresh inside (dried and cut up, they lose all their strength in a few days), cut them into small pieces, but do not wash them. Put the pieces in a small bag and lay or tie it on the affected area and leave it there until the pain has vanished. Often, all pain disappears in just half a day. If the whole back is afflicted you need more roots and a larger bag to place on it. If you are unable or unwilling to stay in bed, bathe the afflicted limb the same day (but not the same half-day) in a fern-root concoction for half an hour.

Drink either a good mulled wine or an elderberry tea at bedtime. A goat's beard (Spiraeae ulmaria) infusion prepared with wine is even better. Continue this treatment for four to six days and you will be cured. However, if your rheumatism is not just a sudden attack but an affliction of many years standing, and perhaps you are already 60 or more years old, take baths in fern-root concoctions or fern-root extracts. As well as this, drink a tea made from birch leaves (Betula alba), goat roots, restharrow (Ononis repens), and goose grass (Galium verum) every day, taking a sip every hour. Thus, you may be cured in three to six weeks, depending on the severity and length of your affliction.

The results sound wonderful, but the procedures seem unattainable, especially if one must get fresh fern roots, and a variety of uncommon herbs. His solution? A factory has prepared his Rheuma-Tea formula that could be purchased in drug stores and Filix, a fern extract made from the fresh fern roots, that can be applied as an embrocation several times daily. These, and other measures aimed at the goal of making herbs more acceptable to busy people, remove the issue (for the herb user) of how to properly identify the herbs, when to collect them, how to dry them, and how to make them into various forms for administration. The more convenient formulations in finished form leave the following questions:

> Else I need to do, along with the herbs that will make the remedy safer or more effective? 5. Is it safe to take the herbs if I have a certain condition (e.g. am pregnant or nursing, am taking certain prescription drugs, etc.)? 6. In this chapter, some general answers to these questions will be provided.

1. Selecting a Remedy

It is normally the task of the medical practitioner to provide a clear diagnosis of what the problem is, giving it a name when available, and revealing, when known, the nature of the pathological processes occurring in the body that need to be addressed. For an individual who leads an essentially healthful lifestyle and who responds to minor ailments by quickly making small corrections, selecting herbs to treat the symptoms that arise may be an easy matter. For those who have been burdened with various ailments since childhood (or, at least, for many years) and those who have squandered good health with bad habits, the situation is more difficult and often requires a professional diagnosis.

With basic diagnostic information in hand, one can select a herbal formula that has effects consistent with the condition to be relieved. Modern herb products that are available over the counter are designed for treating disorders that are not so complex and serious that one needs a prescription by a health professional. The common areas of concern are these: acute, self-limiting infections, such as common cold, rhinitis, and influenza; emotional and nervous disorders, such as mild anxiety, stress, depression, and insomnia; digestive system distress related to eating habits and to the effects of emotions, such as dyspepsia, change in appetite, gas and bloating, diarrhoea, and constipation; aches and pains, such as arthralgia, minor injuries, and muscular tension; and functional disorders that are not extreme, such as mild hypertension, mild diabetes, menstrual disorders, menopausal syndrome, obesity, or mild liver inflammation. People with more serious disorders may also make use of the herbs available over the counter, but should maintain medical monitoring of the disorder and use of appropriate prescribed medical therapies. Thus, for diabetes, Künzle recommended certain herbs for the early stages, but suggested that the herbs could 'help to sustain' the effects of insulin for the advanced cases.

Most often, only one or two remedies are offered (by any one manufacturer) for each of the categories of ailment, thus the consumer is not faced with a difficult decision among many possibilities. Each manufacturer will have their favoured remedy for a particular type of ailment, and selection among the different manufacturers usually is based on one's trust in their product quality rather than the specific ingredients used for a particular ailment. Professional herb prescribers, of which there are scant few available (mainly acupuncturists and naturopathic doctors), have the luxury of selecting among numerous ingredients, formulating a remedy specifically aimed at the needs of a patient and adjusting the formula over time in an attempt to get the most efficacious treatment. Even then, many herb prescribers come to rely on a few trusted formulations that are used for a wide range of disorders in many different people. These trusted formulations typically become a line of manufactured products, such as those prepared on the basis of Künzle's work.

In sum, with the availability of easy-to-use manufactured products that are now labelled with their main indications for use, most people do not have to make any hard decisions in selecting the herbs to use. For those who are better educated about herbs, one can examine not only the use that is described on a package but also the functions of each of the ingredients to determine whether or not a herbal formula is suited to your needs.

2. Dosage of Herbs

Determining the amount of a herb to use has always been a difficult task for herbalists, and approximate quantities are usually cited in the herb guides. For the majority of herbs that have a mild to moderate action, and which are used in the European system (where over-the-counter remedies dominate), the standard amount recommended is in the range of 1-6 g of dried, crude herbs for a one-day dose (in preparation of teas), to be doubled in some cases where rapid action, high body weight, or seriousness of symptoms calls for it.

During the twentieth century, dosage standardisation has become the normal practice. It will be stated, for example, that the dosage of a herb should be 3.0 g for one day. The apparently precise figure may give the impression that there is an exact science of herbal dosage, but that is misleading. What has happened, instead, is that several authorities have agreed that 3 g is a reasonable amount to suggest as efficacious, yet well within the safety limits that have become a central concern. The added decimal point (changing a dosage statement of 3 g to 3.0 g) is only a reflection of the fact that some herbs are recommended in non-integral amounts, such as 4.5 g so that the decimal point is included, but it should not be taken as implying precision.

The dosage indicated in a monograph for a single herb is usually based on the amount of that herb when used by itself. In actual practice, herbs are often used in combinations, sometimes relying on several herbs that have the same basic properties, even overlapping active constituents. In the formulas, the amount of each individual herb is often lower than the amount that is described in the literature for the herb used by itself. A total daily dose of herbs in a formula might range from 6 to 12 g for the over-the-counter type remedies.

When describing the use of herbs, there are often two or more actions attributed to each herb. There may be different dosage requirements for the different actions. For example, if one wishes to get an effect of a herb on the stomach, then the dosage needed is usually quite small. This is because all of the herb ingredients consumed will be in the stomach, the target of its action, in their full dosage at the time it is consumed. By contrast, if one wishes to treat a sinus infection or aching feet, the dosage of the same herb (assuming that this one herb is reputed to treat both the stomach and these other body parts) would usually have to be higher. This is because the herb ingredients will be dispersed throughout the entire bloodstream by the time they reach the part of the body to be affected and will be greatly diluted. Manufactured herbal products usually incorporate a herb into a complex formulation for which only one of the many potential uses of the herbs is being relied upon. Its dosage within the formulation is determined by the herbalist who has designed the herbal mixture so as to address the intended application.

The total dosage of the formula to be taken is suggested on the product package. This dosage is always a conservative recommendation and, unless indicated otherwise, is the amount suggested for an adult. It has to be a suitable dosage for the consumers who have a small body weight, such as a petite woman who might have a weight of only 50 kg (110 lb) or less, and for people who are highly sensitive to things they consume, such as herbs. Therefore, those with higher body weight, some of whom will easily be double this weight, will often do better by taking up to twice the recommended amount. Since it is not possible to list all the variables affecting dosage and the suggestions to adjust for each variable, the label has to reflect the conservative approach. The herb formulas provided to the public are mild ones (the drastic ones are saved for prescription by health professionals or simply give way to the drastic drugs that are heavily regulated). Generally speaking, to keep within safe bounds, one can use one to two times the dosage suggested on package labels. Using less than the recommended amount may prove adequate for some individuals, but will usually result in little therapeutic effect. For teas, they may become a simple beverage rather than a medicinal.

3. Duration of Use

During Künzle's time, and for most of the history of herbal medicine, getting herbs and then preparing them for use was not an easy task. Surely, plants of various types grew nearby, but the right ones might be some distance away or might not be available during the season for which they were needed. Cooking up herbs on today's ranges is far easier than it was in the past, cooking them on kitchen fires. Taking the herbs, or administering them topically, was often an unpleasant experience. Therefore, the rule for duration of herb use was a simple one: just as long as absolutely necessary, no longer. Herbal therapies were often described in terms of curing a disease. A person would be ill, they would take their herbs, their condition would improve, and then they would lead a healthier life.

In the case of his spring tea, Künzle had to remind people of the importance of taking it for at least a week or two. Of course, some serious diseases required longer therapies. Künzle mentions that for persons stricken by consumption (tuberculosis) and already given up on by their physicians (there was no medical cure at the time), some had been cured completely by 'prolonged use' of juice of the chickweed. In modern medical practice, antibiotics have to be administered for months to fully get rid of tuberculosis, and the herbs would likely have taken at least as long. In another instance he recommended wormwood to be used 'over a long period of time' to cure dropsy. In modern practice, leg oedema (formerly called dropsy) is usually treated by diuretics, and these are taken for months. For gout, arthritis, and other serious disorders, Künzle recommended cowslip, but advised (based on the recommendation of Father Kneipp) that it was useful only if used 'for a long period.' The designation 'prolonged use' or 'long period' is necessarily unclear, as the duration will no doubt vary from person to person, but it is determined by when the patient feels that the disease is gone. Compared to the standard duration of use of herbs, which, in *Herbs and Weeds*, usually does not exceed a fortnight (two weeks), such references are to taking herbs for several weeks or months.

Our modern situation has changed greatly. Now that herbal preparations are relatively convenient to use and are readily available all year, most people can take them for a long time. Therefore, the question of duration of taking herbs is no longer limited to as short as possible. Some of the conditions treated by short-term use of herbs are now treated by drugs, either to cure them (e.g. with antibiotics) or allow them to be better tolerated (e.g. with symptom-relieving medicine for cold or flu). However, many diseases that lead people to consider herb therapy cannot be cured; they can only be controlled. The percentage of people living with various cardiovascular diseases (atherosclerosis, hypertension, post-stroke syndrome, and heart failure), chronic pulmonary diseases (such as asthma, chronic obstructive pulmonary disease, and emphysema), cancer, nervous system diseases (including severe cases of attention deficit disorder, bipolar disease, multiple sclerosis, Parkinson's disease, and Alzheimer's disease), hormone-based metabolic disorders (diabetes, hypothyroidism), autoimmune diseases (e.g. arthritis, lupus, and scleroderma), and others is huge. For these people and many others, taking drugs every day is a simple habit, if an undesired but necessary one. Taking herbs every day, then, would seem to have the potential for widespread acceptance.

For many of the medicinal herbs, there is simply no historical experience of taking the herbs for very long periods of time. Whether such a practice would ultimately be helpful or occasionally harmful is not known. There are a few herbs that have been consumed daily for extended time periods and seem to be of benefit or, at the least, of no harm. These include all the kitchen herbs and spices used in various countries and the beverage teas (notably *Camellia sinensis*, the green and black teas, as well as chamomile, peppermint, and ginger), many of which end up in medicinal preparations. So one can say that there is a precedent for using several ingredients of medicinal herb formulas on a daily basis, but there is also some lack of knowledge about the prolonged use for many of the other ingredients. The same situation applies to the drugs that people take. Many of these drugs were developed during recent decades, and the accumulated experience regarding the duration of their use is often limited. We are in uncharted territories when it comes to taking medicinals, be they plant or synthetic drugs, which are now being applied continuously.

Over-the-counter drug products usually carry the following caution: if the condition persists, see your doctor. This is a good suggestion for the use of herbs as well. If the condition continues despite the use of herbs at the proper dosage and for a reasonable period of time (e.g. a few weeks) without obvious improvement, then one should check with a doctor to make sure that the symptoms are not part of something that is quite serious, requiring more aggressive action. Most herbal formulas sold over the counter provide about a five-to-ten-day supply of the herbs, enough to give a reasonable try to see whether or not it will be of help. Sometimes it is enough to completely treat the condition of concern. In most cases, regular use of the herbs over a period of many weeks or even months can be safely undertaken if they have proven helpful at a low dose (e.g. within the package recommendations, perhaps adjusted upwards for body weight as indicated above). If a higher dose is needed in order to get results, then prolonged use should be undertaken with medical supervision. The herbs in Künzle's teas that have come down to us today have been approved by the German Commission E, indicating that there is no harm known from consuming them in the usual manner, which is for several days, weeks, or even a few months.

There are occasional recommendations by well-known herbalists for the daily use of herbs as a preventive against disease. Many people are familiar with the oriental claim, promoted mainly by the Koreans but arising from Chinese tradition, that taking ginseng every day will prevent disease and prolong life. For the most part, Künzle did not recommend daily use of prophylactic herbs for overall health care and, instead, recommended a daily regimen of healthy living (see Chapter 4). One of his main suggestions, in terms of things to consume daily, was to take porridge, which he called 'the food of our ancestors.' Another relatively long-term treatment was the 'fig cure' for chronic constipation, which was based on daily consumption of dried figs that had been soaked in water overnight (drink the water and eat the figs). The same result could be obtained, he said, by using dried pears, prunes, or apricots, though he especially liked the figs because of the small seeds. These treatments were to be carried out for a month or two. He also advised substituting coffee by a beverage product, then available in Switzerland, made from dried figs, called Virgo.

Künzle occasionally recommended that a prophylactic herb regimen be carried out over a long time for specific disorders, but it was not to be on a daily basis. For example, he pointed out that people who were fat, red in the face, and who suffered from vertigo or fainting fits, should beware of suffering a stroke. The vertigo and fainting fits that he referred to were what we today call temporary ischemic attacks (TIAs), which are mini strokes that often precede a potentially fatal stroke (being obese and having a red face are characteristics of people who eat lots of meat and drink lots of alcohol-risk factors for stroke). He suggested that such individuals drink, for three to four days each month, a cup or two of tea made from some species of *Potentilla* (silverweed). As another example, he suggested that painters daily take one to two teaspoons of wormwood extract (boiled in wine and to be drunk rather hot), because this eliminates white lead. Obviously, this would not need to be done when painting jobs were not in progress. Thus, the best way to use herbs is to take them daily over a period of several days to treat a disorder, or take them from time to time to alleviate an acute condition, but don't plan on taking one of them all the time. Let the fruits, vegetables, grains, and beans, carefully prepared and eaten in a relaxed atmosphere be your daily herbs, and utilise the medicinals to assist in times of need. For general health purposes, herbal beverage teas can be used in rotation to get the benefits of numerous herbs.

4. Other Things to Do

Aside from reminding readers of the suggestions in Chapter 4 about a healthy lifestyle, there are only a few additional requirements to point to. The most common adjunct to consumption of herbs to improve health is to use topical treatments. Künzle especially suggested medicinal baths, which could be made, for example, by putting fern root (*Dryopteris filix*) tea into the bathtub or into a foot bath (for gout and other foot pains). The clubmoss (*Lycopodium*, not truly a moss) was suggested for the same applications, but especially for leg cramps, when applied by bath. Similarly, goutwort (*Aegopodium podagaria*) was suggested in hip baths, foot baths, and whole bathtubs for gout, sciatica, and arthralgia. As an alternative to bathing in a solution of the herb extract, one could apply an ointment or liniment with concentrated herb extract to the affected areas. Today, topical application of herbs is often accomplished by using manufactured liniments, essential oils, and creams. For disorders of the limbs, topical applications greatly contribute to the efficacy of any herbal treatment and sometimes stand alone as therapies, especially for those who have sensitive stomachs and don't tolerate the herbs used for limb pains. In addition to topical application of herbs, other treatments applied to the surface of the body may be of help. These include massage (perhaps with medicated oils) and application of heat and cold, as recommended by Father Kneipp's water treatments. Specific exercises might also be given; for example, to deal with constipation or organ prolapse, one might be directed to undertake a series of exercises to tone up the abdominal muscles.

5. Cautions

Herbs have a reputation for being beneficial and lacking harm. For the most part, the gentle herbs included in over-the-counter herbal products fit that description well. Nonetheless, worries about the use of herbs arise from time to time. In particular, there are the concerns of a mother for the well-being of the fetus she carries or the nursing child and then the concerns, more often voiced by the chronically ill and the elderly, of combining herbs with the prescription drugs they have been given. Throughout history, herbs have been used by women during pregnancy to treat related disorders and, at the time of delivery, to ease childbirth; afterwards, they have been used to treat any complications from the delivery. Künzle said that every woman in childbed [after delivery] should drink as much as possible of the herb tea made of lady's mantle (*Alchemilla vulgaris*) to improve the flow of milk. Today, with the knowledge that many substances can adversely affect the fetus and that some powerful drugs can be transferred via the breast milk, many women worry about the potential adverse effects of herbs at this sensitive time. The rule of thumb should be this—If herbs are not really necessary, don't use them and then don't worry. If they are needed, use them modestly and there should still be no need to worry. Keep the dosage on the low side and use the herbs only as long as necessary. Check the literature for cautions about using herbs during pregnancy.

The concern about taking herbs during the time of breastfeeding (which should be for many months, if not a year), appears to be exaggerated. Most healing herbs yield miniscule amounts of their constituents into the milk, and thus the infant receives inconsequential doses. It is advisable to watch out for cases of skin rashes or diarrhoea that might suggest an allergic sensitivity to tiny amounts, but such instances will be very rare. As to the combination of herbs with drugs, there is little known about the interactions. The possibility for adverse consequences is a function of the dosage, and therefore, persons who are concerned about possible interactions are advised, like the pregnant women, to use herbs in modest dosage.

To minimise the potential for interactions, take the herbs and drugs at different times, at least an hour apart. That will not only separate them in the digestive system, but also likely keep the blood levels of each one from reaching their peak at the same time. Studies of herb–drug reactions reported in the medical literature indicate that they are rare and mostly involve one herb (St John's wort, an ingredient in some of the Künzle formulas sold today) and one drug group (anticoagulants, mainly warfarin). In Künzle's time, the issue of combining herbs and drugs didn't arise much. The usual procedure was different than what might arise today. A person would try herbs first, and if they failed to provide adequate results, then the physician would be consulted for drugs or even surgery; or, modern medicine would be tried first, and if that failed, herbs would be resorted as the next attempt. Rather than mixing the two, they would be tried sequentially, with only a few exceptions. As mentioned in the above section on duration of use, the modern situation has presented some unique concerns. Nowadays, people may undertake a drug therapy that has no known end in sight. At the same time, herbs may be desired to treat yet another condition or to attempt to provide additional relief for the same condition as addressed by the drug. It may even be hoped that after using both together for a while, the drug can be deleted. Therefore, the use of herbs and drugs together has become a common consideration. It was reported recently that American seniors (those sixty-five years of age or over) typically receive fourteen prescriptions for drugs each year.

With the rapid advances in medicine, as well as in nutrition, hygiene, and safety practices, resulting in longer life of the people, the probability of using drugs regularly will increase. And, with more people turning to herbs, this means that drugs and herbs will be routinely used together. If you suspect that a herb and a drug that you are taking are incompatible, cease taking the herbs. Otherwise, unless there are reliable warnings against the combinations, the moderate use of herbs taken at times different than the drugs should be considered the norm. In literature, surveys of herb-drug interactions, the incidence rate of such events appears to be very low.

14.5 A Theory of Disease and Healing

Künzle

Künzle recognised that there were numerous causes of disease, and among the concerns he expressed were the inappropriate diets that many people had. But he also had a concept of disease causation that involved the adverse influence of cold. In his book *Comprehensive Guide to Herbal Healing*, there was a chapter entitled 'The healing method of the herbal-priest J. Künzle: the development and simple healing of disease.' Its first section was entitled: 'Most of the problems develop after a cold.' He actually referred both to the common cold and exposure to cold.

He explained it this way:

Most of the disorders develop through the common cold. The cold develops rarely through cold air as many people think, but in a totally different way. In the winter, imagine you have the room heated to 15°C [note: just 59°F, but this is in the mountains in Switzerland, without central heating], while outside it is cold, at -15°C If you let the window open the warmth will go out and the cold will come in. This will take as long as it takes for the inside to become the exact same temperature as the outside. This is what happens when you suffer a cold. The blood has a temperature of 37°C, but the soil has a temperature of 10–20°C: colder than the soil is the stone, colder than the stone is cement, and colder than the cement is the ice. When you stay for a long time with 37 degrees of body temperature on the cold ground, stone, cement, or ice, then the warmth of the body comes down and the cold comes up. The warmth will disappear first from the kidneys, but the kidneys have the work of secreting urine to the bladder which then gets rid of it. Now, if the warmth disappears the kidneys can't work properly anymore, just like the water in the pot can't boil when the fire underneath is too weak. The urine is not produced correctly and too little is excreted. What is supposed to be secreted goes into the blood, where it doesn't belong; the blood wants to get rid of this material and deposits the bad stuff somewhere. These bad substances, mostly uric acids, are usually deposited where the weakest places of the body are.

If the lungs are weak, the uric acid deposits happen there; if there is only a little deposit in the lungs, then there will be phlegm, catarrh, coughing, tightness, asthmatic breathing; or, if there is a lot of deposit, there will be pneumonia, during which there will be almost no urine flow. If those bad substances go into the stomach, then there will be phlegm development in the stomach, causing inflammation and pain in the stomach. If the substances go into the intestines, there will be colon inflammation and tumours. It should be mentioned right away that all inner tumours, despite operation, will come back again and again necessarily, as long as the kidneys, the bladder, and the stool production are not functioning correctly. All tumours will shrink down as soon as these three will work well. This shows the way to healing inner tumours. If the bad substances go into the head, then there will be inflammation of the eyes or the ears, headaches, nervousness, sleeplessness, or encephalitis. Often the blood is secreting the substances through the skin, causing furuncles, lichen planas, blisters, etc. And this type of deposit can produce many pain disorders of the joints when it is deposited there.

When smoke comes out of the fireplace, and you want to stop the smoke, the method for resolving the problem is not to climb on the roof and catch the smoke coming out at the top. No. You know that the smoke comes from the fire in the hearth, so you need to get rid of the fire in the hearth to stop the smoke. Now, in natural medicine, you want to get rid of the fire—you're not jumping after the smoke, namely the diseases of the eyes, ears, teeth, nerves, lungs, or chest, not the manifestations as catarrh, skin disorders, rheumatism, tumors, infections, and so on. You are not just treating the parts of the body in which the disease is expressed, but you go to find the cause of the disorders and you try to get rid of the root of this. The cause, however, is not in the organs and tissues where the disease is expressed acutely, but in the deficient activity of the organs that are intended to get rid of the bad materials, mainly the kidneys, bladder, and intestines. If you want to get rid of this type of disorder thoroughly, you need to first regulate these three organs of excretion. Only then will the increasing additions of bad substances to the weak tissues stop. The old accumulations need to be cleared up. For this there are external and internal remedies.

He then went on to explain the methods of stimulating elimination of the uric acid and other bad substances, which included taking herbal baths and consuming herbal teas. Sweating was considered one of the methods of getting rid of the build-up of uric acid and other substances that were not being adequately secreted by the kidneys. In *Herbs and Weeds*, he mentioned this in his brief explanation of treating 'perspiration of the feet' as follows:

> This is the healthiest illness that exists because all unhealthy substances are eliminated through the soles of the feet. Therefore, it should never be entirely suppressed because this may result in serious, and even incurable, illnesses. These illnesses will continue until the feet perspire again. This will only be achieved with difficulty by many foot-baths with hay blossoms. You may alleviate such perspiration, but *never, never, never by cold footbaths*, but by purifying the kidneys. This is attained by drinking a tea prepared from diuretic herbs.

This recommendation to avoid cold foot baths belongs to the concept of not introducing cold when the kidneys are not working well, one sign of which is excessive foot perspiration. However, he was not recommending simply having lots of sweat pouring out of the body. He considered that night sweating, for example, was very debilitating. Night sweating, according to his thinking, would also reflect the body's attempt to dump its excess toxins. He was not completely opposed to treatments by cold. He considered mild fevers to be a healthy body response to infections, but he thought that high fevers might turn into a dangerous condition, which could be treated, in part, by cold compresses. Thus, for example, he cautioned that when a child is sick and hot or feverish, warm baths and heavy blankets, which simply increase the heat, should be avoided. 'You must wash the child every hour and even more frequently with cold water until the heat has disappeared.' But he did not want to have the body cooled below normal temperature.

The importance of diuresis is also revealed in his explanation of pneumonia as under:

> What causes pneumonia? It is the result of heavy colds; the water stagnates, cannot be expelled and consequently passes into the lungs where it causes immediate inflammation. If you want to avoid pneumonia, drink a tea of holly leaves, quickgrass, or cat's tail as soon as you notice that you cannot pass sufficient water. If the water is not expelled in spite of this treatment, then your bladder is inflamed. In this case, take a hip bath in warm cat's tail decoction for half an hour, which will help to prevent pneumonia. Pleurisy and costal pleura originate from the same source: therefore, recovery will also be achieved as soon as sufficient water is passed.

He recommended, for example, sage to strengthen the kidneys and eliminate large quantities of retained water. Similarly, for influenza, he pointed out that the tea designed for treating this condition (which is now called tea for colds and a slightly different version is now tea for influenza), should be taken throughout the day, and that 'it is most essential that *a lot of water is passed*. If urination does not work in spite of drinking a lot of influenza tea, one has to be on the alert. It means the kidneys are not working as they should.' He recommended, as a therapy, to place cut garlic or onions over the kidneys and keep them there for several hours, saying that 'the kidneys will start to work again and a lot of water will be passed and inflammation of the lungs will certainly be prevented.' In sum, his theory regarding the development of certain diseases (e.g. infections, inflammation, swellings) follows this course: cold → weakens kidney function → the body accumulates water, uric acid, and toxins → weaker organs are affected → fluid and uric acid accumulates in weak organs → inflammation develops in those organs → full disease symptoms are manifest.

The corresponding therapies are as follows: 1). Warm the body and stimulate the kidney function. 2). Drain the excess fluids, along with uric acid and toxins. If, instead of the problem of kidney weakness there is a problem of intestinal stagnation with constipation due to eating too much meat, too much chocolate, not enough fibre, etc., he especially recommended the 'fig cure'.

Many diseases originate from constipation and no medicine whatever will cure them unless constipation has been cured first. Even if the ailment seems to be temporarily cured it will surely break out again. People suffer from constipation when they have a hard and forced stool and no bowel movement for at least one day. The winds which are usually released with the bowel movement rise to the head and cause headaches, ailing eyes, etc. Such people also complain about pressure on the chest, stomach, and abdomen, and a full and anxious feeling. Obstinate constipations will cause ulcers of the stomach and intestines, haemorrhoids, appendicitis, and, in the end often even closing of the stomach and cancer. Stomach and intestinal troubles are often only curable after a good evacuation and after normal bowel movement is achieved.

The simplest, safest, and most efficacious way to have a good bowel movement is a fig cure carried out for a month or two. How do you make this fig cure? Wash five to six common figs in lukewarm water every evening, put them in a glass and cover them with cold water. Eat the figs and drink the water on an empty stomach the next morning. The cure is even more effective when you cut up the figs and leave them in olive oil for a day. Instead of figs you can also take dried pears or prunes in the same way. As is commonly known, figs are full of small seeds. These gradually eliminate all mucus from the stomach and intestines, i.e. the respective membranes are cleaned and thus free again to do their regular task. In case your bowels should move too often after a while, i.e. more than three times daily, stop the fig cure temporarily. For little children, the figs may be chopped finely. People suffering from constipation should avoid chocolate and cocoa like the plague.

In this description, Künzle mentions headaches. He noted several potential types of headaches and treatments. For one type, he had a true nature cure: Persons who have formed a habit of working far into the night, like students learning to excess, scholars, or railway officials who are always surrounded by uproar and turmoil and who can find but very little sleep and remain in this condition for months, often are subject to nervous headaches. Speedwell (*Veronica officinalis*) is sometimes very good for such complaints. But above all, now is the time to take the bull by the horns! Forget all intellectual work. Get away from noise and turmoil, from the office and the town. Go out to the country—as high as possible—and take a great deal of exercise in the fresh air. Do this long enough and until you can sleep soundly again. Choose a restful climatic health resort where you find neither many tourists nor pianos or dogs but many pine trees and murmuring brooks instead. Only such a cure will help to heal this ailment.

Sometimes, remedies for disease are thrust at us, even though we don't realise it. They stand in our way, not like the herbs we normally seek out. Künzle gave an explanation of why one would use both healing herbs and weeds, the basis for his book title. Healing herbs refer mainly to what are normally considered desirable plants—ones that you would purposefully grow in your backyard garden so as to be able to enjoy them or plants that are routinely collected for medicine. As to weeds, those seemingly unwelcome invaders of the garden, footpath, farm, and grassy yard he says as follows:

> Why has God created this large number of weeds which give us all the trouble of pulling them out? Certainly not to annoy us, but because all weeds are healing herbs too. God has strewn them in our paths so that, for better or worse, we shall always have them on hand. Even cats and dogs know this and eat grass from time to time. An old woman, who looked poorly and miserable and was always ailing but still did not die, was advised by an old blacksmith to ask her grey cat, who would certainly know a remedy, for help. The woman observed her cat carefully. She cut some of the same herbs it had eaten, boiled them and drank this tea for some time until she had recovered completely. Now, which is the grass in question? It is dog grass (*Dactylis glomerata*) and cough grass or quick grass (*Agropyrum repens*). Both are ordinary weeds but have been recognised by physicians for two thousand years as excellent remedies for cleaning the kidneys and the bladder and for all urinary affections . . . The most detested weed is the bindweed (*Convulvulus spp.*). It is impossible to exterminate it. Its roots reach down to hell. It always grows anew, encircles all vegetables and presses them down to the earth. But, it is just the bindweed which serves as a wonderful febrifuge.

Also, it calms all internal inflammations (for instance, enteritis). In spring, many fields are literally covered with chickweed (*Stellaria media*) or starweed. In May, and sometimes already in April, these fields are covered with tiny white stellate blossoms. This herb prevents the moisture in the fields from evaporating. Crushed and applied to wounds, it soothes burning; prepared and taken as tea, it cures fevers.

Other fields are covered in field mint (*Mentha arvensis*), which has a strong and aromatic fragrance. This herb is of inestimable value for man and beast. It dissolves all internal tumours, persistent phlegm, etc. . . . The cat's tail—of the horsetail family (*Equisetum spp.*)—proliferates in many fields and is difficult to exterminate. How it has been cursed by enraged weeders who confounded it to hell. But numerous are those who have cursed it and have long since been laid to rest in the churchyard. Had they collected, dried, and used the cat's tail in time, they might still be alive and might have become as old as the ravens of Baschaer, who never make a will before having lived to see ninety springs and winters come and go. Father Kneipp named this weed 'pewter herb' and prescribed it externally . . . Taken internally, cat's tail will cure in a short time—even almost instantly—the most violent haemorrhages and vomiting of blood.

Mistletoe (*Viscum album*) is an importunate parasite weed which is legally pursued, officially eliminated, and prosecuted by the government and the county police. In spite of all this, it is still flourishing in all the twenty-two Swiss cantons. Father Kneipp said that he could not recommend this herb warmly enough to all women because a single cup of mistletoe tea stops haemorrhages and takes care of all disturbances of the circulation of the blood. Thus God, in his love and providence for mankind, has put at our disposal the most wonderful and disdained weeds in our paths, in our hands, and under our feet. Nothing in nature is left to chance; everything comes from the Divine. Never find fault in things you do not really understand The enemy you wish to destroy often proves to be your truest friend. Among Künzle's favoured weeds was meadowsweet. Of it, he noted:

> It is found in greatest abundance in all marshes, ditches, and stagnant water. This disdained parasite weed is a wonderful divine gift because its blossoms heal dropsy when they are

prepared with wine and thus drunk, cure diarrhoea and paralysis in calves, and alleviate rheumatic afflictions of all sorts.

Other favoured herbs include wormwood (*Artemisia absinthium*),
stinging nettles (*Urtica dioica*), male fern (*Dropteris filix*, to be used externally only), lady's mantle (*Alchemilla vulgaris*), St John's wort (*Hypericum
perforatum*), masterwort (*Imperatoria osthruthium*), Benedict's herb (*Geum
urbanum*), crane's bill (*Geranium robertianum*), and plantain (*Plantago
spp.*). These herbs were each explained in his small book as useful for a
variety of ailments. For wormwood, he relayed four cases of remarkable
effects: treating a little girl with pneumonia and also a thirty-year-old
man with that disease; a boy with liver disease that was expected to
kill him; and a woman who suffered blood loss, weakness, loss of appetite, vomiting, and other serious conditions. All of these were said to
be cured by the herbal remedies administered with wormwood as the
key ingredient. He had learnt that some people were already worrying
that the herbs would be endangered by over collection, but he noted:
'They forget that cattle graze the Alps year after year and still the herbs
are not exterminated, but grow denser all the time. This fact is also
proved by persistent roots like masterwort and St. Benedict's herb. As it
is very rarely possible to take out the whole root, the remaining shoots
will survive and the plant will break into leaf again and again.' Indeed,
herbalism has flourished in central Europe during these past decades.

Herbs in the Tea Formulas

The herbs in the tea formulas that were described in the previous
chapter have passed numerous safety evaluations and are considered
by most herbalists as effective ingredients. All of these herbs have
been used for centuries; some of them were already in use during the
ancient Graeco-Roman period of herbalism described in Chapter 2. In
the following pages, there is a brief review of each of the herbs. The
ingredients are these, arranged in alphabetical order:

1	Anise	15	Lemon balm
2	Birch	16	Licorice
3	Boldo	17	Meadowsweet
4	Caraway	18	Orange blossom

5	Chamomile	19	Peppermint
6	Coriander	20	Plantain
7	Echinacea	21	Rosemary
8	Elder	22	Senna leaf
9	Fennel	23	St John's wort
10	Goldenrod	24	Star anise
11	Green tea	25	Thyme
12	Hops	26	Valerian
13	Juniper	27	Yarrow
14	Lavender		

Of these, certain ingredients are included in most of the teas due to their known benefits, good taste, and common use by European herbalists: anise, fennel, hops, lemon balm, licorice, peppermint, and valerian. In particular, peppermint is in all but one of the tea blends (not in Laxative Tea), serving as the basic health tea. It is common practice to have a base ingredient in most blends in other herbal cultures as well: Chinese teas often use ginger, jujube, and licorice as base ingredients, while Indian blends often include myrobalans fruits (a combination of the three), and Indonesian remedies often have turmeric as their base. Here is how Künzle explains the special value of peppermint: All varieties of mint dissolve old residues and eliminate waste matter and obstinate flatulence and are, therefore, used against almost all ailments of man and cattle. Besides, they increase and further the healing power of other herbs. To assist in understanding the therapeutic contributions of the formula ingredients, following is a table of terms used in the herbal literature to describe the actions of herbs.

TERMS USED TO DESCRIBE THE ACTION OF HERBS

Term	Meaning
anodyne	relieves pain
anthelmintic	inhibits intestinal worms
anticattharal	reduces excessive mucus secretions
antidiarrheal	treats diarrhoea, especially chronic condition
antiemetic	reduces nausea and helps prevent vomiting
anti-inflammatory	reduces inflammation (e.g., in arthritis, skin diseases, infections)

Term	Meaning
antipyretic	reduces fever (antipyretic herbs are described as febrifuge)
antirheumatic	relieves joint and muscle pain due to rheumatism (as opposed to injury)
antispasmodic	alleviates muscle contractions
aperient	Produces mild laxative effect
astringent	reduces discharge of fluids (e.g., diarrhea, leukorrhea, copious sputum)
bronchodilator	alleviates wheezing by dilating lung passages
carminative	alleviates gas and bloating
cholagogue	promotes secretion of bile
demulcent	provides soothing effect on mucous membranes (has slippery, coating action)
diaphoretic	promotes sweating, a method of therapy to treat acute infections and fevers
digestive aid	Provides general improvement of digestive function
diuretic	promotes urination, usually in cases of edema
emenogogue	promotes initiation of menstrual bleeding
expectorant	promotes release of sputum
galactagogue	promotes milk production in nursing mothers
Hemostatic	reduces bleeding
hepatoprotective	reduces liver inflammation caused by chemicals, viruses, etc.
hypoglycemic	reduces blood sugar in cases of elevated sugar levels (i.e., diabetes)
hypolipemic	reduces elevated blood lipids (e.g., high cholesterol, high triglycerides)
laxative	promotes bowel movements, usually in cases of constipation
nervine sedative	calming and improving nervous system functions
Refrigerant	has a cooling effect on a non-fever condition, such as experienced on hot days
sedative	calming; usually has prompt effect
stimulant	enlivens nervous system and metabolism
stomachic	improves digestive function of the stomach, improves appetite
tonic	helps overcome weakness
uterine sedative	reduces uterine contractions (i.e., cramping)
uterine stimulant	promotes uterine contractions (i.e., during menstruation)

CHAPTER 15

The Golden Rule in Preventive Health Therapy

15.1 The Therapeutic and Untherapeutic Foods

(The foods that support life and the foods that deplete life)

I n the preventive therapy, we must unedertsatnd the kinds and the nature of the food items that can be therapeutic and those that cannot be so and their preparation and the mood of their eating. There are hosts of other considerations that need our attention. These factors will include such things as the individual's food tolerance level, the age, and the occupation—activties, the food habits, and the lifesytles. Are such patients male or female and are there any related health problem (s). Our attention to these factors will not only affect the clients' daily health, but it will also help to determine the quality of his or her life and how long he or she may live.

Such a statemenet that 'your food is your medicine and your medicine your food', is not wholly correct. This statemenet could be correct when it was made by Ihmotep—the African-Egyptian healer in the year 2890 BC. In modern times, life has become more complex and health care more deversed. In fact, in our experience, it has been discovered that food, although a vital part of the heath care system, cannot on its own be sufficient in the treatement of many complex health abnormalities. Complementary health care practitioners must aim at developing the skills, knowledge, and the senstivity in the determining what food should be combined with what herbal substance (s) for therapeuticvalue and what not. We must be in constant touch with modern research findings about the therapeutic nature of some food products and the herbs. In effect, we must possess thorough knowledge of foods in relation to their nutritive values, their deficiencies, and their resultant effects on human health. If I had my way, all the complementary medicine practitioners must attain proficiency level in their knowledge of applied nurition and Hygiene: personal, material, equipment, and environmental hygiene. These should be in addition to their knowledge of biochemistry, physiology, anatomy, and herbology (the study of herbal medicine). In the quest for preventive health therapy, every practitioner must be challenged to constantly advising and counselling his or her clients to adhere to the following golden rules:

[A]

Meat and Meat Products Food Consumption

These must be properly washed, cleaned, and well cooked. They must be served hot and in a clean plates and dishes. Such cooking practices and the consumption of 'rare done', underdone, and 'medium rare' done of beef must be discouraged and avoided. Special attention must be given to every description of pork or pig meat products. Under no circumstance should pig and pig meat products of any type be eaten underdone or served cold. Fish and fish products must be well cooked and served hot. Fish cake must be well heated before serving for human consumption. It is very important to bear in mind that almost all the cases of food poisoning reported throughout the world are traceable to meat and fish products.

There are many religious bodies that prohibit the consumption of pig and its products. If people must eat pig, they must bear in mind that pig is a mass of worms. Each mouthful of pig meat you eat is not a nutritious food but a mass of small worms, which the naked eye cannot detect. This could be because pigs like to scavenge and will eat any kind of food, including dead insects, worms, rotting carcasses, excreta including their own, garbage, and other pigs. In the sow, the important parasites are the large, white worm ascarids (Ascaris suum) and the red stomach worms. There are three types of stomach worms present in pigs: a thin worm, Hyostrongylus rubidus (the red stomach worm), and thick stomach worms, Ascarops. The red hair-like species is less than 10 mm long but can just be seen by the naked eye. It is found worldwide in the stomach and is a common parasite of outdoor pigs. It is not only the meat and meat by-products that must be give utmost attention, but also vegetables of all kinds meant for human consumption must be seen to be protected against contamination and cross-contamination. The readers may wonder why and how the above points should concern the duties of the complementary health practitioners. Believe me, they do. My research has shown that about 75-80 per cent of all the human sickness or perhaps death is traceable to the consumption of food and beverages. Therefore, following the title of this book, I spare no time in going through all the way. The rest of the chapters in this book will be devoted to and concentrate on the matters concerning foods and beverages. It must be remembered that Imhotep—the ancient 'father of medicine' in Egypt (Kemet) said that our foods should be our medicine and our medicine should be our food. If you reflect over this statement made so many years ago, you will agree that it still holds true to the present day. Any complementary practitioner who pays due attention to this concept will not be misled in his or her practice at all. However, the condition of such foods and the method of their preparation and consumption must be the overriding points.

Between the years 1967-9, I worked as a trainee food production technician in the Dietetics Department at Hammersmith Hospital in North London. There I was able to observe and saw that the orthodox medical practitioners also recognised that certain illnesses must be treated with special kinds of food and dietary therapy. These medically controlled food intakes, can therefore, be described as medicinal. The complementary practitioners must also carry out the study of food, diet, and nutrition along with all other subjects involved in the profession such as herbal chemistry, in order to really understand the basis of herbal constituents, the structures and properties of molecules, phytochemicals and the synergy. The knowledge of biochemistry is also contingent. Our ancient ancestors who brought about the knowledge of medicine, practised traditional medicine through intuition and their natural instinct, but today, this is no longer possible or even feasible at all. We are now in a scientific and technological age; we have nowhere to retreat and have to face reality of the day. The more knowledgeable and more experienced we are in the filed, the more proficient and capable we will become in the versatility of preventive therapy.

It is unfortunate that most of the time one does not hear the modern complementary health practitioners talk about food, nutrition, hygiene, and applied human relations in their practice. The concept of holistic health care must embrace all aspects of human life including social, economic, physical, and psychological well-being. From experience, I have discovered that the application of psychological principles to human relations in any small or big organisation is very vital. In an environment of increasing tense competition of today, health care services should be based on the survival of the best and the fittest. From experience, I have discovered that regardless of diagnosis, the foundation of most health conditions and chronic pains are traceable to one or more of the following:

- Nutritional deficiencies
- Poor diet and poor lifestyle
- Food allergies or sensitivities
- Candida overgrowth and unhygienic conditions
- Environmental toxins
- Depression—family problems
- Lower self-image and lack of confidence
- Loneliness and self-rejection
- Poverty and lacking

Without the application of human cordial relations between the practitioners and the clients during the hours of consultation and counselling, proper and professional therapy will be cut short. The patient's involvement in self-care, is a vital part of the healing process. This will empower the patient to enhance whatever treatment approach is given. Unless the practitioner is willing and prepared to devote sufficient time for each patient and in a relaxed cordial environment, the patient will hardly benefit from any preventive therapy aimed at. It will not be correct to say to the patient, 'Take your depression problem to the psychiatrist who can deal with your mental case of depression.' Or, 'Go to the family problem specialist.' Or go to the night club to end up your loneliness or to the psychologist who can find an answer for the causes of your lower self-image. You see, these answers will automatically defeat the practice of holistic health care. Indeed, it is either that we are properly trained in the field of holistic complementary medicine or we are not, there can be no short cut.

Le us get back to the discussion about the core points of preventing the possible illnesses in the practice of complementary medicine. These requirements must be applicable at both the individual patient's home and at the community institutions. The refrigerators where most precooked or cooked foodstuffs are usually stored must be kept very clean all the time. The individual person(s) involved in the preparation and dishing and serving of any kind of food must, by law, ensure that both their body, their clothes, the service utensils, their uniform, and equipments are cleaned and sterilised at all times. After all, the Royal Society of Public Health and Hygiene has laid down the standards of personal and food Hygiene to be followed by all engaged in the catering for food for human consumption. As a member of that body, I consider that complementary medicine has a direct relationship to the profession of food production and consumption. In societies, basic poverty is endemic, and better information and education on the availability of simple basic food resources are very important.

We Will Not Need Drugs If We Live Right

In fact, the application of drugs in the therapeutic health care came about because people neglect the constant practice and attention to natural order. At the rudiment stages of human development, it was very easy to follow the orderly steps of existence. As the populations increased and living became complex, man began to increase his sense of awareness and expansion in all directions. Both agricultural and industrial revolution in Europe accelerated the development of economic, social, and political movements in all directions. This means that people are no longer living in the same orderly ways as they used to.

The Renaissance was a period of awareness and enlightenment; this period is often referred to as the Age of Enlightenment (or simply the Enlightenment). It is the era in Western philosophy and intellectual, scientific, and cultural life that was centred upon the eighteenth century. This was the beginning of defusing of knowledge in all aspects of life. The old system of doing things began to give way for new order. Commercialisation began to affect everything. The former pattern of food cultivation, harvesting, and procurement became too slow for the accelerated demand. This change also affected the provision of medicine. With this, scientists began to seek faster and speedier ways of treatments. Today, the result of this is referred to as chemical medical treatment with an open knowledge of the side effects. Consequently, we are beginning to look back to the 'dear old traditional health care methods'. The changes affected not only the medical practice but also the food chain. Food chain is the source of all food that is the activity of autotrophy, mainly photosynthesis by plants. The chemical substance produced by man has affected this process. The idea is to accelerate the production of food in response to the need and demand. It is said that such chemical effects has a bearing in the health care problems of mankind.

One of the most important objects of life is how to eat to live because it is food that keeps us here, and it is also food that may take us away. So to regulate the food and beverages we consume is one of the important things of life. To eat one meal a day and nothing between meals is healthy. We do not need drugs if we live right. To live without sickness is a very simple thing to do, if we stop using the thing that makes us sick. We have been made so greedy that it seems almost impossible for us to eat right and live a long life. But it is easy when we learn how to begin it. To eat to live does not mean that one will have a menu of various foods as long as one's arm, from which to choose. You can eat one or two foods such as good bread, pure milk, and dried beans, which will not destroy your life, if you are not able to buy a lot of different foods. This is sufficient to keep you living for many years. Of course, a balanced diet is fine. In it you have plenty of garden vegetables with which you can change your diet, with or without eating that particular vegetables that will make you sick. But, one of the main things to prolong your life is not to eat too frequently, but eat one meal a day. When you get used to eating one meal a day and you feel that you can eat one meal every two days without too many hunger pangs, then do so. Stay off hog flesh and essence. Do not say to me, 'That western man is eating anything, and therefore I do not see them dying so fast.' Remember all that God says you shall not do, but the Western man says you should do. He is a breaker of Divine law by nature and the greatest adversary of the Divine Supreme Being (this is made by nature to be so). As a practitioner, you must tell your clients to eat to live and not live to eat and die. For food keeps us alive and food takes us away, if we do not eat wisely.

A Return to Long Life

'Eat to live' brings about a return to perfection and long life; like Noah and Methuselah, who lived for nearly a thousand years of our calendar year (containing 365 days). Long life is not enjoyed by eating food which will shorten and destroy life. Our stomachs will be worn out in a few years due to the continuation of trying to digest the food that we eat, some of it being the type of food which we should not dare put into our stomachs. Chemical poison in drinks along with a mixture of good and poison foods have been shortening our lives on the average of about 63 1/2 years at the present time. This is a long way from the 600 to 800-900 years of life of our ancestral fathers. If you want a beautiful appearance, eat the proper food and eat one meal a day, then eat one meal every other day. Your children may be able to eat two meals per week. This will put them into centuries as Noah and Methuselah.

Lengthen Your Life

In order to lengthen our lives, we must begin with what we put into us that retains life. There is not a shadow of a doubt that God has taken the proper steps to give us more life in order to have and enjoy the pleasures of life. He said that what we eat keeps us here, and the same will take us away if we are careless. For example, if we eat one-half pound of food a day, At the end of 365 days, we would have eaten 182.5 lb of food per year. But we eat more than this amount. For instance, if we live fifty years, we would eat ffity times this much food, at a half pound of food a day. If we saw 9,000 lb of raw food piled up before us to consume, we would think that this would be a lot of food to go through our bodies. And we would think that it probably would wear us out to eat that much food in our lifetime, although we eat tons of food in our lifetime without knowing it.

If this food is not the proper food to eat, it will wear away our body and cut short three score and ten years of our lives. On the average, people have a lifespan of around sixty-two years. This is a very short life to live on an earth that has been here for trillions of years. And yet, the average of us cannot live for a hundred years under the present system of civilisation. A person who eats like an animal, three or four times a day and all the time between meals, cannot retain a beautiful appearance. Eating three times a day and all the time between meals removes the body's attractiveness in many ways. We eat meat, but yet meat is not good for us. It becomes a habitual tool. This type of food poisons the blood and goes into the flesh and cannot help but transform and destroy the surface of the flesh. Take, for example, a newborn baby. Many times, its beauty lasts for just a short while and then passes away with its growth. Even in our late twenties and early thirties, because of the life that we live and the frequent eating of poison food, our beautiful appearance begins to pass from us so rapidly that by our forties and fifties, it is nearly completely gone. Let us eat one meal a day and try getting the best food that we can to eat: vegetables, fruits, pure fresh milk, and pure wholewheat bread that has been cooked slowly, twice. Doing this will help us live longer and retain our beautiful appearance much longer. Do not get into the habit of eating a lot of greasy food (or if you are already in the habit, stop it). Regardless of whether the grease is from animal flesh or not, our bodies, by nature, are not made to digest and control grease or lots of fat. Thousands of minor ailments disappear from us by eating the proper food and at the proper time, one meal a day. God teaches us never to eat unless we are hungry. Eating when we are not hungry causes these minor ailments. We are forcing the body to digest food before it is calling for this food.

Doctors Falls Victim of the Same Sickness

Eat one meal a day. Eat one meal every two days. Eat one meal every three days. Whatever choice you make, it is going to help you, if you eat the right foods. Those who have been our teachers in everything for four hundred long years did not teach us to eat right, because they were not eating right themselves. And, they, their children and their doctors all live about the same span of life. The span of life for the doctor and his patient is the same. 'Have a long life' is the way we wish others, whether or not we are taught the right way of prolonging our health and lessen our sickness . . . the doctor falls victim of the same sickness and the same diseases as his patients and his span of life is the same as that of his patients. This professes beyond a shadow of a doubt that the doctor's teacher did not teach him right on how to live. It is unfortunate that the modern civilisation does not try to persuade the doctor against alcoholic drinks and eating of the pig and other stale meats of the land and the foods of the sea. The modern civilisation teaches him to eat all the scavengers of the sea that all other civilisations turned down.

How About the Medical Doctors and the Scientists?

If the theologian teachers and scientists of chemicals are indulging in and are not successful in expanding their own lives in what they are offering to us to eat and drink, then why should we follow their ways of life? But we have followed them since we were inducted. The chemical doctors (the pharmaceutical experts) go to the earth to get chemicals to heal themselves and us. These chemicals will soon destroy both. And their bodies were not made to be supported by chemicals for health and longevity. The fact here is that the human body was not made to be drugged.

Please reflect on what you will send down your throat; whether it will be something to keep you here or something to take you away. Some people love a lot of sweet and starchy foods. We should eat a little of both, but never indulge in too much of it. it wills tart sugar boiling your blood. Sugar can be controlled. It is not such a disease that cannot be controlled by your appetite. Just do not indulge in too much sugar. Eat a little bit. If you are a sugar diabetic, stay awayfrom sugar, for sugar will make you diabetic and you will never know that you have it until you indulge in too much of sugary and starchy foods. Eat more protein foods. And eat more fish or that which water produces of life other than scavengers of the water. We have scavengers out there in the water, and we have them on the land. Stay away from that kind of animal or life that lives on nothing but filth itself. And do not be a slave to your eating desires. Be the master of what you should eat and do not allow the desire or hunger to be the master.

Do you think the old patriots who lived 500, 600, 700, 800, 900, and nearly 1,000 years ate such filth? What do you think they ate? They did not eat pig. They did not gobble down all kinds of meats and other foods three times a day. Some of them did not eat but one or two times a whole week. How do you think the people on Mars lived? 'I do not know,' you will say. And, they lived twelve hundred of our earth years. The Bible teaches us, and it is supposed to be from Jesus, that when God comes, he comes to bring you life and take away death and give you more of abundance, plenty. He cannot do it without regulating our eating habits. So this is the way to live a long time.

Best Preventive Practice against Death

It is possible for us to eat many things and we can exist for a while, but if we would like to live as long as we can live, we need proper guidance in the way of teaching us the proper foods to eat to expand our life and keep it expanded. We are really very hesitant in refraining from eating food for any length of time. Why? It is because we are born eating all the food that we can get in our stomachs within one day. There is no regularity in this way of eating. We eat whenever we see some food. We are like pigs that eat all the time whenever they see food. And we are like chickens and other fowl and animals that eat all the time. Eating like this keeps our stomach churning to try to digest the food that we put in it and to pass the food through to our intestines. This soon wears out the digestive juices of our stomach, and we only live as long as the stomach is capable of digesting what we put in to it. There is nothing as naive as believing that our stomach will grind and digest anything we put into it. Just think of what hardship you are putting your stomach to when you do not consider how this junk affects that grinding machine placed in your body (digestive organ system).

We suffer from all kinds of ailments of the body due to our own ignorant way of eating. How many times have you heard people say, when offered food, 'do not wait until you are hungry, eat before you get hungry?' This is a dangerous thing to follow—eating before you get hungry. I have heard many people, and so have you, say that they are eating just because they have not eaten in such a length of time or, 'I missed my breakfast,' or 'I missed my lunch.' They are eating then not because they are hungry, but they are eating because of the time they had set for themselves to eat. Three meals a day, within the short space of eight or ten hours could kill you at a very early age. All foods have a certain percentage of poison in it, and if it is allowed to be increased in a very short while, then that keeps the body housing and storing up poison that it does not need to house. Because we are making an addition to poison that is already there, it makes sense. Sometimes this extra, unwanted food in the body causes pain here and there; and we say that it is something else that it is coming from. It is that big meal you are eat two and three times within eight or ten hours or within twelve hours at the longest. So we kill ourselves. When we get a pain, we run to the doctor for some drug to stop it, or we try to get anything to stop the pain. If we had not found something to stop the pain, then maybe death would have come to us. But seeing and knowing that death comes in the absence of prevention against death, we should try and use the best preventive measure, and that measure is to keep poison out of our bodies by abstaining from keeping our bodies stored with a lot of fresh food for it to digest.

Some Doctors Know

Eat one meal a day or one meal every other day. You may say, 'Oh, I will starve if I eat like that. I have got to have my three meals.' There are even some professional people such as doctors who know that this will prolong your life and theirs too, but they are like us. They were reared under the same teaching, and therefore, they cannot teach you what they themselves do not believe in—how to eat to live. It makes sense to wait such a length of time for our food to digest, and it is good for us. Do not be foolish to use such words as, 'I cannot do that.' We can do many things. There are people known to go without food for forty days and nights. But we have learnt to be ever so eager to spend our language and time in foolishness. We will feel better and we will keep the doctor away—not by an apple (smile), but by prolonging the time between each meal. I keep repeating to you, as others prophesied, that God will come to give you life and more life, abundantly. He cannot give us more life if we hold on to death (eating without any regulation). The very act of eating of one meal a day or one meal every other day makes your beauty and appearance to shine more. You do not need make-up. You are already beautiful by nature. Stay away from all this variety of food and eat common food. Do not try to eat all of that fancy food that has your eyes are attracted to and that your appetite is tempted by. This is not the kind of food that makes you live longer. But it is hard to make people like you move away from that which is wrong and bad for your life. The common food (just milk and bread or just bean soup and bread) is better than all the fancy 'civilisation food' that you may try to eat. Eating good, common food will make you live a long time.

Medical Teaching Based on Three Meals a Day

This world of modern civilisation has hundreds and thousands of ways to tell you and teach you how to eat. Please do not take up the many ways of how to eat—lest you do not have but one way to soon perish. *Eat one meal per day and nothing between meals,* not even the drinking of milk, pops, or juices. You must not eat or drink anything between meals. You must keep your stomach regulated to that one meal, and when you drink enough water to digest that one meal, then do not drink any more water between meals. *Pay no attention* to your doctor saying that you need six to eight glasses of water with one meal per day. What he is telling you goes for three meals per day. All of these medical teachings and administerings are based upon a patient who eats three meals per day. *And* we know what kind of health and sickness we have had with such way of eating. This world offers you a thousand and one different kinds of food to eat. Do not let your eyes destroy your stomach. Eat that which is good and leave alone that which is not good for you. If you try to eat everything that probably is good for your stomach, you will soon have no stomach. The simple food is the food that will give us health and not the food that we spice up with various kinds of spices. Neither is having all those dainty meats, cakes, and pies good for us. They are harder to digest than lamb flesh. Just Look at the advertisement of 'hot dogs'. For a man to hear that some food is named hot dogs, he would not want to eat it. The dog is a very filthy animal for one to name a food after. I do not see how in the world the public gets the idea to buy a food that goes under such a name as the filthy dog. Hot dogs—it is a very cheap food. It is made mostly of scrap beef—something that would not sell if the buyer or the consumer saw it before he bought it made in that fashion. Dog food! Hot dog—just think they buy this all over the world under that name. The most intelligent and delicate eater would not even buy a food that had such a name as 'hot dog'. They have certainly made fools of us. If the food is not 'dog', then why name it 'dog'? One could understand or know the reasnons why food like that was not named something that has a better meaning than give it the name of hot dog. This part of the book is not at all meant to offend many dog lovers. I am talking about associating 'dog' with such a delicious junk food and naming it 'hot dog'. May be that those who are very conversant with the original English history will enlighten us better on the evolution of the name: hot gog.

Very few doctors live up to eighty or ninety years—not to think of living over one hundred years. And they think that they have lived for a long time if they reach a lifespan of eighty or ninety years. They have not been here long enough to know what life is. *Noah* and Methuselah lived almost for a thousand years, but we cannot live one-tenth of that time (hundred years), because we eat the wrong food. The nature of this world (white man) was not to give and prolong our life; it is their nature to shorten our lives, and they have done a good job of it. To destroy life is their very nature. How to eat to live—eat simple food. Do not be reaching for all different kinds of food for they were prepared by the man who wants to commercialise on what you eat. They are interested in commerce. They eat the scavengers of the sea and the scavengers of the earth—reptiles and what not. They have no sense of choice—they will eat anything. Try and resort to what you find in this book and eat to live.

The information in this part of the book is open to the readers to choose whichever style of eating habits they prefer. The primary purpose of this information here is to enable the preventive practitioners to be mindful of how to guide, advise, and nurture their clients about the disease prevention. The relationship between the prcatitioners and the clients should be consultative and suggestive rather than a process of inducement.

15.2 Description of Mosquito

Spread the knowledge of mosquitoes, their habitation, their breeding ground, their behaviour and the diseases they inject into the human body. All these must form part of our knowledge as complementary medical practitioners. We must always advise our patients about the mosquito bites. *If* you are living in the tropical regiono f the world such as Africa, some parts of America, or many parts of Asia, there are special precautions you must take. These will be discussed further in this chapter.

Definition of mosquito:

The word 'mosquito' is Spanish for 'little fly', and its use dates back to about 1583 in North America (Europeans referred to mosquitoes as 'gnats'). Mosquitoes belong to the order *Diptera*, true flies. Mosquitoes are like flies in that they have two wings, but unlike flies, their wings have scales, their legs are long, and the females have a long mouth part (proboscis) for piercing through the skin to suck in their food—the blood.

This female *Anopheles gambiae* mosquito is feeding.

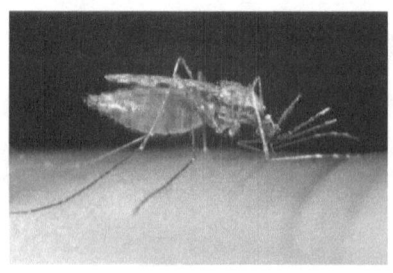

You can see how well-fed this human enemy is. In few minutes, her dining will be completed and she will take off.

A mosquito is an insect. They are in the fly Order Diptera. The females are ectoparasites: they land on warm-blooded animals, pierce a capillary, and inject saliva to stop the blood from coagulating. Then they suck up and eat the blood. In the saliva, there are often deadly microscopic parasites.

The males are nectar-feeders and so are the females. However, in preparation for egg-laying they turn to blood for its protein.

Females cannot lay eggs until they have filled up on enough protein from blood. Then they find a pool of water to lay their eggs in. Mosquitoes lay their eggs in all kinds of water, including water pooled in candy wrappers! The larvae move around near the surface of the water, breathing through air tubes that stick out of the water. They get their food from the water, usually eating algae and other tiny creatures. They like to wiggle around near the surface, which is why some people call them wigglers. The larvae usually enter the pupa stage within a few days or weeks of hatching, depending on the water temperature and the species.

The pupae are called tumblers because they tumble in the water if the water is touched. Tumblers don't eat, but they move around in the water a lot, and like larvae, they breathe from tubes that stick out of the water. The pupa stage is short (only for a few days), and then the mosquito becomes an adult.

Different kinds of mosquitoes like different kinds of blood. Some like human blood, while others like the blood of cows or horses. Sadly, there are so many mosquitoes that almost every mammal has at least one mosquito that likes its blood.

Vectors for Disease

Mosquitoes are a vector (carrier) which carries disease-causing viruses and parasites from person to person. The principal mosquito-borne diseases are the viral diseases such as yellow fever, dengue fever, and malaria carried by the genus Anopheles. Mosquitoes transmit disease to more than seven hundred million people annually in Africa, South America, Central America, Mexico, and much of Asia with millions of resulting deaths.

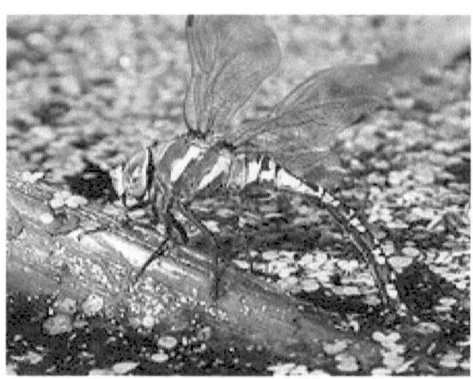

Dragonflies

Dragonflies are natural predators of mosquitoes.

Methods used to prevent the spread of disease or to protect individuals in areas where disease is endemic include the following:

Vector control aimed at mosquito eradication through habitat change: removing stagnant water and other breeding areas, and through use of pesticides, natural predators, and trapping.

Disease prevention through using prophylactic drugs and vaccines, and preventing mosquito bites with insecticides, nets, and repellents.

Water

Standing water, as in a pond or lake, is the main breeding ground. It may or may not be practical to eliminate this water. The water in bird baths can be changed once a week, but one can hardly do that with larger bodies of water. Earlier, the method used to be to spray water with DDT, but that does a lot of damage, and in any event, the mosquito is now highly resistant to the chemical.

Organic Repellents

With increasing reports of the harmful effects DEET has on humans, there has been a gradual move to rely on repellents that are devoid of it, specifically to using repellents that are organic or otherwise are of the kind that have had traditional household purposes prior to their becoming used now as mosquito repellents.

Natural Predators

The dragonfly nymph eats mosquitoes at all stages of development and is quite effective in controlling populations. Some cyclopoid copepods are predators on first instar larvae, killing upto forty Aedes larvae per day. A number of fish eat mosquito larvae, including goldfish, catfish, piranhas, and minnows.

Evolution

The oldest known mosquito with a basically modern anatomy was found in 79-million-year-old Canadian amber from the Upper Cretaceous. An older sister species with more primitive features was found in amber that is 90-100 million years old.

Genetic analyses indicate that the Culicinae and Anophelinae clades may have diverged about 150 million years ago. The Old and New World Anopheles species are believed to have subsequently diverged about 95 million years ago.

Malaria—The Deadly Product of the Tropical Mosquito

In the followoing topics the issue of mosquito is going to be discussed. This is very imporatnt in complementary medicine. The control of the various diseases spread by mosquitoes is critical to the preventive therapy.

How Mosquitoes Work—Mosquito Development—Their Biology

Egg

All mosquitoes lay eggs in water, which can include large bodies of water, standing water (like swimming pools) or areas of collected standing water (like tree holes or gutters). Females lay their eggs on the surface of the water, except for *Aedes* mosquitoes, which lay their eggs above water in protected areas that eventually flood. The eggs can be laid singly or as a group that forms a floating raft of mosquito eggs (see Mosquito Life Cycle for a picture of an egg raft). Most eggs can survive the winter and hatch in the spring.

Identifying Larvae

You can distinguish the larvae of various mosquito species. Anopheles larvae lie parallel to the surface of the water, while larvae of *Aedes* and *Culex* extend down into the water (the air tubes of *Culex* are longer than those of *Aedes*).

Larva

The mosquito eggs hatch into larvae or 'wigglers', which live at the surface of the water and breathe through an *air tube* or *siphon*. The larvae filter organic material through their mouth parts and grow to about 0.5 to 0.75 inches (1 to 2 cm) long. As they grow, they shed their skin (*moult*) several times. Mosquito larvae can swim and dive down from the surface when disturbed (see Mosquito Life Cycle for a Quicktime movie of free-swimming Asian tiger mosquito larvae). The larvae live anywhere from days to several weeks, depending on the water temperature and mosquito species.

Mosquitoes are important

The mosquito larvae and pupae are important food sources for fish in aquatic ecosystems.

Pupa

After the fourth moult, mosquito larvae change into pupae,—or 'tumblers', which live in the water anywhere from one to four days, depending on the water temperature and species. The pupae float at the surface and breathe through two small tubes (*trumpets*). Although they do not eat, pupae are quite active (see Mosquito Life Cycle for a Quicktime movie of free-swimming Asian tiger mosquito pupae). At the end of the pupal stage, the pupae encase themselves and transform into adult mosquitoes.

Adult

Inside the *pupal case*, the pupa transforms into an adult. The adult uses air pressure to break the pupal case open, crawls to a protected area, and rests while its external skeleton hardens, spreading its wings out to dry. Once this is complete, it can fly away and live on the land.

One of the first things that adult mosquitoes do is seek a mate, mate, and then feed. Male mosquitoes have short mouth parts and feed on plant nectar. In contrast, female mosquitoes have a long *proboscis* that they use to bite animals and humans and feed on their blood (the blood provides proteins that the females need to lay eggs). After they feed, female mosquitoes lay their eggs (they need a blood meal each time they lay eggs). Females continue this cycle and live anywhere from many days to weeks (longer over the winter); males usually live only a few days after mating. The life cycles of mosquitoes vary with the species and environmental conditions they are found in.

How Mosquitoes Work: Types of Mosquitoes

There are more than twenty-seven species of mosquitoes in the world, and there are thirteen mosquito genera (plural for 'genus') that live in the United States. Of these genera, most mosquitoes belong to the following three:

- **Aedes**: These are sometimes called 'floodwater' mosquitoes because flooding is important for their eggs to hatch. *Aedes* mosquitoes have abdomens with pointed tips. They include such species as the yellow-fever mosquito (*Aedes aegypti*) and the Asian tiger mosquito (*Aedes albopictus*). They are strong fliers, capable of travelling great distances (up to 75 miles/121 km) from their breeding sites. They persistently bite mammals (especially humans), mainly at dawn and in the early evening. Their bites are painful.
- **Anopheles**: These tend to breed in bodies of permanent freshwater. *Anopheles* mosquitoes also have abdomens with pointed tips. They include several species, such as the common malaria mosquito (Anopheles quadrimaculatus) that spreads malaria to humans.
- **Culex**: These tend to breed in quiet, standing water. Culex mosquitoes have abdomens with blunt tips. They include several species such as the northern house mosquito (*Culex pipiens*). They are weak fliers and tend to live for only a few weeks during the summer months. They persistently bite (preferring birds over humans) and attack at dawn or after dusk. Their bite is painful.

Some mosquitoes, such as the cattail mosquito (*Coquilettidia pertur-bans*), are becoming more prevalent pests as humans are invadingtheir habitats.

Let's examine how mosquitoes live and breed.

Life Cycle and Breeding

Like all insects, mosquitoes hatch from eggs and go through several stages in their life cycle before becoming adults. The females lay their eggs in water, and the larva and pupa stages live entirely in water. When the pupae change into adults, they leave the water and become free-flying land insects. The life cycle of a mosquito can vary from one week to several weeks, depending upon the species (the adult, mated females of some species can survive the winter in cool, damp places until spring, when they will lay their eggs and die.)

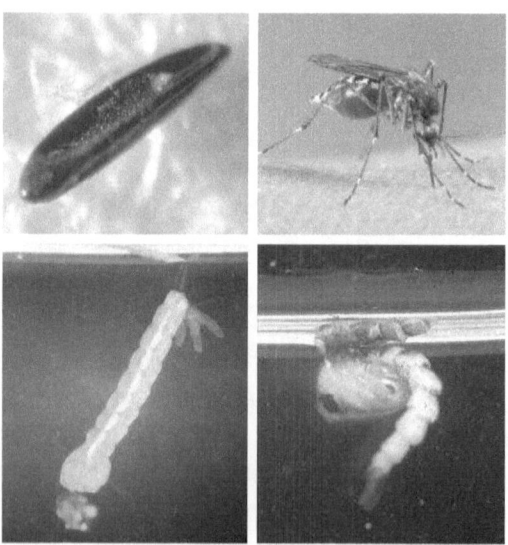

Photos courtesy: Centers for Disease Control and Prevention and USDA/ARS (upper right).

Life cycle of the yellow-fever mosquito (*Aedes aegypti*):

An egg (upper left) laid on the surface of the water hatches into an aquatic larva (lower left). The larva changes into an aquatic pupa (lower right), which then changes into a free-flying adult (upper right). The adult female bites a human to gather blood for laying eggs.

How Mosquitoes Work: Mosquito Bites, Diseases, and Protection

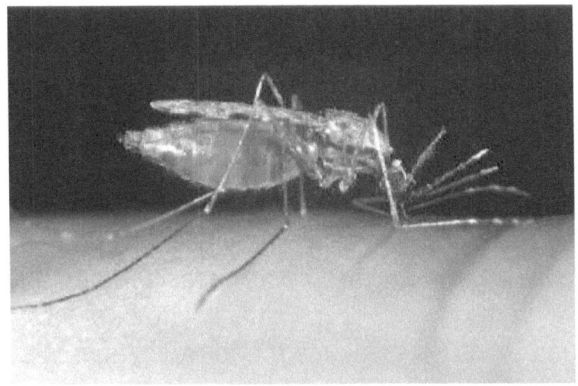

Photo courtesy: Centers for Disease Control and Prevention.
Photographer: Jim Gathany,

This female *Anopheles gambiae* mosquito is feeding. You can see the blood swelling her abdomen.

As mentioned before, only female mosquitoes bite. They are attracted by several things, including heat (infrared light), light, perspiration, body odour, lactic acid, and carbon dioxide. The female lands on your skin and sticks her proboscis into you (the proboscis is very sharp and thin, so you may not feel it going in). Her saliva contains proteins (*anticoagulants*) that prevent your blood from clotting. She sucks your blood into her abdomen (about five microlitrer per serving for an Aedes aegypti mosquito). If she is disturbed, she will fly away. Otherwise, she will remain until she has a full abdomen. If you were to cut the sensory nerve to her abdomen, she would keep sucking until she burst.

After she has bitten you, some saliva remains in the wound. The proteins from the saliva evoke an immune response from your body. The area swells (the bump around the bite area is called a *wheal*), and you itch, a response provoked by the saliva. Eventually, the swelling goes away, but the itch remains until your immune cells break down the saliva proteins. To treat mosquito bites, you should wash them with mild soap and water. Try to avoid scratching the bite area, even though it itches. Some anti-itch medicines such as calamine lotion or an over-the-counter cortisone cream may relieve the itching. Typically, you do not need to seek medical attention (unless you feel dizzy or nauseated, which may indicate a severe allergic reaction to the bite).

Not HIV

The human immunodeficiency virus (HIV) that causes AIDS cannot survive in a mosquito and therefore cannot be transmitted from one person to another through mosquito bites. We thank God for this; otherwise all the tropical African nations would have gone.

- **Diseases**: Mosquitoes can carry many types of diseases that are caused by bacteria, parasites, or viruses. These diseases include:
- **Malaria**: Malaria is caused by a parasite that is transmitted by an *Anopheles* mosquito. The parasite grows in your bloodstream and can produce symptoms that develop anywhere from six to eight days to several months after infection. The symptoms include fever, chills, headaches, muscle aches, and general malaise (similar to flu symptoms). Malaria is a severe disease that can be fatal, but it can be treated with antimalarial drugs. Malaria is prevalent in tropical or subtropical climates.
- **Yellow fever**: Yellow fever no longer occurs in the United States or Europe, but it is prevalent in Africa and parts of South America. It is transmitted by the *Aedes aegypti* mosquito. Yellow fever produces symptoms similar to malaria, but it also includes nausea, vomiting, and jaundice. Like malaria, yellow fever can be fatal. There is no treatment for the disease itself; only the symptoms can be treated. Yellow fever can be controlled by vaccination and mosquito control.
- **Encephalitis**: Encephalitis is caused by viruses that are transmitted by mosquitoes—such as the *Aedes* mosquitoes or *Culiseta* mosquitoes. The symptoms of encephalitis include high fever, stiff neck, headache, confusion, and laziness/sleepiness. There are several types of encephalitis that can be transmitted by mosquitoes, including *St Louis, Western equine, Eastern equine, La Crosse* and *West Nile*. West Nile encephalitis is on the rise in the Eastern United States, which has raised concerns about mosquito control.
- **Dengue fever**: Dengue fever is transmitted by the Asian tiger mosquito, which is native to East Asia and was found in the United States in 1985. It is also transmitted by *Aedes aegypti* in the tropics. Dengue fever is caused by a virus that produces a range of illnesses from viral flu to haemorrhagic fever. It is especially dangerous for children (see Dengue Fever and Dengue Hemorrhagic Fever for more information).

Mosquito Repellents

The best way to reduce mosquito-borne diseases is through mosquito control and personal protection. You can do a few things to reduce the number of mosquito bites that you get while enjoying the outdoors. First, wear clothing that covers most of your body, if temperatures permit. Second, use a mosquito repellent that contains NN-diethyl-meta-toluamide (DEET) at a concentration of 7.5 per cent to 100 per cent. Lower concentrations are sufficient for most outdoor protection, and a 15 per cent concentration is recommended for children. Avon's original Skin-So-Soft is a weak, short-lasting (less than twenty minutes) mosquito repellent, although there are newer Skin-So-Soft formulations that include EPA-recognised insect repellents. Permethrin, an effective pesticide, *is for use on clothing only (Never apply it to your skin, it is a neurotoxin!)*. To learn more about mosquito repellents, see the EPA's How to Use Insect Repellents Safely.

Beyond mosquito repellents and clothing, you can try to control the mosquito population. Mosquitoes need water to breed and will use any source of standing water. If you have a lily pond in your garden, stock it with some fish that will eat the mosquito larvae. Some petroleum oils can be added to water to form a thin surface layer that suffocates the mosquito eggs; however, many of these oils will also suffocate any fish living in the water.

Mosquito Myths

Several natural or man-made products have been touted as mosquito repellents or effective in mosquito control. *Citronella oil*, which is a product of several types of plants that can be made into candles or burnt directly, is an effective mosquito repellent in high concentrations, but individual citronella-producing plants do not make enough oil to effectively repel mosquitoes. Ultraviolet lights (as used in bug zappers) and ultrasonic devices are not effective.

To prevent mosquitoes from entering your home, make sure that all of your window screens are intact.

Finally, there are many commercial pesticides available to kill mosquito larvae and mosquito adults. Many communities conduct large-scale spraying of pesticides containing mallothione to control mosquito populations during the spring and summer, especially in attempts to reduce the spread of West Nile encephalitis. Another option is a device like a Mosquito Magnet, which lures and traps mosquitoes.

Mosquito Summary

Although small in size, mosquitoes have been around for over thirty million years. They have honed their hunting skills over that time and today use chemical, visual, and heat sensors to locate their prey. They use their chemical sensors to detect carbon dioxide and lactic acid from up to a hundred feet away. Certain chemicals in sweat can also trigger their sensors. Their visual sensors aren't very keen, but they can see you moving if you are wearing clothing that contrasts with the background. They use their heat sensors to detect warm-blooded mammals and birds in their vicinity, so they can always locate humans when they are near enough to sense body heat.

There are approximately twenty-seven hundred species of mosquitoes with the majority belonging to three major genera: Aedes (eggs are laid in floodwater areas), Anopheles (eggs are laid in permanent freshwater), and Culex (eggs are laid in quiet, standing water). In terms of development, all mosquitoes start as eggs and hatch into larva or 'wigglers'. As larvae, mosquitoes moult several times until they become pupae or 'tumblers'. As pupae, mosquitoes mature and become adults and begin to mate and feed. After mating, most males die within a few days, whereas the females can live for many weeks, depending on the species of mosquitoes and the environmental conditions present.

Top Five Mosquito Facts

Mosquito is Spanish for 'little fly'. Learn more about mosquitoes. Only female mosquitoes bite. Mosquitoes are attracted to heat, light, perspiration, body odour, lactic acid, and carbon dioxide. Learn more about mosquito bites. Treat mosquito bites by washing them with soap and water. Avoid scratching the bite area by using anti-itch medicines, such as calamine lotion. Learn more about treating mosquito bites. There are many diseases that can be caused by a mosquito bite, including: malaria, yellow fever, encephalitis, and dengue fever Learn more about diseases spread by mosquitoes. There are three basic things you can do to repel mosquitoes: Wear clothing that covers most of your body, use a mosquito repellant that contains NN-diethyl-meta-toluamide (DEET), and eliminate sources of standing water in your area to prevent mosquitoes from breeding. Learn more about mosquito repellants.

Finally

In Europe and in America, some hospitals and medical centres are designated as hospitals or clinics for tropical diseases. Those who must have contracted mosquito diseases like malaria,

15.3 Preventive Therapy and Health Counselling

What we can expect with holistic health counselling—there is very little knowledge or understanding in either the medical field or the mental health field, and many so-called 'mental health' symptoms and 'medical diseases' are really the result of something in an individual's diet, environment, or lack of proper nutrients. Physical illness and psychological symptoms can be triggered off by a variety of dietary, physical, or environmental sources. Food allergy, sensitivity or intolerance, pesticides, common everyday chemicals in your home, nutritional deficiencies, imbalance of nutrients, candida overgrowth, hormonal imbalances, poor diet, and many more factors greatly impact our mental health and physical health. Many psychological and physical symptoms can be alleviated or improved by making simple changes in the diet or environment and lifestyle. Counselling with a holistic health approach looks at the body, mind, and spiritual elements and their interconnection. It examines the underlying causes of the symptoms and encourages a variety of alternative health remedies. There cannot be good mental health by ignoring the physical or spiritual health of the individual and vice versa. Not all conditions, illnesses, or diseases can be completely 'healed', but they can at least be improved drastically. We will, of course, look for healing and seek relief where it exists, but complete healing is a journey that usually consists of time and setbacks. Being healthy does not always mean the 'absence' of disease or illness. It means living and functioning as optimally as possible with your condition—finding harmony and balance in the midst of a storm. We will employ self-care strategies and education that empower you to take control of your own health care plan and be a partner with your health care provider.

Living with Chronic Illness or Chronic Pain

If you live with chronic illness or chronic pain, your life may seem like a roller coaster sometimes. You're likely to deal with a variety of emotional issues on a daily basis. There may be times you need support, encouragement, advice, or education from someone who truly understands. I have first-hand experience in navigating the challenges of chronic illness and chronic pain and understand the impact it can have on your life We may focus of any issue you might have. Coping skills, illness management, symptom management, pain management, relationship issues, sexuality, grieving, coping and adjustment, day-to-day living, acceptance, self-discipline, healing childhood trauma, stress management, etc., etc.

Alternative Mental Health Education

You or someone you love may be living with depression, anxiety, hyperactivity, or other so-called 'mental illnesses' and you would like to find holistic or alternative approaches for relief. Learn how diet, nutrition, and environmental toxins impact your mental health and what to do about it. Conditions such as depression, anxiety, and hyperactivity can be addressed successfully without drugs.

Biochemical Education

Learn how diet, nutrition, and chemicals in our environment affect our mental and physical health and how these factors can create symptoms that appear to be psychological but are actually physical. And how these symptoms can be eliminated or reduced by correcting one's diet and nutrition or by removing chemicals from the environment.

Customised Nutrition

Each one of us is unique biochemically and metabolically. There is no 'one size fits all' vitamin supplement. Your nutritional supplement should be designed specifically for your biochemistry. Use this ground-breaking biochemical test to determine your nutritional needs and create a vitamin supplement created just for you and your body.

Food Sensitivity Testing

Undiagnosed food sensitivity occurs in approximately 80 per cent of the population. It can be at the root of many physical and mental health conditions like depression, anxiety, hyperactivity, irritable bowel, fatigue, arthritis, insomnia, autism, weight gain, fibromyalgia, gastrointestinal distress, earaches, headaches, and many more. With a simple test sent to your home, you can determine your hidden food sensitivities and make drastic improvements in your health.

Candida Education and Support

Candida is a cunning and difficult health condition to manage. It requires a great deal of patience, education, and persistence. Learn how candida impacts your mental and physical health, and get tips and advice on diet, supplementation, treatment options, coping and adjustment, or lifestyle changes.

New Patient Education

Available to those newly diagnosed with fibromyalgia, chemical sensitivities, or chronic fatigue syndrome and would like help and support in learning about all the issues that one will face concerning their illness. Issues such as lifestyle changes, diet, where to find doctors, networking, catalogues, environmental clean-up, coping, etc. can be addressed.

Alcoholism Recovery

As a recovered alcoholic with twenty years of uninterrupted sobriety, I can share with you the reason traditional treatment fails so often and what you need to get sober and stay sober. Learn about alternative treatments for alcoholism that are much more successful than the traditional route.

Weight Management

It's not your fault you're overweight. Learn how factors such as hidden food allergies or sensitivities, thyroid disorders, and common everyday chemicals in your environment trigger your appetite and interfere in proper metabolism, and how you can succeed in maintaining your desired weight.

Professional Consultation

Comprehensive consultation for mental health professionals, public agencies, and health care providers is available to those who are interested in learning about the special and complex needs and issues that one experiences when living with fibromyalgia, chemical sensitivities, or chronic fatigue immune deregulations syndrome. The presentation here should the practitioners to the preventive therapy in all the aspects mentioned above.

CHAPTER 16

16.1 Sexual Therapeutic Preventive Therapy

As a principal part of life, nothing gives an inner joy as sexual play, especially when it is equally enjoyed by both parties. It is because of its therapeutice nature, that I have chosen to present the information in this book. In the countries where the topic of sex is still viewed as a dirty and an inmmoral issue, this book will be banned. But I thank God that the world at large is beginning to become awake!

There are many kinds of health problems associated with sexual matters such as the following: weakness of virility, sex drive weakness, excretion with blood, lack of erection, defection during ejaculation, convulsion of the penis, swelling of the testicle, enlarged testicles, itching of the testicle skin, shrinking of the testicles, ascending of the testicle skin, dropping of the testicles, slackness o f the testicle skin, ulcer of the penis, testicles, and genital area, hard boils on the penis, twitching of the penis, lower sperm count, premature ejaculation, excessive sex drive constant erection of the penis, separation of the peritoneum, hernia of the abdomen and of the groin, and nymphomania.

Any reader of this book interested to be seen for any of the above listed problems or in need of the following products should quote the book reference Number: STP301137 for appointment. To place order, contact us at Beckman Natural Medic: Email: lukeubani@yahoo.com Quote our book ID 301137.

Attention: You no longer have to let Cialis control your life! Now you can enjoy the best sex you've ever had, whenever you want, covered by our money back guarantee! Get Rock-Hard Erections That Stay Hard All Night Long—With Nature's Answer to Cialis!

Who needs all those dangerous side effects just to be able to get it on?

Are you sick of all the side effects and caveats of using Cialis? Wouldn't it be great to be able to have a drink with dinner on a special night? Don't you want to say goodbye to awkward conversations with your doctor?

Then say hello to Orviax, your new male enhancement pill that will let you finally free you from Cialis!

- No prescription needed
- All-natural active ingredients
- No known side effects
- No adverse reactions with alcohol
- Starts working in thirty minutes or less

16.2 The Science of Orviax: The Natural Remedy for Sexual Joy

As a potential Orviax consumer, you have the right to know about the science behind Orviax and why it is a proven solution to erectile dysfunction problems, so you can make an informed choice before you purchase.

Before we can explain the science behind the time-tested ingredients, you need to understand how your body works to provide you with a large, rock-hard erection that will please her all night long.

Your penis is composed of spongy tissue that becomes erect when it is filled with blood. If anything interferes with the blood flow to your penis, it will either not become erect or else will not become as large as it should become. A lack of blood flow will also decrease your libido, which is directly connected to penile response.

Unfortunately, a lot of things can contribute to your penis not getting the blood flow it needs to get the job done. Testosterone gets the process started. If you have a limited amount of testosterone, your penis will not perform up to expectations. Stress, tension, and anxiety can also cause a natural process that limits blood flow to your penis and impedes sexual function.

Finally, poor blood circulation also plays a part in erectile dysfunction, because it makes it harder for your penis to get enough blood to expand to its full potential.

Now, let's look at how our natural herbal compounds help fight these common causes of erectile dysfunction:

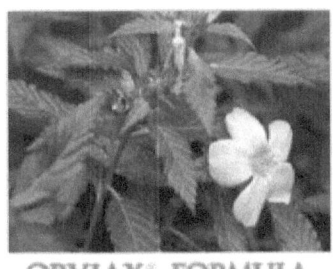

ORVIAX® FORMULA

Damiana

Damiana is a natural nervous system relaxant that fights stress that can inhibit sexual activity. In 1999, a group of researchers in Italy administered damiana to both sexually potent and sexually impotent rats. The extract had no effect on sexually potent rats, but in the others, it increased the percentage of rats achieving ejaculation and made them more sexually active.

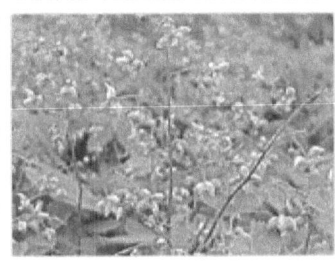

ORVIAX® FORMULA

Epimedium

Epimedium is used to regulate testosterone production and help increase libido. It has been demonstrated to relax rabbit penile tissue by nitric oxide and PDE-5 activity. Like sildenafil (Viagra), icariin, the active compound in epimedium, inhibits the activity of PDE-5, which can reduce testosterone. A recently published Italian study investigated a number of epimedium derivatives and achieved similar results as sildenafil in fighting erectile dysfunction.

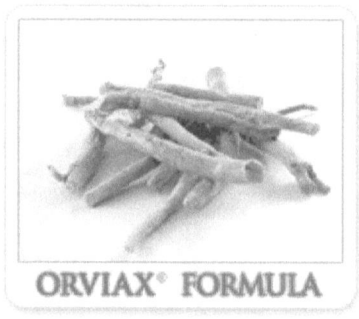

Ashwaganda Root

Ashwagandha is used to fight anxiety that can lead to erectile dysfunction. Sloane-Kettering Hospital reports that 'Ashwagandha is rich in iron; small-scale human studies suggest ashwagandha may promote growth in children and improve hemoglobin level, red blood cell count, and sexual performance in adults. A herbal tea containing ashwagandha was shown to increase natural killer cell activity in healthy volunteers with recurrent coughs and colds. Data also indicate that ashwagandha may be useful in the treatment of anxiety.'

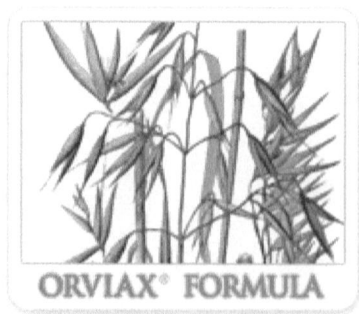

Avena Sativa

Avena sativa has long been used to help increase the breeding rates among horses. Recently, doctors have started exploring if its natural relaxation effects can help humans increase their sex drive as well. Dr Larry

Clapp has studied alternative virility medicines extensively and concludes that avena satvia 'works powerfully to enhance erectile function'.

Dr Ray Sahelian has reported similar findings. Research studies into its overall effect on sexual function in humans are ongoing.

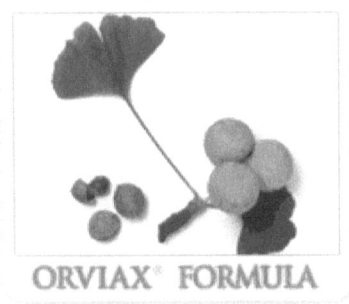

ORVIAX® FORMULA

Gingko Biloba

Ginkgo biloba is known to help reduce stress, boost memory and most importantly, improve blood circulation. University of Maryland Medical Center has reported that 'ginkgo has been shown to be as effective as a prescription medication' in addressing blood flow and circulation problems. The hospital also reported that it helped increase 'social behaviour' and was effective in treating depression (which can lead to erectile dysfunction.)

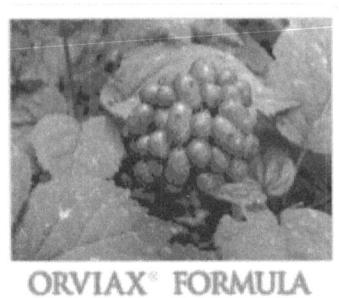

ORVIAX® FORMULA

Korean Ginseng

Korean ginseng is a very well-studied aphrodisiac. A 2002 study by the Southern Illinois University School of Medicine (published in the annals of the New York Academy of Sciences) found that in laboratory animals, Korean ginseng enhanced libido and copulatory performance. The study reported that this was due to the direct effects of ginseng or its ginsenoside (the active ingredient in Korean Ginseng) components on the central nervous system and gonadal tissues. In males, the study found 'ginsenosides can facilitate penile erection'.

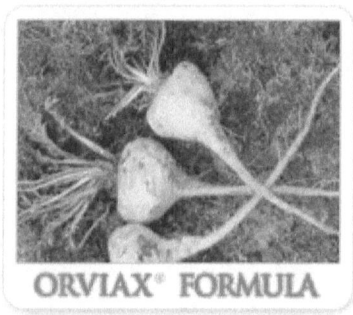

ORVIAX® FORMULA

Maca

Maca has been used as a folk medicine to enhance sexual performance for hundreds of years. In 2002, a double-blind study looked at the effect of four months of treatment with maca tablets on semen quality in nine adult men. Treatment with maca resulted in increased seminal volume, sperm count, and sperm motility. A twelve-week randomised, controlled trial looked at 1,500 mg maca, 3,000 mg maca, or placebo. After eight weeks, there was an improvement in sexual desire in the men taking maca.

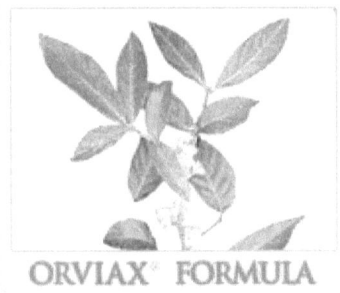

ORVIAX® FORMULA

Muira Puama

Muira Puama is thought to relax the capillaries that bring blood to the penis in order to make it easier to achieve erection. In 1990, at the Institute of Sexology in Paris, France, a clinical study with 262 patients complaining of lack of sexual desire demonstrated muira puama extract to be effective. Within two weeks, at a daily dose of 1–1.5 g of muira puama 4:1 extract, 62 per cent of the patients in the study reported increased libido and improved sexual performance.

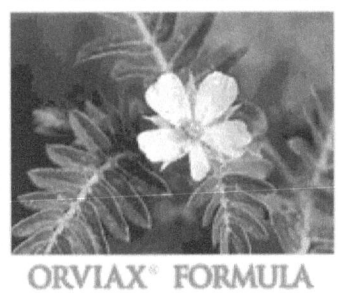

ORVIAX® FORMULA

Tribulus Terrestris

Tribulus Terrestris has been shown to increase testosterone and thus improve male libido. For over thirty years, clinical studies in Bulgaria and Russia have indicated that tribulus increases levels of the hormones testosterone (by increasing luteinising hormone), DHEA, and estrogen, all of which lead to increased sex drive and performance. Preliminary animal studies have found that tribulus heightened sexual behaviour and increased intracavernous pressure. This was attributed to increases in testosterone.

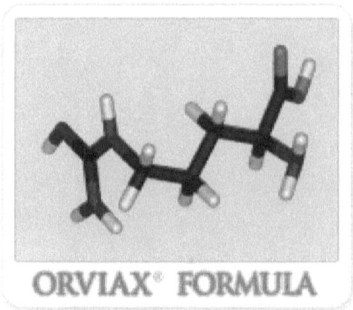

ORVIAX® FORMULA

L-arginine

L-arginine acts similarly to Viagra in the body. Like sildenafil citrate, L-arginine enhances the action of nitric oxide, which relaxes muscles surrounding blood vessels supplying blood to the penis. As a result, blood vessels in the penis dilate, increasing blood flow, which helps maintain an erection. The difference in how L-arginine and Viagra work is that Viagra blocks an enzyme called PDE5 that destroys nitric oxide, and L-arginine is used to make nitric oxide. In one study, fifty men with erectile dysfunction took either 5 g of L-arginine per day or a placebo. After six weeks, more men in the L-arginine group had an improvement compared to those taking the placebo. Our Swiss labs have taken these ingredients from nature and harnessed them into a pill that is making Cialis a thing of the past. Are you ready for a long weekend of satisfying her between the sheets? Order Orviax today!

Use Orviax™ Responsibly

Orviax is an all-natural way for you to get harder easily, achieve bigger, longer-lasting erections, increase your libido and provide your partner with as much sexual satisfaction as possible. It will even help you achieve a larger manly ejaculate load that will impress her and leave her begging for more.

While Orviax is a herbal supplement, it still needs to be used responsibly. Even natural ingredients can be harmful if abused. That's why we feel the responsibility to provide you with a general guide to things you should look out for to make Orviax as risk-free as possible.

- Orviax is only intended to be used by adults. If you are not at least eighteen years of age, Orviax is not for you, and we will not allow you to purchase it.
- Do not use Orviax if you are pregnant or at risk of pregnancy. Some women have attempted to use Orviax to help with their own libido problems even though the product is designed to help male erectile dysfunction. We do not advise you to do so if there is any chance at all that you may be pregnant.
- Only take as directed. The recommended dosage of Orviax is safe and effective for most men. Do not take more than the recommended dose. It is meant to be used as directed.
- If you have any sensitivities to herbal products, consult your physician before taking Orviax. A small number of people may experience allergic reactions to certain herbs. Your doctor can help you determine if Orviax is right for you.

Overall, the risks in using Orviax are very low, particularly when compared to prescription erectile dysfunction medication. Just compare Orviax to the possible side effects of these much more dangerous drugs.

How Does Orviax Compare To Cialis And Other Prescription Erectile Dysfunction Medications?

Getting, controlling, and maintaining rock-hard erections over a long period of time isn't the only thing men love about Orviax. For thousands of our customers, it's all about keeping a secret.

As you already know, most pills that tackle the issue of erectile dysfunction need a prescription. That means a visit to your doctor and a trip to the pharmacy—two more people to add to your list of those who know about your little problem. And with today's health care, there's a paper trail a mile long that anyone from your Human Resources director to your sex partners can just happen to see.

Orviax to the rescue! It's non-prescription, comes in discreet packaging, and is easily overlooked on a credit card statement. But how does Orviax add up to the name-brand prescriptions meds like Cialis?

Drink, Eat, Have Sex And Be Merry—With A Cialis Alternative That Works Even After An Evening Of Fun!

Cialis ads always show frisky couples snuggling up and about to get it on. What they don't show you, however, is those same couples going through hell just to get the timing right so maybe, just maybe, if the stars are aligned, he may be able to get an erection.

That's ridiculous! Who needs the hassle? We all know that a steamy hot moment of passionate sex isn't something you can plan out or negotiate. It should, and usually does, follow an evening of fine dining, maybe some drinks by the fire, or even a shared dessert. With Cialis, you can't eat an hour before you take it, and you are discouraged from drinking at all. And even worse, it can take up to another hour to kick in! Gee! That sounds super romantic! And how embarrassing! There's no way you can hide it from your lady, and it makes you seem like a sick patient, for goodness' sake!

With Orviax, you no longer have to worry about if it's going to work simply because you decided to live your life and have a little fun before turning in for the night. She'll be thrilled by the new spontaneity—she'll never know when you might take her and ravish her next!

Orviax is the Common Sense Alternative to Cialis Customers Are Raving About.

Look, we can show you the charts and list the ingredients and give you the best reasons in the world to choose Orviax for your erectile dysfunction—but the truth is that with something this important, you want to hear how it works in real life, with real men.

Luckily for us, that's not a problem. We get cards, letters, and emails by the bucketful from men who can't wait to tell us how Orviax has changed their lives! Check out just a few:

Harder Erections Guaranteed. What Are You Waiting For?

You know you want to stop the madness and frustration of erectile dysfunction for good. You're ready to satisfy her with hours of great sex and a controllable erection.

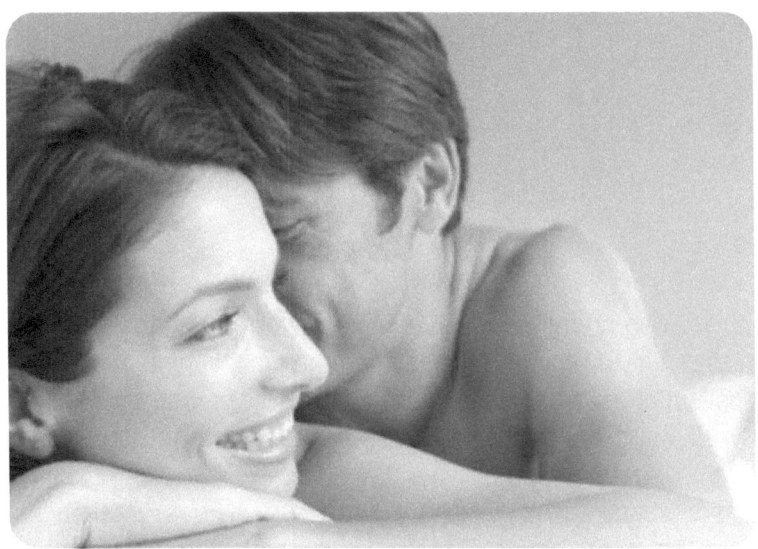

We also know that in today's economy, things like ED pills are the first to get struck from the budget. And if you can't even be sure that Orviax really works, can you justify the expense?

That's why we've created our thirty-day 100 per cent money back guarantee. Simply order Orviax today and try it out this month. If within thirty days you don't see that Orviax is your non-prescription alternative to Cialis, simply send us a note and your unused portion—and we'll refund your money immediately.

That's how confident we are that you'll love the Orviax experience.

Isn't it time you finally took control of your sex life? Don't you want to stop the cycle of embarrassment and weakness that comes with being a Cialis 'patient'? Wouldn't you rather be laughing it up with the love of your life than watching the clock and monitoring your food intake? Look no further. You've found your solution.

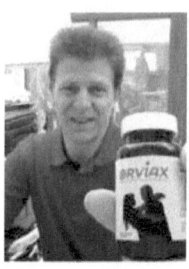

'Having studied many male enhancement web sites I finally decided to give Orviax a try as somehow it seemed the most convincing. Still being skeptical but at the same time optimistic that this product would enhance our love making I ordered a month's supply. I think it is important to understand, that for me anyway, having used Orviax for a month and noticing increased stamina and energy, which was great in itself, I was sure that there was still further improvement to come which was conveyed on the web site. I ordered a further 6 months supply and sure enough, by the end of the second month I was performing like I was in my twenties but with the benefit of experience. My partner and I make love at every opportunity and it seems like we can't get enough of each other. My erections are fuller and firmer and, although I haven't measured my penis I am sure it is bigger, certainly its girth has increased. My partner and I are in our late 40's and we are enjoying our best sexual experiences ever.'

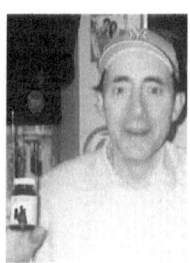

'Hello! I had a lean spell romantically until I met a beautiful lady from Bali in Ireland and after a few dates we went on a hotel break and eventually lay together to make love but I then discovered for the first time in my life I could not perform. I had hints of this beforehand and I was not totally surprised but it did hit me hard (no pun intended) or rather did not hit me 'hard'. I asked her to give me a chance to try solving my 'erectile dysfunction' and to her great credit she did. I got Viagra from my doctor and while it did give me an erection it felt 'unreal' and as a nutritionist I felt a supplement was probably a better option if I could find a good one. I did research on the internet and I found Orviax and i was a bit skeptical at first but on the next y girlfriend I had a 'bullseye' and we had a great lovemaking session in my own bed for added comfort and since then it has been a case of 'hitting the target every time' and it has worked wonders for my confidence every way. Thank you orviax! J.O sullivan, kilkenny, ireland.'

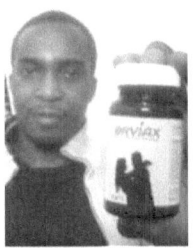

'For the past few months, in addition to my job, I have been heavily involved in physical sports regularly which left me exhausted and greatly reduced my sexual desire and performance. I'm an outgoing single man that loves regularly meeting new women so this exhaustion knocked back my confidence a great deal. So, I decided to use Viagra and other similar products which caused me headaches and dizziness! Luckily, I came across Orviax and now, my sexual drive is way through the roof! The great thing about Orviax is that, it feels so natural, you never remember you've taken any capsules until you feel that erection which I get every time sex pops in my head which is a lot! I get erections I never thought I could achieve and they last as long as my stamina can maintain, which, now is also a lot. Women I've had sex with since using Orviax get very exhausted after sex with me and seem not to be able to get enough of sex with me as they constantly let me know!'

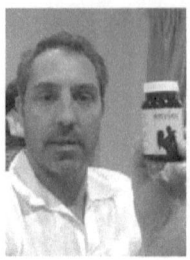

'Dear,

Thanks for the mail and of course the product. Well my story is that me and my girlfriend have been enjoying the benefits of orviax almost daily! Yesss! She just uses me for her twice weekly exercise which thanks to Orviax sure beats going to the gym! You can happily use my picture. Her friends sometimes say she moans too much well the only moaning she does when with me, is whilst biting the my ability to pillow!'

16.3 The Natural Sources of Preventive Therapy for Joints and Bones

It's vital to keep your joints and bones healthy so you can continue to lead an active and independent life. The Easy-Vit joint and bone range has been specially formulated to increase strength and flexibility to protect against long-term damage and joint pain.

Any reader of this book interested to place order for any the above products quote the book reference Number: STP301137. Beckam Natural Medcs, 290A, Lodge Aveneue, Dagenham, Essex, RM8 2HF, United Kingdom. The telephone number to ring is (44) 02082270083, (44) 07733764875, email: lukeubani@yahoo.com

- **Glucosamine Sulphate 2KCL (1,000 mg)**

Glucosamine stimulates the growth of cartilage, protecting your joints from wearing out. Most foods contain very little glucosamine, so it's vital to top up your levels to protect against joint damage and pain. Our glucosamine sulphate tablets provide pure, pharmaceutical grade, sodium-free glucosamine sulphate.

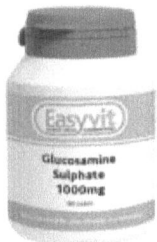

- **Glucosamine Sulphate** 2KCL (1500 mg) Glucosamine stimulates the growth of cartilage, protecting your joints from wearing out. Most foods contain very little Glucosamine so it's vital to top up your levels to protect against joint damage and pain. Our glucosamine sulphate tablets provide pure, pharmaceutical-grade, sodium-free glucosamine sulphate.

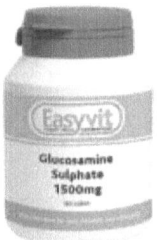

- **Glucosamine Chondroitin and MSM**

Glucosamine is found naturally in your joints and muscles where it plays a role in the smooth working of your cartilage, tendons, and ligaments. We've combined pharmaceutical-grade glucosamine with chondroitin, a compound found naturally in your joints where it helps to attract fluid into the cartilage and MSM (methyl sulphonyl methane), which is essential for building and repairing the connective tissue of joints, tendons, and cartilage.

Each tablet provides: 50 mg Glucosamine Sulphate 2KCl, 10 mg Chondroitin Sulphate, 16 per cent preparation, and 10 mg MSM.

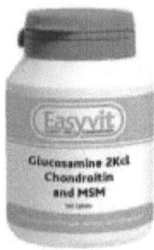

- **High-strength Glucosamine, Chondroitin, MSM, Vit C**

Glucosamine is found naturally in your joints and muscles where it plays a role in the smooth working of your cartilage, tendons and ligaments. We've combined pharmaceutical-grade glucosamine with chondroitin, a compound found naturally in your joints where it helps to attract fluid into the cartilage and MSM (methyl Sulphonylurea Methane), which is essential for building and repairing the connective tissue of joints, tendons and cartilage. As an added bonus, this product now also includes vitamin C.

Each tablet provides: 400 mg Glucosamine Soleplate 2KCl, 100mg Chondroitin Sulphate, 16 per cent preparation, 50 mg MSM, and 60 mg vitamin C.

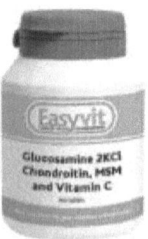

- **Glucosamine and Chondroitin**

This specially formulated glucosamine supplement combines pharmaceutical grade glucosamine sulphate with marine chondroitin. Glucosamine maintains connective tissues, while chondroitin attracts fluid to the cartilage-together they help cushion, lubricate, and strengthen, protecting you against long-term joint damage.

Each tablet provides: 500 mg Glucosamine Sulphate 2KCl and 400 mg Chondroitin Sulphate, 16 per cent preparation.

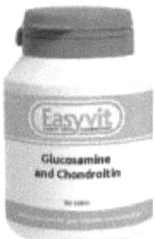

- **High Potency MSM**

MSM (methyl sulphonyl methane) is essential for building and repairing the connective tissue of joints, tendons, and cartilage. It also plays an important part in maintaining tissue found in the skin, lungs, and intestines, helping to protect against allergies. MSM is the fourth most abundant mineral found in the human body.

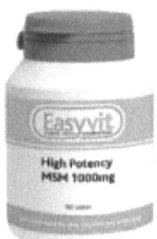

- **Devil's Claw Extract**

This high-strength extract is derived from the fruit of the Devil's Claw and has been used for centuries as a traditional remedy for joint pain. It contains a natural compound called harpagoside, which reduces inflammation in the joints, helping reduce the effects of arthritis.

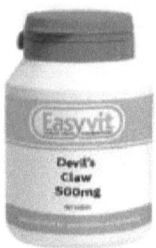

- **Calcium Osteo Formula**

This specially formulated supplement combines calcium and magnesium in one easy tablet. Calcium is vital for strong bones and teeth and is essential in preventing osteoporosis. It also maintains healthy nerve function and aids blood clotting. Magnesium is important to maintain healthy bones and normal muscle function, especially the heart.

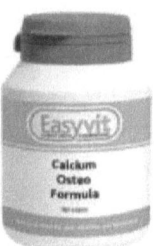

- **Cod Liver Oil**

Cod liver oil has long been a traditional remedy for joint problems as it lubricates them, reducing the friction which can cause pain and inflammation. Its amazing effects don't stop there; it's a rich source of Omega 3, which helps promote good heart function and circulation and is packed with vitamins A and D.

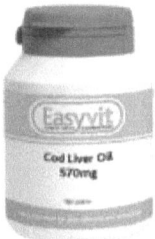

- **Cod Liver Oil (High strength)**

Cod liver oil has long been a traditional remedy for joint problems as it lubricates them, reducing the friction which can cause pain and inflammation. Its amazing effects don't stop there; it's a rich source of Omega 3, which helps promote good heart function and circulation and is packed with vitamins A and D.

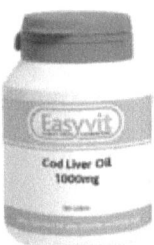

- **Cod Liver Oil and Calcium**

The Omega 3 fatty acids found in cod liver oil are important to maintain a healthy heart, good circulation, and help soothe the discomfort of osteoarthritis. We've combined these benefits with calcium to keep bones and teeth healthy and protect against osteoporosis in one handy supplement.

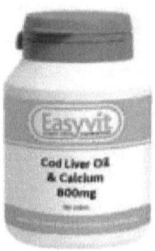

- **Green-lipped Mussel Extract**

Manufactured from the green-lipped mussels, which inhabit the clear waters of New Zealand, this amazing extract reduces the symptoms of osteoarthritis by inhibiting joint inflammation. It may also help alleviate conditions such as asthma, psoriasis, bowel inflammation, and general joint problems.

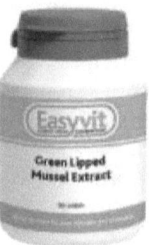

- **Collagen**

If you suffer with painful joints or ligaments then this high-strength supplement can help. Collagen stimulates the growth of new cartilage and reduces joint inflammation and stiffness to relieve the symptoms of arthritis and improve mobility. It can also improve the condition of hair, skin, and nails.

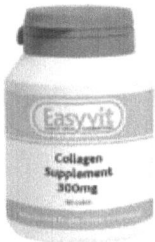

• **Rose Hip Extract**

Rose hip has an anti-inflammatory effect, helping to relieve the symptoms of arthritis and osteoporosis without the unpleasant effects of anti-inflammatory drugs. It is a completely natural plant extract and is high in vitamin C.

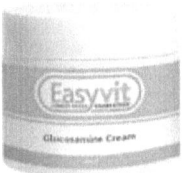

• **Glucosamine Joint Cream**

Apply our high-strength glucosamine cream direct to the site of joint pain or discomfort to maximise its regenerative effects and speed up relief from arthritis or rheumatism. This specially formulated cream also includes five natural essential oils and has anon-greasy base that is easily absorbed.

**Health and Life-sustaining Ingredients in
Each of the above Food Supplements**

Magnesium: Magnesium helps the body to use calcium properly by ensuring it is distributed to those areas where it is most needed: in the bones and nerve cells. Without adequate amounts of magnesium, calcium would be dumped harmfully into the body's soft tissues.

Zinc: Studies have previously shown that men and women with low intakes of zinc have an increased likelihood of getting osteoporosis. Zinc is also an essential mineral with strong antioxidant activity.

Boron: Boron aids in the proper metabolism of the vitamins and minerals involved with bone development. Additionally, although not fully understood, boron appears to affect estrogen and possibly testosterone. Both hormones affect bone health.

Copper: It is required to make connective tissue, which binds one part of the body to another; shores up heart and blood vessels; gives skin its firmness; and bolsters bone strength. Copper's important role in collagen formation, a connective tissue in bones and skin, underscores that copper is vital to build and maintain strong bones.

Vitamin D: Our bodies create vitamin D from the ultraviolet rays in sunshine. Many people living in hot, sunny climates whose diets contain a lot less calcium than the British diet have perfectly adequate amounts of calcium in their bones, blood, and cells because their elevated levels of vitamin D mean they are more efficient at metabolising calcium than we are. So clearly, vitamin D is vital for forming bone matrix.

Vitamin K: According to a study published in the *American Journal of Clinical Nutrition*, women who consume low levels of vitamin K have a greater risk of hip fractures than women who consume high or moderate levels of this nutrient. Since vitamin K also helps heal bone fractures, adequate intake is essential.

CHAPTER 17

The following Electro-complementary Therapeutic Radionics are very useful to the prcatitioners:

Radionic Instruments, Electronic Homoeopathic Research Services and Supplies, Natural Healing Services, Since 1947

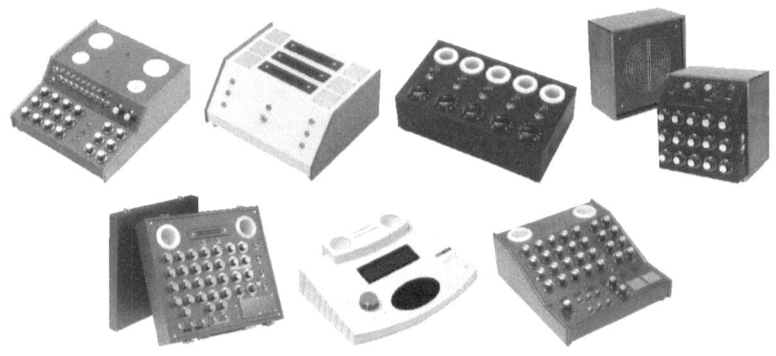

The Radionics and Their Uses in Complementary Health Care

For those practitioners who may be interested in the phamarceutical (manufacturing and production) of any of the products, the above given radionic instruments will be very ideal. The skills in the practical uses of each item will come with the the products.

Radionics is concerned with the context of control fields and 'subtle energies'. The term 'subtle energies' refers in this context to those forms of energy which cannot presently be objectively (physically) measured, because they are signals of very low amplitude which are masked due to the component 'noise' of electrical equipment. In the course of time, however, various subjective methods have been developed, such as radiesthesia, kinesiology, RAC, electro-acupuncture etc., by means of which it is possible to perform reproducible measurements in this context.

17.1 Principles of Radionics

The principles of present-day radionics were laid down by the American doctor, Dr Albert Abrams (1863-1924). In the context of his work in differentiation between various symptoms by means of an automatic, reflex movement of the stomach of a patient, detected by percussion, he discovered an empirically defined arrangement of variable resistances (potentiometer). In this context, the patient was connected via a forehead electrode to the 'input' of a variable resistance box. At the 'output', a healthy person was connected, also via a forehead electrode (test person). On the abdomen of the test person, it was now possible to diagnose the pathology of the patient on the basis of settings of the decade resistance by means of the special knock reflex.

It was not until later that Abrams found that it was not even necessary for the patient himself to be present. It was adequate for him to be replaced by a blood sample (as a 'specimen' or 'proof'). This specimen was poured into a metal cup, which (in place of the patient) was connected to the 'input' of the variable resistance box.

Attribution of Resistance Values to Organs and Symptoms

For example, with this layout, Abrams discovered that cancer can be measured at 50 Ω, gonorrhoea at 52 Ω, etc. If the blood specimen of a cancer sufferer was poured into the metal cup and the variable resistance box set to 50 Ω, on the abdomen of the test person a positive reflex would be obtained. If, on the other hand, for the same patient specimen a setting of 52 Ω (gonorrhoea) was set on the variable resistance box, this positive reflex disappeared (provided that the patient was not also suffering from gonorrhoea). Thus, Abrams developed a series of lists on which organs, symptoms, viruses, bacteria, etc. were allocated to empirically determined resistance values.

With this rate and the variable resistance box, it was thus possible to diagnose a patient on the basis of his blood specimen and to reach conclusions as to the conditions of his organs etc.

The First Medicine Testing

Abrams also found out that this layout made it possible to examine the effect of medicines, particularly in homoeopathy. He poured into the cup containing the patient specimen a corresponding medicine. If this medicine helped the patient with his condition, then the positive reflex on the abdomen of the test person would disappear.

If, for example, the specimen of a malaria patient was poured into the cup and the corresponding value for malaria had been set on the variable resistance box, on the abdomen of the test person a positive reflex would be obtained. If a medicine to cure malaria, such as quinine, was combined with the patient specimen in the cup, then the positive reflex would disappear, i.e. quinine would help this patient to combat malaria.

The Stick Pad Detector

Abrams always required one healthy person to be prepared for his diagnosis, whom he could connect to his apparatus and on whose abdomen he would obtain the corresponding percussion reflex. Since the test person

1) had to be predominantly healthy and
2) had to be paid, the idea of substituting the abdomen of the test person with a latex membrane was arrived at. It was a success! Instead of a percussion reflex, a stick effect on the latex surface (stick pad) was obtained. In the course of time, experiments were performed with various materials for the stick pad. Nowadays, we use acrylic for our equipment.

From Electrical Resistance to Rate

For Abrams and his colleagues, these discoveries could be explained as phenomena of electrically measurable radiation. Abrams set out his explanation of these phenomena in his ERA (Electronic Reaction of Abrams). According to ERA, an imbalance of electrons in the cellular atoms is the cause of all disease.

The term 'Radionics' was then invented by students of Abrams, by combining the two words 'radiation' and 'electronics'. This implies that in radionics it is possible to measure a fine 'radiation' with 'electronic instruments' designed specifically for the purpose.

Abrams' student Ruth Drown was the first to define the radionic instrument as a 'modulator of the life force'. She produced the concept of harmonising the 'de-tuned' life force, using the radionic instrument (see Hahnemann's Homoeopathy). For that reason, her process is also called the 'Homoe Vibra Ray' which implies that it is a 'human vibration radiation'.

Using this fundamentally different interpretation, Drown abandoned the customary unit employed by Abrams for electrical resistance, ohms, after the numerical values, and thereafter called them 'rates'. Cancer was now referred to not as 50 Ohm but rate 50. Thus it became clear for the first time that in this connection, we were concerned with a phenomenon that could no longer be explained by mechanistic physics as employed to date.

Radionic Broadcasting

Ruth Drown was the first person to use the radionic instrument not only for diagnosis but also for therapy. She discovered that this therapy also operated over distance, if a blood specimen of the patient was laid on the instrument. Her explanation of this phenomenon was that the rates exert a background presence in the 'atmosphere' and can be received by a person. The setting of a 'rate' on the instrument would set up a resonance in relation to this rate between the instrument and the patient, and thus increase the person's 'receptivity effect'. She named this process 'Broadcasting', a reference to the radio technology, which was emerging at that time.

Explanatory Models from the Present-Day Viewpoint

The ideas of Ruth Drown are still to be found today in the theory of the 'morphogenetic fields' of the English biologist and philosopher Rupert Sheldrake. Sheldrake works on the assumption that the morphogenetic fields contain all information concerning the structure and form of each organism, including 'inanimate' material. These fields have a holographic structure, which means that the corresponding information is theoretically omnipresent in the universe and can be called up accordingly. The morphogenetic fields are not essentially electromagnetic and are presumably on a plane other than space/time.

The existence of such a plane transcending space/time has even been postulated as an inevitability by some physicists. David Bohm, in this connection, refers to a 'holographic universe' and defines the two areas of existence as having an 'implicit' (folded–up) and 'explicit' (unfolded) order.

The physicist Burkhard Heim believes that in addition to our three spatial dimensions and time as the fourth dimension (= space/time) there exist further transcendent dimensions to which humanity can refer, thanks to the particular characteristics of his awareness. In these higher dimensions (hyperspace) there is information which controls the structure and processes of the lower dimensions via 'synkopes'! This hyperspace thus performs the function of a control field. The interesting feature of Heim's 'quantum field theory' is that it can provide more precise information after the material world (e.g. the mass of electrons) than, for example, quantum theory. Furthermore, the Heim theory also provides information about the intangible world, i.e. the areas which Dr Bruce Copen designated dimension X.

The radionic instrument enables the therapist to call up information specific to the patient from the control fields (dimensions seven and eight according to Heim, Sheldrake's morphogenetic fields) and thus to analyse the underlying causes of disease in a person, animal, or plant. The experienced practitioner knows that he can tune himself via this plane to the patient provided that he/she has a blood or hair specimen of the patient, wherever the patient is, even if they are thousands of kilometres apart. At the same time, deviations can be qualitatively assessed and balanced by radionic therapy.

The Facilities Radionics Offer

To sum up, it can be stated that radionics gives you the possibility of setting up an extensive analysis on the basis of a patient's specimen. In this context, you can take account of the organ status, toxin loading, vitamin and minerals budget, bacteria and viral presence, fungal infections, etc. You can test the appropriate homoeopathic remedy and potency without the use of test sets and assess the correct Bach flower or other flower essences. Furthermore, you have the complete range of colour and precious stone therapy available to you. For this purpose, we have numerous rates available (6,500 rates for organs and symptoms, 30 rates for vitamins, 320 rates for colour, 2,600 rates for homoeopathic remedies, and flower essences, etc.).

The Copen radionic instruments also give you the facility not only of investigating at physical level but also operating at astral and mental levels etc. Depending on the instrument, you have access to six or twelve levels of existence.

With the Electronic Vibro Potentiser (EVP) you can, by radionic means, imprint the specific informational content of any given subject substances in virtually arbitrary potency on carrier substances such as

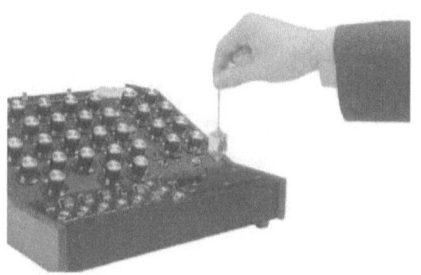

globules (lactose balls), alcohol, etc. [UNPOTENTIZEE TABLETS] The term *potentiser* means to inplant medicine into a susbstance through a electroc vibration. Naturally, Copen radionic instruments also give you the facility for radionic balancing (braodcasting).

Thus, Copen radionics gives you a wide and universally applicable range of facilities for analysis and therapy.

Bibliography

Copen, Bruce: Radionics, Vol. 1
Copen, Bruce: Radionics, Vol. 2
Copen, Bruce: Radionic Computer Handbook

17.2 How Does Radionic Analysis Function

Radionic analysis is produced on the basis of a patient's specimen. The patient's hair or blood is the most suitable for this purpose.

This specimen is placed in the radionic instrument. The therapist then uses a sensor with one hand to move in steps along a list on which the rates for the various organ systems are set out. With the other hand, he performs gentle, circular movements over the stick pad. If the therapist with the sensor arrives at a range in which the patient has a loading (e.g. respiratory tract), he obtains a stick effect on the stick pad.

In our example, the therapist would then set the rate for the respiratory tract on the instrument and test the over-functions/under-functions

(OF/UF) of the patient's respiratory tract. Initially, the stick pad is used to test whether there is an over-function (OF). If no stick reflex is found with over-function, then we turn to under-function (UF). Here, we obtain a stick reflex. It is then possible to test, on a scale from 0 to 9, how powerful the under-function is by gradually changing the values from 0 to 9 and once again simultaneously rubbing the stick pad. When the stick reflex is received, we stop rotating the scale control and can read off the measured value on the scale.

If a high value has been obtained in testing of over-function and under-function, i.e. a value higher than seven, then the details are tested. In our example with the respiratory tract, this would mean that we would be testing the condition of the right-hand lobe of the lung, the left-hand lobe of the lung, the bronchi, etc.

By this means, it is also possible to measure corresponding loadings with fungi, viruses, bacteria, toxins, poisons, etc. In this context, quantitative assessment of loading is always possible to measurement of over-function and under-function.

In place of the stick pad, it is also possible to use the pendulum or the single-hand rod, or other test methods such as kinesiology or RAC etc.

How Does Radionic Balancing Function?

On the basis of information found in the analysis, it is possible to compile a balancing programme. This means that all values which you have tested in OF/UF analysis as being greater than seven are balanced. Furthermore, the corresponding rate is once again set on the instrument (in our example above: it is the rate for the respiratory tract), the specimen (blood or hair) of the patient is placed in the instrument and it is switched to 'balance mode'. It may also be possible for the set rates to be supplemented by homoeopathic remedies or flower essences, which are also placed in the instrument.

The set information is then transferred to the patient by remote action of the patient's specimen, by which means the corresponding energies of the patient are balanced. In the case of instruments with EECS, it is also possible to store complex balancing programmes on card.

Depending on the nature and duration of the illness, a balancing period may last from several minutes to as much as several hours. The number of repeat balancing operations and the intervals between individual balancing operations must also be guided by the nature and duration of the illness.

This is just a brief outline of the features on our instruments. It is not possible to explain all the functions in detail here, but if you have any particular questions please contact our laboratories for further assistance.

For all the enquires about the above listed electro-health care radionic, please contact the following body:

Beckman Natmedics (UK) limited (UK sub-distribotors), 290 A, Lodege Avenue, Dagenham, Essex, RM8 2HF England. Tel (44) (0) 2082270083, (44) 07733764875, email: lukeubani@yahoo.com

17.3 Infectious Disease from Mosquitoes

Infectious disease from mosquitoes must be known and understood in the complementary medicine preventive therapy.

This knowledge is very important, considering the deadly consequences of the diseases transmited by mosquitos bites. All the practitioners engaged in the preventive therapy must acquire the knowledge of how mosquitoes operate. Apart from the epidemic of HIV, malaria fever claims more life than anything else in the troical Africa.

A mosquito is an insect. They are in the fly order Diptera. The females are ectoparasites: they land on warm-blooded animals, including human beings, pierce a capillary, and inject saliva to stop the blood from coagulating. The deadly ones are the females called Anopheles mosquito. Mosquito is a common flying insect that is found throughout the world. Females drink blood and nectar; the males only sip nectar.

How Mosquitoes Work—Mosquito Development

Eggs

All mosquitoes lay eggs in water, which can include large bodies of water, standing water (like swimming pools) or areas of collected standing water (like tree holes or gutters). Females lay their eggs on the surface of the water, except for *Aedes* mosquitoes, which lay their eggs above water in protected areas that eventually flood. The eggs can be laid singly or as a group that forms a floating raft of mosquito eggs (see Mosquito Life Cycle for a picture of an egg raft). Most eggs can survive the winter and hatch in the spring in the temparate regions of the world.

Identifying Larvae:

You can distinguish the larvae of various mosquito species. Anopheles larvae lie parallel to the surface of the water, while larvae of *Aedes* and *Culex* extend down into the water (the air tubes of *Culex* are longer than those of *Aedes*).

Larva

The mosquito eggs hatch into larvae or *wigglers*, which live at the surface of the water and breathe through an *air tube* or *siphon*. The larvae filter organic material through their mouth parts and grow to about 0.5 to 0.75 inches (1 to 2 cm) long; as they grow, they shed their skin (*moult*) several times. Mosquito larvae can swim and dive down from the surface when disturbed (see Mosquito Life Cycle for a Quicktime movie of free-swimming Asian tiger mosquito larvae). The larvae live anywhere from days to several weeks depending on the water temperature and mosquito species.

Mosquitoes are important:

The mosquito larvae and pupae are important food sources for fish in aquatic ecosystems.

Pupa

After the fourth moult, mosquito larvae change into pupae,—or '*tumblers*', which live in the water anywhere from one to four days, depending on the water temperature and species. The pupae float at the surface and breathe through two small tubes (*trumpets*). Although they do not eat, pupae are quite active (see Mosquito Life Cycle for a Quicktime movie of free-swimming Asian tiger mosquito pupae). At the end of the pupal stage, the pupae encase themselves and transform into adult mosquitoes, now ready for action.

Adult

Inside the *pupal case*, the pupa transforms into an adult. The adult uses air pressure to break the pupal case open, crawls to a protected area and rests while its external skeleton hardens, spreading its wings out to dry. Once this is complete, it can fly away and live on the land. The enemy is now about to commence her sexual intercourse.

One of the first things that adult mosquitoes do is seek a mate, mate and then feed. Male mosquitoes have short mouth parts and feed on plant nectar. In contrast, female mosquitoes have a long *proboscis* that they use to bite animals and humans and feed on their blood (the blood provides proteins that the females need to lay eggs). After they feed, females lay their eggs (they need a blood meal each time they lay eggs). Females continue this cycle and live anywhere from many days to weeks (longer over the winter); males usually live only a few days after mating. The life cycles of mosquitoes vary with the species and environmental conditions. In the tropical regions of the world, during the dry seasons, mosquitoes start to diminish and the surviving ones hibernate in stagnant waters in the guters, bushes, and on the trees.

17.4 Types of Mosquitoes

LITTLE FLY:

The word 'mosquito' is Spanish for 'little fly,' and its use dates back to about 1583 in North America (Europeans referred to mosquitoes as 'gnats'). Mosquitoes belong to the order *Diptera*, true flies. Mosquitoes are like flies in that they have two wings, but unlike flies, their wings have scales, their legs are long and the females have a long mouth part (proboscis) for piercing skin.

There are more than 2,700 species of mosquitoes in the world, and there are thirteen mosquito genera (plural for 'genus') that live in the United States. Of these genera, most mosquitoes belong to three:

- **Aedes**—These are sometimes called 'floodwater' mosquitoes because flooding is important for their eggs to hatch. *Aedes* mosquitoes have abdomens with pointed tips. They include such species as the yellow-fever mosquito (*Aedes aegypti*) and the Asian tiger mosquito (*Aedes albopictus*). They are strong fliers, capable of travelling great distances (up to 75 miles/121 km) from their breeding sites. They persistently bite mammals (especially humans), mainly at dawn and in the early evening. Their bites are painful.

- **Anopheles**—These tend to breed in bodies of permanent fresh water. *Anopheles* mosquitoes also have abdomens with pointed tips. They include several species, such as the common malaria mosquito (Anopheles quadrimaculatus), that can spread malaria to humans.

- **Culex**—These tend to breed in quiet, standing water. *Culex* mosquitoes have abdomens with blunt tips. They include several species such as the northern house mosquito (Culex pipiens). They are weak fliers and tend to live for only a few weeks during the summer months. They persistently bite (preferring birds over humans) and attack at dawn or after dusk. Their bite is painful.

Some mosquitoes, such as the cattail mosquito (Coquilettidia perturbans), are becoming more prevalent pests as humans invade their habitats.

Let's examine how mosquitoes live and breed.

Life Cycle and Breeding

Like all insects, mosquitoes hatch from eggs and go through several stages in their life cycle before becoming adults. The females lay their eggs in water, and the larva and pupa stages live entirely in water. When the pupa change into adults, they leave the water and become free-flying land insects. The life cycle of a mosquito can vary from one to several weeks depending upon the species (the adult, mated females of some species can survive the winter in cool, damp places until spring, when they will lay their eggs and die.)

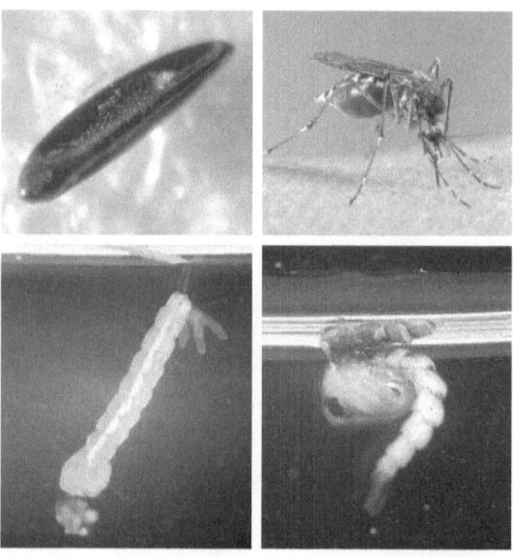

Photos courtesy: Centers for Disease Control and Prevention and USDA/ARS (upper right).

Life cycle of the yellow-fever mosquito (*Aedes aegypti*):

An egg (upper left) laid on the surface of the water hatches into an aquatic larva (lower left). The larva changes into an aquatic pupa (lower right), which then changes into a free-flying adult (upper right). The adult female bites a human to gather blood for laying eggs.

17.5 Mosquito Repellents

The best way to reduce mosquito-borne diseases is through mosquito control and personal protection. You can do a few things to reduce the number of mosquito bites that you get while enjoying the outdoors. First, wear clothing that covers most of your body, if temperatures permit. Second, use a mosquito repellent that contains **NN-diethyl-meta-toluamide** (DEET) at a concentration of 7.5 per cent to 100 per cent. Lower concentrations are sufficient for most outdoor protection, and a 15-per cent concentration is recommended for children. Avon's original Skin-So-Soft is a weak, short-lasting (less than twenty minutes) mosquito repellent, although there are newer Skin-So-Soft formulations that include EPA-recognised insect repellents. **Permethrin**, an effective pesticide, **is for use on clothing only (Never apply it to your skin,**

it is a neurotoxin!). To learn more about mosquito repellents, see the EPA's How to Use Insect Repellents Safely.

Beyond mosquito repellents and clothing, you can try to control the mosquito population. Mosquitoes need water to breed and will use any source of standing water. If you have a lily pond in your garden, stock it with some fish that will eat the mosquito larvae. Some petroleum oils can be added to water to form a thin surface layer that suffocates the mosquito eggs; however, many of these oils will also suffocate any fish living in the water.

Mosquito Myths

Several natural or man-made products have been touted as mosquito repellents or effective in mosquito control. **Citronella oil**, which is a product of several types of plants that can be made into candles or burnt directly, is an effective mosquito repellent in high concentrations, but individual citronella-producing plants do not make enough oil to effectively repel mosquitoes. Ultraviolet lights (as used in bug zappers) and ultrasonic devices are not effective.

To prevent mosquitoes from entering your home, make sure that all of your window screens are intact.

Finally, there are many commercial pesticides available to kill mosquito larvae and mosquito adults. Many communities conduct large-scale spraying of pesticides containing mallothione to control mosquito populations during the spring and summer, especially in attempts to reduce the spread of West Nile encephalitis. Another option is a device like a Mosquito Magnet, which lures and traps mosquitoes.

Mosquitoes and Malaria in Africa

Rechard Mukabana of Kenya has collected empirical data that dispels the myth that bush clearing can control mosquitoes and has assembled crucial evidence that provides a basis for amending a policy that is not practical.

In sub-Saharan Africa, malaria kills more than one million people every year. In many African countries, malaria control guidelines and many school textbooks state that malaria-transmitting mosquitoes can be controlled by clearing bushes from around dwellings—a practice carried out by many rural Africans who believe that mosquitoes rest in bushes.

Unfortunately, this advice is based on recommendations in books produced for the Asian market. Indeed, the advice sometimes dates back to the pre-DDT era in colonial British Borneo that now forms part of Indonesia and Malaysia. As such books are relatively cheap, they are imported into Africa.

However, the mosquito species responsible for the spread of malaria in southeast Asia are different from the primary vector in Africa, Anopheles gambiae. Indeed, female An. gambiae prefer to lay their eggs in open, sunlit pools. By clearing vegetation, rural Africans are inadvertently creating more sunlit pools suitable for the development of An. gambiae larvae.

And is it really true that A. gambiae mosquitoes rest in bushes during the day?

Richard Mukabana of the School of Biological Sciences, University of Nairobi, Kenya, set out to answer this question. He designed a series of experiments to elucidate the behaviour of An. gambiae, the most important local malaria-transmitting mosquito species in Africa, with the aim of identifying simple control procedures that can be implemented in rural areas. In doing so, he has collected empirical data that dispels the bush-clearing myth, and he has assembled crucial evidence that provides a basis for amending a policy that is simply not practical or effective in tropical Africa.

Note: Each year, TWAS offers some 100 research grants of up to US$10,000 to scientists from developing countries for research projects in biology, chemistry, mathematics, and physics. The grants are intended to cover the costs of specialised equipment, essential consumable material, and scientific literature. In 2004, Richard Mukabana of the University of Nairobi, Kenya, was awarded such a grant. This is a report on the research efforts that this grant has supported.

Malaria can also be transmited through the following agents:

1. Pregnant mother to the child in the womb through her blood infected with malaria parasites.
2. Lactating mother via the breast milk to the child.
3. The blood transfusion from a malaria carrier.
4. Through an unhygienic injection neddle.

Malaria Infection in the UK

With travel to long-haul destinations becoming more accessible, UK travellers are increasingly at risk of contracting diseases such as malaria. Travellers need to know the facts. How malaria affects UK travellers:

- Between 1990 and 2009, every year, approximately eighteen hundred British travellers return home with malaria. The UK is one of the biggest importers of malaria in Europe.
- The number of trips made abroad by UK residents was 5.90 million in October 2008.[7]

How dangerous is malaria

- The most severe form of malaria (plasmodium falciparum) accounted for 79 per cent of cases amongst British travellers in 2009.[1]
- Malaria is a preventable infection but can be fatal if left untreated—an average of nine people die each year from malaria in the UK.[1]
- Malaria is transmitted by an infected mosquito. It only takes one bite from an infected mosquito to contract malaria.

How to protect against malaria

You are at risk when travelling to malarious areas if you do not take precautions to prevent yourself from being bitten and also if you do not take antimalarials. You should ideally seek advice from a health care professional eight weeks before you travel but can still seek advice at the last minute. Some advice/protection is better than none.

There are different forms of antimalarials available. Travel clinic will be able to advise on the most suitable one for you.

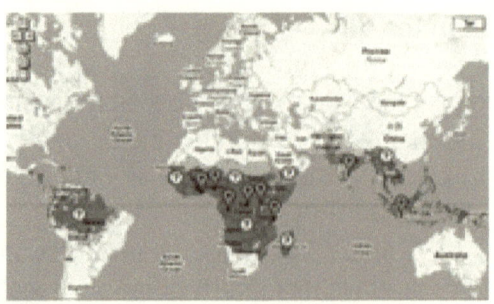

This map should give you an indication of the geographic areas of malarial colony in the world. Wherever you go, enjoy yourself, but make sure you are malaria protected.

CHAPTER 18

The Ancient and Modern Masters in Complementary Medicine

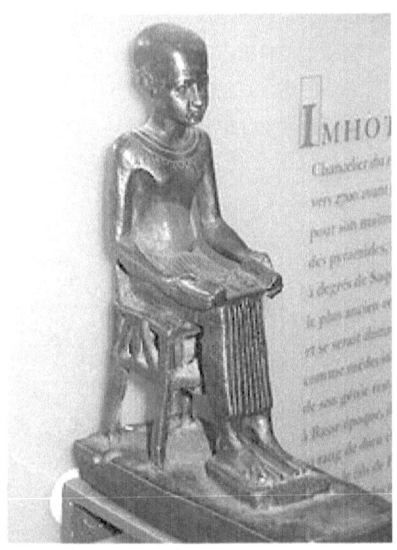

A Statue of Imhotep: The African Father
of Medicine and Healing.

18.1 Imhotep: Ancient Father of healing of Egypt

Imhotep was a high priest in ancient Egypt, and had many other important skills. He was born in Ankhtowe on the sixteenth day of Epiphi. Epiphi is (March), the third month of the Egyptian harvest season. His mother was Khreduonkh and father was Kanofer, an architect. Imhotep also became famous as an architect. After his death, because of his attachment with the god Ptah during his work at Ptah's temple, stories were spread that said that Ptah was his father. As a god, he was often pictured seated, wearing a long kilt robe and a skull cap or a shaven head. He had a papyrus scroll spread on his lap to show his scholarly nature and scribal assistance.

A Step Pyramid

As an architect, Imhotep was most famous because he was the designer of the step pyramid. Before the step pyramid, pharaohs were buried in flat topped structures called mastabas. The term *mastaba* comes from the word meaning bench because they look like the benches most Egyptians placed outside their door. An average mastaba had four walls, a flat top and an underground burial chamber, reached by a vertical shaft or stairwell. There were also a couple of small rooms above the burial chambers containing various items for the afterlife. The step pyramid was actually just a number of mastabas placed one on top of the other, each one smaller than the previous one.

Medical Writer

Imhotep's best-known writings were medical scrolls. He is thought to have written the Edwin Smith papyrus. The papyrus consists of forty-eight injuries of which twenty-seven are head trauma, and six are spine trauma. Here's an example for treatment of a head injury: 'Examination: If thou examinest a man having a wound in his head, while his wound does not have two lips, penetrating to the bone of his skull. (but) not having a gash, thou shouldst palpate his wound (or, thou shouldst lay thy hand upon it); shouldst thou find his skull uninjured, not having a perforation; a split, or a smash in it. Treatment: Thou shouldst bind it with fresh meat the first day (and) treat afterwards with grease, honey (and) lint every day until he recovers wound in the head.'

Becoming a God

Around a hundred years after his death, Imhotep was deified (made into a god). He became the god of medicine and healing. Small temples were built in his honour. People with injuries would sleep near his temple, hoping to be healed. As a god, Imhotep was also worshiped by scribes. Scribes would offer a couple drops of water in libation to him before starting to write. Even when the Greeks took over the town, he was identified with another deified man called Asclepius, and the Greeks continued to honour and build temples for him. This continued until the Arab invasion in North Africa in the seventh century AD Imhotep did many things that boosted Egyptian society to amazing heights. He was the architect that changed Egyptian funeral architecture from mastabas to the phenomenal structures we today call pyramids. As a physician, he healed many people and saved many lives, which after his death led to him becoming a medicine god. If the man who did all these things was a black man, then, we were the originators of medicine and herbal healing. It is our duty to acknowledge and recognise this heritage of ours. Indeed, it will be very folish for us, the Africans, to begin to write or develop our modern traditional medicine witout reference this legendary father of medice—Imhotep. Hippocrates, now referred to by the West as the father of medicine got all his ideas and history from the work of this Egytian-African, Imhotep.

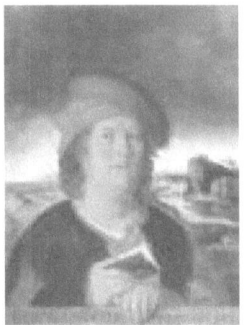

The father of spagyric is Paracelsus (1493-1541),
a great swiss physician, who lived 500 years ago.

18.2 Paracelsus

Paracelsus (11 November or 17 December 1493 in Einsiedeln, Switzerland–24 September 1541) was an alchemist, physician, astrologer, and general occultist. Born Phillip von Hohenheim, he later took up the name Philippus Theophrastus Aureolus Bombastus von Hohenheim, and still later took the title Paracelsus, meaning 'equal to or greater than Celsus', a Roman encyclopedist from the first century known for his tract on medicine.[1]

Biography

Paracelsus was born and raised in the village of Maria Einsiedeln in Switzerland. His father, Wilhelm Bombast von Hohenheim, was a Swabian chemist and physician; his mother was Swiss. As a youth, he worked in nearby mines as an analyst. At the age of sixteen he started studying medicine at the University of Basel, later moving to Vienna. He gained his doctorate degree from the University of Ferrara.[2] His wanderings as an itinerant physician and sometimes journeyman miner [3] took him through Germany, France, Hungary, the Netherlands, Denmark, Sweden, and Russia.

Known portrait of Paracelsus is attributed to Augustin Hirschvogel. Paracelsus rejected Gnostic traditions, but kept much of the Hermetic, neoplatonic, and Pythagorean philosophies from Ficino and Pico della Mirandola; however, Hermetical science had so much Aristotelian theory that his rejection of Gnosticism was practically meaningless. In particular, Paracelsus rejected the magic theories of Agrippa and Flamel; Paracelsus did not think of himself as a magician and scorned those who did, though he was a practising astrologer, as were most, if not all, of the university-trained physicians working at that time in Europe. Astrology was a very important part of Paracelsus's medicine. In his *Archidoxes of Magic*, Paracelsus devoted several sections to astrological talismans for curing disease, providing talismans for various maladies as well as talismans for each sign of the Zodiac. He also invented an alphabet called the alphabet of the Magi, for engraving angelic names upon talismans. Paracelsus pioneered the use of chemicals and minerals in medicine. He used the name 'zink' for the element zinc in about 1526, based on the sharp pointed appearance of its crystals after smelting and the old German word 'zinke' for pointed. He used experimentation in learning about the human body. His hermetical views were that sickness and health in the body relied on the harmony of man, the microcosm, and nature, the macrocosm. He took an approach different from those before him, using this analogy not in the manner of soul-purification, but in the manner that humans must have certain balances of minerals in their bodies and that certain illnesses of the body had chemical remedies that could cure them. (Debus and Multhauf, p. 6-12) He summarised his own views: 'Many have said of Alchemy, that it is for the making of gold and silver. For me such is not the aim, but to consider only what virtue and power may lie in medicines.' (*Edwardes*, p. 47) (also in: Holmyard, Eric John. *Alchemy*. p. 170). Paracelsus gained a reputation for being arrogant and soon garnered the anger of other physicians in Europe. He held the chair of medicine at the University of Basel for less than a year; while there, his colleagues became angered by allegations that he had publicly burnt traditional medical books. He was forced from the city after having legal trouble over a physician's fee he sued to collect. He then wandered through Europe, Africa, and Asia Minor, in the pursuit of hidden knowledge. He revised old manuscripts and wrote new ones, but had trouble finding publishers. In 1536, his *Die grosse Wundartzney* (*The Great Surgery Book*) was published and enabled him to regain fame. He died in 1541 in Salzburg, and was buried according to his wishes in the cemetery at the church of St Sebastian in Salzburg. His remains are now located in a tomb in the porch of the church. After his death, the movement of Paracelsianism was seized upon by many wishing to subvert the traditional Galenic physic, and thus did his therapies become more widely known and used. His motto was 'alterius non sit qui suus esse potest' which means 'let no man that can belong to himself be of another.'

Contributions to toxicology.

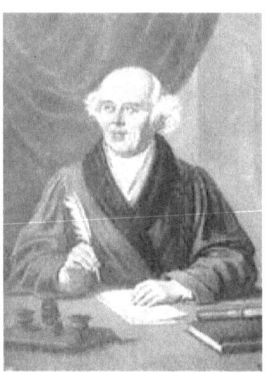

Christian Friedrich Samuel Hahnemann (10 April 1755–2 July 1843), a German physician who created an alternative medicine practice called Homeopathy.

18.3 Christian Friedrich Samuel Hahnemann

Early Life

Christian Friedrich Samuel Hahnemann was born in Meissen, Saxony. His father, along with many other family members, was a painter and designer of porcelain, for which the town of Meissen was famous. As a young man, Hahnemann became proficient in a number of languages, including English, French, Italian, Greek, and Latin. He eventually made a living as a translator and teacher of languages, gaining further proficiency in 'Arabic, Syriac, Chaldaic, and Hebrew. Hahnemann studied medicine for two years at Leipzig. Citing Leipzig's lack of clinical facilities, he moved to Vienna, where he studied for ten months. After one term of further study, he graduated MD at the University of Erlangen on 10 August 1779, qualifying with honours. His poverty may have forced him to choose Erlangen, as the school's fees were lower. Hahnemann's thesis was titled *Conspectus adfectuum spasmodicorum aetiologicus et therapeuticus. [A Dissertation on the Causes and Treatment of Cramps]*

Medical Practice

In 1781, Hahnemann took a village doctor's position in the copper-mining area of Mansfeld, Saxony. He soon married Johanna Henriette Kuchler and would eventually have eleven children. After abandoning medical practice, and while working as a translator of scientific and medical textbooks,[9] Hahnemann travelled around Saxony for many years, staying in many different towns and villages for varying lengths of time, never living far from the River Elbe and settling at different times in Dresden, Torgau, Leipzig, and Köthen (Anhalt), before finally moving to Paris in June 1835.

Creation of Homeopathy and Main Article: Homeopathy

Hahnemann claimed as under that the medicine of his time did as much harm as good:

> My sense of duty would not easily allow me to treat the un-known pathological state of my suffering brethren with these unknown medicines. The thought of becoming in this way a

murderer or malefactor towards the life of my fellow human beings was most terrible to me, so terrible and disturbing that I wholly gave up my practice in the first years of my married life and occupied myself solely with chemistry and writing.[1]

After giving up his practice around 1784, Hahnemann made his living chiefly as a writer and translator, while resolving also to investigate the causes of medicine's alleged errors. While translating William Cullen's *A Treatise on the Materia Medica*, Hahnemann encountered the claim that cinchona, the bark of a Peruvian tree, was effective in treating malaria because of its astringency. Hahnemann believed that other astringent substances are not effective against malaria and began to research cinchona's effect on the human body by self-application. Noting that the drug induced malaria-like symptoms in himself, he concluded that it would do so in any healthy individual. This led him to postulate a healing principle: 'that which can produce a set of symptoms in a healthy individual, can treat a sick individual who is manifesting a similar set of symptoms.' This principle, *like cures like*, became the basis for an approach to medicine which he gave the name 'homeopathy'. He first used the term 'homeopathy' in his essay *Indications of the Homeopathic Employment of Medicines in Ordinary Practice*, published in Hufeland's Journal in 1807.

Development of Homeopathy

Hahnemann tested substances for the effect they produced on a healthy individual and tried to deduce from this the ills they would heal. From his research, he initially concluded that ingesting substances to produce noticeable changes in the body resulted in toxic effects. He then attempted to mitigate this problem through exploring dilutions of the compounds he was testing. He claimed that these dilutions, when prepared according to his technique of succussion (systematic mixing through vigorous shaking) and potentisation, were still effective in alleviating the same symptoms in the sick. Hahnemann began practicing this new technique, which attracted other doctors *c.* 1792.[citation needed] He first published an article about the homeopathic approach in a German language medical journal in 1796. Following a series of further essays, he published in 1810 *Organon of the Rational Art of Healing*, followed over the years by four further editions titled: *The Organon of the Healing Art,* the first systematic treatise and containing all his detailed instructions on the subject. A sixth Organon edition, unpublished during his lifetime, and dating from February 1842, was only published many years after his death. It consisted of a fifth Organon, containing extensive handwritten annotations. (A reading of each edition will demonstrate the extent of the revision and experience-based additions) The Organon is widely regarded as a remodelled form of an essay he published in 1806 called 'The Medicine of Experience', which had been published in Hufeland's Journal. Of the Organon, Dudgeon states it 'was an amplification and extension of his 'Medicine of Experience, worked up with greater care, and put into a more methodical and aphoristic form, after the model of the Hippocratic writings.'

The Coffee Theory

Around the start of the nineteenth century, Hahnemann developed a theory, propounded in his 1803 essay *On the Effects of Coffee from Original Observations*, that many diseases are caused by coffee. Hahnemann later abandoned the coffee theory in favour of the theory that disease is caused by Psora, but it has been noted that the list of conditions Hahnemann attributed to coffee was similar to his list of conditions caused by Psora. The coffee theory has been described as 'a good example both of Hahnemann's superior mental powers and of his occasional tendency to make up a grand theory from scant evidence.'

Later Life

In early 1811, Hahnemann moved his family back to Leipzig with the intention of teaching his new medical system at the University of Leipzig. In accordance with the university statutes, he became a faculty member by submitting and defending a thesis on a medical topic of his choice. On 26 June 1812, Hahnemann presented a Latin thesis, entitled *A Medical Historical Dissertation on the Helleborism of the Ancients*. (Hellebore, a number of species of poisonous flowering plants, related to Buttercup and Magnolia.) Hahnemann continued practising and researching homeopathy, as well as writing and lecturing for the rest of his life. He died in 1843 in Paris, at eighty-eight years of age, and is entombed in a mausoleum at Paris's Père Lachaise cemetery.

Descendants

While there are a few living descendants of Hahnemann's elder sister Charlotte (1752-1812), there is only one known living descendant of Hahnemann himself, Mr Charles Tankard-Hahnemann (seventh generation descendant of Dr Samuel Hahnemann). His father, Mr William Herbert Tankard-Hahnemann (1922-2009), the great-great-great-grandson of Samuel Hahnemann, died on 12 January 2009 (his eighty-seventh birthday) after twenty-two years of active patronage of the British Institute of Homoeopathy. As a young boy, William remembered his mother telling him of her visits to her 'Grand-dad Leo' at Ventnor, Isle of Wight. Later, William Hahnemann knew that this was Dr Leopold Süß-Hahnemann, Dr Samuel Hahnemann's grandson, the only son of his favourite daughter, Amelie (1789-1881). Dr Süß-Hahnemann was the only member of the Hahnemann family to be present at Samuel Hahnemann's funeral, apart from Hahnemann's second wife, Mélanie, in Paris, in 1843, and at his subsequent re-burial in the Père Lachaise Cemetery in east Paris, where only persons of truly notable distinction are interred. Subsequently, Leopold emigrated from France to England, where he practised homoeopathy in London. He retired to the Isle of Wight and died there at the outbreak of World War I, in 1914. Dr Leopold Süß-Hahnemann's youngest daughter, Amalia had two children, Winifred (born 1898) and Herbert. Mr William Tankard-Hahnemann was Winifred's son. Apart from serving as the patron of the British Institute of Homoeopathy, he also had a distinguished career in the City of London and was honoured by being appointed as a 'Freeman of the City of London.'

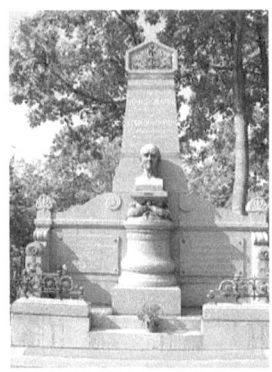

Hahnemann's mausoleum at the Père
Lachaise Cemetery, Paris, France.

His Writings—Hahnemann wrote a number of books, essays, and letters on The Homeopathic Method, Chemistry, and General Medicine as under:

Heilkunde der Erfahrung. Norderstedt 2010, ISBN 3842313268 (in German) Versuch über ein neues Prinzip zur Auffindung der Heilkräfte der Arzneisubstanzen, nebst einigen Blicken auf die bisherigen [Essay on a New Principle for Ascertaining the Curative Powers of Drugs], 1796, http://www.mickler.de/journal/versuch-prinzip-1.htmreprinted in Versuch über ein neues Prinzip zur Auffindung der Heilkräfte der Arzneisubstanzen, nebst einigen Blicken auf die bisherigen, Haug, 1988, ISBN 3776010606 Fragmenta de viribus medicamentorum positivis, a collection of twenty-seven drug 'provings' published in Latin in 1805, *The Organon of the Healing Art* (1810), a detailed delineation of what he saw as the rationale underpinning homeopathic medicine, and guidelines for practice. Hahnemann published the fifth edition in 1833; a revised draft of this (1842) was discovered after Hahnemann's death and finally published as the sixth edition in 1921. *Materia Medica Pura*, a compilation of 'homoeopathic proving' reports, was published in six volumes between vol. I in 1811 and vol. VI in 1827. Revised editions of volumes I and II were published in 1830 and 1833, respectively. *Chronic Diseases* (1828), containing an explanation of the root and cure of chronic disease according to the theory of miasms, together with a compilation of 'homoeopathic proving' reports, which were gathered by Dudgeon, was published in five volumes during the 1830s. *The Friend of Health*, in which Hahnemann 'recommended the use of fresh air, bed rest, proper diet, sunshine, public hygiene,' and numerous other beneficial measures at a time when many other physicians considered them of no value. Asiatic Cholera, in which Hahnemann described cholera as a 'pathogenic' disease caused by 'excessively minute, invisible, living creatures. Hahnemann also campaigned for the humane treatment of the insane in 1792. John Henry Clarke wrote that 'In 1787, Hahnemann discovered the best test for arsenic and other poisons in wine, having pointed out the unreliable nature of the "Wurtemberg Test", which had been in use up to that period.'

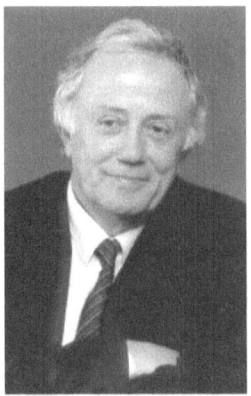

George Vithoulka

18.4 George Vithoulka

George Vithoulkas (born in Athens, 1932) is a teacher and practitioner of homeopathy. He studied homeopathy in South Africa and received a diploma in homeopathy from the Indian Institute of Homeopathy in 1966. Upon receiving his diploma, he returned to Greece, where he practised and began teaching classical homeopathy to medical doctors at what eventually became the Centre of Homeopathic Medicine in Athens. In 1972, Vithoulkas started a Greek homeopathic journal, *Homeopathic Medicine*. In 1976, he organised the first of an annual series of International Homeopathic Seminars. In 1994, he opened the International Academy for Classical Homeopathy on Alonissos, which provides postgraduate training for homeopaths. Vithoulkas has authored a number of books on homeopathy, two of which, *Homeopathy: Medicine of the New Man* and *The Science of Homeopathy*, have been translated extensively, and he is currently writing *Materia Medica Viva*, a homeopathic materia medica or reference work on homeopathic remedies, to reach sixteen volumes when finished. In addition to his books, he has published numerous articles in homeopathic journals and has developed an expert system for homeopaths to use in choosing remedies for their patients. Vithoulkas was a recipient of the Right Livelihood Award in 1996.

Vithoulkas asserts that the paradigm of conventional medicine has been disastrous for the health of mankind, having failed to prevent or cure disease, and that the excessive use of powerful chemical drugs is responsible for a worldwide degeneration of health. In his view, conventional treatments for serious diseases lead to a

18.5 Hippocrates—the Father of Medicine

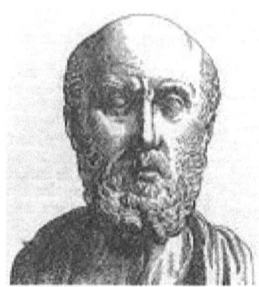

The physician Hippocrates, known as the
'Father of Modern Medicine' 460-370 BC

Ancient Greek Traditional Medicine

A towering figure in the history of medicine was the physician Hippocrates of Kos, considered the 'father of modern medicine'. The *Hippocratic Corpus* is a collection of around seventy early medical works from ancient Greece strongly associated with Hippocrates and his students. Most famously, Hippocrates invented the Hippocratic Oath for physicians, which is still relevant and in use today.

The *Hippocratic Corpus*, is a collection of around seventy early medical works from ancient Greece strongly associated with the ancient Greek physician Hippocrates and his teachings. The first known Greek medical school opened in Cnidus in 700 BC. Alcmaeon, author of the first anatomical work, worked at this school, and it was here that the practice of observing patients was established. Ancient Greek medicine centred around the theory of humours. The most important figure in ancient Greek medicine is the physician Hippocrates, known as the 'Father of Medicine', who established his own medical school at Kos. Hippocrates and his students documented many conditions in the *Hippocratic Corpus*, and developed the Hippocratic Oath for physicians, still in use today. The Greek surgeon Galen was one of the greatest surgeons of the ancient world and performed many audacious operations—including brain and eye surgeries—that were not tried again for almost two millennia. The writings of Hippocrates, Galen, and others had a lasting influence on medieval European medicine and Islamic medicine, until many of their findings eventually became obsolete from the fourteenth century onwards.

Early Influences

Despite their known respect for Egyptian medicine, attempts to discern any particular influence on Greek practice at this early time have not been dramatically successful because of the lack of sources and the challenge of understanding ancient medical terminology. It is clear, however, that the Greeks imported Egyptian substances into their pharmacopoeia, and the influence becames more pronounced after the establishment of a school of Greek medicine in Alexandria. The existence of the Hippocratic Oath implies that this 'Hippocratic' medicine was practised by a group of professional physicians bound (at least among themselves) by a strict ethical code. Aspiring students normally paid a fee for training (a provision was made for exceptions) and entered into a virtual family relationship with their teacher. This training included some oral instruction and probably hands-on experience as the teacher's assistant, since the oath assumes that the student will be interacting with patients. The oath also places limits on what the physician may or may not do ('To please no one will I prescribe a deadly drug') and intriguingly hints at the existence of another class of professional specialists, perhaps akin to surgeons ('I will leave this operation to be performed by practitioners, specialists in this art').

Hippocrates and his followers were the first to describe many diseases and medical conditions. He is given credit for the first description of clubbing of the fingers, an important diagnostic sign in chronic suppurative lung disease, lung cancer, and cyanotic heart disease. For this reason, clubbed fingers are sometimes referred to as 'Hippocratic fingers'. Hippocrates was also the first physician to describe Hippocratic face in *Prognosis*. Shakespeare famously alludes to this description when writing of Falstaff's death in Act II, Scene iii of *Henry V*. Hippocrates began to categorise illnesses as acute, chronic, endemic, and epidemic, and use terms such as, 'exacerbation, relapse, resolution, crisis, paroxysm, peak, and convalescence.' Another of Hippocrates's major contributions may be found in his descriptions of the symptomatology, physical findings, surgical treatment, and prognosis of thoracic empyema, i.e. suppuration of the lining of the chest cavity. His teachings remain relevant to present-day students of pulmonary medicine and surgery. Hippocrates was the first documented chest surgeon, and his findings are still valid. The *Hippocratic Corpus* contains the core medical texts of this school. Although once thought to have been written by Hippocrates himself, today, many scholars believe that these texts were written by a series of authors over several decades. Since it is impossible to determine which may have been written by Hippocrates himself, it is difficult to know which Hippocratic doctrines originated with him.

Asclepieia

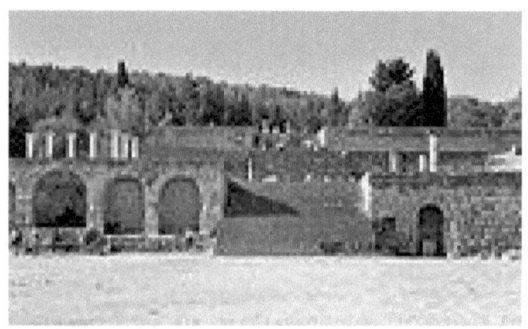

View of the askleipion of Kos, the best preserved instance of an Asklepieion.

Temples dedicated to the healer-god Asclepius, known as Asclepieia (Greek: Ασκληπιεία, sing. Asclepieion Ασκληπιείον), functioned as centres of medical advice, prognosis, and healing. At these shrines, patients would enter a dream-like state of induced sleep known as 'enkoimesis' (Greek: ενκοίμησις) not unlike anaesthesia, in which they either received guidance from the deity in a dream or were cured by surgery. Asclepeia provided carefully controlled spaces conducive to healing and fulfilled several of the requirements of institutions created for healing. In the Asclepieion of Epidaurus, three large marble boards dated to 350 BC preserve the names, case histories, complaints, and cures of about seventy patients who came to the temple with a problem and shed it there. Some of the surgical cures listed, such as the opening of an abdominal abscess or the removal of traumatic foreign material, are realistic enough to have taken place, but with the patient in a state of enkoimesis induced with the help of soporific substances such as opium.[1]

Aristotle

Ancient Greek philosopher Aristotle was the most influential scholar of the living world from antiquity. Though his early natural philosophy work was speculative, Aristotle's later biological writings demonstrate great concern for empiricism, biological causation, and the diversity of life. Aristotle did not experiment, however, holding that items display their real natures in their own environments, rather than in controlled, artificial ones. While in physics and chemistry, this assumption has been found unhelpful, in zoology and ethology it has not, and Aristotle's work 'retains real interest'. He made countless observations of nature, especially the habits and attributes of plants and animals in the world around him, to which he devoted considerable attention in categorising. In all, Aristotle classified 540 animal species and dissected at least 50.

Aristotle believed that intellectual purposes, formal causes, guided all natural processes. Such a teleological view gave Aristotle cause to justify his observed data as an expression of formal design; for example, suggesting that Nature, giving no animal both horns and tusks, was staving off vanity and generally giving creatures faculties only to such a degree as they are necessary. In a similar fashion, Aristotle believed that creatures were arranged in a graded scale of perfection rising from plants on up to man (the *scala naturae* or *Great Chain of Being*.) He held that the level of a creature's perfection was reflected in its form, but it was not foreordained by that form. Yet another aspect of his biology divided souls into three groups: a vegetative soul, responsible for reproduction and growth; a sensitive soul, responsible for mobility and sensation; and a rational soul, capable of thought and reflection. He attributed only the first to plants, the first two to animals, and all three to humans. Aristotle, in contrast to earlier philosophers, and like the Egyptians, placed the rational soul in the heart, rather than the brain. Notable is Aristotle's division of sensation and thought, which generally went against previous philosophers, with the exception of Alcmaeon. Aristotle's successor at the Lyceum, Theophrastus, wrote a series of books on botany—the *History of Plants*—which survived as the most important contribution of antiquity to botany, even into the Middle Ages. Many of Theophrastus' names survive into modern times, such as *carpos* for fruit, and *pericarpion* for seed vessel. Rather than focus on formal causes, as Aristotle did, Theophrastus suggested a mechanistic scheme, drawing analogies between natural and artificial processes, and relying on Aristotle's concept of the efficient cause. Theophrastus also recognised the role of sex in the reproduction of some higher plants, though this last discovery was lost in later ages. The biological/teleological ideas of Aristotle and Theophrastus as well as their emphasis on a series of axioms rather than on empirical observation, cannot be easily separated from their consequent impact on Western medicine.

Frontispiece to a 1644 version of the expanded and illustrated edition of Historia Plantarum (c. 1200), which was originally written around 200 BC

Following Theophrastus (d. 286 BC), the Lyceum failed to produce any original work. Though interest in Aristotle's ideas survived, they were generally taken unquestioningly. It is not until the age of Alexandria under the Ptolemies that advances in biology can be again found. The first medical teacher at Alexandria was Herophilus of Chalcedon, who corrected Aristotle, placing intelligence in the brain, and connected the nervous system to motion and sensation. Herophilus also distinguished between veins and arteries, noting that the latter pulse while the former do not. He did this using the experiment involving cutting certain veins and arteries in a pigs neck until the squealing stopped In the same vein, he developed a diagnostic technique that relied upon distinguishing different types of pulse. He, and his contemporary, Erasistratus of Chios, researched the role of veins and nerves, mapping their courses across the body.

Erasistratus connected the increased complexity of the surface of the human brain compared to other animals to its superior intelligence. He sometimes employed experiments to further his research, at one time repeatedly weighing a caged bird and noting its weight loss between feeding times. Following his teacher's researches into pneumatics, he claimed that the human system of blood vessels was controlled by vacuums, drawing blood across the body. In Erasistratus' physiology, air enters the body, is then drawn by the lungs into the heart, where it is transformed into vital spirit, and is then pumped by the arteries throughout the body. Some of this vital spirit reaches the brain, where it is transformed into animal spirit, which is then distributed by the nerves. Herophilus and Erasistratus performed their experiments upon criminals given to them by their Ptolemaic kings. They dissected these criminals alive and 'while they were still breathing, they observed parts which nature had formerly concealed, and examined their position, colour, shape, size, arrangement, hardness, softness, smoothness, connection.' Though a few ancient atomists such as Lucretius challenged the teleological viewpoint of Aristotelian ideas about life, teleology (and after the rise of Christianity, natural theology) would remain central to biological thought essentially until the eighteenth and nineteenth centuries. In the words of Ernst Mayr, 'Nothing of any real consequence in biology after Lucretius and Galen until the Renaissance.' Aristotle's ideas of natural history and medicine survived, but they were generally taken unquestioningly.

Historical Legacy

Through long contact with Greek culture, and their eventual conquest of Greece, the Romans absorbed many of the Greek ideas on medicine. Early Roman reactions to Greek medicine ranged from enthusiasm to hostility, but eventually the Romans adopted a favourable view of Hippocratic medicine. This acceptance led to the spread of Greek medical theories throughout the Roman Empire, and thus to a large portion of the West. The most influential Roman scholar to continue and expand on the Hippocratic tradition was Galen (d. *c.* 207). Study of Hippocratic and Galenic texts, however, all but disappeared in the Latin West in the early Middle Ages, following the collapse of the Western Empire, although the Hippocratic–Galenic tradition of Greek medicine continued to be studied and practised in the Eastern Roman Empire (Byzantium). After AD 750, Muslim Arabs also had Galen's works in particular translated and thereafter assimilated the Hippocratic-Galenic tradition, eventually making some of their own expansions upon this tradition, with the most influential being Avicenna. Beginning in the late eleventh century, the Hippocratic-Galenic tradition returned to the Latin West, with a series of translations of the Galenic and Hippocratic texts, mainly from Arabic translations but occasionally from the original Greek. In the Renaissance, more translations of Galen and Hippocrates directly from the Greek were made from newly available Byzantine manuscripts. Galen's influence was so great that even after Western Europeans started making dissections in the thirteenth century, scholars often assimilated findings that should have thrown Galen's accuracy into doubt, into the Galenic model. Vesalius' anatomical texts and pictures were, however, a major improvement on Galen's anatomy. William Harvey's demonstration of blood circulation was perhaps the first real blow to Galen's inaccurate ideas about blood circulation. Nevertheless, the Hippocratic-Galenic practice of bloodletting was practised into the nineteenth century despite its ineffectiveness and the extreme riskiness. The Galenic-Hippocratic tradition was only really replaced when the microscope-based studies of Louis Pasteur, Robert Koch, and others demonstrated that disease was not caused by an imbalance of the four humours but rather by micro-organisms such as bacteria.

18.6 African Herbal Medicine

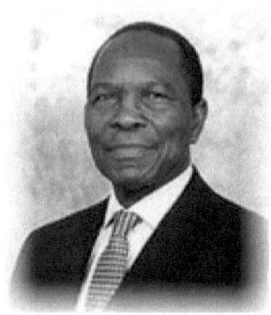

The late Prof. Ssali, the Director of Mariandina
Nutritional Health Products.

The late Dr Ssali was seriously engaged in researching into various ways and methods of preventing modern degenerative diseases. In his country of origin (Uganda) where he worked in many hospitals and universities, he made extraordinary contributions in the health care of the people. The resultant effects of his research findings led to the existence of the famous preventive therapy—mariandina nutritional health products. In all my natural medicine seminars in such countries as Ghana, Ivory Coast, Togo Benin Republic, and Nigeria, Mariandina products was talk of the town. The efficacy and effectiveness of these products made me very proud. I was very much worried over the louder popularity of Dr Ssali's findings—especially when it became very clear that the 'almighty' British Pharmaceutical multinationals were not particularly pleased. They felt embittered that the underdogs were now beginning to compete with their masters. But the franchisee Stogies in Uganda had no clue at all that their nation and the African race had lost a legend in the person of Dr Ssali. However, his legacy will continue to live and flourish! In this book, the full account of Dr Ssali's work is given. We owe it both to Africa and to the generality of mankind to continue from where Dr Ssali had stopped.

'Disease is any type of disorder or body function which is a result of bacterial, viral, fungal infection, degenerative changes in cells and congenital and hereditary' stated Dr Ssali. All can be traced back to some nutritional deficit. All diseases would be eliminated from man if the victim were to be fed on a properly balanced diet right from the moment of conception. The development of a fertilised egg into a fetus depends on the availability of nutrients to power and nourish the developing fetus. These nutrients act as free radical scavengers to protect the body cells from the harmful effects of free radicals that come out of body metabolism. The free radicals are capable of disrupting fetal development. The invasion of body tissues by bacteria, viruses, and fungus is dependent on the absence of enough nutrients to strengthen the immune system, which mops up the organisms. The free radicals are the ones which promote the reproduction of all the invading organisms and in turn the organisms promote the production of free radicals, concluded Dr Ssali.

It is obvious that even congenital or developmental abnormalities can be traced back to nutrition. Nutrition may be affected by the use of toxic substances or drugs that affect cell division, leading to abnormalities and congenital defects. One such chemical is thalidomide and the virus called rubella. All these lead to birth degenerative diseases like diabetes, asthma, and vascular/heart diseases that are all traceable to some nutritional deficit and which causes the cell death in the organs concerned. The pancreas loses the ability to secrete insulin as a result of the degeneration of the cells in the islets of lagerphones. These specialist cells die as a result of a nutrition lacking in vitamins and minerals. Taking white sugar from which molasses containing vitamins and minerals are removed during processing leads to one of the ways by which diabetes develops. When these nutrients are supplied to the person with diabetes, the situation improves rapidly back to normal.

All body cells develop from what are called stem cells in the embryonic stage. A stem cell requires proper nutrition as found in vegetable foods in their original unprocessed state in order to develop with the adult specialised cells as you find in various body organs like the brain, liver, glands, skin, muscle, bones, and intestinal and respiratory tracts. The lack of liberal supplies of these nutrients in fruits and vegetables creates a deficiency in the availability of vitamins like A, B, C, etc.; minerals like iron, zinc, selenium, etc.; and plant hormones; enzymes; and chlorophyll all of which play an important role in the proper development and specialisation of body cells. Examples of congenital defects that can be traced back to nutrition include, heart defects, spinal bifida, missing limbs, hydrocephalus, and many others. A liberal supply of vitamins and minerals are vital in this respect. Infections of the mother during pregnancy include viruses like rubella, which only occurs where antiviral nutrients like vitamin A, C, and E are in short supply. The virus disrupts the proper cell divisions required to complete some body organs like the heart etc.

The immune system, which protects us from all infections, depends on nutrition to produce antibodies and the necessary defence cells like macrophages and lymphocytes. Any deficiency in the necessary nutrients results in weakening of the immune system, which is followed by an invasion of the body by bacteria, viruses, and fungus and even degeneration of body cells. Nutrients help the body to clean itself by mopping up free radicals that we produce during cellular metabolism. These free radicals include hydrogen peroxide, which attacks cell structures if left in position for too long. It can attack vital structures like the cell membrane, the nucleus, and mitochondria. The damage they inflict on the cells is what can cause conditions like diabetes when insulin-secreting cells (islets of langerhans) die in increasing numbers till it results in insulin deficiency called diabetes. When nutrients are replenished, the cells regenerate and diabetes can be cured. The same occurs in other body cells. Cancer occurs because of the destruction of mitochondria, making metabolism using oxidation of glucose impossible for lack of the necessary enzymes in the mitochondria (KREB'S cycle), which power the process. This leads the cells to generate heat energy using fermentation processes and the production of lactic acid. This is the way cancer occurs in body tissues like in the breasts, uterus, lungs, glands, and other tissues.

The cure for cancer must therefore address this anomaly by reconstructing the damaged cell structures and restoring normal body metabolism. Powerful antioxidants, which act as free radical scavengers in the affected parts of the body help the tissue to detoxify itself and prevent further cell damage from free radicals. The oxygen that is released by hydrogen peroxide can attack cell structures and cause the equivalent of iron rust in the body. In situations like these, one requires to drink a lot of water in order to enable the kidneys to excrete those impurities from the blood circulation, where they may continue causing traumatic effects on tissues. Water is an essential part of our nutritional requirements. If the body is denied water supply, it deteriorates rapidly because of dehydration and accumulation of toxic impurities. These impurities that accumulate in tissues cause body damage by depleting the supplies of nutrients from the food taken in daily. The ageing process is perpetuated by this growing nutritional deficit. As we grow, we cut down on our intake of the essential nutrients of vitamins and minerals. The sum total of the nutritional deficiency and chronic dehydration is the progressive ageing process we observe in everyday life. Such a situation where the body cells fail to reproduce themselves as they should by replacing themselves with identical copies is a serious health matter. This is why the hair begins to lose pigmentation and becomes grey and the skin loses its elasticity, eventually becoming rough and wrinkled. This is the reason why cancer incidence increases with age or pollution in the internal and external environment. If we look after ourselves properly by taking a well-balanced diet consisting of unprocessed fresh vegetables and fruits and drink the required amounts of water, then we would be able to maintain our health status close to ideal for many years.

Medicinal herbs are no more than foods with the required nutrients to correct the cellular nutritional deficiency that lead to the diseased state. The use of contraceptive pills, overuse of antibiotics, and smoking are some of the forms of drug abuse that drain heavily on nutrients because of the increased need for detoxification. This is the reason why those who indulge in such practices develop cancer of the breast, lungs, uterus, and prostate. Others develop diabetes, asthma, and blood pressure because of the nutritional deficit created by the increase in the demand for nutrients for the detoxification of free radicals. A disease state like AIDS is a complex manifestation of nutritional deficiencies that include vitamins, minerals, plant hormones, amino acids, and enzymes. The body needs plant ingredients found in leafy vegetables, like chlorophyll, lecithin, and many others. The HIV invades the body by penetrating its cells which are deficient in nutrients and abounding in free radicals. This window of opportunity occurs in all people who indulge in junk foods, drug abuse, overuse of antibiotics, and fizzy drinks with artificial sweeteners. These factors depress the immune system, allowing the virus to successfully establish itself in the body. If the free radicals are regularly mopped up using the free radical scavengers called antioxidants as found in fresh fruit and vegetables, then the virus and cancer cells are eliminated by the power of the immune system.

During sexual union, the male partner ejaculates about 2 ml of semen, which carry the male spermatozoa. This semen also carries with it nutrients to be used by the sperm and the early embryo. To collect these nutrients in the semen, one pint of the male partner's blood is stripped of all these elements which include vitamins, minerals, enzymes, hormones, etc., etc. Repeated ejaculations can deplete the male partner's blood of essential elements required by his immune system. The result of such a situation is to make him vulnerable to infections by viruses and STDs, including HIV. This is the reason why promiscuous males may easily develop AIDS, which means acquired immune deficiency syndrome. Semen is rich in zinc and selenium, both of which are very important for strengthening immunity by providing it with specialised cells called T-helper lymphocytes. These T-helper lymphocytes go through the thymus gland, which prepares them for the battlefield to fight against virus invaders. The thymus gland requires a lot of zinc to do the job. Selenium is needed to make the body's antioxidant called glutathione peroxides. This natural antioxidant is very important in clearing out hydrogen peroxide from the body cells. A diet rich in these nutrients will play an important role in protecting us against all infections and *cancer*. The prostrate gland in the male is the equivalent of the uterus in the *female*. Both these organs are prone to developing cancer if nutrition is deficient in these essential elements among others.

On the other hand, female partners stand to gain the nutrients which are drained out of the male partner's blood. Most of the semen's essential ingredients are absorbed into the female circulation through the birth canal. This provides her with the elements mentioned above for added protection against nutritional-deficiency diseases that come as a result of a weakened immune system. This explanation could account for the survival phenomenon observed among professional female sex workers in Kenya, Uganda, and many other parts of the world. These prostitutes have been found to survive HIV infection despite their risk factors. It has also been observed that these sex workers begin to succumb to HIV/AIDS when they retire from their profession. This would eliminate the original theory that they have a special genetic make-up that protects them against HIV. I am of the opinion that it is the constant liberal supply of essential nutrients that boosts their immunity to the optimum levels capable to resisting STDs.

Herpes Zoster, which is a result of chickenpox virus manifesting itself as blisters on the skin, is another example of the power of the immune system. This virus only surfaces when the body is malnourished and immune deficient. The development of cancer cells starts when the natural killer cells that hunt and destroy them are weakened by poor nutrition. This poor nutrition may be as a result of ingesting overwhelming amounts of toxic substances that require large amounts of nutrients to excrete through the kidneys. If such nutrients are not available, then the immune system is weakened and the natural killer cells fail to cope with the cancer cell development in the tissues. If this is kept up long enough, then the particular site develops cancer. The toxic substances like aspartame (Nutrasweet), contraceptive pills, radioactive materials, alcohol, hydrocarbons, asbestos etc., etc, cause the production of free radicals to rise and stagnate in tissues. This stagnation leads to the damage of cell wall, DNA cross links, and mitochondria structural damage. This DNA damage leads to genetic mutation and cancer changes. The damage to mitochondria structure leads to the failure of the cell to metabolise glucose using oxygen. As a result of this failure, the cell turns to fermentation to produce heat energy with the production of a toxic lactic acid. This is what cancer cells do. They multiply uncontrollably and destroy normal tissues in the neighbourhood. Some of these uncontrollable cells break off and carry their characteristics to other parts of the body as metastasis that spread destruction and death. This process can be halted by providing the tissues with the required nutrients to repair the cellular damage in DNA and mitochondria. These nutrients must also strengthen the immune cells to be capable of destroying the cancer cells. This is possible through the use of herbal nutrients, which contain the necessary ingredients to do the job. This has been achieved in cases of breast cancer, cancer of uterus, melanoma, and other cancers.

Hormone-dependent disorders like diabetes, thyroid gland dysfunction, menopause, libido, and many others can be eliminated by providing these necessary nutrients through diet and, where required, food supplements. Menopause and loss of virility comes because of the progressive reduction in our food intake as we grow older. As a result of eating processed foods like white sugar, white flour, and processed grain where the nutrients are removed and fed to lower animals, we develop deficiency diseases like diabetes, scurvy, eczema, lupus, and asthma. These come about because our body's immune systems have been programmed wrongly because of introducing adverse antigens into the body through vaccinations and inoculations. All these immunity or autoimmune disorders could be corrected by providing the body with the nutrients the body needs to reprogramme the immunity. By providing these supplements, we have been successful in eliminating all symptoms and signs of lupus, asthma, eczema, thyroid gland problems, and so on. Stroke, which is a result of the blocking by blood clots, could be eliminated. The underlying disorder is in the metabolism of cholesterol, leading to partial or complete blockage of a blood vessel. Where there is a blood clot or a ruptured blood vessel and bleeding, you find an accumulation of free radicals and white blood cells in the clot. This pathology needs nutrients to put it right. The cholesterol needs nutrients to facilitate its breakdown into energy. The blood clot and the repair of the damaged blood vessel will be completed by the white blood cells. We have seen this happen in many cases of stroke where paralysis disappeared within weeks or months when the necessary nutrients were provided to the patient. Brain and nerve disorders may develop because of using too much alcohol or a diet deficient in vitamins and minerals. Even psychiatric disorders are a result of the body's failure to make the right nerve transmitters for lack of the proper nutrients. Where these mental problems existed, we provided the patients with nutritional supplements and an improved diet. The result was an improvement or recovery from the dementia of a psychiatric problem.

As a result of the above observations as summarised, the following conclusion was inevitable. The unified field theory of disease and nutrition (establishes) postulates that all disease states have their origin in some form of malnutrition at one stage or another. Even those arising from genetic defects could be attributed to the influence of a mutation that occurred because of a nutritional defect in the diet of the individual, or alternatively, the mutation persisted because of lack of proper nutrition. All disease states, whether they are congenital, infective, and degenerative, have a nutritional factor in their causation and promotion or elimination. Mariandina has a wide spectrum of curative properties that include most of the diseases mentioned above because its formulation includes a wide range of nutrients as was considered essential for the maintenance of optimum nutrition of all types of body cell. The herbs that were selected for inclusion in the Mariandina formulation were those that our research had established to be composed of properties with great nutritional value, which is the basis of their medicinal value and curative properties. The following are the typical examples of the

18.7 Dr Llaila O. Afrika

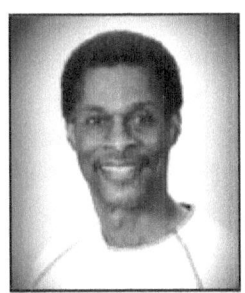

Dr Llaila O. Afrika
Lecturer, Teacher, Historian, Author, Health consultant

Dr Llaila O. Afrika is a lecturer and author. He can help you understand and become aware of natural remedies and treatments. He is a nutritional consultant, massage therapist, historian, certified addictionologist, acupuncturist, writer, and a doctor of naturopathy. He has studied in countries such as Africa, Europe, and of course, America. Dr Afrika believes that each of his clients (from children to the elderly) has been among his many teachers, and he is fully indebted to them all. He lectures on eighty different topics. He contends that good health does not belong exclusively to any culture or race, but is a human right and product of nature. There are many people teaching various aspects of proper nutrition. Good nutrition is important because our food gives us the energy to do the things we have to do and want to do with our lives. How does not eating correctly affect us? The first thing that usually comes to mind is that some people get fat. Getting fat is only one physical manifestation of a certain type of bad nutrition. He has carefully studied both the short- and long-term effects of poor nutrition. This exhaustive analysis can be found in his book, *Nutricide: The Nutritional Destruction of the Black Race*. Originally published in 1993, he has revised and updated it in 2000. He advises us not to eat any meat do and whatever is best or easiest for you. Dr Afrika gives you several examples of the things you can do to get started, but more importantly, he tells us why we should clean up our act.

He encourages us to take any intermediate steps necessary to begin cleaning our body, mind, and spirit of pollutants. It does not matter what you do first to start the healing process. Something must be done. He can help you understand and become aware of natural remedies and treatments. He is a nutritional consultant, massage therapist, historian, certified addictionologist, acupuncturist, writer, and doctor of naturopathy. He has studied in countries such as Africa, Europe, and of course, America. Dr Afrika believes that each of his clients (from children to the elderly) has been among his many teachers, and he is fully indebted to them all. Dr Afrika lectures on eighty different topics. He contends that good health does not belong exclusively to any culture or race, but is a human right and product of nature. There are many people teaching various aspects of proper nutrition. Good nutrition is important because our food gives us the energy to do the things we have to do and want to do with our lives. How does not eating correctly affect us? The first thing that usually comes to mind is some people get fat. Getting fat is only one physical manifestation of a certain type of bad nutrition. Dr Llaila Afrika has carefully studied both the short and long term effects of poor nutrition. This exhaustive analysis can be found in his book 'Nutricide: The nutritional destruction of the Black race'. Originally published in 1993 he has revised and updated it in 2000. Dr Afrika advises us not to eat any meat. He encourages us to take any intermediate steps necessary to begin cleaning our body, mind, and spirit of pollutants. It does not matter what you do first to start the healing process. Something must be done and whatever is best or easiest for you is the step you should take. Dr Afrika gives you several examples of the things you can do to get started but more importantly he tells us why we should clean up our act Dr Afrika is the leading authority on African holistic health in the world and his book *African Holistic Health* is the only best-seller in the subject on the planet.

Hypertension, High Blood Pressure, and Stress

High blood pressure and hypertension are usually caused by a lack of proper nutrition. Improper nutrition weakens the internal organs, immune system, and lowers the organs' abilities to utilise nutrients that feed the body. The body begins to starve because of the loss of proper nutrients. This starvation causes a nutritional deficiency. The nutritionally starved body tries to get more nutrients to pay the debt. Consequently, the body demands more food (nutrients in the blood) by drawing on poor (below-nutrient-level) blood. In order to increase the nutrients the body needs, it must get nutrients from the blood, and so it increases the quantity of blood by increasing the pressure. The increase of pressure is the body's attempt to feed itself. This increase in pressure is the body's last resort to defend itself against the bodily pollutions, gland disorders, free radicals, kidney weakness, hypertension, being overweight, emotional stress, toxemia, deteriorating metabolism, etc., and a foodless food (junk food) diet.

An inflexible vascular system is unable to bring pressure down. The pressure gets high and cannot come down to normal. However, the increased blood pressure fails to nourish the body because the junk foods (fibre-less, enzyme depleted) are depleted of nutrients. This results in hypertension and stress. The blood nutrients can only be supplied by a diet of natural whole foods. Additionally, the blood can have an accumulation of waste floating in it. The waste gets into the veins and arteries, causing them to lose flexibility. The more cellular and chemical waste there is in the blood, the less oxygen and nutrients is available. The pressure is elevated in order to get more nutrients delivered to starved tissue, but instead, this brings more waste and less air. This rise in blood pressure demands more nutrients to sustain the high blood pressure in the blood—which is thick with waste—stresses the heart, and causes a nutritional unpaid debt. This is the case of nutritional suicide as high blood pressure causes high pressure, which in turn causes an extreme nutrient loss called low blood pressure. Subsequently, high and low pressure are caused by disease. The high blood pressure diminishes the ability of the kidneys to filter waste, regulate hormones, aide mineral absorption and cell formation. The kidneys require the temperature and pressure to be normal in order for them to function.

The stress reaction does not cause diseases such as heart disease, arterial hypertension, and nervous disorder. Stress reaction triggers the release of adrenaline. However, wild animals have larger adrenal glands than tamed (domesticated) animals. Consequently, wild animals produce more adrenaline and are under more stress. They do not have disease associated with uncooked foods and processed junk foods. It is the junk food diet and immunosuppressive drugs and malnourishment that cause stress. If stress were the cause of diseases rather than nutrient-poor diet, then black chattel slaves would have died from stress and high blood pressure. It is the nutrient poor health—caused by immunosuppressive drugs (antibiotics, etc.), fiber-less food, cooked food and free radicals (waste)—that causes the disease reaction of hypertension, stress, etc. 80 per cent of all African Americans over the age of forty-five have high blood pressure, 'the silent killer'.

High blood pressure is a major killer of African Americans in particular. Stress, poor diet, alcohol, and drugs are some of the major causes. *Risk factors* for high blood pressure include smoking, alcohol abuse, obesity, a high salt intake, lack of exercise, and stress, along with a family history of hypertension and stroke. *Arteriosclerosis*, or a thickening, hardening, and narrowing of the walls of the arteries is also often associated with high blood pressure. *Drug therapy* like many synthetic drugs, and anti-hypertensive medication has a risk of causing side effects, depending on the person as well as the type of drug being taken. These can include dizziness, nausea, stomach problems, fatigue, impotence, insomnia, loss of appetite, and others. Always speak to your doctor if you are experiencing any of these symptoms.

What about natural Remedies?

There are many well-known *natural remedies* for high blood pressure or hypertension. Conventional medicines usually treat the symptoms of high blood pressure but seldom address the *underlying causes*. Naturopaths recognise that high blood pressure may be a sign or symptom of imbalance in the body. They believe in *removing the causes of high blood pressure* with a combination of lifestyle changes and natural remedies, rather than simply treating the symptoms. *Can herbal remedies and dietary supplements really help?* There is a great deal of scientific evidence to suggest that the use of carefully chosen herbal remedies and dietary supplements can help to lower blood pressure as well as to improve the overall functioning of the heart, arteries, and the entire cardiovascular system. What herbalists have known for centuries has now been clinically proven to be a potentially effective alternative to synthetic blood pressure medication, especially if combined with a healthy diet and regular exercise.

Why Being Black Increases Your Risk of High Blood Pressure

High blood pressure is more common and more severe in black people. But you can still take steps to protect yourself and treat the disease effectively with lifestyle changes and medications. If you're black, pay special attention to your blood pressure—even if you think you're healthy. That's because high blood pressure (hypertension) affects certain groups of people differently than others. And for black people in the United States, high blood pressure often occurs earlier in life, is more severe, and has more complications. If you're black and living in the United States, you're more likely than a person of another culture to develop hypertension and to develop it earlier in your life. And once you have the disease, you're more likely to have severe complications, such as stroke, kidney failure and heart disease. In addition, blacks often don't get treatment until their blood pressure has been high for so long that vital organs are nearly destroyed. Find out why you may be at greater risk of high blood pressure if you're black and what steps you can take to protect yourself.

Thanks to Joanne Katz, ScD, Professor of International Health, Johns Hopkins School of Hygiene and Public Health, Baltimore, MD for contributing to this article. Dr Katz was a co-investigator of the Baltimore Eye Survey, Carbohydrates and Blood Pressure.

R. Hodges, and T. Rebello, *Annals of Internal Medicine*, 1983; 98:838_41.

For treatment and diet instructions, order the high blood pressure DVD or the book *African Holistic Health.*

For diet, order the *Crossover Diet Cookbook.*

Research and Clinical Findings: Böhm K. Choleretic, Action of Some Medicinal Plants. *Arzneimittelforschung,* 1959; 9:376-8.

Drieu K., Preparation and definition of Ginkgo biloba extract, In *Rokan (Ginkgo biloba): Recent Results in Pharmacology and Clinic.* Fünfgeld EW, ed. Berlin: Springer–Verlag, 32-6.

Loew D., Pharmacological and clinical results with Crataegus special extracts in cardiac insufficiency. *ESCOP Phytotelegram,* 1994; 6:20-6

Newall CA, Anderson LA, Phillipson JD. *Herbal Medicines: A Guide for Health–Care Professionals.* London: Pharmaceutical Press, 1996, 206-7.

Petkov V, Manolov P. Pharmacological analysis of the iridoid oleuropein. *Arzneim Forsch/Drug Research* 1972; 22:1476-86.

Simpson D., Buchu-South Africa's amazing herbal remedy. *Scott Med J,* 1998; 43:189-91 [review]

Tauchert M, Ploch M, Hübner W-D. Effectiveness of hawthorn extract LI 132 compared with the ACE inhibitor Captopril: Multicenter double-blind study with 132 patients NYHA stage II. *Münch Med Wochenschr* 1994; 132(suppl): S27–33.

Weikl A, Noh HS, The influence of Crataegus on global cardiac insufficiency, *Herz Gefabe,* 1993; 11:516-24.

Weikl A, Assmus KD, Neukum-Schmidt A, et al. Crataegus special extract WS 1442: Objective proof of efficacy in patients with cardiac insufficiency (NYHA II), *Fortschr Med,* 1996; 114:291-6.

Cathy Wong, Your Guide to Alternative Medicine. Stern, N. and Tuck, M. Pathogenesis of Hypertension in Diabetes Mellitus. *Diabetes Mellitus, a Fundamental and Clinical Test,* 2nd Edition, (Philadelphia; A: Lippincott Williams and Wilkins, 2000) 943-57.

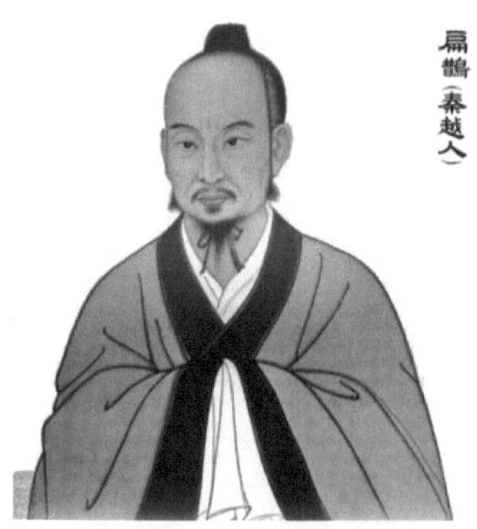

扁
鵲
（秦越人）

PIEN CH'IAO (BIAN QUE 500 BC.
Chinese Physician of the Past
This is one the early founding fathers
of Chinese traditional medicine.

18.8 The System of Chinese Herbal Medicine

The history of Chinese herbal medicine dates back thousands of years to the time of the legendary Chinese Emperor Shen Nong, born in 2737 BC. Considered to be the father of Chinese medicine, he discovered the healing properties of over 365 herbs and other remedies by testing them on himself. The earliest known written version of his Classic Herbal was published in the third century BC.

Over the centuries, many talented doctors added their knowledge and expertise to the expanding body of literature on Chinese herbal remedies and treatments. Zhang Zhongjing, established a system for the diagnosis and treatment of infectious diseases. Sun Simiao, born *c.* AD 581, wrote the first comprehensive encyclopedia of Chinese medicine. His thirty-volume work included over four thousand five hundred formulas, many of which are still in use today.

A prominent figure in Chinese herbal medicine history is renowned physician and naturalist Li Shi Zhen, who lived during the Ming Dynasty from 1518 to 1593. Li's major contribution to Chinese herbal medicine was to completely revise and reorganise the existing literature. His massive *Compendium of Materia Medica* has been translated into many languages and is considered the leading reference work for Chinese herbal medicine.

The goal of traditional Chinese medicine is the prevention of illness by maintaining balance in all aspects of life. This rationale differs from the conventional Western idea of treating symptoms of an existing disease. In the Chinese medical philosophy, the focus is on treating the patient as a whole. Illness is regarded as an imbalance in the patient's body, mind, or spirit. A skilled practitioner of Chinese herbal medicine will choose appropriate herbal formulas to strengthen, nourish, and bring the patient back into balance and harmony.

Chinese herbal medicine has been shown to be effective for a wide variety of acute and chronic conditions, including women's health issues, anxiety and depression, respiratory problems, hypertension, and digestive disorders. Many Chinese herbs are now readily available in the West. A few examples of popular herbs are ginseng, ginger, dong quai, and Ginkgo biloba.

The use of Chinese herbal medicine in the Western world has increased significantly in recent years. People are turning to safe, effective, and time-proven alternative treatments that provide a cure without harmful side effects and often at a much lower cost than pharmaceutical drugs. Traditional Chinese herbal medicine is finally gaining the respect and recognition it deserves in the West.

Everything is one in traditional Chinese medicine: The holistic nature of Chinese medicine is based on the belief that all life is interconnected and that restoring and maintaining balance within the body and all its systems is the key to good health.

The concept of yin and yang theory: Yin and yang theory is all about balance. According to traditional Chinese medicine, balance is essential for healthful living. Therapy: In the practice of

It can be seen from the above information tha the principal aspect of even the Chinese traditional medicine is based on the concept of preventive complementary medicine.

Dedication:

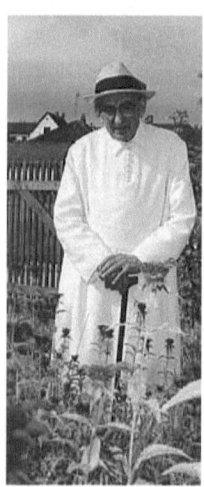

This presentation is dedicated to the Austrian Hermann-Josef Weidinger . . .

Better known as herbal-priest Weidinger, who died on Sunday, 21 March 2004, at the age of eighty-six. He had studied European herbalism in his youth and travelled to China as a missionary in 1938, where he learnt also of their herbal system. He returned from China in 1953. He continued his work as herbalist and proponent of healthy lifestyle, writing some forty books on natural health care. Until recently, he and thirty-seven assistants prepared and prescribed herbal remedies in Karlstein, Austria, at the Paracelsus House Nature Cure Centre.

18.9 About Dr Subhuti Dharmanand

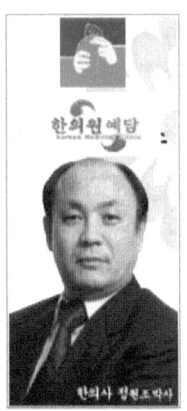

Although Dr Dharmanda cannot be described as one of the founding fathers of traditional medicine, his immense contributions in researching and propagating the modern knowledge of complementary medicine is worthy of press. One hope is that other people involved in natural science from the the developing world should take Dr Dharmanda's work as a challenge and come up with similar endeavours. Otherwise, we would have no choice than to accept all that we are given by the conventional medical science as the ultimate. There is nobody in the West who have carried more than he has done. His research findings have thrown more light into the nature and the uses of various Chinese and other Asian traditional herbal medicine throughout the world. Dr Subhuti Dharmananda received his PhD in biology from the University of California in 1980. He travelled to China several times; the first visit was in 1977 and the most recent in 2001. He has collected a large library of books and journals involved with traditional medicine. In addition to ITM, Dr Subhuti Dharmananda helped initiate People's Herbs Incorporated, All-The-Tea Company, and Dharma Consulting International, and has been a consultant to several major herb companies, including Fmali Herbs (maker of Good Earth Teas), Health Concerns (maker of Chinese Traditionals), and Sen (maker of Sen traditional herbal formulas and other products). He has been an editor, reviewer, and contributor to several journals involved with traditional medicine, including the *International Journal of Oriental Medicine*, and the *Protocol Journal of Botanical Medicine*. Majority of his research findings will be very useful to the preventive therapy both in their application and adequate references.

Left: Statue of Konrad von Gessner (1516-65), a physician in Zurich who specialised in nature studies, cataloguing numerous species and who is considered one of the founders of modern zoology. He liked alpine research and collected numerous mountain plants, with focus on medicinal species.

Right: A medicinal fountain in the park at Hotel Disentiserhof (*c.* 1910), renowned as the strongest therapeutic source of radon in Switzerland. At the time, it was believed that radon, which is radioactive, was a valuable therapy for many diseases.

Covers of the German and English editions of ***Herbs and Weeds***

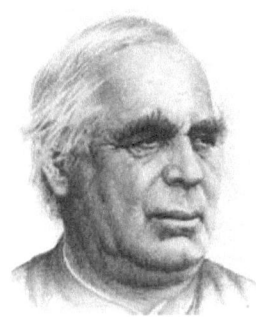

Left: Father Sebastian Kneipp (1821–97), a German Catholic priest who greatly influenced the development of naturopathic medicine. He is probably best known for his recommendations for 'water cures' (applying water of different temperatures and in different ways), which are still utilised today. However, he was also a strong advocate for using herbal remedies and influenced Johann Künzle.

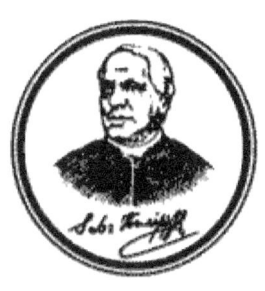

Right: A trademark image for remedies designed by Father Kneipp and manufactured by Oberhausser and Landauer of Wurzburg, Germany.

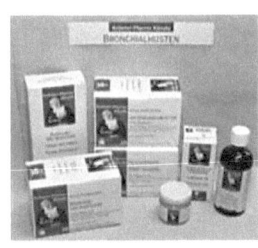

Left: Künzle's products now sold in Europe.

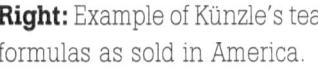

Right: Example of Künzle's tea formulas as sold in America.

Left: Popular photo of Künzle, *c.* 1940.

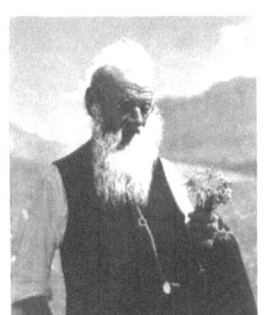

Right: a Grotto established by Künzle around 1912. This is an artificial cave made as a feature of waterfall for arrangement of plantings. When built in modern times, Grotto iis for the display of religious icons or to house an altar.

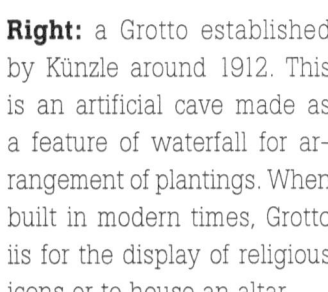

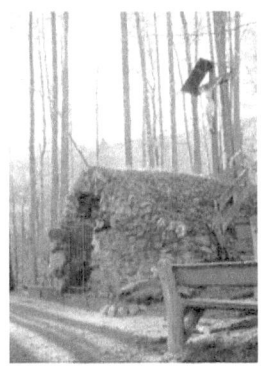

18.10 Dounne Alexander

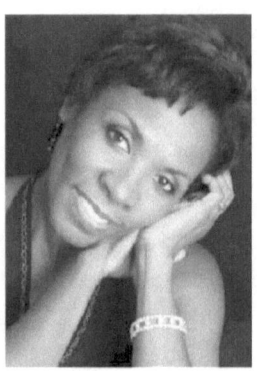

'A Woman on a *Mission*'
Dounne Alexander. MBE, FRSA

Founder of GRAMMA'S® and Joining Hands In Health®—wife, mother, spiritual herbalist, publisher, author, motivational speaker, mentor, health campaigner, and award winning business pioneer. Honoured as a 'true pioneer and visionary' (for her ground-breaking work dedication, determination, and vision . . . in natural health care and business development). Honoured by Queen Elizabeth II—with the MBE Medal in 2007 (for her outstanding service to the British Food Industry). Voted one of the hundred greatest and most influential black people in British history (included in the first official list for the 2000 British millennium history archives, plus her contribution recorded by the BBC and is stored for posterity in the British National Library).

Revolutionising Twenty-first Century Health Care

Long before the invention of synthetic drugs and artificial foods, Dounne's Afro-Caribbean ancestors relied solely on nature for their 'food, cosmetics, and medicine' to maintain lifelong health based on the universal Laws of Life (i.e. love). Dounne [60] is a passionate believer in 'Divine Purpose, Spiritual Consciousness and a strong advocate of traditional self healing'; based on the ancient principle that *natural foods are meant to feed and heal*. For over twenty years, she has been spearheading 'traditional natural health care' emphasising the importance of healing mind, body, and spirit through the provisions of nature—home-cooking and the essential role it plays in maintaining overall (whole body) health. In 1987, she established GRAMMA'S (an ethical herbal-food manufacturing business) specifically to serve this purpose . . . and is the first to integrate 'natural foods with medicinal and culinary herbs' for optimum/sustainable health. In 1994, Dounne discovered *a missing link* in the food chain that healed herself and family pet from terminal cancer and was the inspiration behind her 'Joining Hands In Health' awareness campaign. Through it, she hopes to revolutionise twenty-first century health care by taking 'food and medicine' to the next level. Her ultimate dream is to re-educate and empower everyone to manage their own health, plus join forces with the National Health Service, doctors, health practitioners, and carers to provide cost-effective health-care solutions, as well as integrate animal health and welfare. In 2008, The Minister for Public Health finally approved her extraordinary herbal-products for use in hospitals and hospices. In 2009, The Royal College of Obstetricians and Gynaecologists approved her 'Organic Omega Oils 3, 6, 7, 9' for pregnant women throughout the UK. In 2009, she took up the quest to protect God's healing foods from the clutches of the European Union to safeguard and preserve natural health care for future generations. In November 2009, she was invited to personally present her case to the seven hundred members of the European Parliament in Brussels.

Trail blazer: Dounne has remained a leading light (beacon-of-hope) . . . blazing the trail for natural health care and disadvantaged businesses (women, men, and minorities). Through personal experience, she provides real insight, motivation, and inspiration to people from all walks of life.

She was born (1949) in the beautiful Caribbean Island of Trinidad—as a severely premature baby with a life expectancy of only one month. Thankfully, her late grandmother's strong faith, intuition, tender loving care, and incredible knowledge on the health benefits of natural foods and folklore herbal remedies . . . enabled her to survive against the odds.

As a child, under her grandmother's watchful eyes, she learnt many valuable life lessons . . . steeped in the selfless tradition of sharing information and knowledge with which to benefit others. Being raised in the Caribbean, Dounne experienced an amazing quality of life obtained through living in a pollution-free environment; on a rich diet of natural foods; good, old-fashioned home cooking; home-made herbal remedies;

and on the spiritual belief that the 'universal Creator' has provided abundantly for all our needs through nature. Respecting *Mother Earth* and acknowledging 'food' as their main life-source, her ancestors would and healing' at every stage of its development . . . from tilling the soil; pray for 'blessing planting the seeds; harvesting the crops, through to the final preparation of each meal or remedy. Their belief was simple: 'God is love' and therefore trusted and looked to Him each day for guidance on life. Hence, *traditional self-healing* (i.e. mind, body, and spirit) has always been linked to spirituality. *This was the blueprint that has shaped her life and she later realised that it was also the purpose for which she was sent—to serve.*

By this means, her ancestors were able to maintain *good health* since Creation billions of years ago and only became ill when they disobeyed the laws of life and nature. Dounne explains, 'I was five years old when my great-grandmother (an African spiritual herbalist and midwife) died at the age of 113—from old age and not sickness. She had impeccable memory; excellent eyesight, no age-related conditions, aches, pain, or feebleness, all her own teeth (perfectly strong, clean, and white, using only the hibiscus plant as a natural toothbrush) and was in the best of health. This was considered normal—*sickness* was *rare* in those *days* . . . it was natural to feel *well* all the time. But a generation later, after Western scientists began using us as experimental guinea pigs (i.e. vaccinations and other synthetic drug-medications), my family's "lifespan" fell by over forty years, all dying from chronic illnesses . . . my grandmother (73) from heart disease, grandfather from bowel cancer, my mother (68) from ovarian cancer, father (83) from prostate cancer, plus many, many others.' Dounne believes that by 'abandoning our "faith and trust" in God and His healing foods, we have lost our "Divine connection" with the universe . . . and putting this trust in doctors has resulted in a world where *sickness has now become the norm.'*

'Recognising that scientific interference, lack of education, and misinformation is the root cause of chronic illness, prolonged poor health, and premature death, I chose to follow in my ancestors' footsteps, plus those of the two most respected fathers of medicine—Hippocrates who 2,500 years ago famously quoted "Let thy Food be thy Medicine and thy Medicine be thy Food", and Paracelsus who 500 years ago stated, "All that man needs for health and healing has been provided by God in nature, the challenge for science is to find it". Therefore, GRAMMA'S (named in loving memory of my late grandmother) was established to re-educate and encourage everyone back to a more natural way of life, in order to regain the knowledge of these ancient practices and also experience "self-healing" (first-hand). And in this way restore health, as well as *faith, trust, and respect for* God's healing foods. I hope this will enable everyone to reconnect with the universal power of love and their Divine spiritual consciousness'.

A True Pioneer

She was the first to integrate '*natural foods, medicinal and culinary herbs*' as one complete unit for optimum/sustainable health for both humans and animals, *first* to challenge the laws prohibiting 'health-claims' on natural foods, *first* to initiate health education and awareness campaigns on its healing benefits, *first* to embrace all cultures, animals, and the environment, *first* to initiate major government policy changes for disadvantages in businesses (women, men and minorities).

A National Inspiration

After leaving secondary school at seventeen, Dounne worked for over twenty-two years as a bacteriological and chemical technician and housing manager. She got married in 1971, had two daughters, but by 1986, to escape marital abuse, she took up martial arts and within six months, took back complete control of her life. She moved out of her home into a council flat and started a new life as a single parent. This was the period of Britain's new enterprise culture, and she decided that the best way of securing herself and her children's future would be to start up her own business. As a full-time working mother (on a low income), who has managed to raise her children on nutritious, home-cooked meals, Dounne recognised that the nation was moving into a dangerously unhealthy eating phase of artificial, processed, ready-made meals and junk foods . . . encouraged by manufacturers, retailers, and the government. Foreseeing the long-term damage to present and future generations, she recognised a unique niche in the 'speciality health food market', and six months later, GRAMMA'S was born from the tiny kitchen of her flat. Without any formal business training, experience, qualifications, collateral, or finance, Dounne personally created, designed, packaged, and promoted her now-famous 'Gramma's Herbal Pepper Sauces'. And within three months, she single-handedly negotiated them into Britain's most prestigious department stores Harrods and Fortnum and Mason . . . creating a media frenzy with extensive coverage and was instantly hailed anational inspiration. By the end of that year, her sauces also took pride of place on the shelves of other department stores around the country (Selfridges, Harvey Nichols, Bentalls, Rackhams, Howells, and Kendale Milne). After a two-year difficult battle with British Banks, in 1990, she eventually raised the finance required via the government's Small Firms Loan Guarantee Scheme to establish her first factory. And went on to surpass her natural skills by successfully negotiating her products into the top seven mainstream supermarket chains (Tesco, Safeway—now called Morrisons, Asda, Waitrose, Sainsbury, W. M. Low, Co-op), and stores in Ireland—a feat never before achieved single-handedly by any small British business-owner with the largest national distribution (listings in over seven hundred stores)—thereby, effectively opening the mainstream doors for small businesses in the UK. However, in 1994, after healing her dog from terminal cancer, she realised that the spiritual ethos of GRAMMA'S set her products apart from those on the commercial market, and she decided to withdraw them from the stores and transformed the business into a mail-order service.

- **The First Black Businesswoman** to establish a premium brand, label, and quality foods, plus take 'traditional herbal foods' into the highest levels of the British mainstream markets; raising its profile, quality standards, respect, presentation, and health awareness.

- **Unique Products**—derived from Divine intervention. Dounne has developed the most unique range of extraordinary herbal products, which crosses over all cultural divisions, and are suitable for humans and animals alike and also kind to the environment.

- **American Chilli Institute** (The Hall of Fame)—first to introduce the 'Caribbean Scotch Bonnet Hot Peppers' to the UK's bland palates with the *original ancient hot herbal sauces*—never before commercialised and unique to the world markets. Prior to Dounne's revelations, the British Medical Establishment believed that 'hot peppers' were dangerous to health and therefore discouraged its use in food. So in 1990, Dounne took it upon herself to initiate the first national 'Health Education and Awareness

Campaign' on the nutritional health benefits of hot pepper and spicy foods, and she produced the first detailed literature on its medicinal 'folklore' history. She further gained the backing of renowned British Medical Prof. Irwin Ziment (a leading specialist in respiratory disorders, head of the American UCLA School of Medicine, and author of *Practical Pulmonary Disease*). As a result, 'hot peppers and spicy foods' became the essential ingredient enjoyed today. Dounne's name was then officially recorded in the American Chilli Institute's Hall of Fame—gaining her the respect of many doctors, gourmet connoisseurs, and food lovers alike. However, she received no recognition in Britain. Dounne was the first to reveal that hot peppers were cancer and stomach ulcer preventatives—verified by British and American scientists in 2007 (twenty years later). In 2008, she relaunched her Winter Warming Initiative, using her sauces to help save the lives of vulnerable pensioners (over twenty thousand die each year from cold-related conditions).

- **British Speciality Food Producer**

  Her's was the first black business to gain official 'British business status'; first to carry the Vegetarian Society's approval logo, and the first to obtain Jewish Kosher approval.

- **Eight National Awards**

  1990—Women mean Business; 1990—Black Achievement Award; 1991—runner-up in the British Food Processing Award (the winner was the chairman of the British Food and Drink Federation and second runner-up, the chairman of the British Meat and Livestock Commission); 1992—European Women of Achievement Award; 1993—Honorary Award; 1997—European Federation of Black Women Business-owners Award; 1999—*Voice Newspaper* outstanding Business Award; 1999—Windrush Business Pioneer Award; 2004 Trinidad and Tobago outstanding Service Award.

- **Most Influential British Woman since 1945**

  (Recognised in the BBC's celebrated book—Woman's Hour, in the chapter 'Women Who Led the Way') woman of the year-elected 1991, 1992, 2006, 2007. Fifty most powerful black women in Britain—voted 2007. the royal society of ARTS (FRSA)—a Fellow member in 2004.

- **Patron of Two British Organisations**

- **Face of the Millennium**—1999, after a worldwide search, she was chosen by Oil-of-Olay for their over fifties international advertising campaign.

- **Highest Profiled—over four hundred features on television, radio, magazines and in nineteen books . . .**
     (1988—BBC television series and book *The Perfect Pickle*; 1991—BBC television series and book *Women mean Business*; 1991—*Enterprising Women*; 1991—*Food Lovers London*; 1991—*Food by Post*; 1992 (USA) *Peppers*; 1993—*By Faith and Daring*; 1993—(USA) *Black Women for Beginners*; 1993—*The Food Lovers Guide to Britain*; 1993—*Business Class*; 1994—*The Unemployables*; 1994—*Women In Britain* (British Foreign Office);1995—*Pride of Black British Women*; 1996—(BBC) *Woman's Hour*; 1996—*Roots of the Future*; 1996—*Flavours of the Orient*; 1997—*Black Women Taking Charge*; 1998—*Black Londoners* 1880-1990; 2001—*Portraits of Black Achievement* (for UK schools).

- **Publisher, author, mentor and motivational speaker**—1990, wrote and self-published her first book *The Black Cinderella* (giving a first-hand insight into British banks' insensitivity towards women, start-ups and minority businesses, institutionalised racism and discrimination, lack of financial support and access, ineffective training or legal redress, corrupt insider dealings, plus how the system is deliberately designed to guarantee failure instead of success). She was then headhunted by the 'Shadow Government' as business advisor at cabinet level. Her recommendations for change brought about the appointment of a banking ombudsman for small businesses, plus other major policy changes still benefiting businesses today. In 2001, her second book *A mission of Love*—described as an inspirational masterpiece where she shares her conversations with God and secrets of life, gives an in-depth insight into the causes and solutions of our poor health today and how to become masters of our destiny, plus gives powerful messages for the twernty-first century. It transcends culture, race, class, gender, politics, and religion, explaining what 'life' is all about and giving it a deeper meaning and greater purpose. It has been adopted by Coventry University as a course study text in *leadership, entrepreneurship, personal/ spiritual* development, natural health, and social responsibility, plus used by entrepreneurs as a true insight into 'what it really takes' to become your own boss, especially if you are black, female, and a single parent. Dounne still speaks in schools and universities and privately mentors individuals . . . forever encouraging, motivating, and inspiring others to have faith and believe in themselves; rise above their own expectations; and become the greatest person they can *be* . . . (their authentic *Divine self*). Now at the glorious age of sixty, she says, 'I hope my ongoing work, dedication, determination, and commitment will inspire others to realise that you are never *too old* to be ambitious, to dream, to achieve.'

Dounne Alexander is worthy of press in all ramifications. When I attended her seminar lecture in 1994, I had no doubt in my mind that her health care contributions will reach every corner of the earth. Most of her products will be very useful in applied preventive therapy. Complementary and natural health practitioners should obtain such products, go through the directions, and prescribe them for preventive purposes. When in the year, 2897 BC, the African–Egyptian ancient father of traditional medicine, Imhotep, announced that our foods should be our medicine, he had no idea that his traditional commandment could be taken up by such followers as Hippocrates and company. And this concept has now spread and is being amplified by madam Dounne Alexander in our time. Glory be to God!

18.11 Tibetan Speicialist

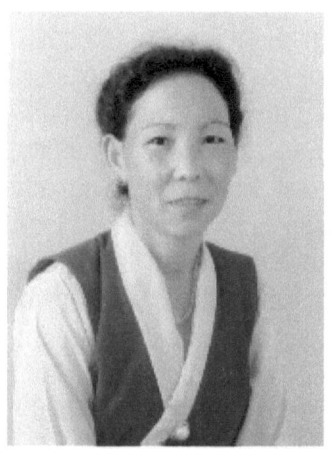

Keyzom Bhutti Phunkyil was conferred the title Amjee upon graduation from the Tibetan Medical and Astrological Institute in Dharamsala, India, in 1972.

She was the chief physician at the Tibetan Medical and Astrological Institute in Darjeeling for twenty-five years until she moved to The United States to join her husband. She now practises in the Boston, Massachusetts area. In 1988, she received the Menrampa degree (T.M.D). In recognition of her dedicated service of over twenty-five years in the field of Tibetan medicine, Amjee Bhutti received the Senior Physician's Award. In 1995, she received The Shiromani Award and in 1997 the Award of Excellence, at the Third and Fifth International Congress, respectively, of the All India board of Alternative Medicines in Calcutta, India. In 1988, the Tibetan government in exile organised a tour to France, Belgium, England, Austria, and the United States for Amjee Bhutti and Dr Tenzin Chodak, senior personal physician to HH the Dalai Lama. In 1990 she was invited to Holland to conduct consultations and clinics. Tibetan medicine has been particularly successful in its treatment of chronic diseases such as rheumatism, arthritis, ulcers, chronic digestive problems, asthma, hepatitis, eczema, liver problems, sinus problems, anxiety, and problems connected with the nervous system. Tibetan herbal—mineral supplements include up to several dozen carefully selected ingredients. These are combined according to classical formulas to balance out all except for a single potency aimed at correcting a specific type of energy imbalance with no side effects.

Further Readings and References

This chapter is devoted entirely for various Readings and Research References.

Reading refereneces of Chinese medicine and the rest of East-Asian medical sciences.

I. The Insitute of Traditional Medicine Library of East Asian Medical Sciences Books and Journals:

The information given by the ITM is placed in this book to enable the interested readers to make references of various East-Asian medical sciences.

The Institute for Traditional Medicine has established a library of medical texts collected over the past twenty-five years. The library project was inspired by the extensive holdings gathered by Joseph Needham and his colleagues at Cambridge University in England and the collection started by Hong-yen Hsu and his associates at the Oriental Healing Arts Institute in California, each of which is comprised of thousands of titles. The institute's more modest project includes four hundred English language books, of which about 160 focus on Chinese herbal medicine and related medical information and theories, which has been the primary focus of ITM's work. There are also a few Chinese language books that are not mentioned in this document, including several large illustrated guides to medicinal materials. ITM has part or all of a collection of certain journals related to Chinese herbs and acupuncture, of which only three have current subscriptions, plus other journals that contain relevant information.

The following pages detail the English language books in the collection, providing for each the name of the book and its author(s), the publication date, publisher, and principal city for the publisher's distribution. The information is presented in the format that ITM has adopted for referencing books. Oriental names of authors have the family name first, but sometimes they are Westernised, placing the family name last (in such case, it is common, though not always the practice, to hyphenate the two personal names).

To make searching for titles easier, the books have been classified as follows:

1. **Materia Medicas** and other books that provide information about the traditional uses of individual medicinal materials.
2. **Formularies** that provide information about the content and applications of numerous traditional formulas, sometimes with modern formulas included.
3. **Historical records**, including translations of traditional texts, analysis of archeological and historical records, and discussions

of the development of traditional Chinese medicine and its cultural context.

4. **Clinical experience** reports (herbal medicine), which represent suggestions for treatments of a large number of different diseases based on the experience of an individual practitioner or a group of practitioners who collaborated in writing about clinical efforts.

5. **Acupuncture and moxibustion** texts. There are dozens of books available on this subject, but many present essentially the same information; ITM's efforts have focused on herbal medicine rather than acupuncture, so this collection is somewhat limited.

6. **Food as medicine** books, depicting Oriental efforts to understand the health impact of foods. Some of these books review the historical developments of food-use in China, with only passing reference to medicine.

7. **General subjects**, including overviews of Asian medicine, special topics within the field of Chinese medicine (including physiology and diagnosis), and general analysis of the application of herbs based on the theoretical framework applied mainly to traditional prescriptions, rather than direct clinical experience of the author(s).

8. **Modern research on herbs**, including analysis of chemical constituents, pharmacology experiments, and clinical trials.

9. **Medical specialties** that are the focus of the books in the library, including cancer, ophthalmology, paediatric disorders, gynaecology, and dermatology.

10. **Translation guides**, dictionaries and books about Chinese characters—their origins, meaning, and uses—that can be used to investigate the implications of Chinese medical and philosophical terms.

11. **Tibetan medicine books**: Tibetan medicine incorporates both Ayurvedic and Chinese medical practices. Tibet has been incorporated into China during this century.

12. **Ayurvedic medicine**: Chinese medicine was partly influenced by the traditional medicine of India, with some of the herbs used by the Chinese coming from India. Like Chinese traditional medicine, Ayurvedic medicine has had a continuous history of theoretical developments, recorded experience, and professional training.

13. **Western medicine**: these are books that are used primarily for the purpose of brief description of disease characteristics and associated therapeutics, or studies of nutrients and herbal active ingredients that do not focus on Chinese herbs.
14. **Journals of Chinese medicine**: these are the journals that present information about Chinese herbs; many of them also contain articles about general Chinese medical subjects and acupuncture.
15. **Other journals**: these are journals that contain relevant information but are not specific to Chinese medicine.

The library is not a comprehensive collection of works on these subjects, partly because there are numerous books and journals that may be popular but do not have any scholarly or scientific orientation, and because others have a very limited scope. This listing includes the primary reference texts and journals used in producing the articles generated at ITM.

To assist practitioners of Chinese medicine in collecting their own library, the books have been given a rating in relation to their value for the study of Chinese medicine. This rating is placed either as a heading or as a code following the book information.

Essential Reading/Reference (ER): Most practitioners of traditional Chinese medicine will find the information in the book of value in improving their background knowledge and capabilities. Only books that have general applications related to the traditional practices are listed as essential; if the book's contents are highly focused on a special subject, the book will usually be classified as advanced reading. Out-of-print books are removed from the essential reading section, even if deemed quite valuable.

Recommended Reading/Reference (RR): The books may cover much the same ground as others that are rated as essential reading, but are less comprehensive or not as detailed. Still, these books may provide some additional insights, perspectives, specialty information, or expanded information that make them quite useful. Or, they may cover a subject of peripheral or more limited interest, but do so in an interesting way.

Advanced Reading/Reference (AR): The books contain information that may be of value for the scholarly pursuit of the field or for the pursuit of a specialty area within the field. Books that may have been designed for general use by practitioners but which fail to attain their goal and those that may require the judgment of well-educated readers to weed through the interpretations (some of which may be incorrect) or through difficult language may be classified as Advanced Reading.

Not Recommended (NR): By comparison with other available books, the books do not provide much useful information for the practice of Chinese medicine (or other fields that shed light on that practice), and/or may be poorly written, and/or is too limited in scope or too out of date to be of value to the majority of practitioners. Books that are of particularly poor quality are not included in this reference list.

Out of Print (OP): The book might only be found in a library, used books store, or by a book search service. The publisher no longer has copies available.

Clearly, there will be substantial differences in opinion about how these books ought to be rated; in fact, it was not always easy to place the books within one of the categories based on the criteria established here. These ratings are largely determined by the perceived ability to obtain information useful for producing the ITM articles about various Chinese medical subjects. Emphasis is placed on such features as: inclusion of quality translation work; comprehensiveness in dealing with the subject at hand; apparent reliability of the information presented; and readability. Sometimes, books containing valuable information may be recommended despite poor readability, and others that have reliable information may be deemed valuable despite lack of comprehensive approach or lack of complete faithfulness of translation. It is possible that a rating will be changed over time; for example, a book that is deemed essential may become out of date (and/or out of print) and may be superseded by another book on the same or similar subject that is better or, at the least, still available.

Generally, books that are well-translated Chinese medical classics and books that are written by Chinese experts with extensive experience will be rated as essential or recommended reading. Books by secondary authors, that is, those who have learnt the subject relatively recently and have rushed ahead to write what they know, are generally not recommended. Health care providers that prescribe Chinese herbs should develop a library that includes most of the essential reading books plus at least one or two of the 'recommended reading' books from each category (at least from those that correspond to their scope of practice). A minimum library of about thirty-five to forty such books in these categories would likely provide the resource information that is essential to conduct a successful practice. The books listed in the following pages that are not out of print may be obtained either directly from the publisher or from one of the many distributors of Oriental medical books, including the following:

Redwing Book Company: 44 Linden St., Brookline, MA, 02146 (general supplier of natural healing books).

Eastwind Books and Arts: 633 Vallejo St., San Francisco, CA, 94133 (selected Chinese medical books).

Oriental Healing Arts Institute: 1945 Palo Verde Ave., Long Beach, CA, 90815.

Blue Poppy Press: 1775 Linden Ave. Boulder, CO, 80304 (mainly their own publications).

Institute for Traditional Medicine: 2017 SE Hawthorne, Portland, OR, 97214

(ITM publications plus several books rated here as Essential, Recommended, or Advanced).

18.12 Materia Medicas and Guides to Individual Herbs

The most comprehensive guides to individual herbs with traditional indications and uses described are *Thousand Formulas and Thousand Herbs*, volume 1 (listing 1,000 items); *Oriental Materia Medica* (765 items); *Chinese Herbal Medicine Materia Medica* (470 items); and *Chinese-English Manual of Common-Used Herbs in Traditional Chinese Medicine* (350 items). All of these present accurate and useful information though only one, *Chinese Herbal Medicine Materia Medica*, was written by Westerners and is accepted as a teaching text at American colleges of Oriental medicine. All of these guides will prove useful to practitioners, as they have notably differing presentation styles and some differences in content even for individual herbs. *Oriental Materia Medica* is relied upon extensively for the ITM literature and contains most of the herbs that are important to know, so it is listed as an essential reference. Most of the other items in this section of the library present only a relatively small selection of herbs and present more limited information (and are therefore not recommended) or specialised information (and are deemed advanced reading) about the herbs.

Essential Reading/Reference

Hsu HY, et al., *Oriental Materia Medica: A Concise Guide*, 1986; Oriental Healing Arts Institute, Long Beach, CA.

Recommended Reading/Reference

Bensky D and Gamble A, *Chinese Herbal Medicine: Materia Medica*, 1993; Eastland Press, Seattle, WA.

Huang Bingshan and Wang Yuxia, *Thousand Formulas and Thousand Herbs of Traditional Chinese Medicine*, vol. 1, 1993; Heilongjiang Education Press, Harbin.

(OP) Ou Ming (chief editor), *Chinese-English Manual of Common-Used Herbs in Traditional Chinese Medicine*, 1989; Joint Publishing Co., Hong Kong.

Advanced Reading/Reference

Ling Yeouruenn, *A New Compendium of Materia Medica*, 1995; Science Press, Beijing.

Perry LM, *Medicinal Plants of East and Southeast Asia*, 1980; MIT Press, Cambridge, MA.

(OP) Pharmacopoeia Commission of PRC, *Pharmacopoeia of the PRC*, (English edition) 1988 People's Medical Publishing House, Beijing.

(OP; 1995 edition is available) Sionneau P, *Pao Zhi: An Introduction to the Use of Processed Chinese Medicinals*, 1995; Blue Poppy Press, Boulder, CO.

Smith FP and Stuart GA, *Chinese Medicinal Herbs*, 1973; Georgetown Press, San Francisco, CA.

Yen Kunying, *Illustrated Chinese Materia Medica*, (2 vol.), 1986; Southern Materials Center, Inc., Taipei.

Zhang Enquin (ed. in chief), *English–Chinese Rare Chinese Materia Medica*, 1990; Publishing House of Shanghai College of Traditional Chinese Medicine, Shanghai.

18.13 Formularies and Guides to Formulation

Books of formulas can be divided into three broad categories: those with the traditional formulas that are studied in China; the formulas that are used by Kanpo doctors in Japan (and similarly in Taiwan), which are mainly a subset of the former with a few items rarely discussed in China; and the patent formulas, which include traditional and modern prescriptions that are manufactured by a large number of commercial enterprises. The principal books of Chinese herbal formulas and Kanpo formulas that are relied on at ITM are from the same publishers and are companion volumes to the Materia Medica guides mentioned above. In order from largest number of traditional formulas down, *Thousand Formulas and Thousand Herbs*, volume 2, *Chinese Herbal Medicine: Formulas and Strategies*, and *Chinese-English Manual of Common-Used Prescriptions in Traditional Chinese Medicine. Commonly Used Chinese Herbal Formulas with Illustrations Companion Guide* offers over four hundred formulas that are mainly those used by Japanese Kanpo and Taiwanese practitioners. The older patent medicine guides are not very useful due to the rapidly changing availability of the patents, changing and inaccurate labelling (relied upon by Western authors of the guides), and limited information about the formulation and uses. The new book by Fratkin resolves some of these problems, at least for now. Of the formula guides, only *Chinese Herbal Medicine: Formulas and Strategies* is listed as essential reading because of the presentation of a large number of formulas along with extensive descriptions for many of them.

Essential Reading/Reference

Bensky D and Barolet R, *Chinese Herbal Medicine: Formulas and Strategies*, 1990; rev. ed., Eastland Press, Seattle, WA.

Recommended Reading/Reference

Dong Zhilin and Jiang Jingxian, *100 Famous and Effective Prescriptions of Ancient and Modern Times*, 1990; China Ocean Press, Beijing.

(OP)Fratkin J, *Chinese Herbal Patent Medicines: The Clinical Desk Reference*, 2001; Shya Publications, Boulder, CO.

Geng Junying, et al., *Practical Traditional Chinese Medicine and Pharmacology: Herbal Formulas*, 1991; New World Press, Beijing.

Hsu HY and Hsu CS, *Commonly Used Chinese Herb Formulas Companion Handbook*, 1997; Oriental Healing Arts Institute, Long Beach, CA.

Hsu HY and Hsu CS, *Commonly Used Chinese Herb Formulas with Illustrations*, 1980; rev. ed., Oriental Healing Arts Institute, Long Beach, CA.

(OP; replaced by above title) Huang Bingshan and Wang Yuxia, *Thousand Formulas and Thousand Herbs of Traditional Chinese Medicine*, vol. 2, 1993; Heilongjiang Education Press, Harbin.

(OP) Ou Ming, *Chinese-English Manual of Common-Used Prescriptions in Traditional Chinese Medicine*, 1989; Joint Publishing Co., Hong Kong.

Naeser M, *Outline Guide to Chinese Herbal Patent Medicines in Pill Form*, 1990; Boston Chinese Medicine, Boston, MA.

Songnong (chief editor), *Chinese Medicated Liquor Therapy*, 1996; Beijing Science and Technology Press, Beijing.

Zhu CH, *Clinical Handbook of Chinese Prepared Medicines*, 1989; Paradigm Publications, Brookline, MA.

Practitioners of Chinese herbal medicine are expected to be familiar with the *Nei Jing* (which has two component parts, *Su Wen* and *Ling Shu*) and with the *Shang Han Lun* (also having two parts, *Shang Han Lun* and *Jin Gui Yao Lue*); additionally, it is helpful to be aware of one or more works of famous physicians, such as Li Dongyuan (aka Li Gao). Translation of these ancient texts is no easy matter. Chinese writing tends to be quite succinct and readers (especially translators) often read into the text things that may or may not have been intended by the original author(s). Often, the book that is being translated has already been modified from the original by Chinese authors who not only copied the text, but made corrections, rearrangements, and interpretations. Despite some concerns about the translations, one volume each of the *Nei Jing* components have been rated as essential reading, and one volume each of the *Shang Han Lun* have been rated as recommended reading. Most others are either not recommended or are suggested only for those undertaking advanced studies; the exception is the unique work by Zhang Xuchun translated by Paul Unschuld under the title *Forgotten Traditions of Ancient Chinese Medicine*, which, I believe, provides valuable insights into the thinking about traditional Chinese medicine and the forces that shape it, and has been rated as essential reading (made easier by having available an inexpensive paperback version).

Essential Reading/Reference

Maoshing Ni, *The Yellow Emperor's Classic of Medicine: A New Translation of the Neijing Suwen with Commentary*, 1995; Shambhala, Boston, MA.

Unschuld PU, *Forgotten Traditions of Ancient Chinese Medicine*, 1990; Paradigm Publications, Brookline, MA.

Wu Jingnuan (translator), *Ling Shu, or The Spiritual Pivot*, 1993; Taoist Center, Washington, D.C.

Recommended Reading/Reference

Chen Ping (editor in chief), *History and Development of Traditional Chinese Medicine*, 1999; Science Press, Beijing.

Hsu HY and Peacher WG (editors), *Shang Han Lun: The Great Classic of Chinese Medicine*, 1981; Oriental Healing Arts Institute, Long Beach, CA.

Hsu HY and Wang SY (translators), *Chin Kuei You Lueh*, 1983; Oriental Healing Arts Institute, Long Beach, CA.

Hsu HY and Wang SY, *The Theory of Feverish Diseases and Its Clinical Applications*, 1985; Oriental Healing Arts Institute, Long Beach, CA.

Unschuld PU, *Medicine in China: History of Pharmaceutics*, 1986; University of California Press, Berkeley, CA.

Unschuld PU, *Medicine in China: A History of Ideas*, 1985; University of California Press, Berkeley, CA.

Yang Shouzhong and Li Jianyong (translators), *Li Dongyuan's Treatise on the Spleen and Stomach*, 1993; Blue Poppy Press, Boulder, CO.

Zhu Ming, *The Medical Classic of the Yellow Emperor*, 2001; Foreign Languages Press, Beijing.

Advanced Reading/Reference

Chace C and Zhang Tingliang, *A Qin Bowei Anthology*, 1997; Paradigm Publications, Brookline, MA.

Nakayama S and Sivin N, (editors), *Chinese Science: Explorations of an Ancient Tradition*, 1973; MIT Press, Cambridge, MA.

(OP) Needham J, *Science and Civilisation in China*, vol. 2, 1974; Cambridge University Press, London.

Unschuld PU, *Introductory Readings in Classical Chinese Medicine*, 1988; Kluwer Academic Publishers, Dordrecht, Holland.

Unschuld PU, *Medicine in China: Nan-Ching*, 1986; University of California Press, Berkeley, CA.

Unschuld PU, *Medicine in China: Historical Artifacts and Images*, 2000; Prestel Verlag, Munich.

Wong KC and Wu LT, *History of Chinese Medicine*, 1973; AMS Press, Inc., New York.

(OP) Yang Shouzhong (translator), *Extra Treatises based on Investigation and Inquiry (Gezhi Yulun)*, 1994; Blue Poppy Press, Boulder, CO.

Yang Shouzhong (translator), *The Heart Transmission of Medicine*, 1997; Blue Poppy Press, Boulder, CO.

Yang Shouzhong, *Master Hua's Classic of the Central Viscera*, 1993; Blue Poppy Press, Boulder, CO.

Yang Shouzhong (translator), *The Divine Farmer's Materia Medica*, 1997; Blue Poppy Press, Boulder, CO.

Yang Shouzhong and Chace C, *The Systematic Classic of Acupuncture and Moxibustion*, 1994; Blue Poppy Press, Boulder, CO.

Zhang Zhongjing, *Synopsis of Prescriptions of the Golden Chamber*, 1987; New World Press, Beijing.

Zhang Zhongjing, *Treatise on Febrile Diseases Caused by Cold with 500 Cases*, 1993; New World Press, Beiji.

It became common practice in China for physicians to compile suggestions of treatments—herbal formulas—based on what was done in their own practice or what was generally done at a hospital facility. These books may be compiled by experienced physicians or by young practitioners who report on what they have learnt from their teachers. Frequently, these books are laid out according to disorder (a favoured pattern is to deal with disorders of the body from top to down, then general metabolic disorders, and then deal with specialty areas, such as gynaecology, paediatrics, and 'surgical problems'). There is a brief description of the aetiology and manifestation of the disease, traditional subcategories (e.g. liver fire, spleen weakness, liver/kidney deficiency), and one or more recommended formulas. In some books, a case study is presented, and this case usually shows that the prescription given to the patient is not the same as the one that has just been recommended in the book, but, rather, a derivative or modification. Unfortunately, it is difficult to rate any of these as essential reading, as they rarely provide sufficient insight, but some are recommended because the information presented appears to be a reliable reflection of modern Chinese practice.

Recommended Reading/Reference

Shang Xianmin, et al., *Practical Traditional Chinese Medicine and Pharmacology: Clinical Experiences*, 1990; New World Press, Beijing.

Yan Wu and Warren Fischer, *Practical Therapeutics of Traditional Chinese Medicine*, 1997; Paradigm Publications, Brookline, MA.

Zhang Enquin, *Clinic of Traditional Chinese Medicine*, 1990; Publishing House of Shanghai College of Traditional Chinese Medicine, Shanghai.

Advanced Reading/Reference

Fruehauf H and Dharmananda S, *Treatment of Difficult and Recalcitrant Diseases with Chinese Herbs*, 1997; ITM, Portland, OR.

Maciocia G, *The Practice of Chinese Medicine*, 1994; Churchill Livingstone, London.

Shao Nianfang, *The Treatment of Knotty Diseases with Chinese Acupuncture and Chinese Herbal Medicine*, 1990; Shandong Science and Technology Press, Jinan.

Wang Qi and Dong Zhilin, *Modern Clinical Necessities for Traditional Chinese Medicine*, 1990; China Ocean Press, Beijing.

18.14 Acupuncture and Moxibustion

The books included here fall into three broad categories: first, books that list each point (somewhat like the materia medica guides do for herbs) and present the relevant information; these books often also attach some information about treatment strategies; second, specialty books that deal with a particular type of therapy: ear acupuncture, scalp acupuncture, moxibustion, etc.; third, books that are organised according to treatment of diseases (in these, it is assumed that the acupuncturist already knows about the individual points and the various treatment methods). For a book to be recommended, it must present both reliable standard and extensive information; there are plenty of books available that offer information that does not tie in to any standard theories or practices (the book is often highly personal) and several that provide too little detail to be of much use other than as a quick reminder for those who have learnt the field very well (in which case, the book is probably not needed). Since acupuncture is usually practised only after extensive training, the value of these books is to provide additional insights that might have been missed or forgotten.

Essential Reading/Reference

Ellis A, Wiseman N, and Boss K, *Fundamentals of Chinese Acupuncture*, 1988; Paradigm Publications, Brookline, MA.

Qiu Maoliang (Man. ed.), *Chinese Acupuncture and Moxibustion*, 1993; Churchill Livingstone, London.

Recommended Reading/Reference

Chen Ken and Cui Yonquiang, *Handbook to Chinese Auricular Therapy*, 1990; Foreign Language Press, Beijing.

Cheng Xinnong (chief editor), *Chinese Acupuncture and Moxibustion*, 1987; Foreign Languages Press, Beijing.

Deadman P and Mazin AK, *A Manual of Acupuncture*, 1998; Journal of Chinese Medicine Publications, East Sussex, England.

Ellis A, Wiseman N, and Boss K, *Grasping the Wind*, 1989; Paradigm Publications, Brookline, MA.

Mingching Zhu, *Zhu's Scalp Acupuncture*, 1992; Eight Dragons Publishing, Hong Kong.

O'Connor J and Bensky D (translators), *Acupuncture: A Comprehensive Text,* 1981; Eastland Press, Seattle, WA.

Yu Huichan and Han Furu, *Golden Needle Wang Leting,* 1996; Blue Poppy Press, Boulder, CO.

Zhang Enquin (editor in chief), *Chinese Acupuncture and Moxibustion,* 1990; Publishing House of Shanghai College of Traditional Chinese Medicine, Shanghai.

Zhang Ru and Dong Zhilin, *Modern Clinical Necessities for Acupuncture and Moxibustion,* 1990; China Ocean Press, Beijing.

Advanced Reading/Reference

Kong Yaoqi, Ren Xingsheng, and Lu Shoukang, *The Acupuncture Treatment for Parlaysis,* 1996; Science Press, Beijing.

Ross J, *Acupuncture Point Combinations: The Key to Clinical Success,* 1995; Churchill Livingstone, London.

Zhang Ruifu, Wu Xifen, and Wang NS, *Illustrated Dictionary of Chinese Acupuncture,* 1986; Sheep's Publication, U.S.A., San Francisco, CA.

Mingching Zhu, *A Handbook for Treatment of Acute Syndromes by Using Acupuncture and Moxibustion,* 1992; Eight Dragons Publishing, Hong Kong.

Medical Publishing House, Beijing.

18.15 Food as Medicine

In China, the border between foods and medicines is indefinite. The principles of therapy governing herbs are the same as those governing foods. Therefore, the study of food from the Chinese perspective is valuable to those who prescribe herbs. The books listed here have very diverse nature; for example, *The Food of China* and *Food in Chinese Culture* are academic studies of the historical introduction and reliance on various foods with only passing mention of their medicinal value, while most of the other books are about using the foods for specific healing actions.

Recommended Reading/Reference

Chang Chaoliang, et al., *Vegetables as Medicine*, 1989; The Ram's Skull Press, Kuranda, Australia. (OP)

Dai Yinfang and Liu Chengjun, *Fruit as Medicine*, 1986; The Ram's Skull Press, Kuranda, Australia. (OP)

Lu HC, *Chinese System of Food Cures*, 1986; Sterling Publishing Co. Inc., New York.

Ni MS, *The Tao of Nutrition*, 1987; College of Tao and Traditional Chinese Healing, Los Angeles, CA.

Advanced Reading/Reference

Anderson EN, *The Food of China*, 1988; Yale University Press, New Haven, CT.

Chang KC, *Food in Chinese Culture*, 1977; Yale University Press, New Haven, CT.

Zhang Enquin (ed. in chief), *Chinese Medicated Diet*, 1988; Publishing House of Shanghai College of Traditional Chinese Medicine, Shanghai.

18.16 General

Essential Reading/Reference

Maciocia G, *The Foundations of Chinese Medicine*, 1989; Churchill Livingstone, London.

Recommended Reading/Reference

Chace C and Zhang Tingliang, *A Qin Bowei Anthology*, 1997; Paradigm Publications, Brookline, MA.

Chen Zelin and Chen Meifang, *A Comprehensive Guide to Chinese Herbal Medicine*, 1992; Oriental Healing Arts Institute, Long Beach, CA.

Fruehauf H, *Five Organ Networks of Chinese Medicine*, 1998; ITM, Portland, OR.

Katpchuk TJ, *The Web That Has No Weaver: Understanding Chinese Medicine*, 1983; St. Martins Press, New York.

State Administration of Traditional Chinese Medicine, *Advanced Textbook on Traditional Chinese Medicine and Pharmacology*, (4 vol.) 1995-6; New World Press, Beijing.

Wang Qi and Dong Zhi Lin, *New Practical Syndrome Differentiation of T.C.M.*, 1992; China Ocean Press, Beijing. (OP)

Xu Xiangcai (chief editor), *The English-Chinese Encyclopedia of Practical Traditional Chinese Medicine*, (21 vols.) 1989; Higher Education Press, Beijing.

Advanced Reading/Reference

Chen Zelin and Chen Meifang, *The Essence and Scientific Background of Tongue Diagnosis*, 1989; Oriental Healing Arts Institute, Long Beach, CA.

Hsu HY and Peacher WG, *Chen's History of Chinese Medical Science*, 1978; Oriental Healing Arts Institute, Long Beach, CA.

Kleinman A, Kunstadter P, et al., *Culture and Healing in Asian Societies*, 1978; Schenkman Publishing Company, Cambridge, MA.

Larre C and de la Vallée ER, *Rooted in Spirit: The Heart of Chinese Medicine*, 1995; Station Hill Press, Barrytown, NY.

Larre C, Schatz J, and de la Vallée ER, *Survey of Traditional Chinese Medicine*, 1986; Traditional Acupuncture Institute, Columbia, MD.

Leslie C (editor), *Asian Medical Systems*, 1976; University of California Press, Berkeley, CA.

Sionneau P, *Dui Yao: The Art of Combining Chinese Medicinals*, 1997; Blue Poppy Press, Boulder, CO.

Hillier SM and Jewell JA, *Health Care and Traditional Medicine in China 1800-1982*, 1983; Routledge and Kegan Paul, London.

(OP) Hsu HY, *How to Treat Yourself with Chinese Herbs*, 1980; Oriental Healing Arts Institute, Long Beach, CA.

Hyatt R, *Healing with Chinese Herbs*, 1990; Healing Arts Press, Rochester, VT.

Toyohiko Kikutani, *Combined Use of Western Therapies and Chinese Medicine*, 1987; Oriental Healing Arts Institute, Long Beach, CA.

Liu Zhengcai, *The Mystery of Longevity*, 1990; Foreign Language Press, Beijing.

Ross J, *Zang Fu: The Organ Systems of Traditional Chinese Medicine*, 1989; Churchill Livingstone, London.

Sivin N, *Traditional Medicine in Contemporary China*, 1987; University of Michigan, Ann Arbor, MI.

Unschuld PU, *Chinese Medicine*, 1998; Paradigm Publications, Brookline, MA.

Wiseman N, and Ellis A, *Fundamentals of Chinese Medicine*, 1985; Paradigm Pub., Brookline, MA.

18.17 Modern Research on Herbs

Chemical, pharmacological, and clinical evaluation of herbs has been a major thrust of work in China (and other Asian countries, notably Japan) for fifty years. Additionally, during the past twenty years or so, Western researchers have taken up this subject. A difficulty with relying on books for this type of information is the rapidity with which they become outdated. The quality and type of research being conducted has improved greatly in recent years; this makes reliance on earlier and poorer quality research less useful. Still, while some areas of research are highly active, others are quite slow to show progress, so compilations of research in one place, as in some of these books, is a handy way to access it. Many of these books are already out of print, because research-oriented texts are usually produced in a single, small-print run. For practitioners who prescribe the herbs, these books will generally prove to be advanced reading; they are especially helpful to those who teach on the subject of research or who plan to conduct research. More up-to-date information is obtained from journals, though there are very few of them presenting full research reports in English. Unlike medical journals, these books always contain abstracted information, and it is sometimes difficult to evaluate the validity and applicability of the reported findings.

Recommended Reading/Reference

Zhu YP, *Chinese Materia Medica: Chemistry, Pharmacology, and Applications*, 1998; Harwood Academic Publishers, Amsterdam.

Chang HM and But PPH (editors), *Pharmacology and Applications of Chinese Materia Medica*, (2 vols.), 1986; World Scientific, Singapore. *[OP; replaced by above title]*

Advanced Reading/Reference

Dong Zhilin and Yu Shufang, *Modern Study and Application of Materia Medica*, 1990; China Ocean Press, Beijing. (OP)

Hsu HY, Chen YP, and Hong Ming, *The Chemical Constituents of Oriental Herbs*, 1982; Oriental Healing Arts Institute, Long Beach, CA.

Chang HM, et al., *Advances in Chinese Medicinal Materials Research*, 1985; World Scientific, Singapore. (OP).

Ko R and Au A, *1997-1998 Compendium of Asian Patent Medicines*, 1998; California Department of Health Services, Sacramento, CA. (OP).

Tang W and Eisenbrand G, *Chinese Drugs of Plant Origin*, 1992; Springer-Verlag, Berlin. (OP).

Ying Jianzhe, Mao Xiadan, et al., *Icones of Medicinal Fungi from China*, 1987; Science Press, Beijing. (OP).

Zhou Jinhuang, et al., *Recent Advances in Chinese Herbal Drugs-Actions and Uses*, 1991; Science Press, Beijing. (OP).

18.18 Medical Specialities

Individuals seeking treatment by Chinese medicine often prefer to have a specialist trained in their particular area of concern. In the West, there is little specialisation, but the need for detailed knowledge in several fields remains. Examples of specialisations that appear in the literature are dermatology, rheumatology, ophthalmology, gynaecology, and paediatrics. These books usually have the same basic characteristics as those described above under the heading 'Clinical Experience.' Cancer treatment with herbs is a major area of clinical practice in China and is of growing interest to Westerners. There has been a substantial change in emphasis in China, from use of herbs to treat cancer to use of herbs as an adjunct to cancer therapies. The book *Treating Cancer with Chinese Herbs* is an example of one reporting on treatments with herbs alone, while *Cancer Treatment with Fu Zheng Pei Ben Principle* is an example of one that is limited to addressing adverse effects of modern cancer therapies. Some of these books are guides to the individual herbs that may be used for either of these purposes, such as *Anticancer Medicinal Herbs*. To be recommended reading, the book must present extensive information about the herbs or substantial details about treatment strategies; due to the fact that these books involve specialisation, none have been rated as essential reading.

Cancer

Recommended Reading/Reference

Chang Minyi, *Anticancer Medicinal Herbs*, 1992; Hunan Science and Technology Publishing House, Changsha.

Pan Mingji, *Cancer Treatment with Fu Zheng Pei Ben Principle*, 1992; Fujian Science and Technology Publishing House, Fujian. (OP)

Advanced Reading/Reference

Hsu HY, *Treating Cancer with Chinese Herbs*, 1990; Oriental Healing Arts Institute, Long Beach, CA.

Jia Kun, *Prevention and Treatment of Carcinoma in Traditional Chinese Medicine*, 1985; The Commercial Press, Hong Kong.

Ou Ming, et al., *An Illustrated Guide to Antineoplastic Chinese Herbal Medicine*, 1990; The Commercial Press, Hong Kong.

Shi Lanling and Shi Peiquan, *Experience in Treating Carcinomas with Traditional Chinese Medicine*, 1992; Shandong Science and Technology Press, Shandong.

Pan Mingji, *How to Discover Cancer Through Self-Examination*, 1992; Fujian Science and Technology Publishing House, Fujian.

Sun Chiyuan, *A Probing into the Treatment of Leukemia with Traditional Chinese Medicine*, 1990; Hai Feng Publishing Company, Hong Kong.

Zhang Daizhao, *The Treatment of Cancer by Integrated Chinese-Western Medicine*, 1989; Blue Poppy Press, Boulder, CO.

Dermatology

Li Lin, *Practical Traditional Chinese Dermatology*, 1995; Hai Feng Publishing Company, Hong Kong.

(RR)Liang Jianhui, *A Handbook of Traditional Chinese Dermatology*, 1988; Blue Poppy Press, Boulder, CO.

(AR) Shen Dehui, Wu Xiufen, and Wang N, *Manual of Dermatology in Chinese Medicine*, 1995; Eastland Press, Seattle, WA.

(NR) Xu Xiangcai (chief editor), *The English-Chinese Encyclopedia of Practical Traditional Chinese Medicine*, (vol. 16: Dermatology), 1991; Higher Education Press, Beijing. [RR]

Gerontology

Liu Zhengcai, *The Mystery of Longevity*, 1990; Foreign Languages Press, Beijing. (AR)

Yan Dexin, *Aging and Blood Stasis: A New TCM Approach to Geriatrics*, 1995; Blue Poppy Press, Boulder, CO. (AR)

Infections and Feverish Diseases

Hou Jinglun, et al. (editors), *Traditional Chinese Treatment of Infectious Diseases*, 1997; Academy Press, Beijing. (AR)

Wen JM and Seifert G, *Warm Disease Theory*, 2000; Paradigm Publications, Brookline, MA. (RR)

Paediatrics

Cao Jiming, Su Xinming, and Cao Junqi (editors), *Essentials of Traditional Chinese Pediatrics*, 1990; Foreign Language Press, Beijing. (RR)

Xu Xiangcai (chief editor), *The English–Chinese Encyclopedia of Practical Traditional Chinese Medicine*, (vol. 13: Pediatrics), 1991; Higher Education Press, Beijing. (RR)

Xiao Shuqin, Zhang Xiwen, et al., *Pediatric Bronchitis: Its TCM Cause, Diagnosis, and Treatment*, 1991; Blue Poppy Press, Boulder, CO. (AR)

Gynaecology/Urology

Furth C, *A Flourishing Yin: Gender in China's Medical History, 960–1665*, 1999; University of California Press, Berkeley, CA. (AR)

Lin A, *A Handbook of TCM Urology and Male Sexual Dysfunction*, 1992; Blue Poppy Press, Boulder, CO. (NR)

Shibata Y and Wu J, *Kampo Treatment for Climacteric Disorders*, 1997; Paradigm Publications, Brookline, MA. (AR)

Xu Xiangcai (chief editor), *The English–Chinese Encyclopedia of Practical Traditional Chinese Medicine*, (vol. 12: Gynecology), 1990; Higher Education Press, Beijing. (RR)

Neurology

Cheung CS, Lai YK, and Kaw UA, *Mental Dysfunction as Treated by Traditional Chinese Medicine*, 1981; Traditional Chinese Medicine Publisher, San Francisco, CA. (OP)

Ophthalmology

Xu Xiangcai (chief editor), *The English–Chinese Encyclopedia of Practical Traditional Chinese Medicine*, (vol. 17: Ophthalmology), 1994; Higher Education Press, Beijing. (RR)

Kovacs J and Unschuld PU, *Essential Subtleties on the Silver Sea*, 1998; University of California Press, Berkeley, CA. (AR)

Orthopaedics, Traumatology, and Rheumatology

Xu Xiangcai (chief editor), *The English–Chinese Encyclopedia of Practical Traditional Chinese Medicine*, (vol. 14: Orthopedics and Traumatology), 1992; Higher Education Press, Beijing. (RR)

Vangermeersch C and Sun Peilin, *Bi-Syndromes*, 1994; SATAS, Belgium. (AR)

18.19 Translation Guides

This section includes a wide range of books about Chinese characters, as well as some books that are specifically about Chinese medicine. Although practitioners of Chinese medicine can rely on dictionaries that translate terms from Chinese to English and English to Chinese, a knowledge of the basic Chinese characters may aid in deeper understanding of the concepts.

Recommended Reading/Reference

Anonymous, *Learner's Chinese-English Dictionary*, 5th edn, 1984; Nanyang Siang Pau and Umum Publisher, Singapore.

Lindqvist C, *China: Empire of Living Symbols*, 1991; Addison-Wesley Publishing Co., NY.

Wiseman N, *English-Chinese, Chinese-English Dictionary of Chinese Medicine*, 1995; Foreign Languages Press, Beijing.

Advanced Reading/Reference

Fazzioli E, *Chinese Calligraphy: From Pictograph to Ideogram: The History of 214 Essential Chinese/Japanese Characters*, 1986; Abbeville Press, NY.

Li Leyi, *Tracing The Roots of Chinese Characters: 500 Cases*, 1993; Beijing Language and Culture University Press, Beijing.

Liao SJ (editor), *Chinese-English Terminology of Traditional Chinese Medicine*, 1981; Hunan Science and Technology Press, Hunan.

Tan Huaypeng, *Fun with Chinese Characters: The Straits Times Collection* (3 volumes), 1980-3; Federal Publications, Hong Kong.

Wang Hongyuan, *The Origins of Chinese Characters*, 1993; Sinolingua, Beijing.

Wieger L, *Chinese Characters: Their Origin, Etymology, History, Classification, and Signification*, 1965; Dover Publications, NY.

Wilder GD and Ingram JH, *Analysis of Chinese Characters*, 1974; Dover Publications, NY.

Wiseman N, and Boss K, *Glossary of Chinese Medical Terms and Acupuncture Points*, 1990; Paradigm Publications, Brookline, MA.

Wiseman N and Ye Feng, *A Practical Dictionary of Chinese Medicine*, 1998; Paradigm Publications, Brookline, MA.

Xie Zhufan and Huang Xiokai (editors), *Dictionary of Traditional Chinese Medicine*, 1984; Commercial Press, Hong Kong.

18.20 Tibetan Medicine

Tibetan medicine is an integration of four traditions: Ayurvedic medicine and Buddhism from India, the pre-Buddhist shamanism that existed in Tibet, and Chinese medicine. Many of these books are difficult to obtain and provide limited information. However, for those who wish to know Tibetan medicine, a study of several of the books, especially those listed here as recommended reading, will provide a good overview.

Recommended Reading/Reference

Clifford T, *Tibetan Buddhist Medicine and Psychiatry: The Diamond Healing*, 1984; Samuel Weiser, Inc., York Beach, ME.

Norbu D, *An Introduction to Tibetan Medicine*, 1976; Tibetan Review, New Delhi.

Rapgay L, et al., *Mind and Mental Health in Tibetan Medicine*, 1988; Potala Publications, New York.

Tsarong TJ, *Fundamentals of Tibetan Medicine*, 1981; Tibetan Medical Centre, Dharamsala, India.

Advanced Reading/Reference

Baker IA, *The Tibetan Art of Healing*, 1997; Thames and Hudson, London.

Clark B, *The Quintessence Tantras of Tibetan Medicine*, 1995; Snow Lion Publications, Ithica, NY.

Dash VB, *Tibetan Medicine, with Special Reference to Yoga Sataka*, 1985; Library of Tibetan Works and Archives, New Delhi.

Dhönden Y, *The Ambrosia Heart Tantra*, 1977; Library of Tibetan Works and Archives, New Delhi.

Rapgay L, *The Art of Tibetan Medical Urinalysis*, 1986; Tibetan Holistic Medical Series, Dharamsala, India.

Rechung Rinpoche, *Tibetan Medicine*, 1976; University of California Press, Berkeley, CA.

Tsarong TJ, *Handbook of Traditional Tibetan Drugs*, 1986; Tibetan Medical Publications, West Bengal, India.

Out of Print

Dhönden Y and Kelsang J, *Tibetan Medicine (Series No. 6)*, 1983; Library of Tibetan Works and Archives, New Delhi.

Kilty G, *Tibetan Medicine (Series No. 7)*, 1984; Library of Tibetan Works and Archives, New Delhi.

Molvray M, *Tibetan Medicine (Series No. 11)*, 1988; Library of Tibetan Works and Archives, New Delhi.

Lobsang Rapgay, *Tibetan Medicine (Series No. 3)*, 1981; Library of Tibetan Works and Archives, New Delhi.

18.21 Ayurvedic Medicine

Ayurvedic medicine differs markedly from Chinese medicine, but there are some areas of overlap: both systems were codified around the same time in civilisations at similar stages of development; both systems have many herbs in common; and both systems have strong emphasis on the value of food as medicine, the use of traditional formulations, and the application of physical exercises (e.g. yoga in India and taiji in China), and physical therapies (e.g. massage in India and acupuncture in China). The problem with Ayurvedic medicine that also plagues Chinese medicine is that there are so many books produced that are not very true to the tradition. However, unlike Chinese medicine, which has a large and growing profession in the West, Ayurveda is mostly taught to laypersons outside of India, so the demand for rigorous training is less. This has some effect on the quality of publications. Only two books have been deemed essential reading: *Ayurveda: Life, Health, Longevity* (for background on the entire field of Ayurvedic medicine) and the *Indian Materia Medica*, which has a good overview of the individual herbs from the traditional viewpoint (it was written more than seventy-five years ago, though republished more recently), with mention of many valued herb combinations.

Essential Reading/Reference

Nadkarni KM, *Indian Materia Medica*, (2 vol.), 1976; Popular Prakashan Put. Ltd., Bombay.

Svoboda R, *Ayurveda: Life, Health, and Longevity*, 1992; Penguin Books, India, New Delhi.

Recommended Reading/Reference

Harish Johari, *Ayurvedic Massage*, 1996; Healing Arts Press, Rochester, VT.

Verma V, *Ayurveda: A Way of Life*, 1985; Samuel Weiser, Inc., York Beach, ME.

Advanced Reading/Reference

Kaviratna AC and Sharma P (translators), *Caraka-Samhita*, Second Revised Edition (5 volumes), 1996; Indian Books Centre, Delhi.

Kutumbiah P, *Ancient Indian Medicine*, 1962; Orient Longman Ltd., Bombay. (OP)

Svoboda R, *Prakruti: Your Ayurvedic Constitution*, 1989; Geocom, Albuquerque, NM.

Svoboda R and Lade A, *Tao and Dharma: Chinese Medicine and Ayurveda*, 1995; The Lotus Press, Twin Lakes, WI.

Zysk K, *Asceticism and Healing in Ancient India*, 1991; Oxford University Press, New York.

18.22 Western Herbs and Western Medicine

When patients present their Western diagnosis, it is important for the practitioner of traditional medicine to understand it, be able to discuss the matter within certain limits, and, as may be necessary, explain the traditional treatment in relation to the Western diagnosis and treatment. Western medicine includes general understanding of diagnosis and treatment, as presented in guides and encyclopedias, and reference to specific treatment methods, including drugs, nutritional supplements, and herbs. Books that have been found valuable for ITM presentation of information about disorders are listed here.

Essential Reading/Reference

Berkow R (editor in chief), *The Merck Manual* (17th edn), 1997; Merck & Co., Rahway, NJ.

Recommended Reading/Reference

Boik J, *Natural Compounds in Cancer Therapy*, 2001; Oregon Medical Press, Princeton, MN.

Clayman CB (editor), *AMA Encyclopedia of Medicine*, 1989; Random House, New York.

Grieve M, *A Modern Herbal*, 1971; Dover Publications, New York.

Murray M and Pizzorno J, *Encyclopedia of Natural Medicine*, 1990; Prima Publishing, Rocklin, CA.

Rybacki JJ and Long JW, *The Essential Guide to Prescription Drugs*, 1997; HarperPerennial, New York.

Werbach M, *Foundations of Nutritional Medicine*, 1997; Third Line Press, Tarzana, CA.

Werbach M, *Healing Through Nutrition*, 1993; HarperCollins, New York.

Werbach M, *Nutritional Influences on Illness*, Second Edition, 1993; Third Line Press, Tarzana, CA.

Werbach M, *Nutritional Influences on Mental Illness*, Second Edition, 1999; Third Line Press, Tarzana, CA.

Advanced Reading/Reference

Blumental M, et al., *The Complete German Commission E Monographs*, 1998; American Botanical Council, Austin, TX.

Blumental M, Goldberg A, and Brinckman J, *Herbal Medicine: Expanded Commission E Monographs*, 2000; American Botanical Council, Austin, TX.

Cody V, Middleton Jr., E, and Harborne JB (editors), *Plant Flavonoids in Biology and Medicine*, 1987; Alan R. Liss, Inc., New York.

Goth A, *Medical Pharmacology*, 1984; C.V. Mosby Co., St. Louis, MO.

Eake CD, *An Historical Account of Pharmacology to the Twentieth Century*, 1975; Charles C. Thomas, Springfield, IL.

Morton JF, *Major Medicinal Plants: Botany, Culture, and Uses*, Charles C. Thomas, Springfield, IL.

Tyler VE, Brady LR, and Robbers JE, *Pharmacognosy*, 1976; Lea & Febiger, Philadelphia, PA.

18.23 Journals of Chinese Medicine

Publishing a journal is an arduous task, and it is especially difficult when the number of subscribers is small (most journals of Chinese medicine number their subscribers only in the hundreds) and when the number of excellent reports is also small (few practitioners of Chinese medicine have received training that would lead to production of high-quality reports). As a result, there are relatively few journals, and most of them have a short publication life. Following are the journals that have been received at ITM, either by subscription or donation. Though none are of such high quality as to be deemed essential reading, practitioners of Chinese medicine ought to have at least two research oriented journals, and (of the ones still available for subscription) the ones used most at ITM are *Journal of Traditional Chinese Medicine*, the *International Journal of Oriental Medicine*, and the *Journal of Integrated Traditional and Western Medicine.*

Recommended Reading/Reference

Bulletin of the Oriental Healing Arts Institute (published 1976–88; back issues available from Oriental Healing Arts Institute, Long Beach, CA). (OP)

International Journal of Oriental Medicine (published since 1989; Oriental Healing Arts Institute, Long Beach, CA).

Journal of the American College of Traditional Chinese Medicine (published 1982-9; back issues available from the American College of TCM, San Francisco, CA). (OP)

The Journal of Traditional Chinese Medicine (published since 1981; 18 Beixincang, Dongzhimen Nei, Beijing 100700).

Advanced Reading/Reference

Abstracts of Chinese Medicine (published 1987–96; Medicinal Materials Research Center, Chinese University of Hong Kong, Shatin, N.T., Hong Kong; back issues not available). (OP)

Chinese Journal of Integrated Traditional and Western Medicine (Beijing; English language publication since 1995; Press: 1 Caochang, Xiyuan, Beijing 100091, China).

18.24 Other Journals

Although not devoted to Chinese medicine or even to natural medicine, the *Journal of the American Medical Association* (JAMA) is strongly recommended for practitioners of Chinese medicine so that the latest advances in knowledge of medicine can be viewed. JAMA has recently published several articles on alternative medicine and provided clinical study reports about nutritional supplements and herbs.

Recommended Reading/Reference

Herbalgram (American Botanical Council, P.O. Box 201660, Austin, TX 78720).

Journal of the American Medical Association (515 N State St., Chicago, IL 60610).

Advanced Reading/Reference

Journal of Naturopathic Medicine (Journal Management Group, Ten Morgan Ave., Norwalk, CT 06851). *Protocol Journal of Botanical Medicine* (published 1995–7; P. O. Box 108, Harvard, MA 01451). (OP)

Chapter 19

Bibliography

I owe profound thanks to many scientists, doctors, nutritionists, homoeopaths, naturopaths, herbalists and all other natural medicine practitioners. My special regards to NSA, the producers of the famous Juice Plus Products including the researchers of various professional medical articles published by the Institute of Optimum Nutrition. Also I must thank Dr Llaila Afrika who is one the principal naturopathic doctors of our time for his contributions in this book. The following references have guided my completion of this book:

- *Health and Disease* by Baser Dave, Alasdair Gray & Cliffside. Published by the Open University Press Buckingham.
- *A Manual of Traditional and Complementary Medicine* by Dr. HCA Vogel. Published by Mainstream Publishers (The nature doctor).
- *The Vitamin Bible* by Dr. Earl Mendel. Published by Arlington Books, London.
- *How to Eat to Live* by Elijah Muhammad. Published by the Nation of Islam USA.
- *The Organ of Medicine* by Dr. Samuel Hahneman. Published by Victor.
- *Homeopathy and Human Evolution* by Martin Miles. Published by Winter Press, London.
- *Signs and Symptoms of Vitamin Deficiency* by Dr. Leonard Mervin. Published by Anberwood Publishing Limited.
- *Family Medical Encyclopaedia* by Heart Corporation, London.
- *Healing with Herbal Justice* by Sigrid Gusher.
- 'Tomorrow's Medicine' by *Optimum Nutrition Magazine,* 1998.
- *Homoeopathy Up-date Magazine.* Published by Jain Publishing Ltd. India.

- *Homoeopathy International* by UK Homoeopathic Medical Association, London.
- *Healthy Way Magazine* by Bio-force UK Limited.
- *Guide to Homoeopathy* by Dr. Anne Clover.
- *What Is the Alternative?* by Hazel Courtney.
- *Health Guardian Magazine* by Health guardian Publishers Limited (UK).

Resource Articles Used in Reference of These Document Reviews on Garlic:

Chang HM and But PPH, *Pharmacology and Applications of Chinese Materia Medica,* 1986; volume 1, pages 84-93 (with 57 references), World Scientific, Singapore.

Tang W and Eisenbrand G, *Chinese Drugs of Plant Origin,* 1992; pages 79-86 (with 35 references), Springer Verlag, Berlin.

Recent Articles

The following articles were published during the five years prior to the current paper and were used as sources of information presented here.

Desponded RG, et al., Inhibition of Mycobacterium avium complex isolates from AIDS patients by garlic, *Journal of Antimicrobial Chemotherapy,* 1993; 32: 623-6.

Guo NL, et al., Demonstration of the antiviral activity of garlic extract against human cytomegalovirus in vitro, *Chinese Medical Journal,* 1993; 106 (2): 93-6.

Guo NL, et al., Inhibitory effect of garlic extract on cytomegalovirus, *Journal of Beijing Medical University,* 1990; 22(2): 152.

Morioka N, et al. A protein fraction from aged garlic extract enhances cytotoxicity and proliferation of human lymphocytes mediated by interleukin-2 and concanavalin A, *Cancer Immunology and Immunotherapy,* 1993; 37: 316-22.

Nagae S, et al., Pharmacokinetics of the garlic compound S-allylcysteine, *Planta Medica*, 1994; 60(3): 214-17.

Lachmann G, et al. The pharmacokinetics of S35 labeled garlic consituents alliin, allicin, and vinyldithiine, *Arzneimittelforschung*, 1994; 44(6): 734-43.

Yang CS, Wang ZY, and Hong JY, Inhibition of tumor genesis by chemicals from garlic and tea, *Advances in Experimental Medical Biology*, 1994; 354: 113-22.

Gwilt PR, et al. The effect of garlic extract on human metabolism of acetaminophen, *Cancer Epidemiological Biomarkers*, 1994; 3(2): 155-60.

Feng DJ, Zheng SL, and Wang ZQ, Cytoprotection of garlic juice on gastric lesion produced by HCL in rats, *Acta Universitatis Medicinae*, 1990; 19(2): 115-17.

Hu PJ and Wargovich MJ, Protective effect of diallyl sulfide, a natural extract of garlic, on MNNG-induced damage of rat glandular stomach mucosa, *Chinese Journal of Oncology*, 1990; 12 (6): 429-31.

Weber ND, et al. In vitro virucidal effects of Allium sativum extract and compounds, *Planta Medica*, 1992; 58: 417-23.

Reeve VE, et al., A garlic extract protects from ultraviolet B radiation-induced suppression of contact hypersensitivity, *Photochemistry and Photobiology*, 1993; 58(6): 813-17.

Abdullah TH, Kirkpatrick DV, and Carter J, Enhancement of natural killer cell activity in AIDS with garlic, *Deutsche Zeitschrift Onkologie*, 1989; 21: 52-3.

Earlier Works

Several articles in older journals (before 1989) present valuable insights into the constituents and effects of garlic administration.

Liu DH, Clinical Observation on Beixin No. 1 in the treatment of tuber-culosis sinus, *Zhongjiyikan*, 1986; 21(2): 121-3.

Zhang LP, et al. Analysis of the major constituents of garlic essential oil, *Chinese Traditional Patent Medicine*, 1989; 11(5): 35.

Hanafy MS, et al., Effect of garlic on lead contents in chicken tissues, *Deutsch Tierarztl Wochenschr*, 1994; 101(4): 157-8.

El-Mofty MM, et al., Preventive action of garlic on aflatoxin B1-induced carcinosgenisis in the toad Bufo regularize, *Nutrition and Cancer*, 1994; 21(1): 95-100.

Gao YM, Xie JY, and Piao YJ, Ultra structural observation of intratumoral Europhiles and macrophages induced by garlic oil, *Journal of Chinese and Western Integrated Medicine*, 1993, 13 (9): 546-8.

Fronting RA and Bulmer GS., In vitro effect of aqueous extract of garlic on the growth and viability of Cryptococcus neoformans, *Mycopathologia*, 1978; 70: 397-405.

Tsai Y et al., Antiviral properties of garlic: In vitro effects on influenza B, herpes simplex I, and coxsackie viruses, *Antimicrobial Agents in Chemotherapy*, 1985; 27(4): 485-6.

Rao RR, et al., Inhibition of Mycobacterium tuberculosis by garlic extract, *Nature*, 1946; 157.

Nagai K, Experimental studies on the preventive effect of garlic extract against infection with influenza virus, *Japanese Journal of Infectious Diseases*, 1973; 47:321.

Prasad G and Sharma VD, Efficacy of garlic treatment against experimental Candidiasis in chicks, *British Veterinary Journal*, 1980; 136:448-51.

Moore GS and Atkins RD, The fungicidal and fungi static effects of an aqueous garlic extract on medically important yeast-like fungi, *Mycological*, 1977; 69: 341-8.

Ziment I, Possible mechanisms of action of traditional Oriental drugs for bronchitis, *Advances in Chinese Medicinal Materials Research* (Chang HM, et al. editors), World Scientific

References

Chronic Disease in Minority Populations Centers for Disease Control and Prevention, (1994) Centers for Disease Control and Prevention, Office on Smoking and Health, Unpublished data, 1995. Tobacco Use Among U.S. Racial/Ethnic Groups-U.S. Department of Health and Human Services. African Americans, American Indian and Alaska Natives, Asian Americans and Pacific Islanders, and Hispanics: A Report of the Surgeon General. Atlanta: U.S. Department of Health and Human Services, Centers for Disease Control and Prevention, 1998. Cigarette Smoking Rates May Have Peaked Among Younger Teens: The University of Michigan. 1997 (press release), December 18, 1997.

Tobacco Use Among High School Students—United States, 1997 Centers for Disease Control and Preventio, *Morbidity and Mortality Weekly Report,* 1998; (46): 433-40.

Cigarette Smoking Among Adults—Centers for Disease Control and Prevention. United States, 1993, *MMWR,* 1994; (43): 925-9.

Smoking Cessation During Previous Year Among Adults—Centers for Disease Control and Prevention-United States, 1990 and 1991, *MMWR,* 1993; (42): 504-7.

Cigarette Advertising and Black-White Differences in Brand Preference, K.M. Cummings, G. Giovino, A.J. Mendicino, *Public Health Reports,* 1987

Target Tobacco Markets—J.L. Stoddard, Johnson, CA. Boley. T. Cruz, S. Sussman, Outdoor Advertising in Los Angeles Minority Neighbors. American Journal of Public Health, 1997 (87): 1232-3.

Minority Issues. Tobacco Use: An American Crisis. H. Freeman, J.L. Delgado, C.E. Douglas, Final Report of the Conference (January 1993).

The Effect of Dietary Sucrose on Blood Lipids, Serum Insulin, Platelet Adhesiveness and Body Weight in Human Volunteers—Postgraduate Medicine Journal. S. Scanto, and J. Yudkin, 1969

Metabolic Changes Induced by Sugar in Relation to Coronary Heart Disease and Diabetes. By J. Yudkin, Nutrition and Health 1987.

Diabetes, Coronary Thrombosis and the Saccharine Disease: By T. Cleave, and G. Campbell, (Bristol, England: John Wright and Sons, 1960).

Carbohydrates and Blood Pressure. Annals of Internal Medicine. By Hodges, R., and Rebello, T.

Effects of Dietary Sugars on Metabolic Risk Factors Associated with Heart Disease. Nutritional Health S. Reiser 1985. Dr. Afrika.ublishing, Singapore. 1985: 193-202 Recommended Reading/References: chines, other Asian TM and others.

References

Unschuld PU, *Medicine in China: Historical Artifacts and Images*, 2000; Prestel Verlag, Munich.

Maoshing Ni, *The Yellow Emperor's Classic of Medicine: A New Translation of the Neijing Suwen with Commentary*, 1995; Shambhala, Boston, MA.

Yang Shouzhong (translator), *The Divine Farmer's Materia Medica*, 1997; Blue Poppy Press, Boulder, CO.

Hsu HY and Peacher WG (editors), Shang Han Lun: The Great Classic of Chinese Medicine, 1981; Oriental Healing Arts Institute, Long Beach, CA.

Hsu HY and Wang SY (translators), *Chin Kuei You Lueh*, 1983; Oriental Healing Arts Institute, Long Beach, CA.

Huang Bingshan and Wang Yuxia, *Thousand Formulas and Thousand Herbs of Traditional Chinese Medicine*, vol. 2, 1993; Heilongjiang Education Press, Harbin.

Bensky D and Barolet R, *Chinese Herbal Medicine: Formulas and Strategies*, 1990; rev. ed., Eastland Press, Seattle, WA.

Unschuld PU, *Forgotten Traditions of Ancient Chinese Medicine*, 1990; Paradigm Publications, Brookline, MA.

Chen Keji, The effect and abuse syndrome of ginseng, *Journal of Traditional Chinese Medicine*, 1981; 1(1): 69-72.

Smith FP and Stuart GA, *Chinese Medicinal Herbs*, 1973; Georgetown Press, San Francisco, CA.

Chang HM and But PPH (editors), *Pharmacology and Applications of Chinese Materia Medica*, (2 vols.), 1986; World Scientific, Singapore.

Chang HM, et al., *Advances in Chinese Medicinal Materials Research*, 1985; World Scientific, Singapore.

Siegel RK, Ginseng abuse syndrome, *Journal of the American Medical Association*, 1979; 241(15): 1614-15.

Blumenthal M, Debunking the 'ginseng abuse syndrome', *Whole Foods*, 1991; March: 89-91.

Hsu HY, et al., *Oriental Materia Medica: A Concise Guide*, 1986; Oriental Healing Arts Institute, Long Beach, CA.

Pharmacopoeia Commission of PRC, *Pharmacopoeia of the PRC* (English edition), 1988; People's Medical Publishing House, Beijing.

Tang W and Eisenbrand G, *Chinese Drugs of Plant Origin*, 1992; Springer-Verlag, Berlin.

Zhu YP, *Chinese Materia Medica: Chemistry, Pharmacology, and Applications*, 1998; Harwood Academic Publishers, Amsterdam.

Liberti LE and Der Marderosian A, *Evaluation of commercial ginseng products*, Journal of Pharmaceutical Science 1978; 10:1487-9.

Han KH, et al., Effects of red ginseng on blood pressure in patients with essential hypertension and white coat hypertension, *American Journal of Chinese Medicine*, 1998; 26(2): 199-209.

Bae HW, editor, *Korean Ginseng*, 1978; Seoul: Korea Ginseng Research Institute.

Hou JP, *Ginseng: The Myth and the Truth*, 1978; Wilshire Book Company, North Hollywood, CA.

Dharmananda S, Panax ginseng: A clinical study of its effects on risk factors of cardiovascular diseases, *Bulletin of the Oriental Healing Arts Institute*, 1983; 8(1): 1-13.

Unschuld PU, *Medicine in China: History of Pharmaceutics*, 1986; University of California Press, Berkeley, CA.

Zhang Enquin (editor in chief), *English-Chinese Rare Chinese Materia Medica*, 1990; Publishing House of Shanghai College of Traditional Chinese Medicine, Shanghai.

Yuan Jinqi, et al., 116 cases of coronary angina pectoris treated with powder composed of ginseng, notoginseng, and succinum, *Journal Traditional Chinese Medicine*, 1997;17(1): 14-17.

Qiu Ruixiang, He Jingbo, Effects of Xin Mai Tong Capsule on vasoregulatory peptides in the patients of coronary heart disease, *Journal Traditional Chinese Medicine*, 2000; 20(4): 251-3.

Attele AS, et al., Antidiabetic effects of Panax ginseng berry extract and the identification of an effective component, *Diabetes*, 2002; 51(6): 1851-8.

Ling Yourun, *A New Compendium of Materia Medica: Pharmaceutical Botany and Chinese Medicinal Plants*, 1995; Science Press, Beijing.

Ou Ming (chief editor), *Chinese-English Manual of Common-Used Herbs in Traditional Chinese Medicine*, 1989; Joint Publishing Co., Hong Kong.

Sandberg F, The analytical problems involved in the ginseng products on the ginseng market, In *Proceedings of the 2nd International Ginseng Symposium*, 1978; Korea Ginseng Research Institute, Seoul, Korea; pp. 41-2.

Vogler BK, Pittler MH, Ernst E, The efficacy of ginseng: a systematic review of randomised clinical trials, *European Journal of Clinical Pharmacology*, 1999; 55: 567-75.

Boik J, *Natural Compounds in Cancer Therapy*, 2001; Oregon Medical Press, Princeton, MN.

Bremer K, Chase MW, Stevens PF, The angiosperm phylogeny group: an ordinal classification for the families of flowering plants, *Annals of the Missouri Botanical Garden*, 1998; 85(4): 531-53.

Soldati F, Sticher O, HPLC separation and quantitative determination of ginsenosides from Panax ginseng and Panax quinquefolium and ginseng drug preparations, *Planta Medica*, 1980; 39: 348-67.

Li CP, Li RC, An introductory note to ginseng, *American Journal of Chinese Medicine*, 1973; 1(2): 249-61.

Bahrke MS, Morgan WP, Evaluation of ergonogenic properties of ginseng: an update, *Sports Medicine*, 2000; 29(2): 113-33.

Gu Chifan, The experience of application of ginseng in the newborn baby, *Manuscript (personal communication)*, 1987; Oct 11.

Hou JP, The chemical constituents of ginseng plants, *Comparative Medicine East and West* 1977; 5(2): 123-45.

Chuang WC, et al., A comparative study on commercial samples of ginseng radix, *Planta Medica*, 1995; 61: 459-65.

Vuksan V, et al., American ginseng reduces postprandial glycemia in nondiabetic subjects and subjects with type 2 diabetes mellitus, *Archives of Internal Medicine*, 2000; 160: 1009-13.

Xiao Peigen, Chen Keji, Recent advances in clinical studies of Chinese medicinal herbs, *Phytotherapy Research*, 1988; 2(2): 116-32.

Chang YS, Lee JY, Kim CW, The effect of ginsenoside-triol on the postoperative recovery in gynecological patients, In *Proceedings of the 2nd International Ginseng Symposium*, 1978; Korea Ginseng Research Institute, Seoul, Korea, pp. 79-84.

Awang DVC, The neglected ginsenosides of North American ginseng, *Journal of Herbs, Spices, and Medicinal Plants*, 2000; 7(2): 103-9.

Furth C, *A Flourishing Yin: Gender in China's Medical History, 960-1665*, 1999; University of California Press, Berkeley, CA.

Cao H, But PPH, Hu SY, The ginseng plants: commercial products and quality assessment, *Chinese Journal of Integrated Traditional and Western Medicine*, 1997; 3(4): 306-10.

Wang R, Ren SJ, Lien EJ, Chemical and clinical investigations of ginseng: a survey, *International Journal of Oriental Medicine*, 1999; 24(2): 57-84.

Zhu Weigang, et al., Effects of ginseng polysaccharides on immunologic functions in mice, *Bulletin of Hunan Medical University*, 1991; 16(2): 107-10.

Tanaka OM, Kasai RJ, Morita TN, Chemistry of ginseng and related plants: recent advances, *Abstracts of Chinese Medicine*, 1986; 1(1): 130-52.

Brown DJ, *Herbal Prescriptions for Better Health*, 1996 (2nd edition 2002); Prima Publishing, Rocklin, CA.

Zhao XZ, Antisenility effect of ginseng rhizome saponin, *Chinese Journal of Integrated Traditional and Western Medicine*, 1990; 10(10): 586-9.

Unschuld PU, *Introductory Readings in Classical Chinese Medicine*, 1988; Kluwer Academic Publishers, Dordrecht, Holland.

Dixon P, *Ginseng*, 1976; Gerald Duckworth and Company, London.

Hedady L, *Asian Health Secrets*, 1996; Three Rivers Press, New York.

Chen SE, Sawchuk RJ, Staba EJ, Pharmacokinetics of ginseng compounds, In *Proceedings of the 2nd International Ginseng Symposium*, 1978; Korea Ginseng Research Institute, Seoul, Korea; pp.55-6.

Saito HS, Lee YM, Pharmacological properties of Panax ginseng root, In *Proceedings of the 2nd International Ginseng Symposium*, 1978; Korea Ginseng Research Institute, Seoul, Korea; pp.109-14.

Shoji J, Recent advances in the chemical studies of ginseng, In Chang HM, et al., (editors), *Advances in Chinese Medicinal Materials Research*, 1985; World Scientific, Singapore, pp. 455-69.

Meier B, et al., Quantitative analysis of ginseng by HPLC, In Chang HM, et al., editors. *Advances in Chinese Medicinal Materials Research*, 1985; World Scientific, Singapore, pp. 471-84.

Bradley P, editor, *British Herbal Compendium: A Handbook of Scientific Information on Widely Used Drug Plants*, 1992; British Herbal Medicine Association, London.

Hu SY, Knowledge of ginseng from ancient records, *Journal of the Chinese University of Hong Kong*, 1977; 4(2): 285-305.

Hall T, Lu ZZ, et al., Evaluation of consistency of the standardized Asian ginseng product in the ginseng evaluation program, *Herbalgram*, 2001; 52, 31-45

Anonymous, *Learner's Chinese-English Dictionary*, 5th edn, 1984; Nanyang Siang Pau and Umum Publisher, Singapore.

Lindqvist C, *China: Empire of Living Symbols*, 1991; Addison-Wesley Publishing Co., NY.

Wiseman N, *English-Chinese, Chinese-English Dictionary of Chinese Medicine*, 1995; Foreign Languages Press, Beijing.

Advanced Reading/Reference

Fazzioli E, *Chinese Calligraphy: From Pictograph to Ideogram: The History of 214 Essential Chinese/Japanese Characters*, 1986; Abbeville Press, NY.

Li Leyi, *Tracing The Roots of Chinese Characters: 500 Cases*, 1993; Beijing Language and Culture University Press, Beijing.

Liao SJ (editor), *Chinese-English Terminology of Traditional Chinese Medicine*, 1981; Hunan Science and Technology Press, Hunan.

Tan Huaypeng, *Fun with Chinese Characters: The Straits Times Collection* (3 volumes), 1980-3; Federal Publications, Hong Kong.

Wang Hongyuan, *The Origins of Chinese Characters*, 1993; Sinolingua, Beijing.

Wieger L, *Chinese Characters: Their Origin, Etymology, History, Classification, and Signification*, 1965; Dover Publications, NY.

Wilder GD and Ingram JH, *Analysis of Chinese Characters*, 1974; Dover Publications, NY.

Wiseman N, and Boss K, *Glossary of Chinese Medical Terms and Acupuncture Points*, 1990; Paradigm Publications, Brookline, MA.

Wiseman N and Ye Feng, *A Practical Dictionary of Chinese Medicine*, 1998; Paradigm Publications, Brookline, MA.

Xie Zhufan and Huang Xiokai (editors), *Dictionary of Traditional Chinese Medicine*, 1984; Commercial Press, Hong Kong.

TIBETAN MEDICINE

Tibetan medicine is an integration of four traditions: Ayurvedic medicine and Buddhism from India, the pre-Buddhist shamanism that existed in Tibet, and Chinese medicine. Many of these books are difficult to obtain and provide limited information. However, for those who wish to know Tibetan medicine, a study of several of the books, especially those listed here as recommended reading, will provide a good overview.

Recommended Reading/Reference

Clifford T, *Tibetan Buddhist Medicine and Psychiatry: The Diamond Healing*, 1984; Samuel Weiser, Inc., York Beach, ME.

Norbu D, *An Introduction to Tibetan Medicine*, 1976; Tibetan Review, New Delhi.

Rapgay L, et al., *Mind and Mental Health in Tibetan Medicine*, 1988; Potala Publications, New York.

Tsarong TJ, *Fundamentals of Tibetan Medicine*, 1981; Tibetan Medical Centre, Dharamsala, India.

Advanced Reading/Reference

Baker IA, *The Tibetan Art of Healing*, 1997; Thames and Hudson, London.

Clark B, *The Quintessence Tantras of Tibetan Medicine*, 1995; Snow Lion Publications, Ithica, NY.

Dash VB, *Tibetan Medicine, with Special Reference to Yoga Sataka*, 1985; Library of Tibetan Works and Archives, New Delhi.

Dhönden Y, *The Ambrosia Heart Tantra*, 1977; Library of Tibetan Works and Archives, New Delhi.

Rapgay L, *The Art of Tibetan Medical Urinalysis*, 1986; Tibetan Holistic Medical Series, Dharamsala, India.

Rechung Rinpoche, *Tibetan Medicine*, 1976; University of California Press, Berkeley, CA.

Tsarong TJ, *Handbook of Traditional Tibetan Drugs*, 1986; Tibetan Medical Publications, West Bengal, India.

AYURVEDIC MEDICINE

Ayurvedic medicine differs markedly from Chinese medicine, but there are some areas of overlap: both systems were codified around the same time in civilizations at similar stages of development; both systems have many herbs in common; and both systems have strong emphasis on the value of food as medicine, the use of traditional formulations, and the application of physical exercises (e.g., yoga in India and taiji in China), and physical therapies (e.g., massage in India and acupuncture in China). A problem with Ayurvedic medicine that also plagues Chinese medicine, is that there are so many books produced that are not very true to the tradition. However, unlike Chinese medicine, which has a large and growing profession in the West, Ayurveda is mostly taught to laypersons outside of India, so the demand for rigorous training is less. This has some effect on the quality of publications. Only two books have been deemed essential reading: **Ayurveda: Life, Health, Longevity** (for background on the entire field of Ayurvedic medicine) and the **Indian Materia Medica**, which has a good overview of the individual herbs from the traditional viewpoint (it was written more than 75 years ago, though republished more recently), with mention of many valued herb combinations.

Essential Reading/Reference

Nadkarni KM, *Indian Materia Medica*, (2 vol.), 1976; Popular Prakashan Put. Ltd., Bombay.

Svoboda R, *Ayurveda: Life, Health, and Longevity*, 1992; Penguin Books, India, New Delhi.

Recommended Reading/Reference

Harish Johari, *Ayurvedic Massage*, 1996; Healing Arts Press, Rochester, VT.

Verma V, *Ayurveda: A Way of Life*, 1985; Samuel Weiser, Inc., York Beach, ME.

Advanced Reading/Reference

Kaviratna AC and Sharma P (translators), *Caraka-Samhita*, Second Revised Edition, (5 volumes), 1996; Indian Books Centre, Delhi.

Kutumbiah P, *Ancient Indian Medicine*, 1962; Orient Longman Ltd., Bombay. (OP)

Svoboda R, *Prakruti: Your Ayurvedic Constitution*, 1989; Geocom, Albuquerque, NM.

Svoboda R and Lade A, *Tao and Dharma: Chinese Medicine and Ayurveda*, 1995; The Lotus Press, Twin Lakes, WI.

Zysk K, *Asceticism and Healing in Ancient India*, 1991; Oxford University Press, New York.

HERBS AND WESTERN MEDICINE

When patients present their Western diagnosis, it is important for the practitioner of traditional medicine to understand it, be able to discuss the matter within certain limits, and, as may be necessary, explain the traditional treatment in relation to the Western diagnosis and treatment. Western medicine includes general understanding of diagnosis and treatment, as presented in guides and encyclopedias, and reference to specific treatment methods, including drugs, nutritional supplements, and herbs. Books that have been found valuable for ITM presentation of information about disorders are listed here.

Essential Reading/Reference

Berkow R (editor in chief), *The Merck Manual* (17th edn), 1997; Merck & Co., Rahway, NJ.

Recommended Reading/Reference

Boik J, *Natural Compounds in Cancer Therapy*, 2001; Oregon Medical Press, Princeton, MN.

Clayman CB (editor), *AMA Encyclopedia of Medicine*, 1989; Random House, New York.

Grieve M, *A Modern Herbal*, 1971; Dover Publications, New York.

Murray M and Pizzorno J, *Encyclopedia of Natural Medicine*, 1990; Prima Publishing, Rocklin, CA.

Rybacki JJ and Long JW, *The Essential Guide to Prescription Drugs*, 1997; HarperPerennial, New York.

Werbach M, *Foundations of Nutritional Medicine*, 1997; Third Line Press, Tarzana, CA.

Werbach M, *Healing Through Nutrition*, 1993; HarperCollins, New York.

Werbach M, *Nutritional Influences on Illness*, Second Edition, 1993; Third Line Press, Tarzana, CA.

Werbach M, *Nutritional Influences on Mental Illness*, Second Edition, 1999; Third Line Press, Tarzana, CA.

Advanced Reading/Reference

Blumental M, et al., *The Complete German Commission E Monographs*, 1998; American Botanical Council, Austin, TX.

Blumental M, Goldberg A, and Brinckman J, *Herbal Medicine: Expanded Commission E Monographs*, 2000; American Botanical Council, Austin, TX.

Goth A, *Medical Pharmacology*, 1984; C.V. Mosby Co., St. Louis, MO.

Leake CD, *An Historical Account of Pharmacology to the Twentieth Century*, 1975; Charles C. Thomas, Springfield, IL.

Morton JF, *Major Medicinal Plants: Botany, Culture, and Uses*, Charles C. Thomas, Springfield, IL.

Tyler VE, Brady LR, and Robbers JE, *Pharmacognosy*, 1976; Lea & Febiger, Philadelphia, PA.

JOURNALS OF CHINESE MEDICINE

Publishing a journal is an arduous task, and it is especially difficult when the number of subscribers is small (most journals of Chinese medicine number their subscribers only in the hundreds) and when the number of excellent reports is also small (few practitioners of Chinese medicine have received training that would lead to production of high quality reports). As a result, there are relatively few journals, and most of them have a short publication life. Following are the journals that have been received at ITM, either by subscription or donation. Though none are of such high quality as to be deemed essential reading, practitioners of Chinese medicine ought to have at least two research oriented journals, and (of the ones still available for subscription) the ones used most at ITM are Journal of Traditional Chinese Medicine, the International Journal of Oriental Medicine, and the Journal of Integrated Traditional and Western Medicine.

Recommended Reading/Reference

Bulletin of the Oriental Healing Arts Institute (published 1976-88; back issues available from Oriental Healing Arts Institute, Long Beach, CA). (OP)

International Journal of Oriental Medicine (published since 1989; Oriental Healing Arts Institute, Long Beach, CA).

Journal of the American College of Traditional Chinese Medicine (published 1982-9; back issues available from the American College of TCM, San Francisco, CA). (OP)

The Journal of Traditional Chinese Medicine (published since 1981; 18 Beixincang, Dongzhimen Nei, Beijing 100700).

Advanced Reading/Reference

Abstracts of Chinese Medicine (published 1987-96; Medicinal Materials Research Center, Chinese University of Hong Kong, Shatin, N.T., Hong Kong; back issues not available). (OP)

Chinese Journal of Integrated Traditional and Western Medicine (Beijing; English language publication since 1995, Press: 1 Caochang, Xiyuan, Beijing 100091, China).

American Journal of Chinese Medicine (published since 1974; P.O. Box 555, Garden City, New York 11530).

The Journal of Chinese Medicine (published since 1981; 22 Cromwell Road, Hove, Sussex BN3 3EB, England).

Oriental Medicine (published since 1991; 3723 N. Southport, Chicago, IL).

OTHER JOURNALS

Although not devoted to Chinese medicine or even to natural medicine, the Journal of the American Medical Association (JAMA) is strongly recommended for practitioners of Chinese medicine so that the latest advances in knowledge of medicine can be viewed. JAMA has recently published several articles on alternative medicine and provided clinical study reports about nutritional supplements and herbs.

Recommended Reading/Reference

Herbalgram (American Botanical Council, P. O. Box 201660, Austin, TX 78720).

Journal of the American Medical Association (515 N State St., Chicago, IL 60610).

Advanced Reading/Reference Journal of Naturopathic Medicine (Journal Management Group, Ten Morgan Ave., Norwalk, CT 06851).

Protocol Journal of Botanical Medicine (published 1995-7; P.O. Box 108, Harvard, MA 01451). (OP)

AN EPILOGUE

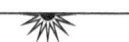

THE PREVENTIVE THERAPY IN COMPLEMENTARY
MEDICINE
AUTHOR'S DESCRIPTION OF THE BOOK—4,000.

This book is a product of many hard days and nights of efforts, and the fruit of many supporting endeavor. It is a multi-purpose coverage of various traditional medicine systems existing in many parts of the world. The principal objective is to project the practice of preventive therapy in the body of complementary medicine. In his philosophical application of homeopathy as part of natural medicine, Dr. Frederick Christian Hahnemann, warned us about the tendency to derail into the practice of orthodoxy. By this he meant, the concept of applying medicine up—on—medicine to every indication of health imbalance without our reflection on the possible alternative approach of remedying the problem. Our knowledge of the natural self-healing process inherent in the human body has not influenced our practice in the complementary therapy. From experience, if it has, it is only in a lesser degree. But most books on complementary medicine have not indicated this facts.

The primary purpose of the present book is to expose both the students of complementary medicine and the practitioners to the validity and the importance of preventive therapy. "The saying is that prevention is always better than cure". This book is not just another text on the principle of complementary medicine nor is it an instruction manual. It is rather a reference book essential for the efficient practice of preventive' therapy in complementary medicine. It must form an important book of reference to both students and practitioners of natural medicine no matter the aspect involved.

The major aim of the book is to draw the attention of the Complementary Healthcare Practitioners towards the urgent need for us to begin to re-evaluate in greater detail, our Healthcare Remedial Treatment. Our approach must now focus principally, on Functional complimentary Medicine based on the philosophy of "holism" with preventive therapy as a cardinal point of attention. For some of the complementary practices, the pattern has been "orthodoxy" in approach. For example, setting up a Clinic or Health Centre with the expectation of sick people trooping in and out for treatment. This "Never Ending" expectation of people with illness, in fact, negates the concept of holistic medicine. In our quest for complementary preventive therapy, we must aim at "Natures' Material Medical."

The book have drawn attention of the practitioners to food commodities, their procurement, their storage, their preparation for human consumption, absorption and bio-utility in the body(the application for the sustenance of life. It also emphasized the crucial importance of nutrition and nutrients, dietary supplements-vitamins and mineral substance.

Research have shown that the people of African origin whose major sources of diets were indigenous commodities, free from chemical, derived their balance nutrients and protection from their foods. Usually, they have high degree of resistance to disease, high degree of immune system and lived healthier and longer life. These food commodities in their biochemistry possess therapeutic properties for maintaining good health with no side effects or addiction. Most of natural remedies derive their ingredients from such foods products. The book expressely outlined various foods derived from the African indigenous soils as sources of prevention of some western based illnesses.

TYPICAL EXAMPLES OF SUCH FOOD AFRICA COMMODITIES:

Yam and Coco Yam.-Unripe Plantain.-Unripe Banana. Unripe Pawpaw–Coco yam Leaves.—Sweet Potato and their Leaves.-Green and Red Pepper.—Cassava and Cassava Leaves. Tropical Water Mellon and their Seeds. Egusi Oil and their Seeds.-Pumpkins and their seeds. Tropical Water Leaves.—Ugu and their Seeds. Uha-Leaves. Ewedu , Okwuru; Ogbono and their Oil. Tropical Chicken-Natural Breed and their eggs, and Gene Fowl.-Tropical Red Ginger, Tropical Garlic and Tropical Red Onion. Tropical Snail and Wooden Dried Bush Meat. Okazi.-Ngalangala, Ehuru, Achi and ukpo; Nchuawa, Ugbogro. Adu. Nkwu.Eruru.Mbusu. Abuba-Eke [Piton Oil.] Akide, Odudu, Ukpara and Grass Hopper, Grass Cutter-Bush Meat.-Nzu and many more Tropical African Food commodities which I am not able to mention here. Anybody who tells you that any of the above listed items including the red oil from African palm tree is unhealthy, must substantiate this claim with independent-unbiased research evidence. The book has also shown that an effective practice of modern African traditional medicine must be based on the following principles:

- Prevention and treatment.
- Regeneration of the body defence mechanism.
- The effective ejection of waste from the body.
- The creation of harmony and balance within the body.
- The prevention of low-sperm counts in men and increase vitality.
- The stabilization of food intake and nutrients.
- The prevention of fibroid in female.

WESTERN ILLNESSES COMMON AMONG AFRICAN MALE

- Weakness of vitality-low sexual drive
- Lack of erection and low sperm count.
- Defection during ejaculation on the increase
- Swelling of the Testicle.
- The itching and shrinking of the Testicle
- Penis ulcer, twitching of the penis.
- Excessive Sex Drive and Constant Erection
- Nymphomania syndrome.
- Sexual transmitted Diseases including HIV Aids.

- Diseases transmitted through Oral Sex-parasitic worm and many more.

WESTERN ILLNESSES COMMON AMONG AFRICAN WOMEN

- Excessive Menstrual flow on the increase.
- Excessive Vaginal secretion on the increase.
- Vaginal itching and excessive vaginal wetting on the increase.
- Low sexual drive and sexual Frigidity on the increase.
- Painful Menstrual flow on the increase.
- Abnormal Vaginal odour on the increase.
- Ulcer and wound of the womb on the increase.
- Deviation on the mouth and protrusion of the womb on increase.
- Haemorrhoid-Pie and Boils of the womb on increas
- Inclination of the womb to one side on the increase.
- Cancer and strangulation of the womb on the increase.

THE WESTERN CIVILIZATION DISEASES

This is a new attention to otherwise an old problem. The arrival of western system of life did not only affect both the economic and social life of the Africans, it also brought with it a profound change in the food and health care system of the people. The principal aim of this topic in the book is to draw attention to various common illnesses affecting both female, men, old and young people of African origin. Among all other races of the world, Africans are found to be the only people who have "swallowed" (especially, the negative aspects) of the so called modern western civilization with an accelerated high speed. But this blind high speed has brought with it an uncountable health-care disaster to us. Indeed, it is very hard today to find any African community where heart attack does not exist, where cancer is not known. African community where there is no obesity, Blood Pressure, Men and women sex organ diseases. An African community where such a new killer diseases as

HIV Aid have not visited. The following are the old and New Common illnesses so rampant among Male and female of African origin:-

- Blood Pressure-generally on the increase.
- The diseases of unhealthy food brand loyalty on increase.
- Psychosomatic Illnesses on the increase.
- Eczema disorder on the increase.
- Hair loss disorder on the increase.
- Parasitic infection of the colon on increase.
- Cross infection though bi-sexual syndrome on increase.
- An imperial imprint trauma increasingly reproducing its self.
- Mental poisoning caused by racism and deprivation bitterness— all on the increase.
- Acute Inner restlessness and depression on increase.
- Drunkenness and Drug addiction on the increase.
- An uncontrollable sexual urge/Nymphomania syndrome on the increase.

EXAMPLES OF PSYCHOSOMATIC & PSYCHOLOGICAL HEALHT IMBALACE ARE AS FOLLOWS:

- Mental Torment.
- Unknown Fear of self and fear of others.
- Weak-willed.
- Subservience syndrome.
- Easley discouraged syndrome.
- Self-hatred and self-rejection syndrome
- Easley over whelmed.
- Sense of hopelessness.
- Simplicity of Heart syndrome.
- Over Zealous Hospitality syndrome
- Lack of inner joy-as the fruit of human spirit and creativity.
- Evil and negative effects derived from human skin colour hatred.
- Racial discrimination syndrome
- The Negative effects of Colonial based education.

- Evil danger of abject poverty syndrome
- The effects of chemical cosmetics.
- The effects of Fatigue and Tension-stress.
- The Fear of being charmed by an enemy syndrome
- The effects of Negative thoughts and feelings.
- Negative memories of the past experiences.
- The phobia of being hunted by demons of the forests and empty buildings.
- The phobia of being possessed by an invincible beings of a female Spirit living in the Sea called Mammy-Water
- Bleached Skin color syndrome
- The feeling of inadequacy called Inferiority complex syndrome
- The danger of Superiority complex-from reversed racism
- Cross-cultural Racism Syndrome. (Tribalism)
- Drug addiction-syndrome.
- The negative syndrome of loneliness and rejection syndrome
- The effects of Negative words—lack of confidence in self.
- The negative behavior inherent from our imperial imprint legacy syndrome.
- Multiple effects of skin color discrimination.
- Fratricidal syndrome.

The book also presents pertinent information on the therapeutic health therapy. On mind and body therapy and on the nourishment of human soul therapy. It explained the behavior of mosquito-how it breads, how it transmit disease and how it can be controlled. The general conclusion rests on the effective and efficient of preventive therapy in complementary medicine.

AUTHOR BIO

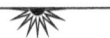

The Author
Dr. Lumumba Umunna Ubani
Bsc. MBA. PhD. ND. HOM. PGD. Ed

Born in Umuaghara, Ogbe, Imo State of Nigeria, Dr. Ubani came to Britain in at a tender age in 1963. Like most self-made Africans from humble families of ordinary means, he did all sorts of odd jobs to finance his education. He attended Vauxhall College in West London and Wands worth college in South London for his GCE ordinary and Advanced Levels. He attended Hendon College of Technology in North London; Elizabeth Gaskell college of Education in Manchester England. He earned Higher Diploma in Hospitality and Institutional Management. Pursuing further interest, he studied at the London College of Naturopathic Medicine and obtained PGD in Homeopathy and African Traditional Medicine.

Dr. Ubani further went to the universities of New Hampshire and Western Colorado in the United States and obtained Bsc; MBA and PhD with special interest in Hospitality and Tourism Human Behavior. He has carried out an independent Research Study in various African countries to survey the effects of imperial imprint legacy among the African Citizenry. And in the Hospitality, Tourism and Human Relations Management in the continent of Africa

He has had extensive experience and exposure in various areas of education, administration, commerce and industry. He had worked in America, in Britain, in Nigeria, Ghana and in Ivory Coast. As a senior Principal Lecturer, he headed the Department of Hospitality and Tourism

Dr. Lumumba Umunna Ubani

Management at the Federal Polytechnic in Kogi state Nigeria. He was in charge of Medicament Naturel Africain Clinique in Abidjan. He is the director of Beckman Naturopathic Medicine Limited in Britain. He is a consultant on Tourism Management and Human Resources Development. Dr. is a speaker on various aspects of African Life: The Afrikan family and the place of African women in History. He is a guest speaker at the Big Interview on the Black History Month at the OBE on-going Television Show.

Dr. Ubani is the founder and the Rector of the Afrikan Institute. He has been the co-ordinator of Anglo-African Cultural Society in Britain for more than five years. He is the author of Preventive Therapy in Complementary Medicine; He is also The Author of the African Mind Reconnection and Spiritual Reawakening.

INDEX

Alexander, Dounne   15, 688-93, 695

Alhacen see Ibn al-Haytham

Ali ibn Abbas al-Majusi   447, 459

Ali ibn Sahl Rabban al-Tabari   446, 472

alkaloids   152, 185-6, 192, 424, 429, 562, 564

allelochemicals   192

allicin   136, 140, 143, 145, 147-8, 154-9, 375, 381-2, 729

alternative medicine   23

America, health crisis in   34-5, 37, 39

American School of Naturopathy 125, 542

amino acids   163, 280

Ammar ibn Ali al-Mawsili   465, 467, 474

An Hao Natural Health Care Clinic 276-7

anthroposophical medicine   199-202

Archidoxes of Magic (Paracelsus) 656

Aristotle   536, 666-9

aromatherapy   209-10, 212-13

aromatic prescriptions   305-8, 310, 312-18

arthritis   205-6

Asclepieia   666

Asclepieions   483, 666

Asclepius   64, 480, 655, 666

ashwagandha   62, 208, 618

Asian Health Secrets (Hadady)   429, 737

Atharvaveda   229

atherosclerosis   113, 132, 136, 139-40, 142-3, 155, 307, 313, 377, 573

Attenborough, David   329-30

Avalokitesvara   350

Avena Sativa   618

Avenzoar see Ibn Zuhr

Avicenna see Ibn Sina

avocados   161-2

Ayurveda   7, 23, 33, 109, 116, 187, 189, 193, 198, 224-9, 231-2, 234-9, 248, 349-50, 720-2, 739-41

B

Badianus Manuscript   188

Bag of Pearls, A (Institute of Traditional Medicine)   277

Baijnath, H.   99

Bencao Congxin (Wu Yiluo)   388

Bencao Gangmu (Li Shizhen)   353, 358, 415-16, 420

Bencao Tujing (Su Song)   218, 220

Bencao Yanyi Buyi (Zhu Danxi)   322

Bharadwaja   231

Bhavamisra   231

Bhushan, Patwardhan   240

Bimaristans   445

bioaccumulation   117

BioDisc   127

Bircher-Benner, M.   46

Blaim, Adolf   552

Bohm, David   641

Boik, J.   428, 723, 735, 742

Book of Healing, The (Ibn Sina)   447

Book of Optics (Ibn al-Haytham) 452, 465

Book of Plants (Al-Dinawari)   471

Book of the Elite (Gaubari)   458

Book on Poisons (Ibn Wahshiya) 327